Surgery of the Hip Joint

Second Edition

Volume I

Surgery of the Hip Joint

Second Edition

Volume I

Edited by Raymond G. Tronzo

With contributions by Henry Vernon Crock, D. Robert V. Dickens, Victor H. Frankel, Barry J. Greenberg, Walter B. Greene, Michael Harty, Robert D. Heath, Walter A. Hoyt Jr., G. Dean MacEwen, Arne Melby III, Michael B. Millis , John A. Ogden, Peter D. Pizzutillo, James W. Pugh, Eduardo Salvati, W. John Sharrard, Raymond G. Tronzo, Dennis R. Wenger, and Alfred R. Shands. Jr.

With 361 halftone and 248 line illustrations

Springer-Verlag
New York Berlin Heidelberg Tokyo

Raymond G. Tronzo, Chief, Orthopaedic Surgery, Humana Hospital, West Palm Beach, Florida. *Address correspondence to* Palm Beach Joint Replacement Center, 1114 North Olive Avenue, West Palm Beach, Florida 33401, U.S.A.

Medical Illustrators: Steven P. Gigliotti, P.O. Box 67, Broomall, Pennsylvania 19008, U.S.A.; Beth Ingraham, Director, Orthopedic Resource Center, Children's Hospital Medical Center, Boston, Massachusetts 02115, U.S.A.; John A. Ogden, M.D., Chief of Staff, Tampa Unit, Shriners Hospital for Crippled Children, 3500 East Fletcher Avenue, Tampa, Florida 33612, U.S.A.

Library of Congress Cataloging in Publication Data
Main entry under title:
Surgery of the hip joint.
Bibliography: p.
Includes index.
1. Hip joint—Surgery. I. Tronzo, Raymond G.
[DNLM: 1. Hip joint—Surgery. WE 860 S961]
RD549.S87 1984 617'.581 84–1450

Surgery of the Hip Joint was originally published in 1973 © Lea and Febiger.

Softcover reprint of the hardcover 2nd edition 1984

Typeset by Kingsport Press, Kingsport, Tennessee, U.S.A.

9 8 7 6 5 4 3 2 1

ISBN-13: 978-1-4612-9745-1 e-ISBN-13: 978-1-4612-5224-5
DOI: 10.1007/978-1-4612-5224-5

This book is dedicated to those teachers who showed us how;
to those students at all levels who challenged us to learn more;
and to those patients whose comfort brought us our rewards.

Preface

The first edition of *Surgery of the Hip Joint* has had certain measures of success. Its cover won the Outstanding Award for art at a publishers trade show. A year later it was translated into Spanish for exposure to the vast world of the Spanish speaking peoples. As I traveled through Europe, it was repeatedly a pleasant surprise to have the book recognized as an authoritative reference. This was a great tribute to the experts whose diligent efforts made it all possible. Apparently the book has stood the test of time to judge from the many inquiries and constructive comments made toward urging us on to write a second edition.

It was not an easy task to gather another cadre of authorities to update our knowledge of the hip joint. People who have earned respected positions in their field are unavoidably burdened with a busy schedule, so a chapter in this text must be appreciated as coming from someone devoted to giving up some of his precious time for the sake of sharing his knowledge with peers and students.

As we struggled along, it became obvious that the book should be divided into three volumes, because outdated concepts had to be scrapped if an up-to-date text were to be offered. Time passed so rapidly that total hip arthroplasties would not become stabilized because of a never-ending parade of implant designs with increasing bioengineering considerations. More recently the bone-cement interface has become a major source of failure which has ushered in a new era of biological bonding of the implant. Consequently, three divisions of the book have evolved. Volume I covers basics plus children's diseases of the hip, Volume II is devoted to adult hip problems and all of their surgical management with the notable exception of total hip arthroplasties, which will be explored comprehensively as a separate surgical procedure in Volume III.

Only the first three chapters have been retained because they reviewed basic material and had been written so well the first time that they deserved to be left alone. Everything else is either entirely new or has undergone major revision. In essence, then, *Surgery of the Hip Joint, 2nd edition,* is a new text.

The main focus of the book has remained the same: a comprehensive treatise on the surgical treatment of conditions of the hip joint. "There are many ways of skinning a cat" is most applicable to orthopedic surgery. Each author has been charged with giving an overview of the options and then presenting the reader with the reasons for his personal surgical approach to the problem at hand. Although this book has been used in the courtroom as a reference to support various positions, the views as stated represent only one man's opinion. They are not the last word on what is right and what is wrong.

Finally, two axioms are humbly offered. Oftentimes we as surgeons become obsessed with the mechanics of a single implant while losing sight of the principles of the operation. We, therefore, must be masters of the operation, not slaves to any device. Furthermore, we must realize that the success of any given operation will depend on whether the skill of our hands matches the quickness of our minds.

Preface to the First Edition

While hand surgery must be shared with hand surgeons, foot surgery with podiatrists, fractures with general surgeons, and spine surgery with neurosurgeons, hip surgery is clearly becoming the exclusive domain of orthopedic surgeons. With the drama surrounding total hip arthroplasties, new careers are being carved out for the hip surgeon. Hip clinics are sprouting up and hip fellowships are being offered for super-subspecialty training. Indeed, hip centers are being built; although Mr. Charnley currently has the only bona fide hip center, at Wrightington, England, more will surely be established elsewhere.

Certainly the hip joint deserves all this attention. It is not only the largest joint in the body but is the site of major diseases in patients of all ages from infancy to senility. It has become the crossroads in orthopedics where clinician and basic researcher meet. Biomaterials and biomechanics were just emerging areas until their meteoric growth resulting from the complex search for the ideal artificial hip joint.

Much is being learned from the intense research surrounding the hip joint. Few problems have as yet been solved, but the future holds promises for many breakthroughs. There are signs, too, of a more aggressive surgical attack against crippling deformities. Orthopedists are increasingly inventive about new surgical procedures and are willing to treat lesions early in the evolution of the disease. With careful planning, it is hoped that this new approach will bring about happy solutions to problems rather than create new ones.

Interestingly enough, there are few books devoted to the vital hip region. Most that have been published were focused on a specific area. The need for a comprehensive text is unchallenged.

The attempt to be realistically comprehensive, up to date and authoritative has been formidable. It could not have been done alone, for no individual alive is knowledgeable enough to be a single author. What has been gathered together here, then, is a group of surgeons who come closest to being "the experts" in given areas because of heir devoted interest. Overlapping has been kept to a minimum, and each author was asked to be generally comprehensive only in the sense of presenting meaningful material to the reader. The final mode of treatment was to be individualized; no one was to defend a middle ground but was urged to provide a personalized view of what he felt to be successful.

Finally, the theme of the book, as its title, was to be *Surgery of the Hip Joint,* with little emphasis on the theoretical or medical aspects of hip diseases. A notable exception to this is the chapter on soft-tissue lesions, which was included only as a means of keeping the surgical conditions in their proper perspective.

It is hoped that the book's audience will be orthopedic surgeons, both young and old, who need a global reference for the surgical management of hip disorders.

Contents

Contributors

Henry Vernon Crock, A.O., M.D., M.S., F.R.C.S., F.R.A.C.S.
Professorial Associate, St. Vincent's Hospital, University of Melbourne; Senior Orthopaedic Surgeon, St. Vincent's Hospital, University of Melbourne, Fitzroy, Victoria, Australia.

D. Robert V. Dickens, M.B., B.S., F.R.A.C.S
Orthopaedic Surgeon, Royal Children's Hospital, Melbourne, Victoria, Australia.

Victor H. Frankel, M.D.
Professor of Orthopaedic Surgery, Mount Sinai School of Medicine, New York, New York; Director, Department of Orthopaedic Surgery, Hospital for Joint Diseases Orthopaedic Institute, New York, New York, U.S.A.

Barry J. Greenberg, M.D.
Assistant Professor of Orthopaedics, Northeastern Ohio University College of Medicine; Senior Orthopaedic Staff, Akron City Hospital, Akron, Ohio, U.S.A.

Walter B. Greene, M.D.
Associate Professor of Orthopaedic Surgery and Pediatrics, Department of Surgery, The University of North Carolina School of Medicine; Attending Surgeon, North Carolina Memorial Hospital, Chapel Hill, North Carolina, U.S.A.

Michael Harty, M.A., M.CH., F.A.R.C.S. (Eng.)
Professor of Anatomy and Orthopaedic Surgery (Anatomy), University of Pennsylvania School of Medicine, Philadelphia, Pennsylvania, U.S.A.

Robert D. Heath, M.D.
Director (Retired), Department of Orthopedics, Geisinger Medical Center, Danville, Pennsylvania, U.S.A.

Walter A. Hoyt, Jr., M.D.
Professor, Orthopaedic Surgery, Northeastern Ohio University College of Medicine; Past Chairman, Department of Orthopedics, Akron City Hospital; Past Chairman, Department of Orthopedics, Children's Medical Center of Akron, Akron, Ohio, U.S.A.

G. Dean MacEwen, M.D.
Professor of Orthopaedic Surgery, Jefferson Medical College of Thomas Jefferson University; Medical Director, Alfred I. duPont Institute, Wilmington, Delaware, U.S.A.

Arne Melby, III, M.D.
Associate Professor, Northeastern Universities College of Medicine, Rottstown, Ohio; Junior Staff, Akron City Hospital; Senior Staff, Children's Hospital Medical Center of Akron, Akron, Ohio, U.S.A.

Michael B. Millis, M.D.
Instructor in Orthopaedic Surgery, Harvard Medical School; Associate in Orthopaedic Surgery, Children's Hospital Medical Center and Brigham and Women's Hospital, Boston, Massachusetts, U.S.A.

John A. Ogden, M.D.
Professor of Orthopaedic Surgery, University of South Florida; Chief of Staff, Shriners Hospital for Crippled Children, Tampa, Florida, U.S.A.

Peter D. Pizzutillo, M.D.
Pediatric Orthopaedist and Clinical Assistant Professor of Orthopaedic Surgery, Thomas Jefferson University Hospital, Philadelphia, Pennsylvania; Director of Medical Education, Alfred I. duPont Institute, Wilmington, Delaware, U.S.A.

James W. Pugh, PH.D.
Associate Professor of Orthopaedics, Mount Sinai School of Medicine of The City University of New York; Adjunct Professor of Bioengineering, The Cooper Union School of Engineering; Adjunct Associate Professor of Engineering Technology, The City College of The City University of New York; Adjunct Associate Professor of Occupational Health and Safety, The Center for Safety, New York University; Director, Division of Bioengineering, Hospital for Joint Diseases Orthopaedic Institute, New York, New York, U.S.A.

Eduardo A. Salvati, M.D.
Chief of Hip Clinic, The Hospital for Special Surgery, Cornell University Medical Center; Clinical Professor of Surgery (Orthopedics), Cornell University Medical College; Attending Orthopedic Surgeon, The Hospital

for Special Surgery and The New York Hospital, New York, New York, U.S.A.

Alfred R. Shands, Jr., M.D.
Formerly Medical Director Emeritus, Alfred I. duPont Institute, Wilmington, Delaware, U.S.A.

W. John Sharrard, M.D., CH.M., F.R.C.S.
Senior Orthopaedic Surgeon, University Hospitals of Sheffield, England; Consultant Orthopaedic Surgeon, Sheffield Children's Hospital and Royal Hallamshire Hospital, Sheffield, England.

Raymond G. Tronzo, M.D.
Chief, Orthopaedic Surgery, Humana Hospital, West Palm Beach, Florida, U.S.A.

Dennis R. Wenger, M.D.
Associate Professor of Orthopaedic Surgery, University of Texas Health Science Center at Dallas; Assistant Chief of Staff, Texas Scottish Rite Hospital, Dallas, Texas, U.S.A.

Fundamentals in Hip Surgery

CHAPTER 1

Historical Milestones in the Development of Modern Surgery of the Hip Joint

ALFRED R. SHANDS, JR.

In presenting the historical milestones in the development of modern surgery of the hip joint, two questions first must be answered: (1) What conditions most frequently require surgery? (2) What surgery is most often performed? The etiologies of hip conditions are traumatic, congenital, developmental, and infectious, in that order. Infections, both pyogenic and tuberculous, frequent before the days of antibiotic therapy, now are seldom seen except where adequate medical care is lacking. In adults the traumatic conditions, such as fracture of the neck of the femur and dislocation of the hip, are the most common. However, in the elderly, an osteoarthritis requiring surgery is more frequently observed than in past years. In children congenital dislocation, acetabular dysplasia, and slipping of the upper femoral epiphysis are the types of conditions most often requiring surgery.

A complete history of the development of all types of hip surgery would be inappropriate for a short historical chapter of this type; thus, as the title indicates, only the important milestones in the development of the most frequent surgery now employed will be given, while other procedures which the author considers most significant in reaching these milestones will be mentioned.

As to the surgery most often performed, the author presents the following ten groupings:

1. Upper femoral osteotomy
2. Pin and plate fixation of fractures
3. Reconstruction operation
4. Arthroplasty
5. Hip replacement, partial or complete
6. Shelf operation and pelvic osteotomy
7. Cheilotomy and acetabuloplasty
8. Hip resection
9. Arthrodesis
10. Surgical approaches and soft-tissue operations.

Upper Femoral Osteotomy

The beginning of major surgery of the hip in America was in the year 1826, when John Rhea Barton,[15] of Philadelphia (Fig. 1–1), performed a femoral osteotomy between the greater and lesser trochanters (Fig. 1–2) to secure motion in an ankylosed hip. The operation was on a sailor with a hip joint ankylosed in adduction, internal rotation, and flexion due to an old fracture with an infection. The operation resulted in a pseudarthrosis, and the procedure took seven minutes. After the sixth week there was active motion which remained for six years, and then all motion was lost. The patient died of pulmonary tuberculosis ten years after the operation; however, he carried on his work as a trunkmaker until his death. This operation is considered by some to have been the first successful arthroplasty.

In 1822 Anthony White,[180] of London, performed a subtrochanteric osteotomy on a 9-year-old boy for a deformity. In 1835 Bouvier,[20] of Paris, performed the first subtrochanteric osteotomy for the treatment of congenital dislocation of the hip, while in 1854 Langenbeck,[91] in Germany, introduced subcutaneous osteotomy of the

Editor's Note: Even though this chapter was written 10 years ago, it remains a masterpiece.

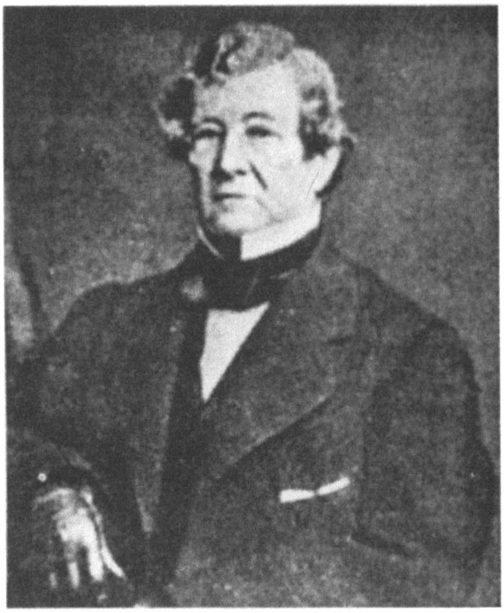

FIG. 1–1. John Rhea Barton, 1794–1871. (From Thompson, F. R.: John Rhea Barton. Clin. Orthop., 6:3, 1955.)

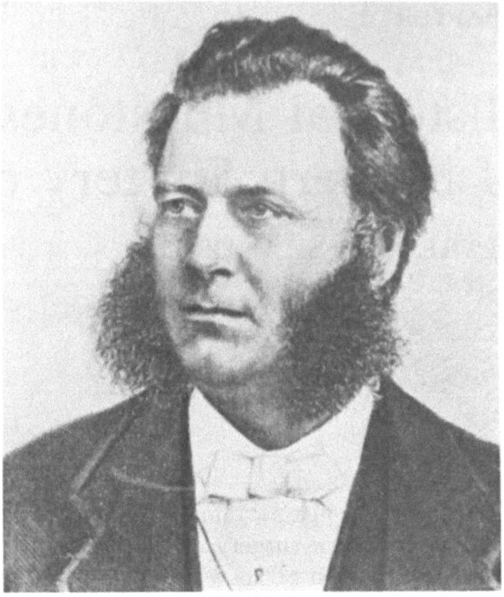

FIG. 1–3 Lewis A. Sayre, 1820–1900. (Courtesy of the New York Academy of Medicine.)

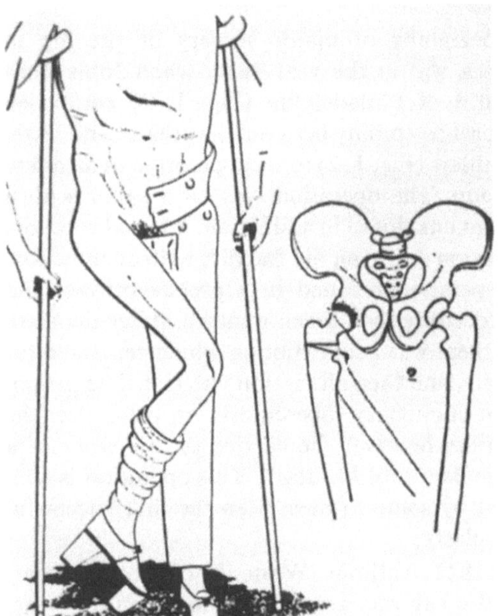

FIG. 1–2 Photograph of drawing of patient of John Rhea Barton showing patient before operation and site of high femoral osteotomy. (From Thompson, F. R.: John Rhea Barton. Clin. Orthop., 6:3, 1955.)

femur, which was followed with similar operations in England by Brodhurst[24] in 1865 and William Adams[3] in 1869. In 1863 Sayre[149] reported (Fig. 1–3) an osteotomy for ankylosis of the hip by removing a block of bone which, he stated, was a modification of the first osteotomy performed by Dr. Rhea Barton. The title of his paper was "A New Method for Artificial Hip Joint in Bony Anchylosis," indicative of an arthroplasty. In 1872 Gant,[54] who became well known for the subtrochanteric osteotomy which bore his name, reported his first operation. Displacement osteotomies for osteoarthritis of the hip and ununited fracture of the neck of the femur were popularized by McMurray[108] (Fig. 1–4) in 1936, with his report on an oblique displacement osteotomy (Fig. 1–5). In 1944 Leadbetter[96] described a cervical axial displacement osteotomy (Fig. 1–6) in which an osteotomy was done in the same axial line of the neck at the junction of the middle and inner thirds and the base of the greater trochanter; the lower neck and femoral shaft were displaced medially beneath the head of a point within the lower acetabular rim, in many ways similar to the McMurray osteotomy.

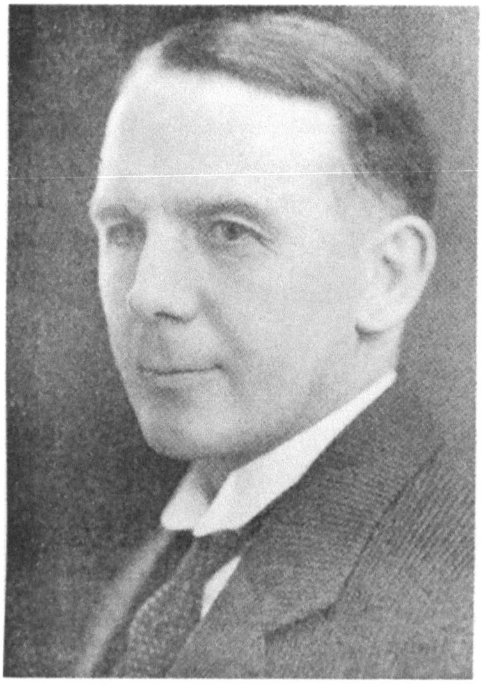

FIG. 1–4 Thomas Porter McMurray, 1888–1949. (From J. Bone Joint Surg., 31B:618, 1949. Used by permission of The Journal of Bone and Joint Surgery.)

Previous to this, upper femoral osteotomies, with the distal fragment displaced and driven into the acetabulum for stability, had been described by Von Baeyer [13] in 1918 and Lorenz [101] in 1919. The Lorenz procedure was called the "bifurcation operation" (Fig. 1–7) and was a modification of the Kirmission [85] procdure first reported in 1894. These were done mainly to secure stability in the old unreduced congenital dislocation. In 1922 Schanz [151] (Fig. 1–8) reported his low subtrochanteric abduction osteotomy (Fig. 1–9) to secure better stability for the old hip fracture and for the unreduced congenital dislocation; the operation at once became very popular.

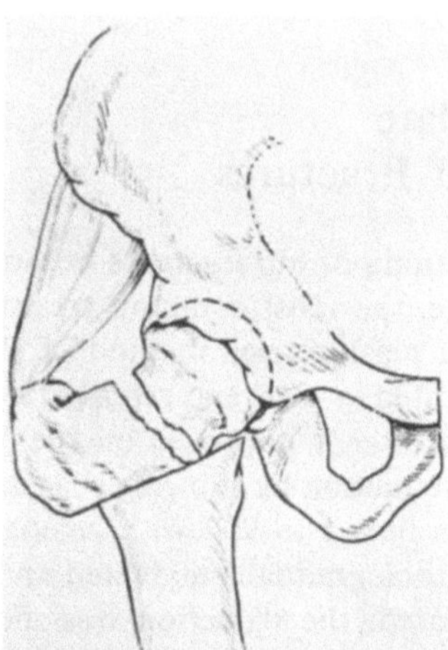

FIG. 1–5 McMurray osteotomy. (From Colonna, P. C.: *Principles of Orthopaedic Surgery*, rev. ed. Boston, Little, Brown, 1960.)

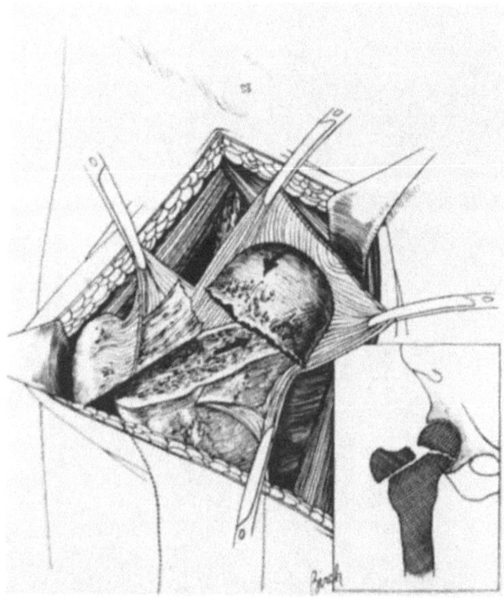

FIG. 1–6. Leadbetter cervical-axial osteotomy. (From Leadbetter, G. W.: Cervical-axial osteotomy of the femur, a preliminary report. J. Bone Joint Surg. 26:713, 1944. Used by permission of the Journal of Bone and Joint Surgery.)

In 1935 Pauwels,[137] who had worked with Schanz, described an adduction osteotomy at the intertrochanteric level (Fig. 1–10). His theoretical work has been adapted by modern day hip surgeons, Müller, Bombelli, and Muttlemeier. There is a resurgence in interest in his "varus" osteotomy today with the increasing failure rate of total hip replacement in younger patients. Milch [115] in 1941 described his "pelvic support" abduction osteotomy with a resection of the head. Pauwels and Milch both made significant contributions to this field of surgery. In 1947 J. A. Dickson [46] described a geometric high femoral osteotomy (Fig. 1–11) for both an ununited fracture of the hip and osteoarthritis. This operation had considerable merit, as an exact amount of bone determined from the roentgenogram prior to surgery could be removed to secure the necessary degree of abduction. In the ununited fracture of the neck, the osteotomy

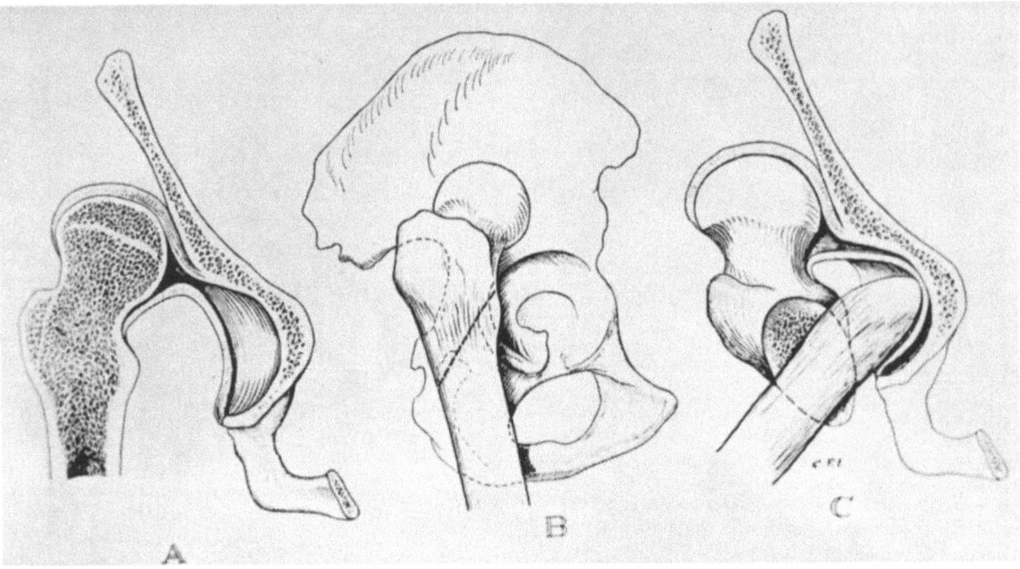

FIG. 1–7 Lorenz bifurcation operation. (From Campbell, W. C.: *Operative Orthopaedics*, 1st ed. St. Louis, Mosby, 1939.)

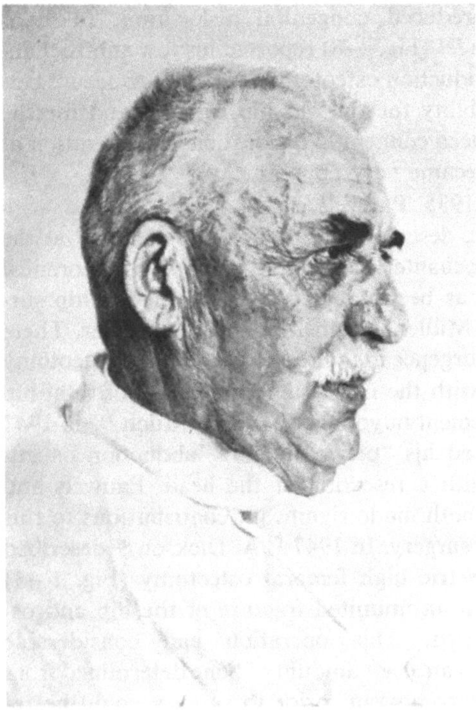

FIG. 1–8 Alfred Schanz, d. 1931, of Dresden, Germany.

was supplemented with multiple bone grafts across the fracture site.

In 1943 Blount [18] and in 1944 A. T. Moore [121] each described an excellent blade plate for the fixation of the high subtrochanteric osteotomy; these were significant contributions because they added internal fixation for early ambulation.

Pin and Plate Fixation of Fractures

Before the pinning of hip fractures became a general procedure, the most common treatment was the abduction plaster spica method of Whitman, first demonstrated in 1902 and reported in 1904.[181] In 1927 Leadbetter [95] improved on the Whitman technique of reduction by showing that if the fractured hip was flexed to 90° with strong upward traction, and then gradually abducted and forcibly internally rotated, the reduction was more accurate and, hence, more stable. This did a great deal to standardize the manipulative reduction. The Whitman abduction cast with the Leadbetter reduction certainly should be considered a milestone

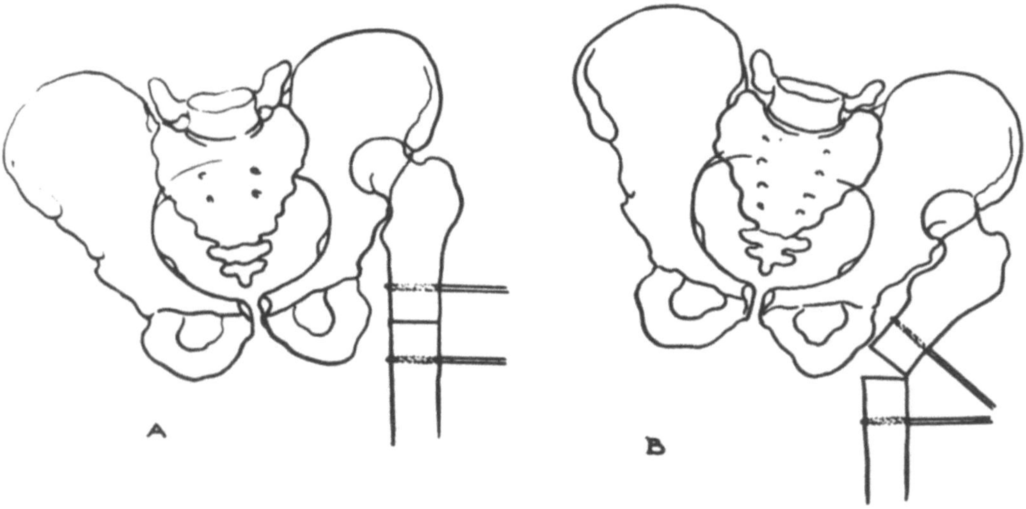

FIG. 1–9 Schanz osteotomy for congenital dislocation of the hip. (From Hass, J.: Congenital Dislocation of the Hip. Springfield, Charles C Thomas, 1951. Used with permission.)[70]

in the treatment of fractures of the hip before nailing was generally accepted as the preferable treatment.

A fracture of the neck of the femur has always been one of the most common fractures to be followed by nonunion, but after Smith-Petersen (Fig. 1–12) in 1925 first demonstrated the use of a triflange nail for fixation of the fragments after reduction, and the principle of pin fixation became generally accepted, nonunions in most clinics were reduced by at least 50% and the whole picture of the treatment of the hip fracture rapidly changed. Smith-Petersen and associates [157] first published a report of this nailing procedure in 1931.

In 1932 Johannsen,[80] of Göteberg, Sweden, and Wescott,[179] of Roanoke, Virginia, introduced a cannulated triflange nail which made possible the use of a guidewire in the insertion of the nail, thus ensuring a more accurate nailing. In 1934 A. T. Moore[118] reported the use of three and, later, four parallel threaded pins (Fig. 1–13) inserted through the fractured neck and into the head after reduction. He stated that this method resulted in better fixation of the fracture fragments with less damage to the circulation than that with one

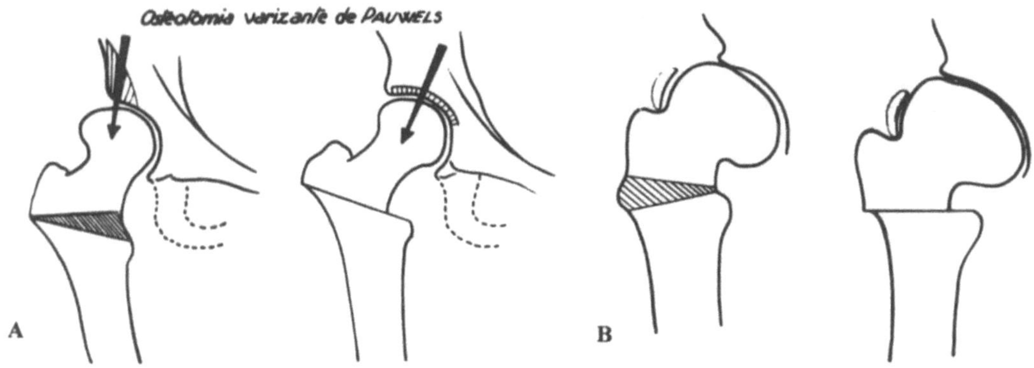

FIG. 1–10 Pauwels' osteotomies. **A** Varus. The diagram shows how the weight-bearing area and weight-bearing axis are changed by osteotomy in coxa vara. **B** Valgus. The diagram shows improvement in congruity of joint surfaces produced by this osteotomy in coxa valga. (From Ottolenghi, C. E., and Frigerio, E.: Intertrochanteric osteotomies in osteoarthritis of the hip; fundamentals, indications, techniques, and results. J. Bone Joint Surg., 44A:865, 1962. Used with permission of The Journal of Bone and Joint Surgery.)

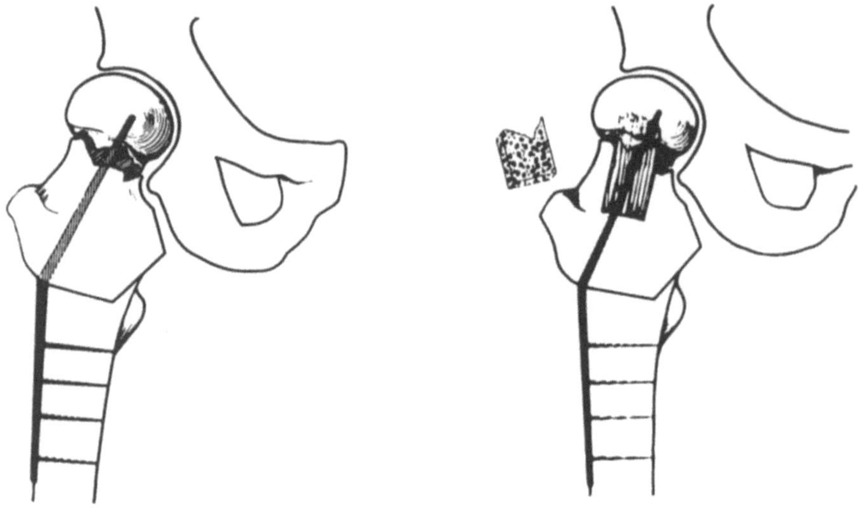

FIG. 1–11 Dickson's geometric osteotomy. (From Dickson, J. A.: The high geometric osteotomy with rotation and bone graft, for ununited fractures of the neck and of the femur. J. Bone Joint Surg., 29:1005, 1947. Used with permission of The Journal of Bone and Joint Surgery.)

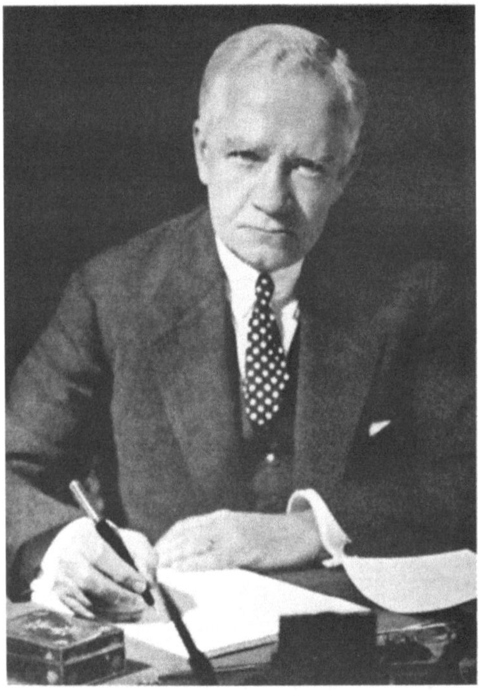

FIG. 1–12 Marius N. Smith-Petersen, 1886–1953. (From J. Bone Joint Surg., 35A:1043, 1953. Used with permission of The Journal of Bone and Joint Surgery.)

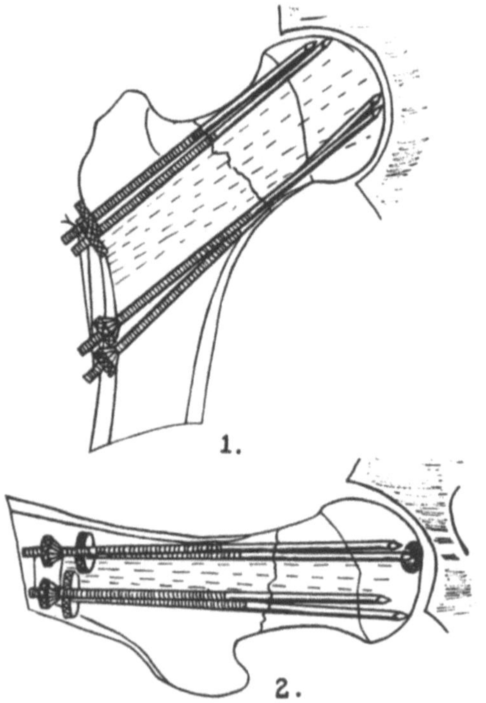

FIG. 1–13 Moore pins. (From Moore, A. T.: "Hip joint fracture, a mechanical problem," Instructional course lectures of the American Academy of Orthopaedic Surgeons, Vol. 10, p. 43, 1953.)

triflange nail. Following the publications of Smith-Petersen,[157] Wescott,[179] Johannsen,[80] and Moore,[118] many others adapted the internal-fixation principle to fractures of the neck of the femur and there were reports on many other types of nails, screws, and screw bolts for greater stability.

The use of a nail or screw for hip fractures was not new, for as early as 1878 in Germany Langenbeck [93] and König [87] used a nail. In 1897 Nicolaysen [132] treated hip fractures with pins in conjunction with a hip spica. Davis [41] in 1900 and Da Costa [39] in 1907, both of Philadelphia, used an ordinary wood screw, as did Martin [112] of New Orleans in 1920. Soon after the introduction of the triflange nail, Thornton [172] in Atlanta and Jewett [79] in Orlando, Florida, added a plate to the outer end of the nail and fixed it to the femoral shaft with screws, while Neufeld [167] of Los Angeles produced a V-shaped nail with a plate which was fixed to the shaft with screws. These were used in trochanteric fractures as well as fractures of the neck. The real *milestone,* however, in the treatment of the hip fracture was the contribution of Smith-Petersen, which changed the accepted treatment from the Whitman-Leadbetter reduction and abduction plaster spica method to pin fixation.

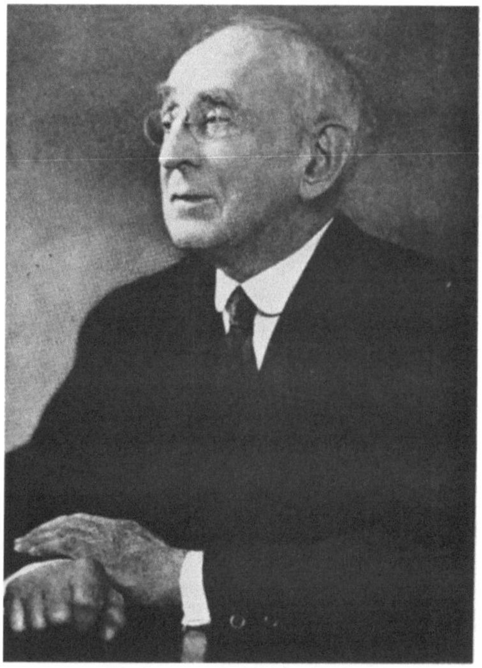

Fig. 1–14 Elliott G. Brackett, 1860–1943. (From J. Bone Joint Surg. 25:245, 1943. Used with permission of The Journal of Bone and Joint Surgery.)

Reconstruction Operations

In 1917 Brackett [21] (Fig. 1–14) described a reconstruction operation for nonunion of the neck of the femur which consisted of hollowing out the femoral head and placing the upper end of the femur in this hollowed-out head after the greater trochanter had been transplanted with its attached abductor muscles lower down on the shaft (Fig. 1–15). Whitman [182] (Fig. 1–16) in 1921 described total removal of the head and neck, and then placing the upper end of the femur in the acetabulum after the greater trochanter with the abductor muscles attached had been transplanted lower down on the shaft (Fig. 1–17), as in the Brackett operation. This operation was performed for both an ununited fracture of the neck of the femur and a painful arthritis of the hip. The operation of Whitman was extremely popular in France up to 1950, when the two Judets [82] first reported successful results with the use of their short-stem prosthesis. In 1932 Magnuson,[110] of Chicago, described a modified Brackett operation and in 1935 Colonna [36] a modified Whitman operation. In the

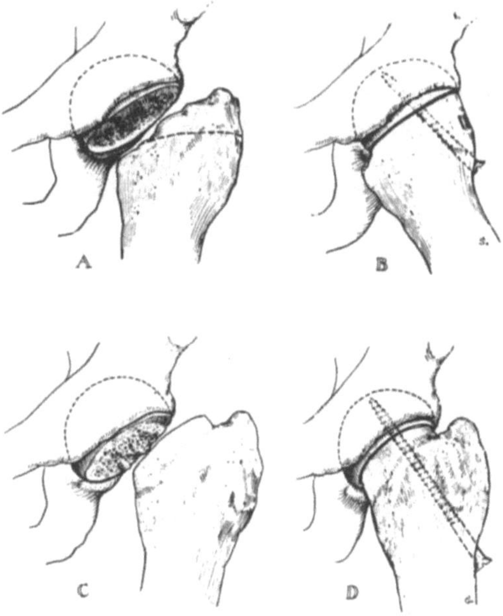

Fig. 1–15 Brackett reconstruction operation. **A** and **B** If neck is completely absorbed, denuded trochanter is placed in excavated head. **C D** If neck is well preserved, fracture surface is freshened and placed in concavity of head of femur. (Figs. 1–15, 1–17 from Boyd, H. B.: Delayed union and non-union of fractures. In Crenshaw, A. H., ed.: Campbell's Operative Orthopaedics, 5th ed. St. Louis, The C. V. Mosby Co., 1971.)

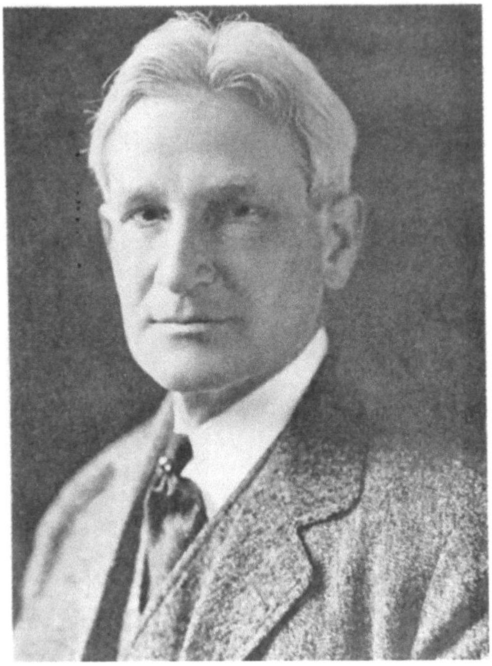

FIG. 1–16 Royal Whitman, 1857–1946. (From J. Bone Joint Surg., 28:891, 1946. Used with permission of The Journal of Bone and Joint Surgery.)

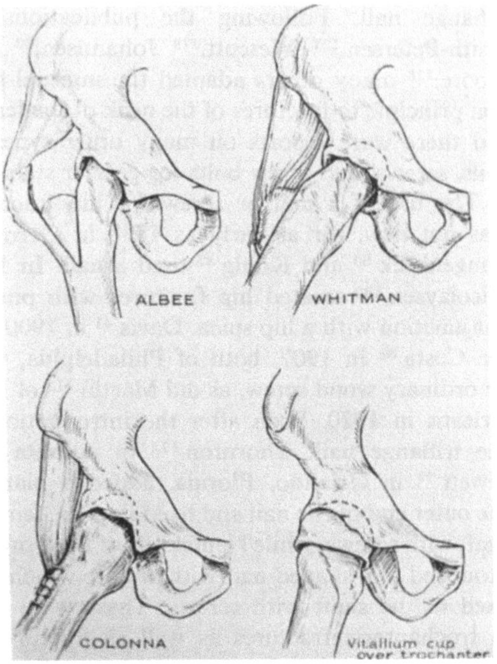

FIG. 1–18 Reconstruction operations for ununited fractures of the neck of the femur. (From Colonna, P. C.: *Principles of Orthopaedic Surgery,* rev. ed. Boston, Little, Brown, 1960.)

Colonna procedure, the abductor muscles were transplanted down the shaft of the femur and the whole upper end of the femur with the greater trochanter placed in the acetabulum (Fig. 1–18). Many other reconstruction operations, such as those of Luck[102] and P. D. Wilson,[187] have been reported. Some were followed by very good results; however, the degree of success depended largely on the after-care.

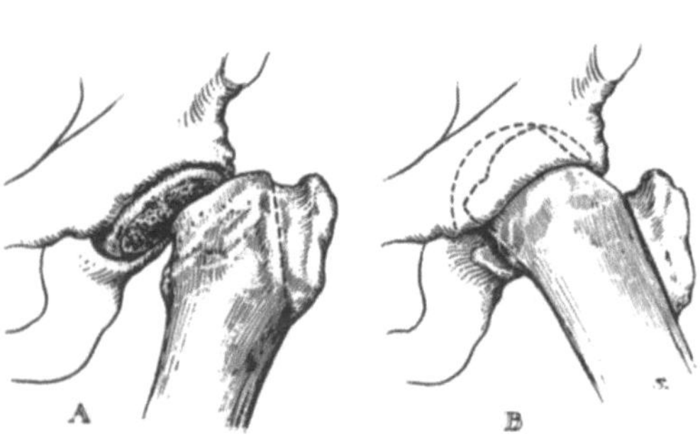

FIG. 1–17 Whitman reconstruction operation. (From *Campbell's Operative Orthopaedics,* 4th ed. St. Louis, Mosby, 1963.) **A** Line of division of trochanter with attachments of abductor muscles. **B** Head removed, neck reduced into acetabulum, abductor muscles attached at lower level on femur.

As early as 1915, Albee [4] (Fig. 1–19) described both the successful use of a tibial graft through the greater trochanter and into the head to secure union in the ununited hip fracture and an unusual reconstruction operation (Fig. 1–18). Henderson [73] reported the use of a fibula graft for nonunion of the neck of the femur. For the painful hip, Sir Robert Jones[81] created a pseudarthrosis by performing an osteotomy through the middle third of the neck, removing the greater trochanter with its muscle attachments and attaching this to the outer end of the inner fragment (Fig. 1–20). This became known as the Jones pseudarthrosis operation. However, the greatest credit for the development of hip reconstruction should be given to Brackett.

Arthroplasty

In the development of arthroplasty, the idea of inserting interposing material after an osteotomy of the ankylosed joint is credited to a well-known general surgeon with orthopedic leanings,

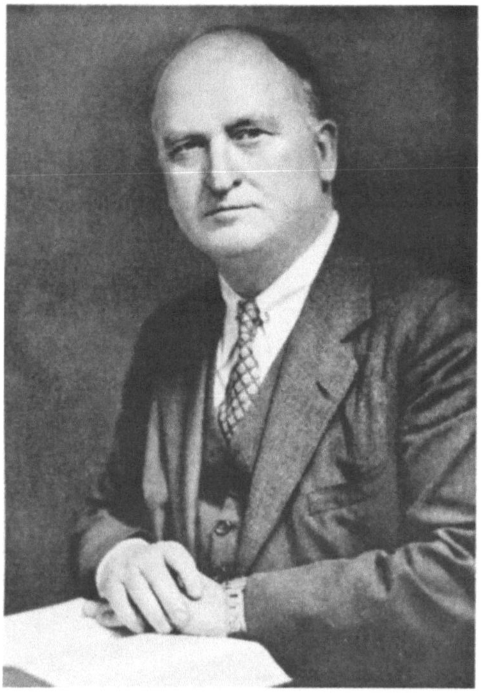

FIG. 1–19 Fred H. Albee, 1876–1945. (From J. Bone Joint Surg., 27:345, 1945. Used with permission of The Journal of Bone and Joint Surgery.)

Carnochan [29] of New York. In 1840 he put a block of wood between the raw bony surfaces after resection of the neck of the mandible in an ankylosed jaw. In 1860 Verneuil,[176] of France, pioneered in the use of soft parts as interposing material: first muscle and then fat and fascia. In 1885 the renowned Ollier [135] became interested in soft parts as interposing material. In 1902 Murphy [128] used muscle flaps, fascia covered with fat, and fascia alone as interposing material; he developed many of the reaming instruments for arthroplasty used today. Murphy's publications were followed by renewed interest in fascial arthroplasty of the hip on the part of Lexer [98] (1908) and Payr [139] (1910) in Germany. In 1955 whole-thickness skin was reported as an interposing material in arthroplasties by Kalle Kallio,[83] of Finland. However, Loewe,[100] as early as 1913, had reported using skin as an interposing material.

The great advance in arthroplasty of the hip came in 1923, when Smith-Petersen [159] first used a glass cup to cover the reshaped head of the femur. The cups were originally of ordinary glass, but this was found to be unsuitable because of breaking. A viscaloid material which was a form of Celluloid was used next, but this material caused too much foreign-body reaction. In 1933 Pyrex glass was used, then Bakelite in 1937, and, finally, Vitallium in 1938 (Fig. 1–21). In 1957, two years after Smith-Petersen had died, his assistant Aufranc [10] reported 82% good or satisfactory results in 1000 hips operated upon at the Massachusetts General Hospital with the Smith-Petersen Vitallium cup technique.

Those who were best known for their work on hip arthroplasties in the period 1910 to 1930, and whose writings and experiences had a great deal to do with the ultimate development of satisfactory techniques, were: Baer [12] (Fig. 1–22) of Baltimore (1918), who used the chromicized submucosa of a pig's bladder as an interposing material, commonly called "Baer's membrane" (Fig. 1–23); Putti [143,144] (Fig. 1–24) of Bologna, Italy (1921); Campbell [27] (Fig. 1–25) of Memphis (1926); and MacAusland [104] of Boston (1929)—all of whom used fascia lata as an interposing material. The results of arthroplasties of the hip reported by these pioneers were generally good, but those of other joints, with the exception of the jaw, were not.

Two other procedures spoken of as arthroplasties should be mentioned, one by Colonna [37] and the other by J. R. Moore; [124] however, neither of these involved the creation of motion in a partial or completely ankylosed joint. In 1936 Colonna [37] described a procedure for an unstable congenital dislocation of the hip which consisted of deepening the acetabulum, covering the head with the capsule and then placing the head in the acetabulum. This has been spoken of as the Colonna arthroplasty (Fig. 1–26) for congenital dislocation. In 1948 J. R. Moore[124] described what he called a cartilage cup arthroplasty for ununited fracture of the neck of the femur which was, in many ways, similar to the Brackett reconstruction operation. The *milestone* in arthroplasty, however, was undoubtedly the Smith-Petersen cup arthroplasty, which has a selected place today in adolescent problem cases.

Hip Replacement

In 1940 Bohlman, of Baltimore, and A. T. Moore,[120] of Columbia, South Carolina, inserted a stainless-steel prosthesis for the replacement of the whole upper third of the shaft of the femur,

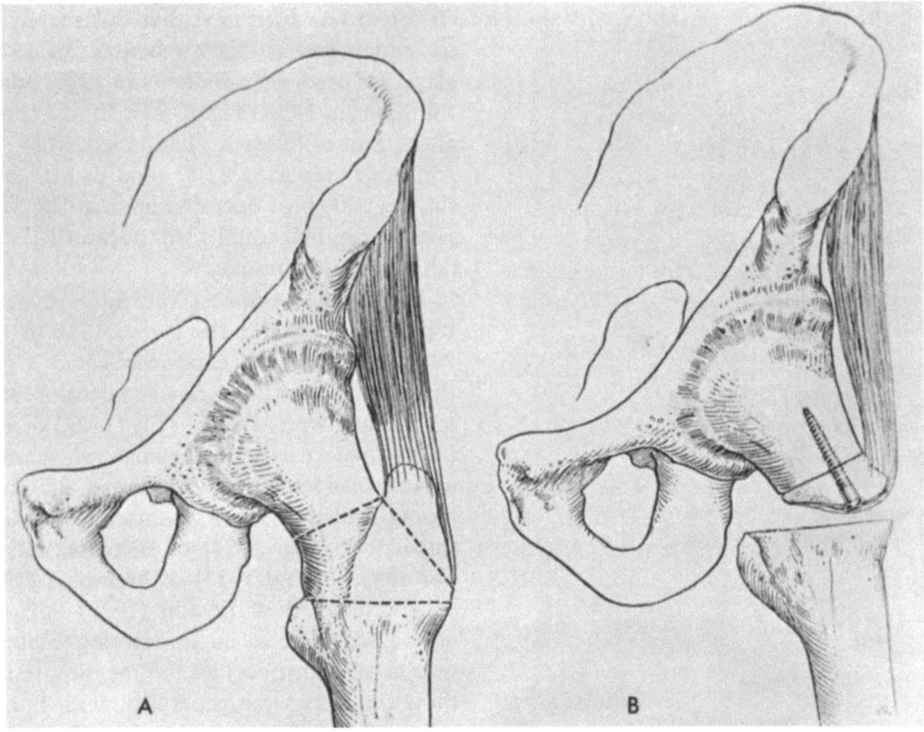

Fig. 1–20 Jones pseudarthrosis operation for ankylosis of the hip. (From Campbell, W. C.: *Operative Orthopaedics,* 1st ed. St. Louis, Mosby, 1939.) **A** Bone within dotted line completely excised. **B** Trochanter fixed to neck of femur with metal screw, interposing attachment of abductor muscles between shaft and trochanter.

including the head and neck (Fig. 1–27). Reported in 1943, this was performed on a patient of Moore's with a large malignant giant-cell tumor. After resection, the 12-inch prosthesis, designed by Bohlman, was attached to the shaft of the remaining femur. The operation was quite successful and enabled the patient to walk for thirteen months without pain before he died of heart disease. It was the first time such a procedure had been done and was a significant development in hip surgery.

When the Judet brothers [82] in 1950 reported 300 cases in which a short-stem acrylic hip prosthesis had been used, a tremendous worldwide interest was created in the problem. Their first cases had been performed 3.5 years before being reported. After removal of the head and distal portion of the neck, the stem of the prosthesis was inserted through a hole in the remaining neck to the outer cortex below the greater trochanter. The original Judet prosthesis was made of methyl methacrylate, but later nylon and other materials, including Vitallium and stainless steel, were used. Thirty or more different types of hip prostheses were developed in a very short period of time, some with a short and others with a long stem, inserted into the medullary cavity of the upper shaft. In 1951 Peterson [142] reported a short-stem stainless-steel prosthesis which was fixed with a flange to the outer side of the shaft of the femur with screws. The long-stem prosthesis soon proved to be most successful and the one of choice. Two types of long-stem prostheses developed in the United States became popular, one in 1950 by Fred Thompson,[168] of New York, and the other in 1952 by A. T. Moore.[122] Moore's prosthesis, which had fenestrations in the upper stem, was called a self-locking prosthesis, because cancellous bone was placed in the fenestrations of the stem for bone attached to the cortex on either side, thus locking the prosthesis in place. In 1954 Lippmann,[99] of New York, described a well-conceived long-stem transfixion hip prosthesis, which in many ways was superior to the other prostheses but never became popular. However, before the long-stem

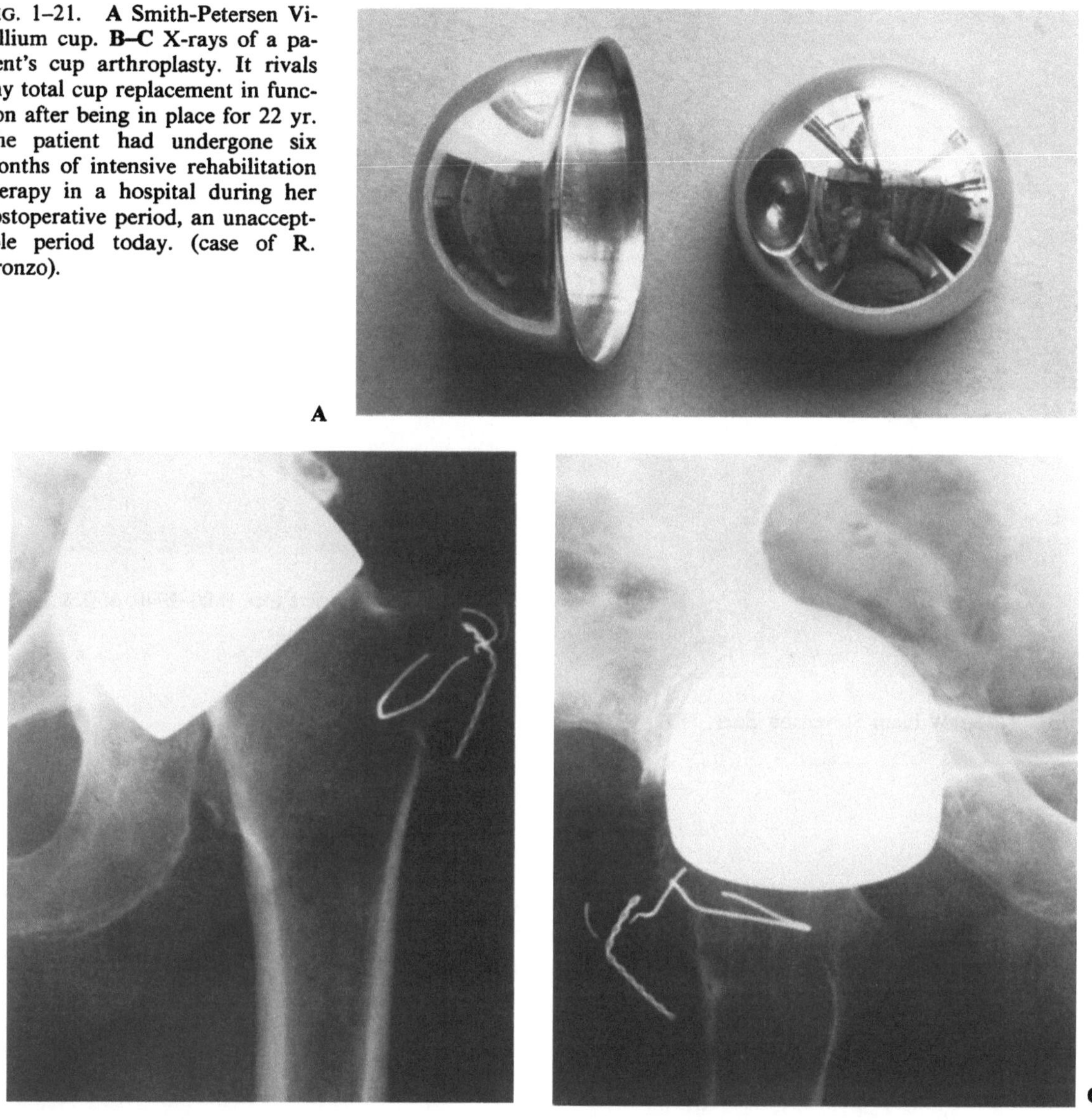

FIG. 1–21. **A** Smith-Petersen Vitallium cup. **B–C** X-rays of a patient's cup arthroplasty. It rivals any total cup replacement in function after being in place for 22 yr. The patient had undergone six months of intensive rehabilitation therapy in a hospital during her postoperative period, an unacceptable period today. (case of R. Tronzo).

prosthesis proved its superiority over the short stem, two unusually named prostheses were described: one in 1951 by McBride,[105] of Oklahoma City, the "door knob" prosthesis, which had a long tapered, threaded stem which went into the medullary cavity of the shaft, and the other by J. E. M. Thomson,[171] of Lincoln, Nebraska, the "light bulb" prosthesis, which had a short stem.

It should be mentioned that, before the Judet short-stem prosthesis was used in France, Delbet [44] in 1919 had used a reinforced rubber prosthesis and in 1927 Hey Groves,[64] of England, an ivory femoral head prosthesis. In giving the milestones of hip replacement, mention should be made of Venable and Stuck [175] whose work in the 1930s demonstrated the nonreactive qualities in the tissues of the metal Vitallium, a light metal with sufficient strength to meet the demands of prostheses and which can be shaped as desired. It was soon found suitable for nails, cups, and all types of prostheses.

The real advances in the development of partial hip replacement are the Bohlman-Moore replacement in 1940; the Judets' short-stem acrylic prosthesis in 1950; and the Thompson and Moore long-stem prostheses in the early 1950s.

In recent years total hip replacement has been widely used and popularized by McKee and

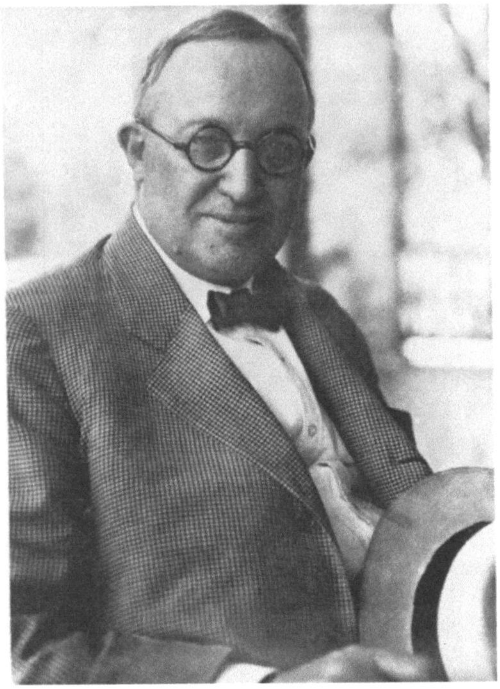

FIG. 1–22 William Stevenson Baer, 1872–1931.

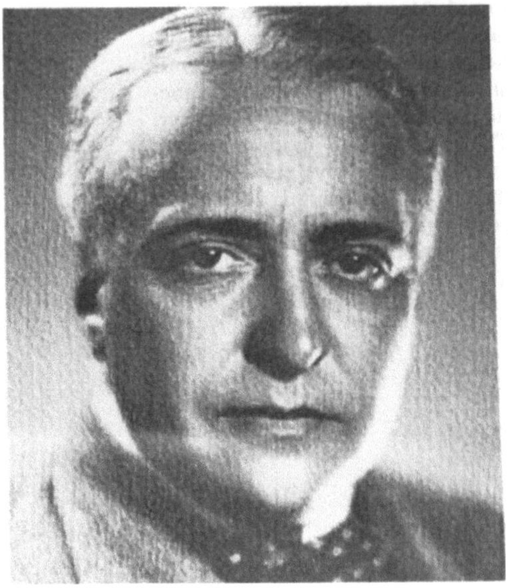

FIG. 1–24 Vittorio Putti, 1880–1940, of Bologna, Italy.

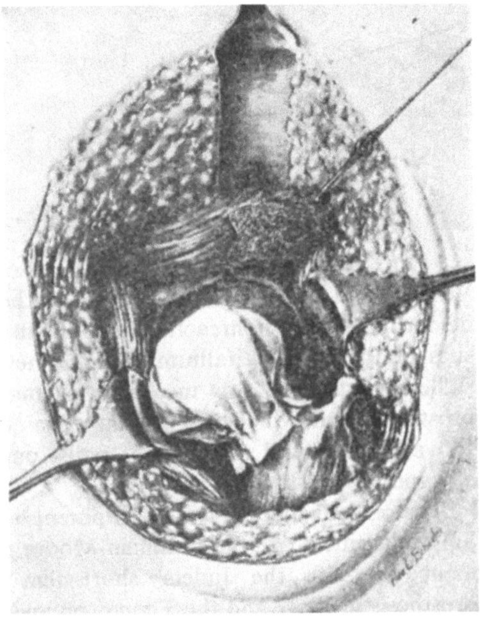

FIG. 1–23 Arthroplasty of the hip with Baer membrane. (From Baer, W. S.[12])

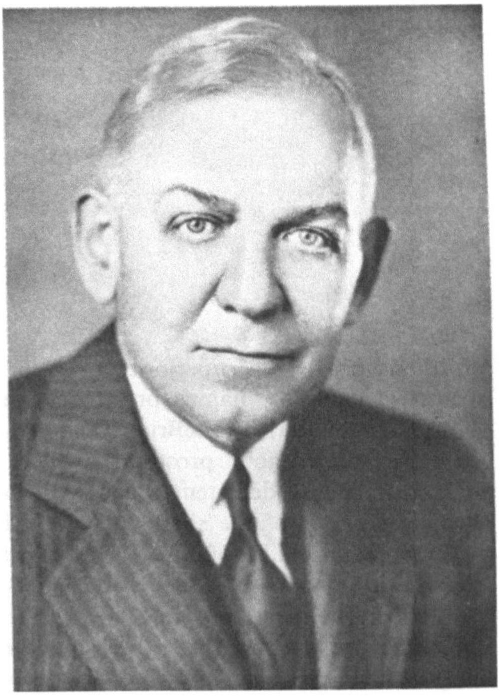

FIG. 1–25 Willis C. Campbell, 1880–1941. (From J. Bone Joint Surg., 23:716, 1941. Used with permission of The Journal of Bone and Joint Surgery.)

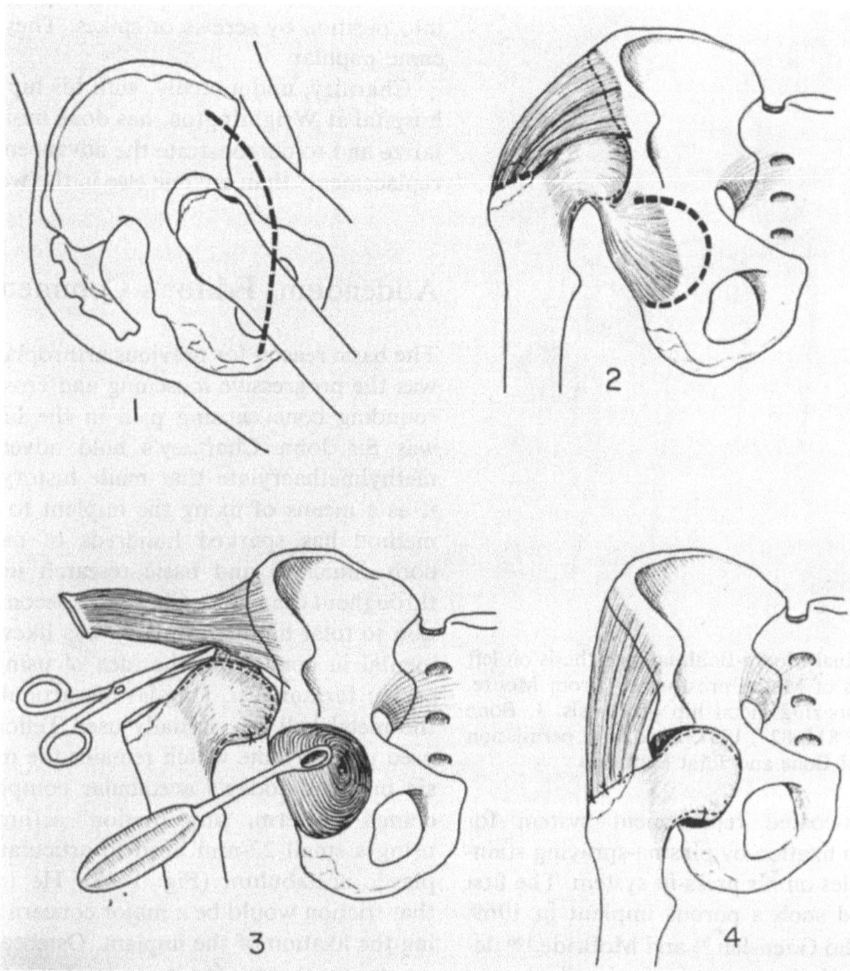

FIG. 1–26 Colonna's arthroplasty for congenital dislocation of the hip. (Used with permission from Colonna, P. C.: Surgery, Gynecology, and Obstetrics 63:71–781.)

Farrar [107] and Charnley, [31] of England. In this, an acetabular portion is fixed into the pelvis and a stem prosthesis into the shaft of the femur. This procedure is now beginning to prove its superiority over partial hip replacement.

The first total hip replacement was said to have been performed by Gluck [61] in 1890 and consisted of an ivory ball-and-socket joint in which a cement type of material was used. In 1938 Wiles [183] described the first stainless-steel total hip replacement used at the Middlesex Hospital in London. He is considered to have been the originator of the idea for the present-day total hip replacement, but according to his report in 1950 his replacement was never very satisfactory. The total hip prosthesis of McKee and Farrar,[107] of Norwich, England (1951), consists of a metal acetabulum cup and a Thompson prosthesis of a chrome-cobalt alloy while that of Charnley,[31] of Whittington, near Manchester, England, consists of an acetabular cup of a plastic material of high-density polyethylene. Both are rigidly attached into the acetabulum with cold curing acrylic cement. The Charnley procedure is spoken of as a "low friction" arthroplasty. (See Fig. 1–28.)

In 1966 Ring [145] described a total hip replacement procedure in which a Moore prosthesis was used for the femur with a metal acetabular cup screwed into the pelvis. It was the first comprehensive system for cementless (press-fit) fixation. Tronzo's prosthetic system was similar except that the cup was eccentric—it has peripheral spikes to stop rotation, which plagued the screwed-in cup of Ring (Fig. 1–29). Tronzo pioneered the first

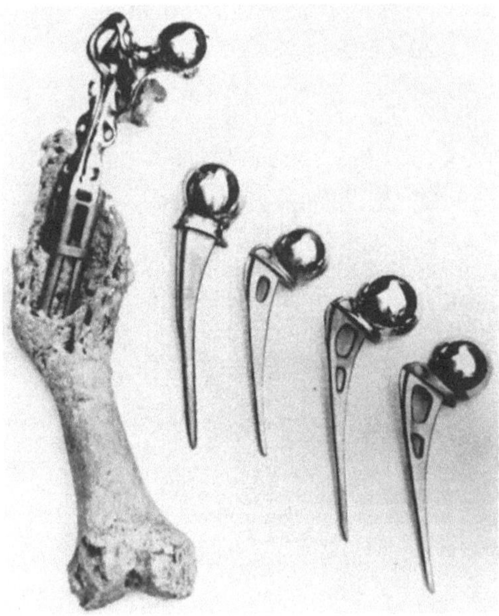

FIG. 1–27 Original Moore-Bohlman prosthesis on left and early models of Moore prostheses. (From Moore, A. T.: The self-locking metal hip prosthesis. J. Bone Joint Surg., 39A: 811–827, 1957. Used with permission of The Journal of Bone and Joint Surgery.)

human porous-coated replacement system for boney ingrowth fixation by plasma-spraying stainless steel particles on his press-fit system. The first human received such a porous implant in 1969.

Urist,[174] as did Gaenslen [51] and McBride,[106] developed an acetabular cup prosthesis which was used with a reshaped head as in a Smith-Petersen cup arthroplasty. These acetabular cups were fixed into position by screws or spikes. They never became popular.

Charnley, undoubtedly, with his hip clinic and hospital at Wrightington, has done more to popularize and to demonstrate the advancement in hip replacements than anyone else in the world today.

Addendum: Editor's Comment

The basic reason for previous arthroplasties to fail was the progressive loosening and erosion of surrounding bone causing pain in the hip joint. It was Sir John Charnley's bold adventure with methylmethacrylate that made history. He used it as a means of fixing the implant to bone. The method has sparked hundreds of papers from both clinicians and basic research investigators throughout the world. Charnley's second contribution to total hip arthroplasty was likewise monumental in conceiving the idea of using a plastic socket for smooth, long-lasting articulation with the metal ball. He initially used Teflon but then used polyethylene which remains the material basic in all of today's acetabular components. He coined the term, "low friction" arthroplasty, by using a small 22-mm head to articulate with the plastic acetabulum (Fig. 1–28). He initially felt that friction would be a major concern in preserving the fixation of the implant. Osteotomizing the greater trochanter for its reattachment under improved tension was a further basic tenet of Charnley.

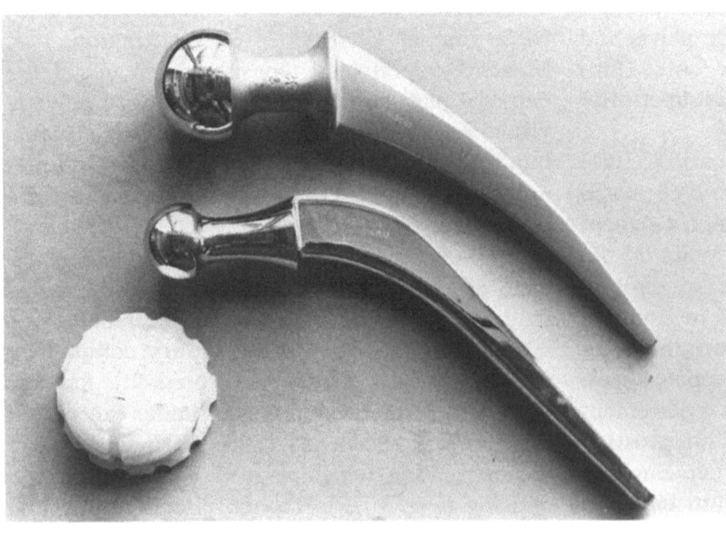

FIG. 1–28. The lower prosthesis and its cup is the Charnley with its low-friction 22-mm head. For comparison the Müller prosthesis is shown with its 32-mm head.

FIG. 1–29. The Tronzo prosthetic system.

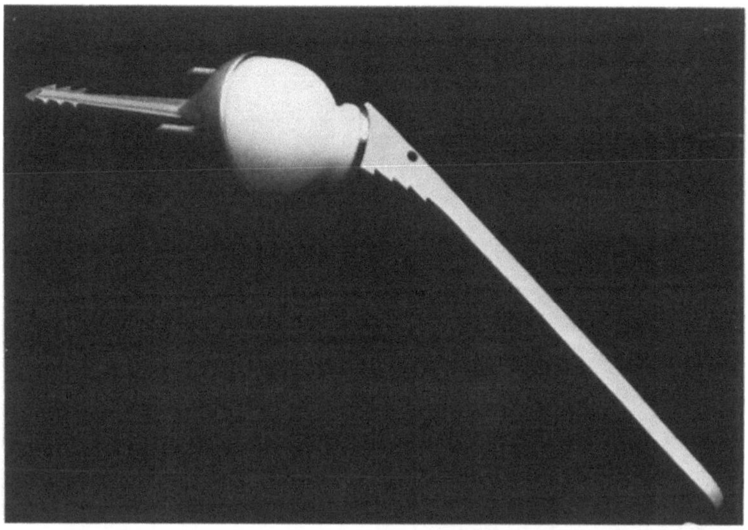

Time has shown that neitherthe 22-mm head nor osteotomy of the greater trochanter is necessary to the success of a total hip replacement, although there are still many devotees of these concepts.

Sir John Charnley (Fig. 1–30) passed away August 5, 1982 in Manchester, England. He left an indelible mark and will be missed by all of us.

Professor Maurice Müller has contributed enormously to the study and development of total hip arthroplasty. He opposed the Charnley concept of a 22-mm head and the need for osteotomizing the greater trochanter. His prosthesis is a 32-mm head inserted without removing the greater trochanter. He was able to create improved tension of the abductors by having his prosthesis manufactured with different neck lengths which was not available with the Charnley device. He showed that friction between the head and acetabulum was not critical. The smaller 22-mm head had the inherent capacity of dislocating. The Müller 32-mm head was made larger so that it would inherently be more stable. It became more popular than the Charnley (Fig. 1–28). Professor Müller's lectures in clinics both in Switzerland and elsewhere have been attended by thousands of orthopedic surgeons.

Dr. Frank Stinchfield (Fig. 1–31) made a significant contribution to the comprehensive study of hip problems by founding the Hip Society in 1968 which led to the creation of another organization called the International Hip Society. Through his endeavors, the Hip Society has become a forum for both basic and clinical research. It has become the podium for advancement of total hip arthroplasty through presentations of papers at the annual Academy of Orthopedic Surgeons Meeting and their subsequent publication in the Proceedings of the Hip Society. All forms of hip problems, both pediatric and adult, are likewise presented at this widely attended meeting.

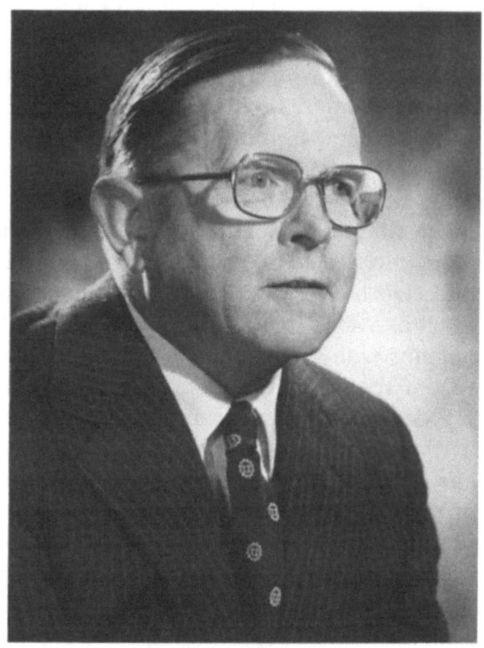

FIG. 1–30 Sir John Charnley, C.B.E., F.R.S., F.R.C.S.

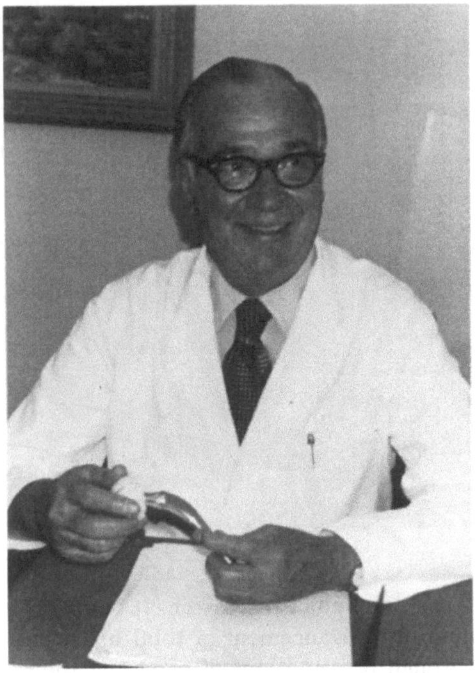

FIG. 1–31 Frank E. Stinchfield, M.D., F.A.C.S.

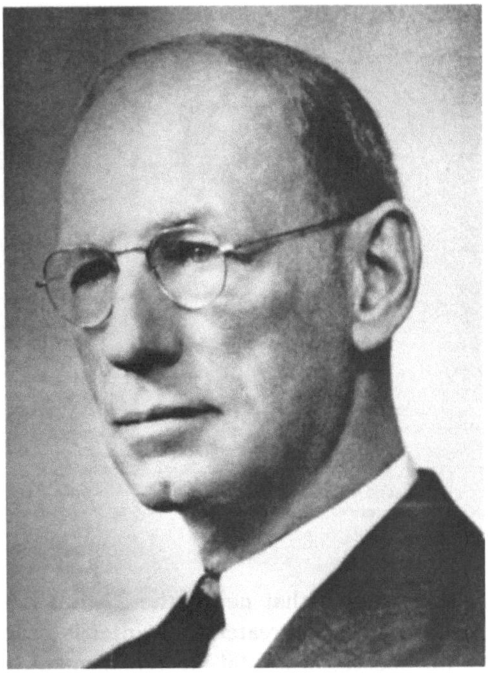

FIG. 1–32 A. Bruce Gill, 1876–1965.

Shelf Operation and Pelvic Osteotomy

It was early appreciated that an unstable hip could be given a certain amount of stability for weight bearing if a shelf or buttress of bone was created at the upper rim of the acetabulum to prevent the head from going upward with walking. In 1891 König [88] and in 1909 Jackson Clarke [35] constructed a bony block by turning down a flap of bone from the ilium over the head of the femur. Albee,[7] as early as 1913, placed tibial bone grafts into the pelvis above the upper rim of the acetabulum to act as a shelf or bony block which, in 1917, he combined with a semicircular bone flap turned down from the ilium. Compere and Phemister [38] in 1935 described a similar procedure. In 1923 Spitzy [163] used a wide strong tibial graft driven into the pelvis for the same purpose. Somewhat similar procedures were described by Lance [89] in 1925 and Ghormley [55] in 1931.

In 1922 Fairbank [47] was the first to perform a shelf operation for a congenital dislocation of the hip. In 1935 Gill [58] (Fig. 1–32) reported a plastic reconstruction of the acetabulum which proved to be, in his hands, one of the most successful procedures of any shelf operation (Fig. 1–33). In 1939 Nachlas [131] also described a shelf operation, which he named a "bucket-handle" procedure, which was an acetabuloplasty.

In 1955 Chiari,[33] of Vienna, first reported a pelvic osteotomy in order to secure a more stable coverage of the head. The osteotomy was performed above the upper acetabulum (Fig. 1–34). This was followed with descriptions of pelvic osteotomies by Pemberton,[140] of Salt Lake City, in 1960 and Salter,[146] of Toronto, in 1961. This operation is now an accepted procedure and represents another milestone in the development of hip surgery.

Cheilotomy and Acetabuloplasty

Operations for the relief of pain in osteoarthritis and other conditions of the hip by removing spurs and excess bone about the acetabulum and head of the femur have been performed for many years. The procedure is called cheilotomy. The hip considered suitable for a cheilotomy usually shows pain on weight bearing with limitation of abduction and internal rotation. Baer, of Johns Hopkins

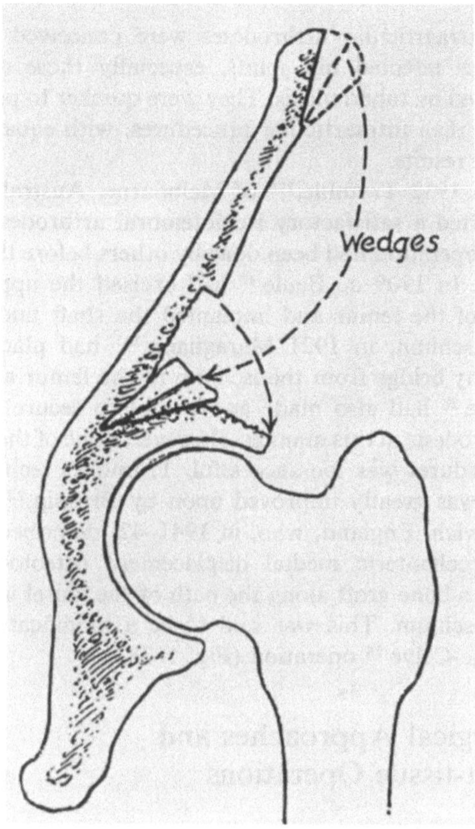

FIG. 1–33 Gill shelf operation. (From Campbell, W. C.: *Operative Orthopaedics*, 1st ed. St. Louis, Mosby, 1939.)

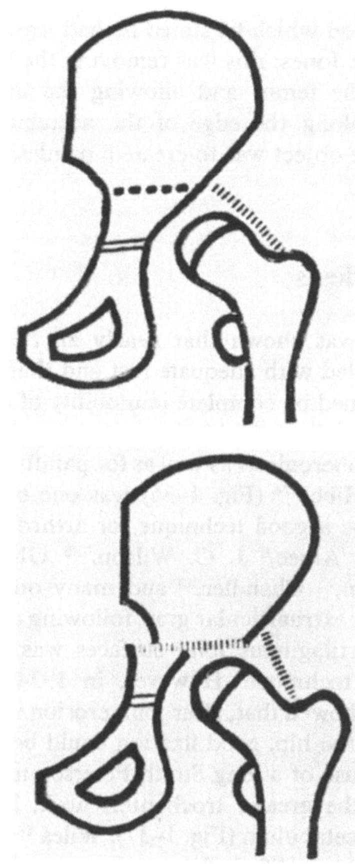

FIG. 1–34 The diagrammatic description of Chiari pelvic osteotomy. After the extraarticular separation of the pelvic girdle and the medial displacement of the hip joint, a strong acetabular roof results without bone grafting. The gluteal musculature alters its direction of pull and improves its efficiency. (From Chiari, K.: Zeitschrift für Orthopaedic und ihre Grenzgebiete 87:14–26, 1955. With permission from F. Enke Verlag, Stuttgart.)

in the 1920s, when the writer was one of his residents, did many of these procedures which he called "hip reconstruction operation." In the Baer procedure the head was dislocated, all rough edges, osteophytes, and spurs about the acetabulum and head of the femur were removed, and the head was replaced, sometimes trimmed to a smaller size as for a cup arthroplasty. The results were not uniformly good, but in a few instances were spectacular. In 1933 Hey Groves [65] wrote about cheilotomy, but before that time Murphy,[129] of Chicago, had performed these operations. In 1936 Smith-Petersen [158] described the removal of the anterior portion of the acetabulum done for the pain associated with malum coxae senilis, an old slipped upper femoral epiphysis, an intra-pelvic protrusion of the head (protrusio acetabuli), and an old coxa plana. It was hoped that the operation might result in the permanent relief of pain in these cases, but the long-term end-results were not encouraging.

Hip Resection

One of the oldest hip operations is resection of the head of the femur for tuberculosis. This was first done by Anthony White,[180] of London, in 1821. In 1852 a well-known general surgeon, Bigelow [17] of Boston, performed the first hip resection for tuberculosis in America, and in 1854 Sayre,[148] of New York, performed the second; however, it was Sayre who popularized the procedure over a period of 30 years, during which time he performed 70 hip resections.[150] In 1861 Fock [48] did the same for arthritis, but an unstable hip resulted. In 1945 Girdlestone,[60] of Oxford, described an operation which he stated he had learned from Sir Robert Jones; this was removing the head and neck of the femur and allowing the upper end to glide along the edge of the acetabulum and ilium. The object was to create a painless, mobile, false joint.

Arthrodesis

When it was shown that nearly all tuberculous joints healed with adequate rest and that this was best obtained by complete immobility of the joint, an arthrodesis of the hip became a popular procedure for tuberculosis as well as for painful arthritis. In 1926 Hibbs [74] (Fig. 1–35) was one of the first to describe a good technique for arthrodesis, followed by Albee,[6] J. C. Wilson,[185] Ghormley,[55] Henderson,[71] Chandler,[30] and many others (Fig. 1–36). An extraarticular graft following an erosion of the cartilaginous joint surfaces was the most common technique. However, in 1934 Watson-Jones[178] showed that, after joint erosion in osteoarthritis of the hip, good fixation could be obtained with the use of a long Smith-Petersen nail driven through the greater trochanter, neck, head, and into the acetabulum (Fig. 1–37). Wiles [183] reported in 1958 a modified Watson-Jones technique in which an extraarticular graft is added.

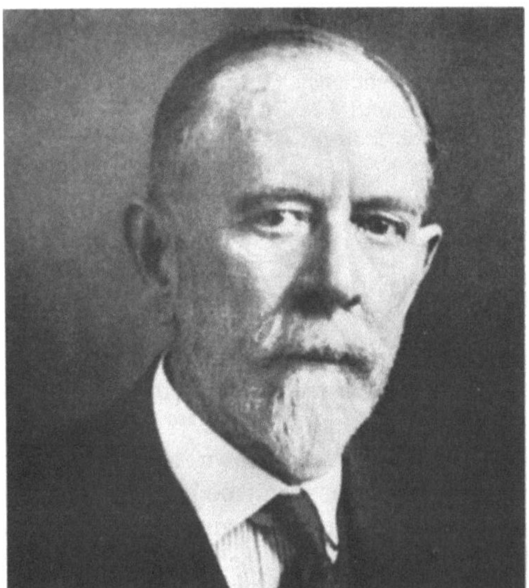

FIG. 1–35 Russell A. Hibbs, 1869–1932. (From Smith, A. D.: *The New York Orthopaedic Hospital. A Century of Progress in Orthopaedic Surgery.* Privately published.)

Extraarticular arthrodeses were conceived to bypass infected hip joints, especially those destroyed by tuberculosis. They were quicker to perform than intraarticular procedures, with equally good results.

In 1932 Trumble,[173] of Melbourne, Australia, reported a satisfactory ischiofemoral arthrodesis. The operation had been done by others before this time. In 1909 de Beule [43] had excised the upper end of the femur and implanted the shaft under the ischium; in 1921 Maragliano [111] had placed a bony bridge from the ischium to the femur and Calvé [25] had also made an attempt to secure an arthrodesis in this manner. However, none of these procedures was too successful. Trumble's technique was greatly improved upon by Brittain,[22] of Norwich, England, who, in 1941–42, described a subtrochanteric medial displacement osteotomy with a bone graft along the path of the chisel into the ischium. This was said to be a modification of the Calvé [25] operation (Fig. 1–38).

Surgical Approaches and Soft-tissue Operations

Good and effective surgery in any part of the body, and particularly in the hip joint, is dependent in a large measure on the exposure of the structures to be operated upon, hence the great importance of the surgical approach. The two approaches used more often now (their development might be considered milestones in modern hip surgery) are the Smith-Petersen[156] anterior iliofemoral incision and the Gibson[56] posterolateral incision. However, many other approaches give an excellent exposure, such as the lateral U incision of Ollier [135] (1892), long used by many surgeons, the lateral incision of Watson-Jones,[177] and the posterior curved incision of Kocher [86] (1907) and Langenbeck [93] (1874). Gibson's incision, developed from those of Langenbeck [93] and Kocher,[86] was first described in 1950, but had been used by Gibson [56] routinely for 35 years before that time. Smith-Petersen [156] first described his incision in 1917; it was developed from the approaches of Bardenhauer,[14] Sprengel,[165] Larghi,[94] and Hueter.[75] In addition, Luck [103] in 1955 described a transverse anterior approach which had considerable merit for intertrochanteric reconstruction of the hip for ununited fracture of the neck of the femur.

In presenting the development of hip surgery,

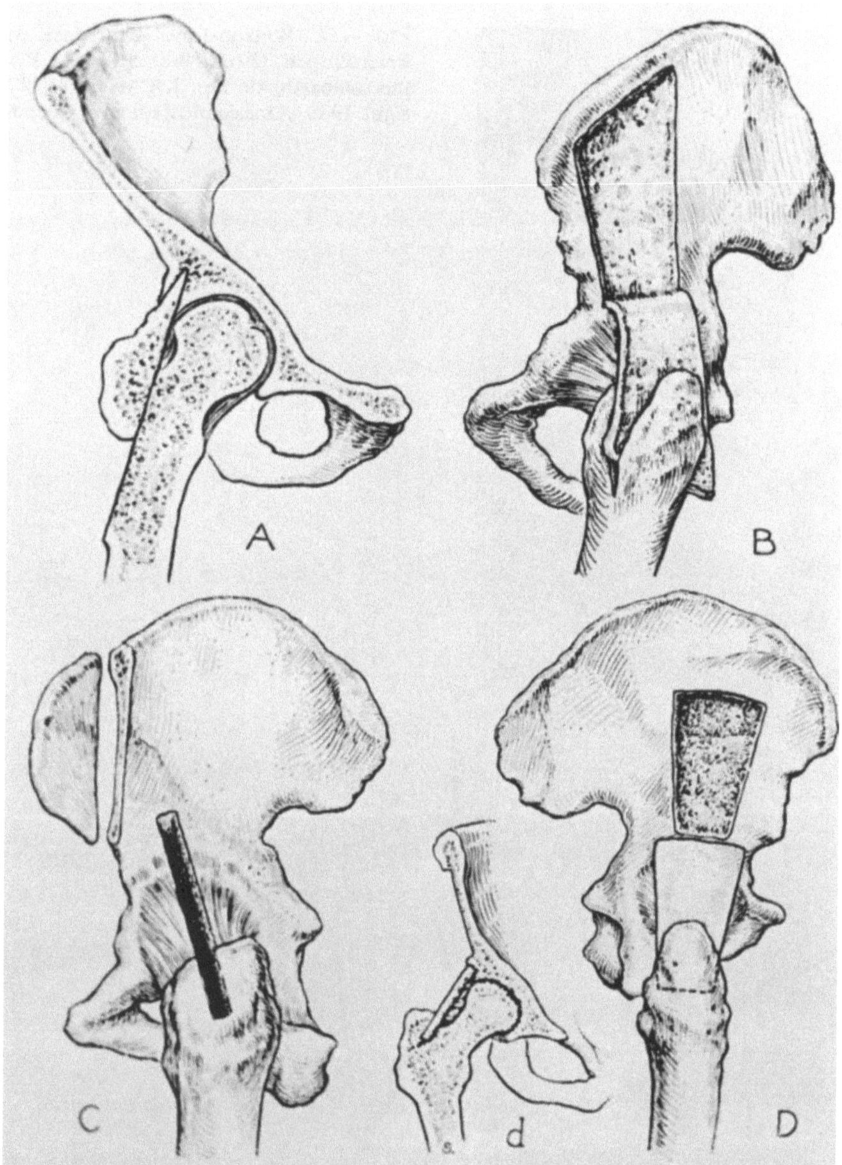

FIG. 1–36 Hip arthrodeses. **A** Hibbs. **B** J. C. Wilson. **C** Ghormley. **D** Henderson. (From Campbell, W. C.: *Operative Orthopaedics*, 1st ed. St. Louis, Mosby, 1939.)

mention should be made of fasciotomies and a few of the other soft-tissue procedures about the hip which were commonly done in the days when poliomyelitis was prevalent. Of the polio deformities requiring surgery, flexion deformity of the hip was by far the most frequently observed. In 1914 Soutter [161] described a fasciotomy for a flexion contracture; this involved stripping the fascia lata and associated flexor muscles subperiosteally from the anterior superior spine and crest of the ilium and allowing these structures to slip down the side of the pelvis to be attached at a distal site. In 1925 Campbell [26] described an operation for the same, transferring the anterior superior spine and anterior portion of the iliac crest with the muscles attached to a lower level on the ilium. Both of these were excellent procedures, usually allowing full extension of the hip. There were many other operations described for the purpose of correcting a hip flexion deformity, but the Soutter and Camp-

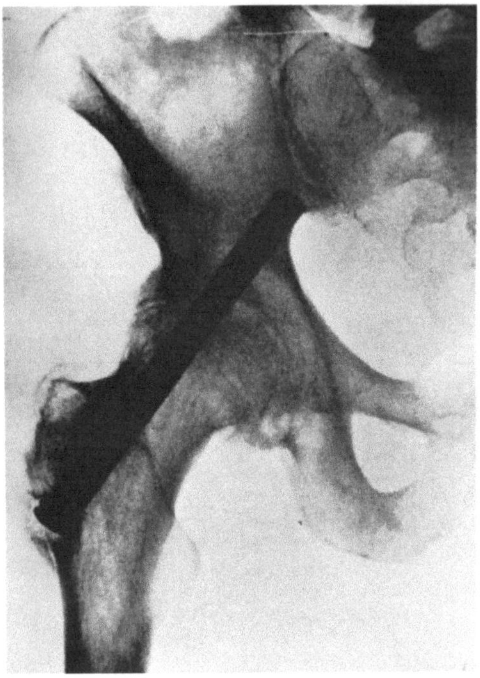

FIG 1–37 Watson-Jones arthrodesis with long Smith-Petersen nail. (From Watson-Jones, R.: Arthrodesis of the osteoarthritic hip. J.A.M.A., 110:279, 1938. Copyright 1938, American Medical Association.)

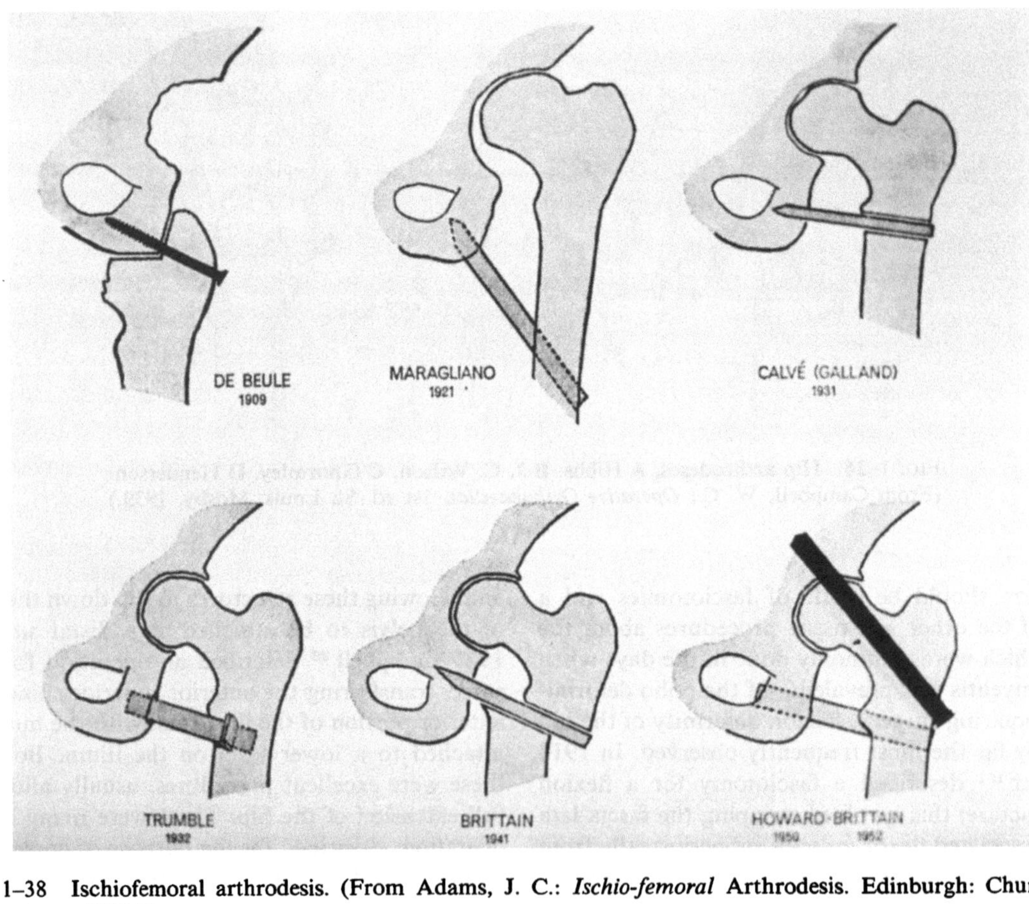

FIG 1–38 Ischiofemoral arthrodesis. (From Adams, J. C.: *Ischio-femoral* Arthrodesis. Edinburgh: Churchill-Livingstone, 1966.)[2]

bell procedures soon became the most popular.

To decrease the backward swaying on walking due to a gluteus maximus paralysis, F. D. Dickson [45] in 1927 described the transference of the origin of the tensor fasciae latae with its bony attachment posteriorly into the posterior superior spine of the ilium and the adjacent portion of the iliac crest. For the same condition, Ober [133] in 1927 described an operation freeing the lower attachment of the erector spinae muscles, and attaching to this a long strip of fascia lata which was passed over the gluteus maximus and fixed into the femur at the gluteus maximus insertion.

For hip instability, particularly in polio, and in an occasional dislocation when a bone block is not indicated, operations have been described for reefing the capsule of the hip; however, none of these has proven satisfactory for any length of time. In polio and spina bifida with a paralysis of the gluteus medius or of this muscle and the gluteus maximus, an operation to increase stability was described in 1952 by Mustard; [130] the iliopsoas muscle is transferred to the greater trochanter. In 1964 Sharrard [155] described a posterior iliopsoas transplantation which he had first done in 1958 for recurrent dislocation of the hip, mostly in patients with meningomyelocele; his results were very encouraging. These two operations are both significant in the development of soft-tissue hip surgery.

Conclusions

This chapter has given some of the more important milestones of history as the writer sees them, although he recognizes that others might not consider them the most significant. Obviously had it not been for the thinking and doing of those of the past, hip surgery would not be as far advanced as it is today. To these pioneers, we in modern orthopedics owe a great debt of gratitude. Much has been accomplished in perfecting better operations and techniques, and the road to the future holds promise for a great deal more with image intensifiers in the operating room to facilitate more precise surgery.

Bibliography

Note: The bibliography contains references to all articles mentioned in the text and also references to many significant articles and books which have not been mentioned. It is the author's belief that anyone further interested in the development of hip surgery and wishing to learn more than is contained in this chapter can find satisfactory references here.

Bibliography

1. Adams, J. C.: A reconsideration of cup arthroplasty of the hip with a precise method of concentric arthroplasty. J. Bone Joint Surg., 35B:199–208, 1953.
2. Adams, J. C.: *Ischio-femoral Arthrodesis.* Edinburgh: Churchill-Livingstone, 1966.
3. Adams, W.: Remarks on the subcutaneous division of the neck of the thigh-bone as compared with other operations for rectifying extreme distortion at the hip joint with bony anchylosis. Brit. Med. J., 2:673–676, 1870.
4. Albee, F. H.: The bone graft peg in the treatment of fractures of neck of femur. Ann. Surg., 62:85–91, 1915.
5. Albee, F. H.: Treatment of ununited fracture of the neck of the femur. Surg. Gynec. Obstet., 49:810–817, 1929.
6. Albee, F. H.: Extra-articular arthrodesis of the hip for tuberculosis. Ann. Surg., 89:404–426, 1929.
7. Albee, F. H.: *Injuries and Diseases of the Hip.* New York, Paul B. Hoeber, 1937.
8. Albee, F. H.: The kinesiological lever in reconstruction operations on the hip. J. Bone Joint Surg., 22:406, 1940.
9. Allis, O. H.: *An Inquiry into the Difficulties Encountered in the Reduction of Dislocations of the Hip.* Philadelphia, Dorman, 1896.
10. Aufranc, O. E.: Constructive hip surgery with Vitallium mold. A report on 1000 cases of arthroplasty of the hip over a 15-year period. J. Bone Joint Surg., 39A:237–248, 1957.
11. Aufranc, O. E.: *Constructive Surgery of the Hip.* St. Louis, Mosby, 1962.
12. Baer, W. S.: Arthroplasty with the aid of animal membrane. Amer. J. Orthop. Surg., 16:1–29, 94–115, 171–199, 1919.
13. Baeyer, von H.: Operative Behandlung von nicht reponierten angeborenen Huftverrenkungen. Munchen. Med. Wschr., 65:1216, 1918.
14. Bardenhauer: Referred to in Campbell, W. C.: *Operative Orthopedics,* 4th ed. St. Louis, Mosby, 1963.
15. Barton, J. R.: On the treatment of ankylosis, by the formation of artificial joints. N. Amer. Med. Surg. J., 3:279–292, 1827.
16. Bick, E. M.: *Source Book of Orthopaedics,* 2nd. ed. Baltimore, Williams & Wilkins, 1948.

17. Bigelow, H. J.: Resection of the head of the femur. Amer. J. Med. Sci., 24:90, 1852.
18. Blount, W. P.: Blade-plate internal fixation for high femoral osteotomies. J. Bone Joint Surg., 25:319–339, 1943.
19. Bohlman, H. R.: Replacement reconstruction of the hip. Amer. J. Surg., 84:268–278, 1952.
20. Bouvier, S. H. V.: Luxations congenitales de la hanche. Bull. Acad. Med. (Paris), 3:759, 1838.
21. Brackett, E. G.: Fractured neck of the femur; operation of transplantation of the femoral head to trochanter. Boston Med. Surg. J., 192:1118–1120, 1925.
22. Brittain, H. A.: Ischiofemoral arthrodesis. Brit. J. Surg., 29:93–104, 1941.
23. Brittain, H. A.: *Architectural Principles in Arthrodesis.* Edinburgh, Livingstone, 1942.
24. Brodhurst, B. E.: *The Deformities of the Human Body. A System of Orthopaedic Surgery, being a Course of Lectures Delivered at St. George's Hospital.* London, Churchill, 1871.
25. Calvé, J.: Ischiofemoral arthrodesis. Quoted by Galland in 1931 in Adams, J. C.: *Ischiofemoral Arthrodesis.* Baltimore, Williams & Wilkins, 1966.
26. Campbell, W. C.: Transference of the crest of the ilium for flexion contractures of the hip. Southern Med. J., 16:289, 1925.
27. Campbell, W. C.: Arthroplasty of the hip; an analysis of 48 cases. Surg. Gynec. Obstet., 43:9–17, 1926.
28. Campbell, W. C.: The physiology of arthroplasty (Sir Robert Jones Lecture). J. Bone Joint Surg., 13:223–245, 1931.
29. Carnochan, J. M.: Arch. Med., 284, 1860 and Clin. Orthop., 44:74, 1966 (see ref. 170).
30. Chandler, F. A.: Hip-fusion operation. J. Bone Joint Surg., 15:947–952, 1933.
31. Charnley, J.: Total prosthetic replacement of the hip. Physiotherapy, 53:407–409, 1967.
32. Charry, R.: *The Resection Angulation of the Hip.* Paris, Deren & Cie, 1964.
33. Chiari, K.: Ergebnisse mit der Beckenosteotomie als Pfannendach-plastik (Results of pelvic osteotomy as of the shelf method of acetabular roof plastic). Z. Orthop., 87:14-26, 1955.
34. Chiari, K.: The operative treatment of congenital dislocation of the hip. Wien Med. Wschr., 107:1020–1022, 1957.
35. Clarke, J. J.: Congenital dislocation of the hip joint: the ultimate results of the manipulative operation, and a note on a new operation for relapsed cases. Lancet, 2:925–296, 1909.
36. Colonna, P. C.: A new type of reconstruction operation for old ununited fracture of the femoral neck. J. Bone Joint Surg., 17:110–122, 1935.
37. Colonna, P. C.: An arthroplastic procedure for congenital dislocation of the hip, a two-stage procedure. Surg. Gynec. Obstet., 63:771–781, 1936.
38. Compere, E. L., and Phemister, D. B.: The tibial peg shelf in congenital dislocation of the hip. J. Bone Joint Surg., 17:60–72, 1935.
39. Da Costa, J. C.: Nailing of a fracture of the neck of the femur. Referred to in Wilson, H. A.: Amer. J. Orthop. Surg., 5:351, 1907–08.
40. d'Aubigne, R. M., and Postel, M.: Functional results of hip arthroplasty with acrylic prosthesis. J. Bone Joint Surg., 36A:451–475, 1954.
41. Davis, G. G.: An operation for ununited fracture of the neck of the femur. Univ. Med. Mag. Philadelphia, 13:507, 1900.
42. Davis, G. G.: The operative treatment of intracapsular fracture of the neck of the femur. Amer. J. Orthop. Surg., 6:481–483, 1908–09.
43. DeBeule, F.: La resection de la hanche suivie de fixation de l'extremite superieure du femur a la tuberosité ischiatique. J. Chir. Ann. Soc. Belge Chir., 9:173–176, 1901.
44. Delbet, P.: Resultat eloigne dun visage pour fracture transcervicale du femur. Bull. Soc. Chir. Paris, 45:305, 1919.
45. Dickson, F. D.: An operation for stabilizing paralytic hips, a preliminary report. J. Bone Joint Surg., 9:1–7, 1927.
46. Dickson, J. A.: The high geometric osteotomy with rotation and bone graft, for ununited fractures of the neck of the femur. J. Bone Joint Surg., 29:1005–1018, 1947.
47. Fairbank, H. A. T.: Late results of treatment of congenital dislocations of the hip. Brit. J. Surg., 10:24–37, 1922.
48. Fock, C.: Bemerkungen und Erfahrungen über die Resection im Hüftgelenke. Arch. Klin. Chir., 1:172, 1861.
49. Ford, E.: *Observations on the Disease of the Hip Joint.* London, Dilly, 1794.
50. Frankel, V. H.: *The Femoral Neck: An Experimental Study of Function, Fracture Mechanism, and Internal Fixation.* (Uppsala, Almqvist & Wiksells, 1960.) Springfield, Thomas, 1960.
51. Gaenslen, F. G.: The acetabular prosthesis. Discussion of paper of McBride, E. D.: The flanged acetabular replacement prosthesis. Arch. Surg., 83:726–278, 1961.
52. Gaenslen, F. G.: The Schanz subtrochanteric osteotomy for irreducible dislocation of the hip. J. Bone Joint Surg., 17:76–87, 1935.
53. Galland, M.: Les arthrodeses ischio-femorales. Rev. Orthop., 36:285–296, 1950.
54. Gant, F. J.: Subcutaneous osteotomy below the trochanters. Brit. Med. J., 2:606, 1879.
55. Ghormley, R. D.: Use of the anterior superior

spine and crest of the ilium in surgery of the hip joint. J. Bone Joint Surg., 13:784–798, 1931.
56. Gibson, A.: Posterior exposure of the hip joint. J. Bone Joint Surg., 32B:183–186, 1950.
57. Gibney, V. B.: *The Hip and Its Diseases.* New York, Bermingham, 1884.
58. Gill, A. B.: Plastic construction of an acetabulum in congenital dislocation of the hip—the shelf operation. J. Bone Joint Surg., 17:48–59, 1935.
59. Girdlestone, G. R.: Arthrodesis and other operations for tuberculosis of the hip. In: *The Robert Jones Birthday Volume.* Cambridge, Oxford University Press, 1928.
60. Girdlestone, G. R.: Pseudarthrosis. In: Discussion on the treatment of unilateral osteoarthritis of the hip. Proc. Roy. Soc. Med., 38:363–268, 1945.
61. Gluck, T.: Autoplastik- transplantation- implantation von Fremdkörpern. Klin. Wschr., 27:421–427, 1890.
62. Godoy-Moreira, F. E.: A special stud-bolt screw for fixation of fractures of the neck of the femur. J. Bone Joint Surg., 22:683–697, 1940.
63. Groves, E. W. H.: Arthroplasty. Brit. J. Surg., 11:234–250, 1923.
64. Groves, E. W. H.: Some contributions to the reconstructive surgery of the hip. Brit. J. Surg., 14:486–517, 1927.
65. Groves, E. W. H.: Surgical treatment of osteoarthritis of the hip. Brit. Med. J., I:3–5, 1933.
66. Haboush, E. J.: Biomechanics of femoral nail and nailplate insertions in fractures of the neck of the femur. Bull. Hosp. Joint Dis., 14:125–137, 1953.
67. Haboush, E. J.: A new operation for arthroplasty of the hip based on biomechanics, photoelasticity, fast-setting dental acrylic, and other considerations. Bull. Hosp. Joint Dis., 14:242–277, 1953.
68. Harmon, P. H.: Arthroplasty of the hip for osteoarthritis utilizing foreign body cups of plastic. Surg. Gynec. Obstet., 76:347–365, 1943.
69. Hass, J.: Extra-artikulare Ankylosierung der Hufte. Zbl. Chir., 49:1466, 1922.
70. Hass, J.: *Congenital Dislocation of the Hip.* Springfield, Ill., Thomas, 1951.
71. Henderson, M. S.: Combined intra-articular and extra-articular arthrodesis for tuberculosis of the hip joint. J. Bone Joint Surg., 15:51–57, 1933.
72. Henderson, M. S.: Internal fixation of fractures of the neck of the femur. Arch. Surg., 35:419–430, 1937.
73. Henderson, M. S.: Ununited fracture of the neck of the femur treated by the aid of the bone graft. J. Bone Joint Surg., 22:97–106, 1940.
74. Hibbs, R. A.: A preliminary report of twenty cases of hip joint tuberculosis treated by an operation devised to eliminate motion by fusing the joint. J. Bone Joint Surg., 24:522–533, 1926.
75. Hueter, C.: *Grundriss der Chirurgie* (General Surgery), 7 editions. Leipzig, Vogel, 1880–1892.
76. Jakobsson, A.: The shelf operation; an evaluation of results in congenital dysplasia, subluxation and dislocation of the hip joint. Acta Orthop. Scand., Suppl. 15, 1954.
77. Jergesen, F., and Abbott, L. C.: A comprehensive exposure of the hip joint. J. Bone Joint Surg., 37A:798–808, 1955.
78. Jewett, E. L., Albee, F. H., Jr., Powers, E. J., and Stanford, F. D.: Treatment of all fractures of the femoral neck and trochanteric region with the original one-piece flanged nail. J. Int. Coll. Surg., 18:313–328, 1952.
79. Jewett, E. L.: One-piece angle nail for trochanteric fractures. J. Bone Joint Surg., 23:803–810, 1941.
80. Johansson, S.: On operative treatment of medial fractures of neck of femur. Acta Orthop. Scand., 3:362–392, 1932.
81. Jones, Sir R.: *Orthopaedic Surgery of Injuries.* London, Oxford University Press, 1921.
82. Judet, J., and Judet, R.: The use of an artificial femoral head for arthroplasty of the hip joint. J. Bone Joint Surg., 32B:166–173, 1950.
83. Kallio, K. E.: Skin arthroplasty of the hip joint. Acta Orthop. Scand., 26:327–328, 1957.
84. Keith, Sir A.: *Menders of the Maimed.* London, Frowde, 1919.
85. Kirmisson, E.: De l'osteotomie soustrochanterienne appliqueé a certains cas de luxation congenitale de la hanche. Rev. Orthop., 5:137–146, 1894.
86. Kocher, T.: *Text-book of Operative Surgery,* (English translation from 4th German ed.). London, Black, 1911.
87. König, F.: See Von Langenbeck.[93]
88. König, F.: Bildung einer knocherner Hemmung fur den Gelenkkopf bei kongenitalen Luxationen. Zbl. Chir., 17:146, 1891.
89. Lance, M.: Le traitement palliatif des luxations congenitales inveterées de la hanche. Rev. Orthop., 12:557, 1925.
90. Lance, M.: In: *Traité de Chirurgie Orthopedique* (Ombredanne, L., and Mathieu, P., eds.) Paris, Masson, 1937.
91. Langenbeck, B. Von: Die subcutane Osteotomie. Deutsch. Klin. Zeit. für Beobachtungen aus deutschen Kliniken und Krankenhausern, 6:327–335, 1854.
92. Langenbeck, B. Von: *Uber die Schussfracturen der Gelenke und ihre Behandlung.* Berlin, Hirschwald, 1868.
93. Langenbeck, B. Von: Verh. Deutsch. Ges. Chir., 7:92, 1878.

94. Larghi, X: Referred to in Campbell, W. C.: *Operative Orthopedics*, 4th ed. St. Louis, Mosby, 1963.
95. Leadbetter, G. W.: A treatment for fracture of the neck of the femur. J. Bone Joint Surg., 15:931–940, 1933.
96. Leadbetter, G. W.: Cervical-axial osteotomy of the femur, a preliminary report. J. Bone Joint Surg., 26:713–720, 1944.
97. Lexer, E.: *Die gesamte Wiederherstellungchirurgie*. Leipzig, Barth, 1931.
98. Lexer, E.: Über Gelenktransportation. Med. Klin. Berlin, 4:817–820, 1908.
99. Lippmann, R. K.: The transfixion hip prosthesis, observations based upon 5 years of use. J. Bone Joint Surg., 39A:759–785, 1957.
100. Loewe, O.: Über Hautimplantation an Stelle der freien Faszien-plastik. München. Med. Wschr., 60:1320, 1913.
101. Lorenz, A.: Über die Behandlung der irreponiblen angeborenen Hüftluxationen und der Schenkelhalspseudoarthrosen mittels Gabelung (Bifurkation des oberen Femurendes). Wien Klin. Wschr., 32:997, 1919.
102. Luck, J. V.: A reconstruction operation for pseudarthrosis and resorption of the neck of the femur. J. Iowa Med. Soc., 28:620–622, 1938.
103. Luck, J. V.: A new transverse anterior approach to the hip. J. Bone Joint Surg., 37A:534–536, 1955.
104. MacAusland, W. R., and MacAusland, A. R.: *The Mobilization of Ankylosed Joints by Arthroplasty*. Philadelphia, Lea & Febiger, 1929.
105. McBride, E. D.: A femoral head prosthesis for the hip joint. J. Bone Joint Surg., 34A:989–996, 1952.
106. McBride, E. D.: The flanged acetabular replacement prosthesis. Arch. Surg., 83:721–728, 1961.
107. McKee, G. K., and Watson-Farrar, J.: Replacement of arthritic hips by the McKee-Farrar prosthesis. J. Bone Joint Surg., 48B:245–259, 1966.
108. McMurray, T. P.: Ununited fractures of the neck of the femur. J. Bone Joint Surg., 18:319–327, 1936.
109. McMurray, T. P.: Fracture of the neck of the femur treated by oblique osteotomy. Brit. Med. J., I:330–333, 1938.
110. Magnuson, P. B.: The repair of ununited fracture of the neck of the femur. J.A.M.A., 98:1791–1794, 1932.
111. Maragliano, D.: Nuovi punti di appoggio chirurgico nelle lussazioni vere da coxite. Chir. Organi Mov., 5:225–247, 1921.
112. Martin, E. D., and King, A. C.: New method of treating fractures of the neck of the femur. New Orleans Med. Surg. J., 75:710–715, 1923.
113. Martin, E. D.: Fractures of the neck of the femur. Int. J. Med. Surg., 46:301–306, 1933.
114. Michele, A. A.: *The Iliopsoas*. Springfield, Ill., Thomas, 1962.
115. Milch, H.: The "pelvic support" osteotomy. J. Bone Joint Surg., 23:581–595, 1941.
116. Milch, H.: *Osteotomy of the Long Bones*. Springfield, Ill., Thomas, 1947.
117. Milch, H.: The resection-angulation operation for hip-joint disabilities. J. Bone Joint Surg., 37A: 699–717, 1955.
118. Moore, A. T.: Fracture of the hip joint (intracapsular); a new method of skeletal fixation. J. S. Carolina Med. Assoc., 30:199–205, 1934.
119. Moore, A. T.: Fracture of the hip joint. Surg. Gynec. Obstet., 64:420–436, 1937.
120. Moore, A. T., and Bohlman, H. R.: Metal hip joint, a case report. J. Bone Joint Surg., 25:688–692, 1943.
121. Moore, A. T.: Blade-plate internal fixation for intertrochanteric fractures. J. Bone Joint Surg., 26:52–62, 1944.
122. Moore, A. T.: Metal hip joint: new self-locking Vitallium prosthesis. Southern Med. J., 45:1015–1019, 1952.
123. Moore, A. T.: The self-locking metal hip prosthesis. J. Bone Joint Surg., 39A:811–827, 1957.
124. Moore, J. R.: Cartilaginous-cup arthroplasty in ununited fractures of the neck of the femur. J. Bone Joint Surg., 30A:313–330, 1948.
125. Moret, M.: Contribution a l'étude du traitement chirurgical des luxations de la hanche invéterées par la constitution d'une butée osteoplastique. Thesis, Paris, 1925 (No. 507, from S.G.O. Index, Vol. VII, 1928).
126. Müller, M. E.: *Die Huftnahen Femurosteotomien*. Stuttgart, Thieme Verlag, 1957.
127. Murphy, J. B.: Ankylosis; arthroplasty—clinical and experimental. J.A.M.A., 44:1573–1582, 1671–1678, 1749–1756, 1905.
128. Murphy, J. B.: Arthroplasty. Ann. Surg., 57:593–647, 1913.
129. Murphy, J. B.: Bony lipping of the right acetabular margin and of the neck of the femur following a metastatic arthritis-arthroplasty of the hip cheilotomy. Surg. Clin. J. B. Murphy, 4:239–246, 1915.
130. Mustard, W. T.: Iliopsoas transfer for weakness of the hip abductors. J. Bone Joint Surg., 34A: 647–650, 1952.
131. Nachlas, I. W.: Acetabuloplasty for dislocation of the hip. Southern Med. J., 32:565–571, 1939.
132. Nicolaysen, J.: Lidt om diagnosen og behandlingen af fractura colli femoris. Nord. Med. Ark., 8:1–19, 1897.
133. Ober, F. R.: An operation for the relief of paraly-

sis of the gluteus maximus muscle, J.A.M.A., 88:1063, 1927.
134. Ollier, L.X.E.L.: *Traite des Resections et des Operations Conservatrices qu'on peut Pratiquer sur le Systeme Osseus.* Paris, Masson, 1885.
135. Ollier, P.: Lateral "U" approach to the hip. In: *Campbell's Operative Orthopedics,* 4th ed. St. Louis, Mosby, 1963; Paris, Traite des Resections, 1892.
136. Osborne, R. R.: The approach to the hip-joint. Brit. J. Surg., 18:49–52, 1930.
137. Pauwels, F.: *Der Schenkelhalsbruch, ein mechanisches Problem.* Stuttgart, Enke, 1935.
138. Payr, E.: Blütige Mobilisierung versteifter Gelenke. Zbl. Chir., 37:1227, 1910.
139. Payr, E.: Uber die operative Mobilisierung ankylosierter Gelenke. Munchen. Med. Wschr., 57: 1921–1927, 1910.
140. Pemberton, P. A.: Rotation of the acetabular roof for treatment of congenital dysplasia of the hip. Trans. 8th Cong. Soc. Int. Chir. Orthop. Trauma, 255–264, 1960.
141. Pemberton, P. A.: Pericapsular osteotomy of the ilium for treatment of congenital subluxation and dislocation of the hip. J. Bone Joint Surg., 47A:65–86, 1965.
142. Peterson, L. T.: The use of a metallic femoral head. J. Bone Joint Surg., 33A:65–75, 1951.
143. Putti, V.: La mobilizzazione chirurgica delle anchilose del ginocchio. Chir. Organi Mov., 1:1–70, 1917.
144. Putti, V.: Arthroplasty. J. Orthop. Surg. 3:421–430, 1921.
145. Ring, P. A.: Complete replacement arthroplasty of the hip by the Ring prosthesis. J. Bone Joint Surg., 50B:720–731, 1968.
146. Salter, R. B.: Innominate osteotomy in the treatment of congenital dislocation and subluxation of the hip. J. Bone Joint Surg., 43B:518–539, 1961.
147. Sandison, C: Fractures of neck of femur. Piedmont Hosp. Bull., 10:28–35, 1937.
148. Sayre, L. A.: Exsection of the head of the femur and removal of the upper rim of the acetabulum for morbus coxarius. New York J. Med., 14:70–82, 1855.
149. Sayre, L. A.: A new method for artificial hip-joint in bony anchylosis, two cases. Trans. Med. Soc. New York, 111–127, 1863.
150. Sayre, L. A.: Exsection of the head of the femur for morbus coxarius. Med. Rec. New York, 6:281, 1871–72.
151. Schanz, A.: Uber die nach Schenkelhalsbruchen zuruckbleibenden Gestveringen. Deutch. Med. Wschr., 51:730–732, 1925.
152. Schanz, A.: *Praktische Orthopadie.* Berlin, Springer, 1928.
153. Senn, N.: Fractures of the neck of the femur, with special reference to bony union after intracapsular fracture. Trans. Amer. Surg. Assoc., 1:333, 1881–83.
154. Senn, N.: The treatment of fractures of the neck of the femur by immediate reduction and permanent fixation. J.A.M.A., 13:150–159, 1889.
155. Sharrard, W. J. W.: Posterior iliopsoas transplantation in the treatment of paralytic dislocation of the hip. J. Bone Joint Surg., 46B:426–444, 1964.
156. Smith-Petersen, M. N.: A new supra-articular subperiosteal approach to the hip joint. Amer. J. Orthop. Surg., 15:592–595, 1917.
157. Smith-Petersen, M. N., Cave, E. F., and Van Gorder, G. W.: Intra-capsular fractures of the neck of the femur; treatment by internal fixation. Arch. Surg., 23:715–759, 1931.
158. Smith-Petersen, M. N.: Treatment of malum coxae senilis, old slipped upper femoral epiphysis, intrapelvic protrusion of the acetabulum, and coxa plana by means of acetabuloplasty. J. Bone Joint Surg., 18:869–880, 1936.
159. Smith-Petersen, M. N.: Arthroplasty of the hip, a new method. J. Bone Joint Surg., 21:269–288, 1939.
160. Smith-Petersen, M. N.: Evolution of mould arthroplasty of the hip joint. J. Bone Joint Surg., 30B:59–73, 1948.
161. Soutter, R.: Fasciotomy of the hip. Boston Med. Surg. J., 11, 1914.
162. Soutter, R.: *Technique of Operations on the Bones, Joints, Muscles, and Tendons.* New York, Macmillan, 1917.
163. Spitzy, H.: Kunstliche pfannendachbildung, Benutzung von Knochenbolzen zur temporaren Fixation. Z. Orthop. Chir., 43:284, 1924.
164. Sprengel, O.: Zur operativen Nachbehandlung alter Huftresectionen. Beitr. z. wissensch. Med. Festschrift 69th . . . d. Versammd. deutsch Naturf. u. Aerzte. . . . edited by Rudolf Beneke. Braunschweig, 1897, pp. 51–82.
165. Sprengel, O.: Referred to in Campbell, W. C.: *Operative Orthopedics,* 4th ed. St. Louis, Mosby, 1963.
166. Strange, F. G.: *The Hip.* Baltimore, Williams & Wilkins, 1965.
167. Taylor, G. M., Neufeld, A. J., and Jansen, J.: Internal fixation for intertrochanteric fractures. J. Bone Joint Surg., 26:707, 1944.
168. Thompson, F. R.: Vitallium intramedullary hip prosthesis; preliminary report. New York J. Med., 52:3011–3020, 1952.
169. Thompson, F. R.: Two and a half years' experience with a Vitallium intramedullary hip prosthe-

sis. J. Bone Joint Surg., 36A:489–502, 1954.

170. Thompson, F. R.: An essay on the development of arthroplasty of the hip. Clin. Orthop., 44:73–82, 1966.

171. Thomson, J. E. M.: A prosthesis for the femoral head; a preliminary report. J. Bone Joint Surg., 34A:175–182, 1952.

172. Thornton, L.: The treatment of trochanteric fracture femur: Two new methods. Piedmont Hosp. Bull., 10:21–37, 1937.

173. Trumble, H. C.: A method of fixation of the hip joint by means of an extra-articular bone graft. Aust. New Zeal. J. Surg., 1:413–420, 1932.

174. Urist, M.: The principles of hip-socket arthroplasty. J. Bone Joint Surg., 39A:786–810, 1957.

175. Venable, C. S., Stuck, W. G., and Beach, A.: The effects on bone of the presence of metals; based upon electrolysis; an experimental study. Ann. Surg., 105:917–938, 1937.

176. Verneuil, A.: De la creation d'une fausses articulation par section ou resection partielle de l'os maxillaire inferieur, comme moyen de remedier a l'ankylose vraire ou fausse de la machoire inferieure. Arch. Gen. Med., 15:174, 1860.

177. Watson-Jones, R.: Lateral approach to the hip joint. In: *Campbell's Operative Orthopedics,* 4th ed. St. Louis, Mosby, 1963.

178. Watson-Jones, R., and Robinson, W. C.: Arthrodesis of the osteoarthritic hip joint. J. Bone Joint Surg., 38A:353–377, 1956.

179. Wescott, H. H.: A method for the internal fixation of transcervical fractures of the femur. J. Bone Joint Surg., 16:372–376, 1934.

180. White, A.: Obituary. Lancet, 1:324, 1849.

181. Whitman, R.: A new treatment for fracture of the neck of the femur. Med. Rec., 65:441–447, 1904.

182. Whitman, R.: The reconstruction operation for ununited fracture of the neck of the femur. Surg. Gynec. Obstet., 32:479–486, 1921.

183. Wiles, P.: The surgery of the osteo-arthritic hip. Brit. J. Surg., 45:488–497, 1958.

184. Wilson, H. A.: Treatment of ununited fractures of the neck of the femur by use of coin silver nails. Amer. J. Orthop. Surg., 5:339–353, 1907–08.

185. Wilson, J. C.: Extra-articular fusion of tuberculous hip joint. Calif. West. Med., 27:774–776, 1927.

186. Wilson, J. C.: Operative fixation of tuberculous hips in children; end result study of 33 patients from the orthopaedic department of the Children's Hospital. J. Bone Joint Surg., 15:22–47, 1933.

187. Wilson, P. D.: Trochanteric arthroplasty in the treatment of ununited fractures of the neck of the femur. J. Bone Joint Surg., 29:313–327, 1947.

CHAPTER 2

Physical Diagnosis of the Hip

ROBERT D. HEATH

History

In attempting to make a diagnosis in a patient with disease involving the hip joint, an accurate and complete history is of paramount importance. One must determine the duration of the disability. Was the onset acute or gradual? Was it secondary to trauma? Is pain a significant factor? Where is the pain located? When is the pain present? What intensifies it? What relieves it? Does it radiate? Have there been systemic signs of infection? The answers to these questions help in differentiating the cause of the patient's problem.

It is important to determine the presence or absence of pain since some problems are characteristically painful (traumatic problems, infectious problems, arthritic problems, neoplasms), and some are characteristically painless (congenital dislocation of the hip, congenital coxa vara, Charcot joints). It is also important to know when the pain is present. Patients with degenerative arthritis often are worse after a period of activity and are frequently benefited temporarily by inactivity. Patients with osteoid osteomas have a relatively constant type of pain not significantly aggravated by position or activity, and usually relieved by aspirin. The pain arising from many types of neoplasms and chronic infections is frequently worse at night.

The hip joint has three nerve supplies: the obturator nerve, the sciatic nerve, and the femoral nerve. Consequently, pain arising from a problem in the hip joint may be felt about the hip anteriorly, posteriorly, medially or laterally, or it may be referred along the pathway of any of the three nerves which supply the joint. Many patients with hip problems will have no pain in the area of the hip, but will complain of all of their pain around the anterior aspect of the knee due to reference down the obturator nerve. Patients have been mistakenly treated for knee problems when the actual source of the trouble is the hip joint.

It is necessary to be familiar with other systems which may produce pain in the same area as does hip disease. Lesions involving the lower lumbar vertebrae and the sacrum frequently refer pain into the posterior hip area, and those involving the upper lumbar vertebrae into the anterior thigh. Certain types of hernias and abdominal problems may cause pain in the inguinal area and proximal thigh. Pain in the buttock and anterior thigh may be of vascular origin. Pain brought on by walking a short distance and relieved by cessation of walking suggests the possibility of vascular, inadequacy.

The patient's age is important. Certain hip problems are seen only in children and only during certain age periods in childhood or adolescence. Other problems are seen only in later life (Table 2–1).

Much significant information can be obtained from past medical history. A previous traumatic dislocation of the hip, or fracture of the femoral neck, should suggest the possibility of aseptic necrosis or traumatic arthritis. A past history of chronic alcoholism, gout, lupus erythematosus, or steroid therapy over a long period suggests the possibility of idiopathic aseptic necrosis as a cause of disability. Knowing that a patient has sickle-cell anemia should make the examiner suspicious of an infarct when there are complaints of hip disability. A known past history of diabetes, syringomyelia or tabes dorsalis should make one consider a Charcot joint in a patient with a painless

TABLE 2–1 Hip Problems Related to Age

Disease	Age	Limp	Pain	Stable	Systemic Signs	Leg Shortening
Congenital dislocation of hip	Infancy→	Yes	Not in young	No	No	Yes
Toxic synovitis	2–10	Yes	Yes	Yes	Mild	No
Perthes disease	2–12	Yes	Usually mild	Yes	No	Not early
Congenital coxa vara	Infancy→	Yes	Not in young	No	No	Yes
Acute septic arthritis	Infancy→	Yes	Yes	Yes	Yes	No
Osteomyelitis, femoral neck	Infancy→	Yes	Yes	Yes	Yes	No
Old septic arthritis with destroyed head	Infancy→	Yes	±	±	No	Yes
Avulsed anterior superior spine or lesser trochanter	12–16	Yes	Yes	Yes	No	No
Slipped femoral capital epiphysis	10–16	Yes	Yes	Usually, except acute slip	No	Yes
Osteoid osteoma, femoral neck	5–30	±	Yes	Yes	No	No
Malignancy	Any age	±	Yes	Yes	No	No
Arthritis, rheumatoid	Any age	±	Usually	Usually	±	May be apparent shortening
Arthritis, degenerative	40→	±	Usually	Usually	No	May be apparent shortening
Neurotrophic joint	40→	Yes	No	No	No	Usually
Aseptic necrosis	Any age	Yes	Yes	Yes	No	Not significant

unstable hip. A past history of Perthes disease, slipped capital femoral epiphysis, or a congenital dislocation of the hip may be the cause of degenerative arthritis in later life.

The type of examination required for a patient with a chronic problem differs from that required for a patient with an acute traumatic or infectious problem. A good history helps not only in making an accurate preliminary diagnosis but also in directing the physician toward the appropriate type of physical examination.

Examination of the Hip

Chronic Problems

Be familiar with the landmarks about the hip. The anterior superior iliac spine is superficial and easily palpated. From this point the iliac crest can be palpated to its termination at the posterior superior iliac spine. The iliac tubercle can be felt about two inches behind the anterior superior iliac spine. The greater trochanter of the femur is approximately a hand's breadth below the iliac tubercle, and the top of the trochanter is about level with the upper margin of the symphysis pubis. The pubic tubercle is about one inch lateral to the symphysis pubis and can usually be palpated. The inguinal ligament stretches from the anterior superior spine to the pubic tubercle. The ischial tuberosity is covered with the bulky gluteus maximus when the thigh is in extension, but can be easily felt if the hip is flexed 90°. The head of the femur is located just below the inguinal ligament halfway between the anterior superior iliac spine and the symphysis pubis. The femoral artery can also be palpated at this point. Nelaton's line and Bryant's triangle have some clinical use (Fig. 2–1).

Go about the examination systematically. It is worthwhile for the physician to develop his own routine as to sequence in the examination. This contributes to efficiency, and minimizes the possibility of overlooking part of the examination. The following paragraphs have proved their value and are a suggestion as to sequence.

Have the patient stand. By inspection and pal-

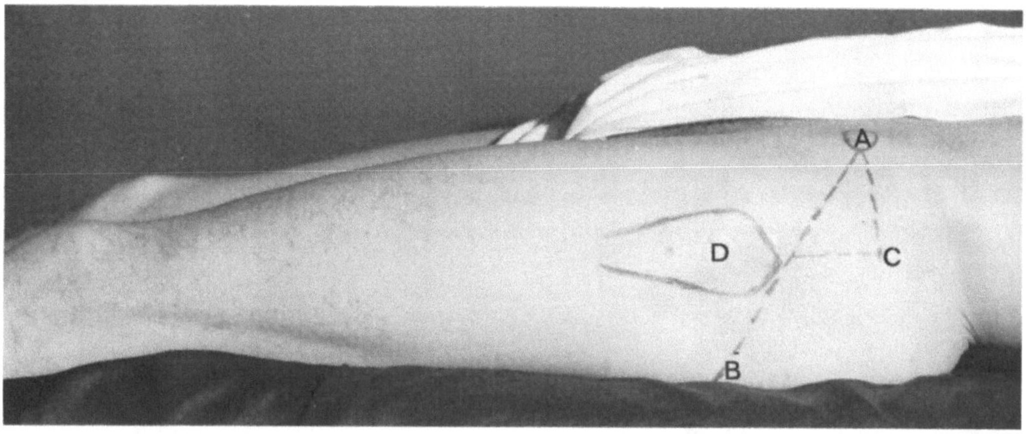

FIG. 2–1 *A* represents the anterior superior iliac spine; *B* the ischial tuberosity; and *D* the greater trochanter. *AB* is known as Nelaton's line. Normally, the greater trochanter should be on or below this line. In hip dislocations and coxa vara, however, it will be above the line. Bryant's triangle is formed by lines *AD, DC,* and *AC.* When the patient is lying supine, Bryant's triangle is formed by a perpendicular dropped from the anterior superior iliac spine, by a line joining the trochanter and the anterior superior iliac spine, and by a line extending from the tip of the trochanter to the perpendicular dropped from the anterior superior iliac spine. In any condition allowing upward displacement of the femur, the base of the triangle is shortened.

pation compare the level of the iliac crests and the anterior superior iliac spines. A unilateral elevation of the iliac crest or the anterior superior spine may indicate a fixed lumbar scoliosis, a fixed adduction or abduction deformity of a hip, or a true inequality of leg length. Determine if both knees are in full extension and both feet flat on the floor. In the presence of mobile hip joints and a mobile spine, an actual difference of approximately 1½ inches in leg length may be hidden without the patient's assuming an equinus foot stance on the side of the short leg. If the patient is seen to be standing on the toes of one foot, first eliminate the existence of a fixed equinus deformity by having the patient place his foot in dorsiflexion. In the absence of a fixed equinus deformity but with the iliac crest elevated on the side of the apparent equinus deformity, consider a fixed adduction deformity of the hip on the side with the high iliac crest, a fixed abduction deformity on the opposite side, or a fixed lumbar scoliosis. If the patient stands with both feet flat, with one iliac crest higher than the other and the opposite knee flexed, consider the same possibilities. With a fixed adduction deformity of the hip, the patient must either stand with the adducted side crossing his normal leg or may compensate by raising the pelvis on the side of the fixed adduction. This raising of the pelvis is the mechanism by which the apparent shortening of the extremity is produced. With a fixed abduction deformity, the leg will appear relatively longer. The pelvis has to tilt upward on the opposite side; therefore that leg appears shorter, and the patient has to stand on the toes of that extremity. A fixed lumbar scoliosis as a cause of pelvic tilt can easily be detected by having the patient bend his trunk to the right and left and noticing the difference in the range of motion (Figs. 2–2 to 2–5).

Look for abnormal prominences about the hip. A patient with a congenital dislocation of the hip will usually have an abnormal prominence in the buttock and an increased lordosis. The greater trochanter will appear prominent in a patient with a coxa vara. Obvious atrophy of the gluteal muscles, scars, or incisions should be noted.

Stability of the hip is then checked. A function of normal abductor muscles is to stabilize the pelvis in its relationship to the greater trochanter of the femur when weight is borne on one leg. For example, if a patient with normal abductor muscles stands on his right leg and raises the left foot off the floor, the left iliac crest should rise slightly. If, for any reason, there is weakness of the abductor muscle mechanism of the right hip, the iliac crest on the left side will drop, indicating that the abductor muscle cannot maintain the normal relationship between the pelvis and the femur (Fig. 2–6).

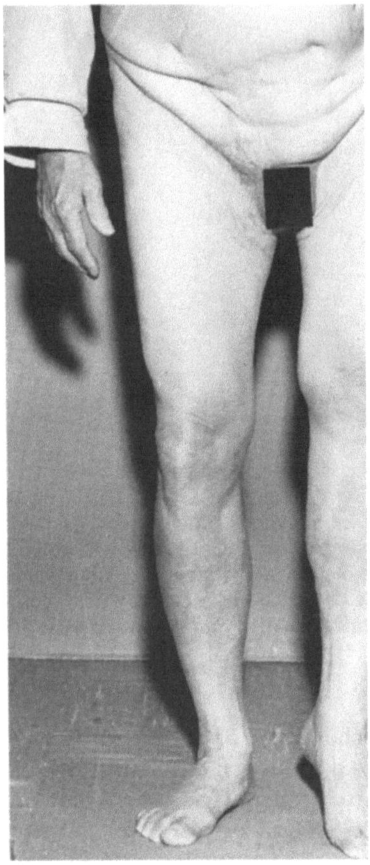

FIG. 2–2 This patient has a fixed adduction deformity of the left hip. He is compensating for the adduction deformity by raising the pelvis on the left side. This produces an apparent shortening, so that he has to stand on the toes of the left foot.

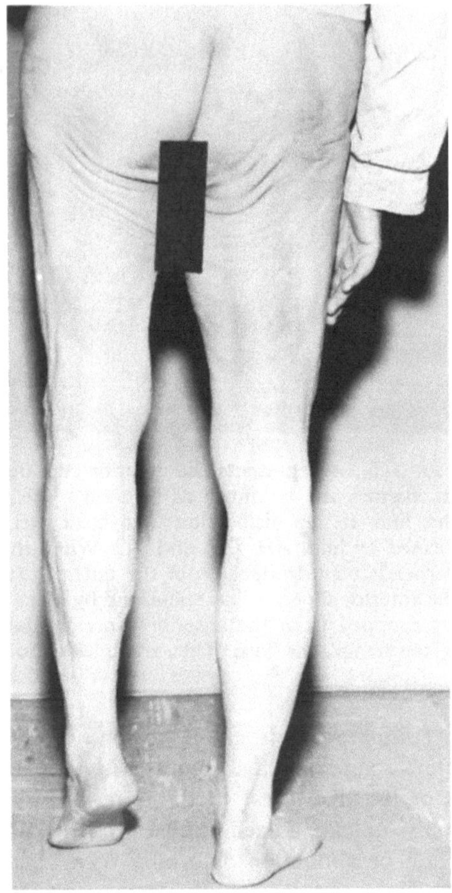

FIG. 2–3 The same patient as in Figure 2–2, seen from the rear.

Abductor muscle weakness is seen in paralytic diseases such as poliomyelitis or muscular dystrophy. It is also present in any condition in which the origin and insertion of the abductor muscles are brought close together, thereby diminishing the strength of these muscles. This occurs in unreduced congenital dislocations of the hip, coxa vara, and in conditions resulting in absorption of the femoral neck. This test for stability has been known as the Trendelenburg test. It has been called positive when evidence of instability exists and negative when the hip appears stable. According to Ducroquet,[2] this phenomenon actually was first described by Duchenne de Boulogne in 1867 in his book *Physiology of Movement.* The exact terms of his description were "The functional difficulty which has struck me the most in individuals in whom the gluteus medius and minimus were atrophied, is the inclination of the pelvis on the opposite side when they were standing on the damaged limb. Then, being unable to straighten the pelvis, they inclined their trunk considerably to the side which reposed on the ground in order to bring it back to the line of gravity." Trendelenburg[4] discovered "The true cause of limping in congenital dislocation to be atrophy of the gluteus medius and minimus leading to fall of the pelvis. The reason for this fall is that the abductors of the weight bearing thigh can no longer support the pelvis horizontally, due to the dislocation, or the change in direction of the muscles or atrophy increasing with the age of the dislocation." Ducroquet suggested

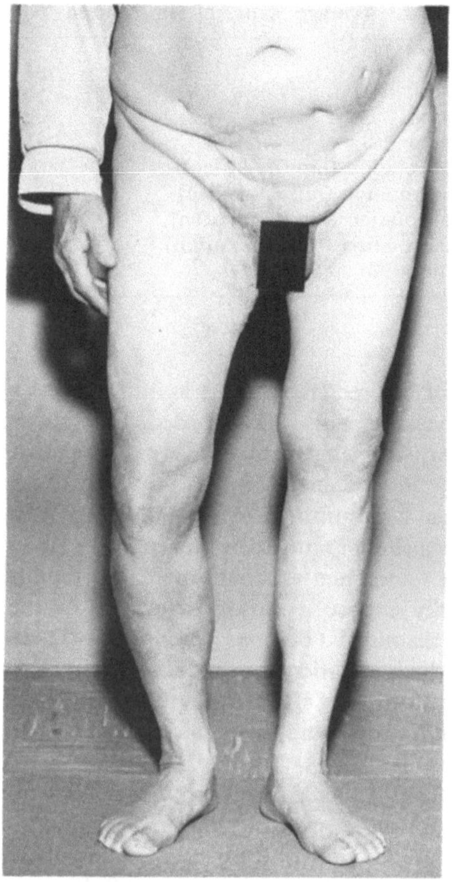

FIG. 2–4 The same patient as in previous two figures. Instead of standing on the toes of the adducted side, the patient may stand with the knee on the normal side in a flexed position.

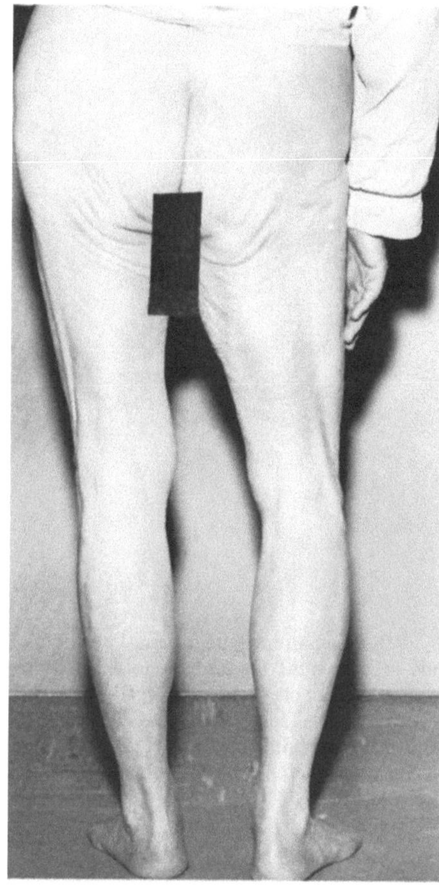

FIG. 2–5 The same patient in the position shown in Figure 2–4, seen from the rear.

that the Trendelenburg limp should be known as the limp of Duchenne de Boulogne.

The range of back motion is then examined and the relative flexibility of the spine determined. If back motion produces the type of pain of which the patient complains, lesions of the spine must be considered as possible causes for the symptom. Remember, however, that flexion and extension of the spine are accompanied by flexion and extension of the pelvis in relation to the femoral head. It will be difficult at times to determine whether the pain originates in the spine or in the hip joint. This is particularly apt to be true in the early stages, before significant loss of hip motion or associated signs of spine abnormalities occur.

The presence of a limp is observed by having the patient walk. The complaint of pain on weight bearing is noted. Several types of gaits are seen in patients with hip problems. One of these is the antalgic gait (antalgic meaning analgesic). The patient tends to hold the leg in a protective position which will insure the least irritation of the joint. In early stages of hip-joint inflammation this position is usually one of moderate flexion, abduction, and external rotation. The patient will also spend as little time as possible bearing weight on the side of the sore limb, and when walking will hop rapidly from the sore limb. The gluteus medius gait is one of instability. When weight is borne on the side with the weak abductor muscles, the pelvis drops on the opposite side and the shoulders incline toward the side of the weak hip in order

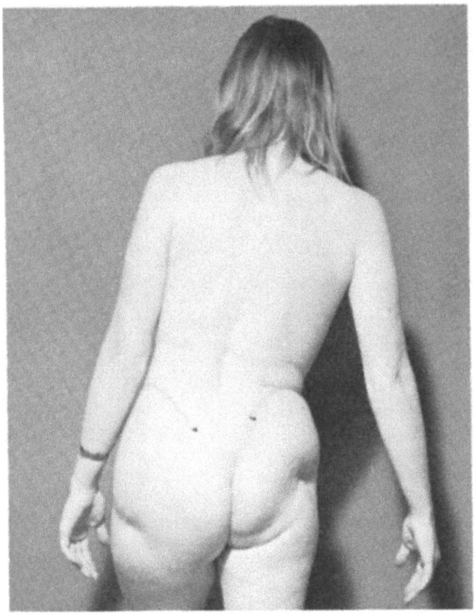

FIG. 2–6 When a patient with normal abductor muscles stands on her right leg and raises the left foot off the floor, the left iliac crest should rise slightly (negative Trendelenburg test). This patient has weakness of the abductor muscle mechanism of the right hip; therefore, the iliac crest on the left side will drop (positive Trendelenburg test).

to aid balance. If the weakness exists on both sides, the patient will have a typical "duck waddle." The reader is referred to Ducroque [2] for an excellent analysis of gaits.

Have the patient sit on the side of the examining table to check patellar and Achilles reflexes. Extend the knees to see if there is evidence of significant hamstring spasm. Then have the patient lie supine. Check for areas of tenderness and any palpable masses. Tenderness is commonly found over the area of the femoral head and over the greater trochanter. Tenderness over the greater trochanter is seen in patients with calcareous tendonitis, simple tendonitis, fibrositis and sometimes primary hip-joint disease. It is not possible as a rule to detect the presence of an effusion in the hip joint by palpation. The presence of femoral and pedal pulses is then determined.

The range of motion of both hips is recorded. Unless care is exercised in this examination, many errors can be made. The patient must be on a firm table, not a soft bed, if accurate measurements are expected. The analysis of end-results of many

TABLE 2–2 Average Range of Hip Motion

Flexion	135°
Extension	30°
Abduction	45°
Adduction	30°
Internal rotation (hip 0° flexion)	35°
External rotation (hip 0° flexion)	45°
Internal rotation (hip 90° flexion)	45°
External rotation (hip 90° flexion)	45°
Abduction (90° flexion)	65°

types of hip reconstructions is futile unless accurate measurements are recorded. One should be familiar with the normal average range of hip motion [3] (see Table 2–2).

When determining the range of flexion of a hip, the opposite hip must be flexed fully upon the patient's abdomen and held there. This will automatically expose a flexion deformity of the hip being examined (Thomas test, Fig. 2–7). If this is not done, a patient can hide approximately 30° of fixed flexion of the hip (Fig. 2–8). If no flexion deformity exists, the hip is said to be in a position of 0° of flexion.

The hip is then carried through as wide a range of flexion as is possible; the knee is flexed 90°. If it has been possible to flex the hip 120°, the range of flexion is recorded as 0–120°. If one begins with a fixed flexion deformity of 20°, and there is flexion beyond this point to 100°, the range of flexion is recorded as 20–100°. This method automatically records fixed flexion deformities as well as giving the range of available flexion in the simplest way (Figs. 2–9 to 2–11).

The range of abduction and adduction is next determined. To do this properly, it is essential that the pelvis be level and locked in position. A simple way to do this is to abduct the normal leg its maximum amount and maintain this position by flexing the knee and locking it over the side of the examining table (Fig. 2–12). Check the iliac crests and the level of the anterior superior iliac spines. The leg is then carried into maximum abduction and adduction (Figs. 2–13, 2–14). The range of these motions can be determined fairly accurately, if the normal hip is locked in maximum abduction, without being misled by motion of the pelvis. If the hip is not locked, however, it is difficult to recognize even mild fixed adduction or abduction deformities.

Let us say that we recognize a fixed adduction

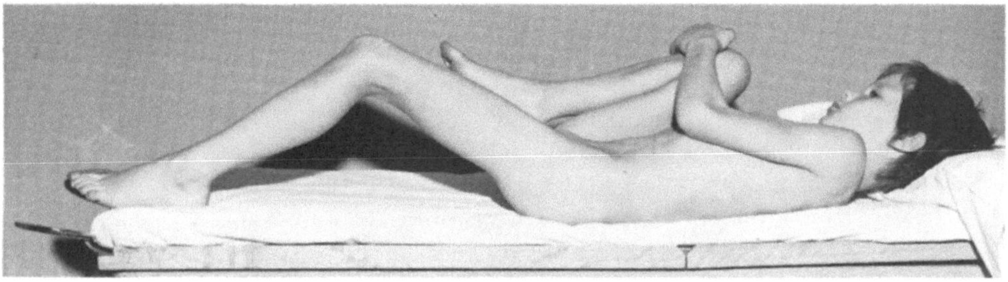

FIG. 2–7 When examining the range of flexion of a hip, the opposite hip must be flexed fully upon the patient's abdomen and held there. This will automatically expose a flexion deformity of the hip which is being examined (Thomas test). Be certain the back is straight, not hyperextended.

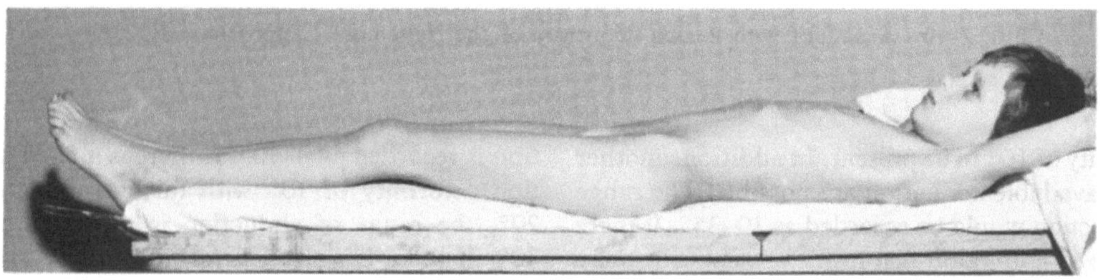

FIG. 2–8 If the opposite hip is not flexed upon the patient's abdomen, it is possible to hide approximately 30° of fixed flexion. The above patient hid the flexion deformity of her left hip by increasing her lumbar lordosis.

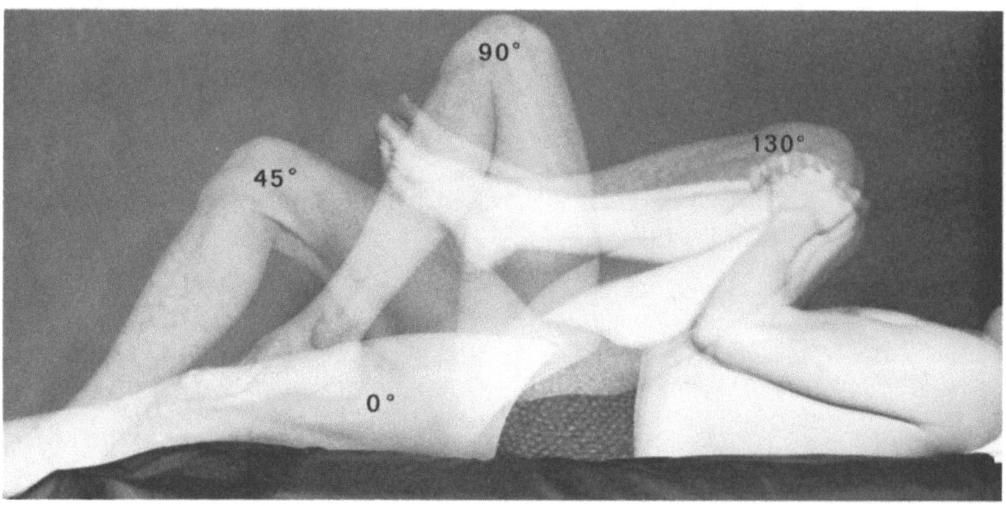

FIG. 2–9 The range of flexion is recorded in degrees, beginning with 0° as neutral flexion and extension, and progressing to 120° or 130° at full flexion.

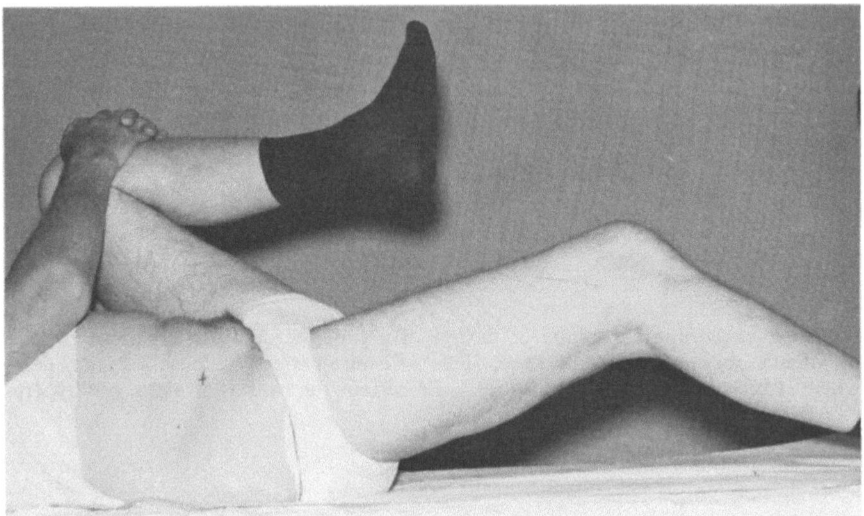

FIG. 2–10 A patient with flexion deformity of the right hip of approximately 20°.

deformity of 10° to be present. In addition, another 15° of available adduction are possible. The range of adduction would be recorded as 10–25°. If there is no fixed adduction deformity present, but there are 30° of available adduction, the range of adduction is recorded as 0–30°. If there is a fixed abduction deformity of 10° with further abduction of 20°, the range of abduction is recorded as 10–30°. If there is a fixed deformity in any range of motion and further motion is not possible in that

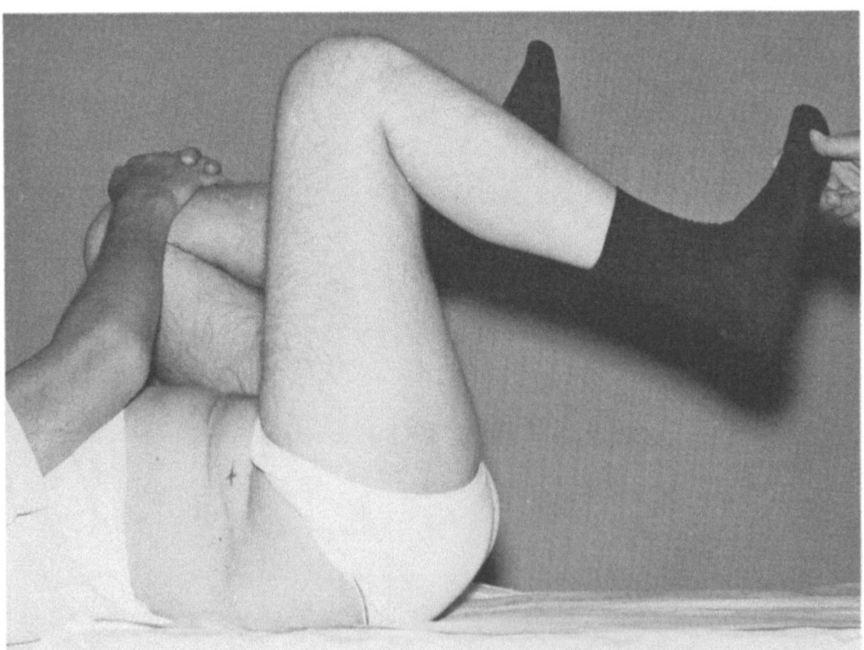

FIG. 2–11 The same patient at maximum flexion, 90°. His range of flexion is recorded as 20–90°.

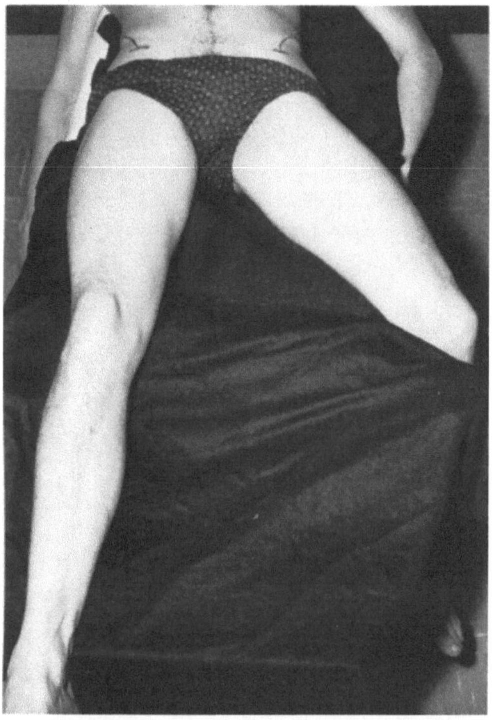

FIG. 2–12 To eliminate pelvic motion when checking abduction and adduction, first abduct the normal leg fully, then lock it over the side of the examining table. Check the symmetry of the anterior superior iliac spines and iliac crests.

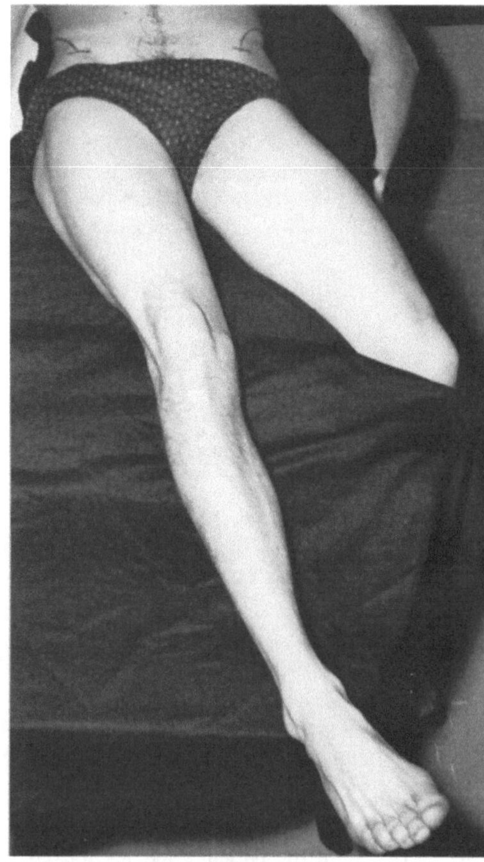

FIG. 2–13 The range of adduction is carried out. Locking the normal leg in maximum abduction does not completely prevent pelvic motion when the opposite leg is carried through a range of adduction. Motion of the pelvis must be watched and palpated.

direction, it may be recorded as: adduction, 15° fixed deformity or external rotation, 10° fixed deformity.

Record the range of internal and external rotation with the hip in a position of 90° flexion and then examine the range of abduction in the same position. This motion is commonly limited in early stages of hip-joint disease (Figs. 2–15, 2–16).

Leg length should then be measured by determining the distance from the anterior superior iliac spine to the medial malleolus; at best, however, this is a crude method.

Internal and external rotation with the hips in 0° of flexion can be obtained with the patient supine or prone. A more accurate measurement is reached with the patient prone; this may not be possible, however, in patients with bilateral hip disease or who are elderly.

In the prone position, flex the knees to 90°. To check internal rotation of the hips, keep the knees together and rotate the legs outward. The angle formed by the two legs aids in recognizing any difference in internal rotation. The hips are then externally rotated by crossing the legs, and the degree of external rotation is estimated. For accuracy, the end of the femur rather than the foot should be held when rotating the legs. This is particularly important in a child. The laxity existing in the average child's knee will add probably 20° to the apparent hip rotation if the foot is held during the maneuver. This is especially true when one is checking a child for the origin of a toe-in or toe-out gait (Figs. 2–17 to 2–19). The subtle differences in hip rotation in a patient with an early slipped capital femoral epiphysis are more apt to be detected if rotations are carried out with the patient in a prone position.

The range of hip extension is recorded by raising the thigh upward without increasing the lum-

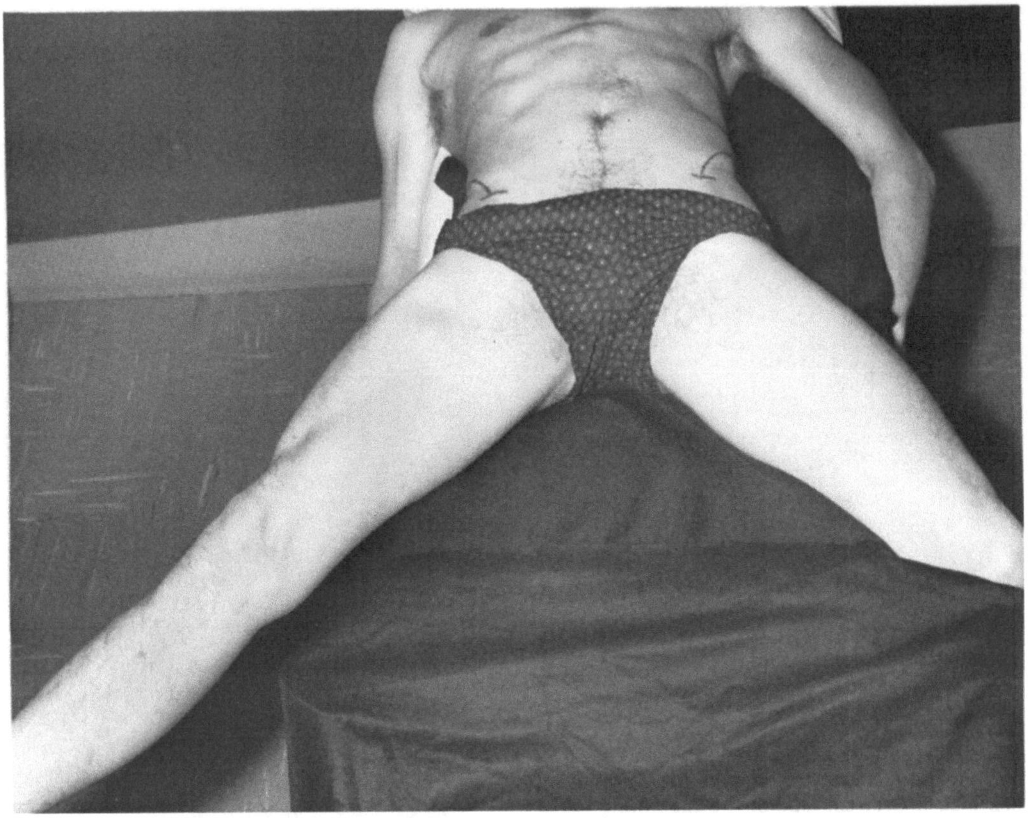

FIG. 2–14 With the patient's left leg locked in maximum abduction, the range of abduction of the right hip is carried out without having to worry about pelvic shifting.

bar lordosis. To do this accurately, have the opposite thigh flexed over the end of the examining table. This eliminates the lordosis before the range of extension is begun.

If there is any indication to check for contracture of the iliotibial band, have the patient lie on one side with the bottom thigh flexed to eliminate lumbar lordosis. The upper leg is then abducted and extended while the knee is flexed 90° (Fig. 2–20). The upper leg is then allowed to come toward the examining table (Fig. 2–21). If there is a contracture of the iliotibial band or fascia lata,

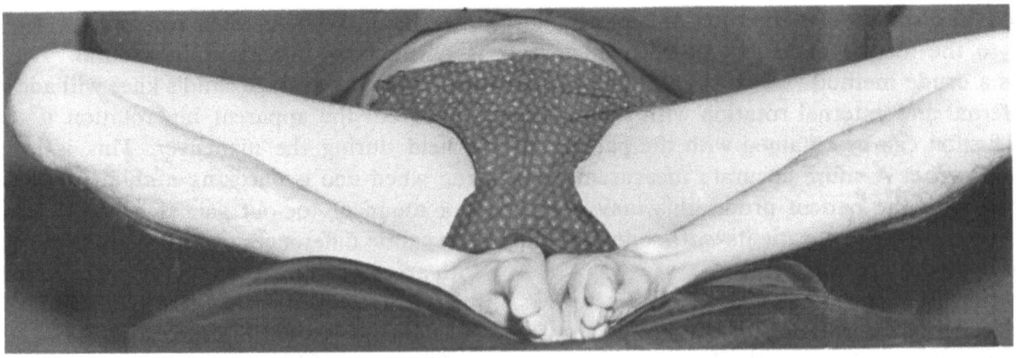

FIG. 2–15 The normal range of flexion abduction is approximately 65°.

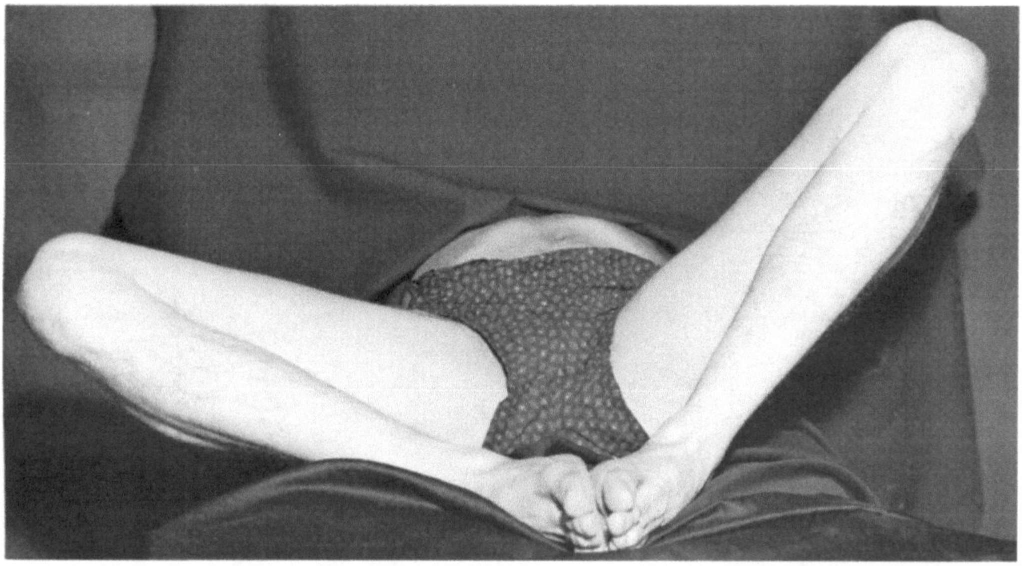

FIG. 2–16 Flexion abduction of the left hip is limited, as easily seen by comparing the two legs. This is one of the motions lost early in hip disease.

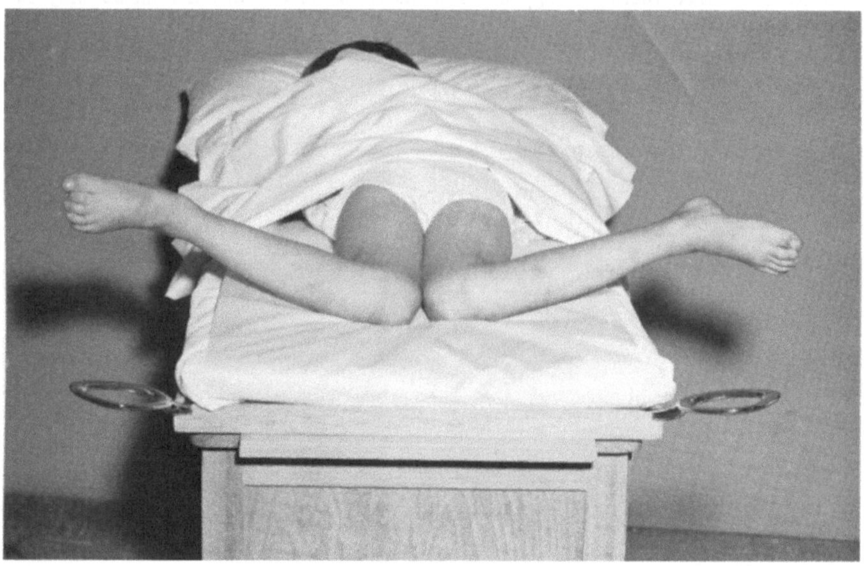

FIG. 2–17 Examining internal rotation of the hips. If there is a significant difference between the two, it will be easily recognized by comparing the angle formed by the two legs.

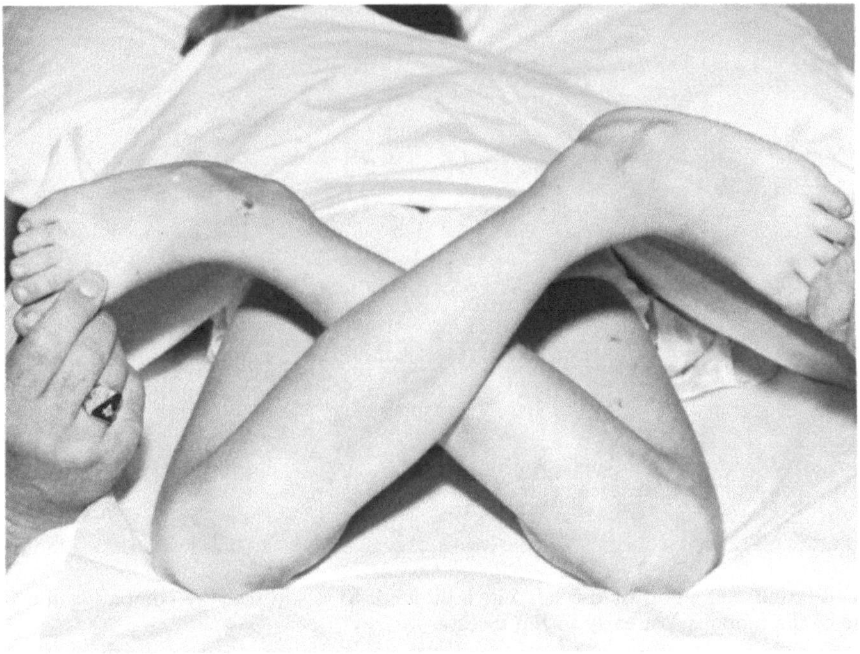

FIG. 2–18 External rotation of the hips is noted by crossing the legs. If pressure is applied to the feet, there will appear to be more external rotation than actually exists, due to knee laxity.

A
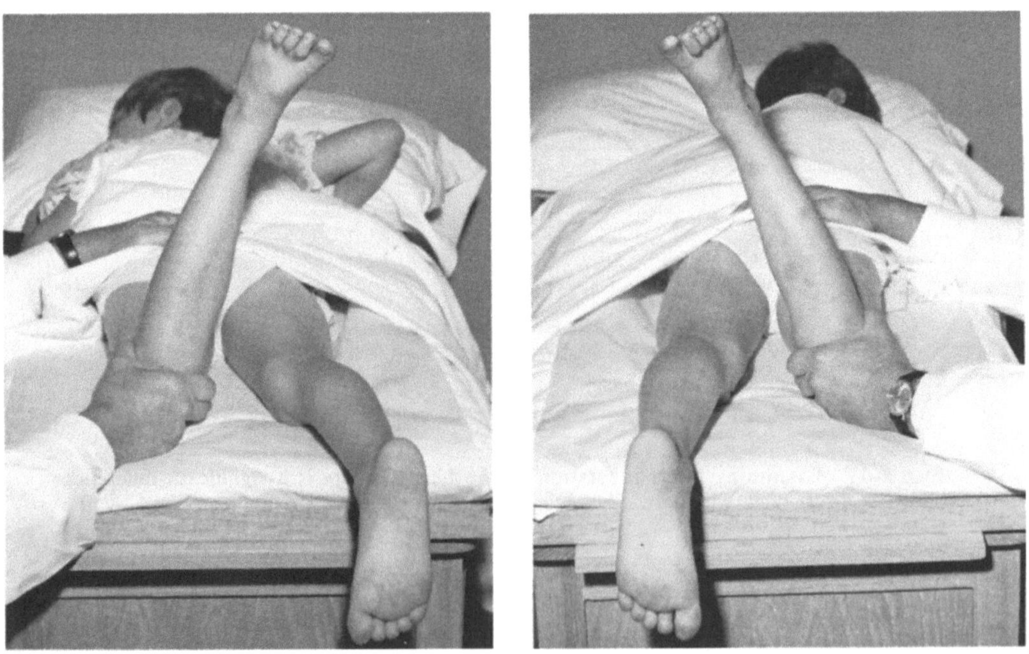
B

FIGS. 2–19 **A** and **B** The child in preceding two figures is being examined by holding the end of the femur rather than the foot. It will be seen that much less external rotation is obtained when this is done. This is an accurate method.

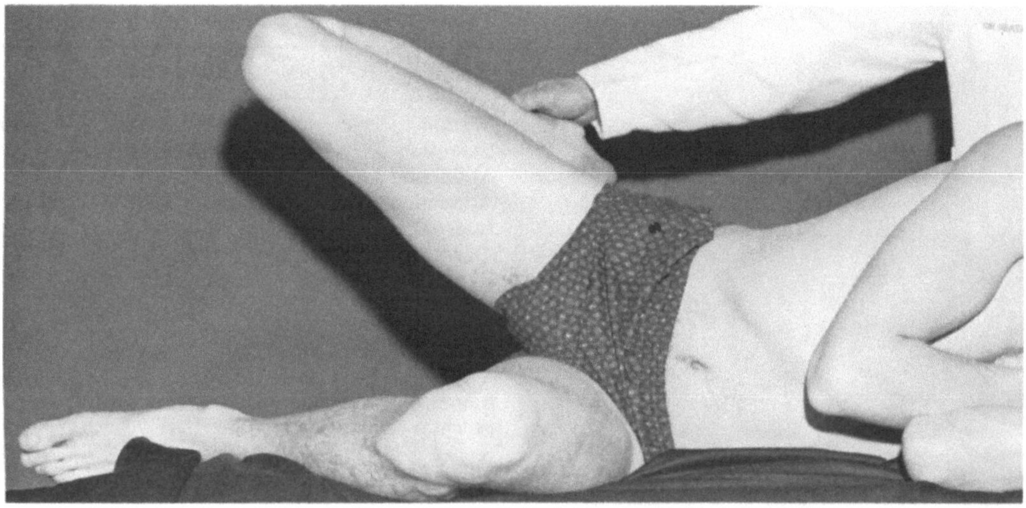

FIG. 2–20 Ober test for contracture of the fascia lata. The bottom leg is flexed to a right angle to eliminate lordosis. The upper leg is abducted and extended with the knee in a position of 90° flexion. The upper leg is then allowed to drop to the examining table. If it will not come toward the examining table, contracture of the fascia lata is indicated.

the thigh will remain in a position of abduction. This is known as the Ober test and probably has its greatest application in neuromuscular conditions.

It is helpful to record the motions in chart form (Table 2–3).

Always be gentle in determining a range of hip motion. Unnecessary pain will irritate the patient and he will voluntarily restrict motion.

Traumatic Problems

In a patient with a history of acute trauma, a rapid, correct diagnosis is essential. An accurate record of motion is unnecessary. Motion is checked to see if it produces pain, or if it is grossly limited. The history, the age of the patient, the mechanism of injury, and the appearance of the patient provide useful clues in arriving at the diag-

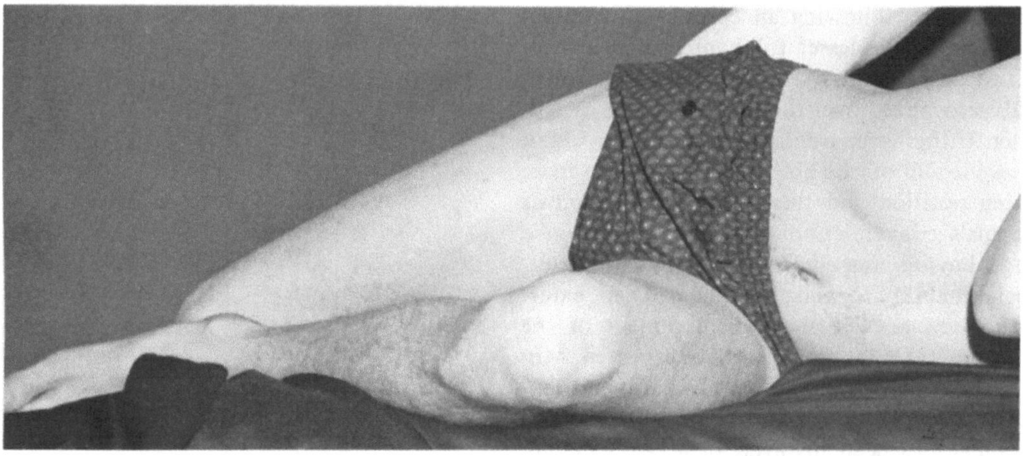

FIG. 2–21 The Ober test is negative. The leg has been brought to the examining table, indicating that the fascia lata is not contracted.

TABLE 2–3 Suggested Chart of Hip Motion

	Right Hip	Leg Hip
Flexion	0–120°	10–80°
Extension	0– 30°	0°
Abduction	45°	0°
Adduction	30°	10–30°
Internal rotation (extension)	35°	0–10°
External rotation (extension)	45°	0–30°

For office or hospital records, keep hip motions in chart form. A glance at the above chart shows that the right hip motion is normal and left hip motion is fairly limited. Progress of a patient is easily followed in this way.

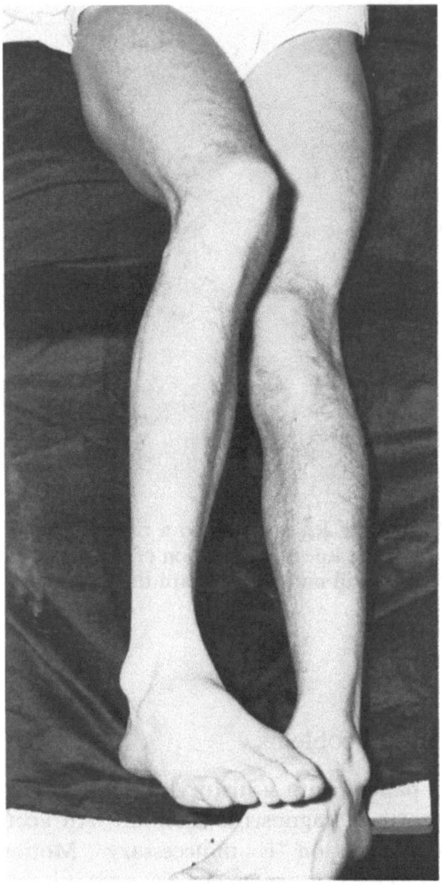

FIG. 2–22 Typical deformity of traumatic posterior dislocation of the hip is shortening, adduction, and internal rotation.

nosis. For example, in a teen-ager with acute pain in the hip area following an episode of running, an avulsion of the lesser trochanter or of one of the iliac spines would seem likely. Tenderness would be localized over the involved spine or trochanter. If the lesser trochanter has been avulsed, the patient will not be able to flex his thigh from a sitting position and there may be ecchymosis in Scarpa's triangle (Ludloff's sign). Again, in a teenager having jumped from a height, with resulting pain, inability to walk, and a shortened, externally rotated leg, an acute displacement of the femoral capital epiphysis would be suspected. Motion in these cases is painful and limited, and tenderness is found over the anterior hip area. When the patient has been involved in a car accident, and if a leg appears shortened, adducted, and internally rotated, a posterior dislocation of the hip would appear likely (Fig. 2–22). If the leg appears mildly abducted and externally rotated, with marked swelling and cyanosis of the entire lower extremity, an anterior dislocation of the hip is likely. The swelling and cyanosis are secondary to pressure on the femoral vein.

In the older age groups, think of a fracture of the femoral neck or of the intertrochanteric area

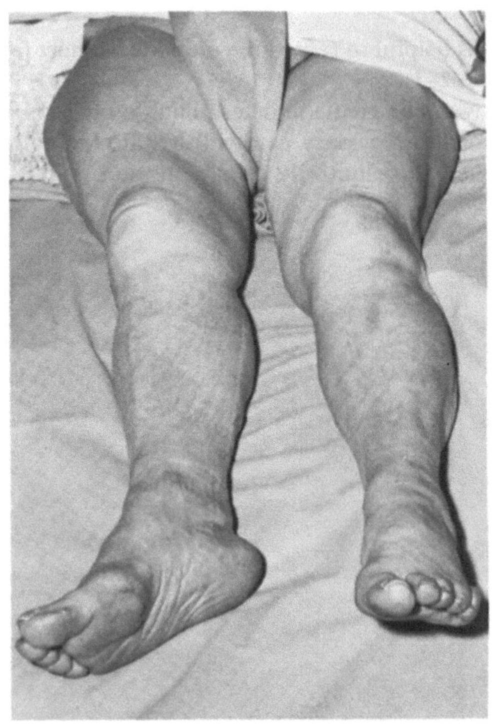

FIG. 2–23 Fracture of the right hip. The leg is shortened and externally rotated.

of the femur if the extremity appears short and externally rotated following a fall (Fig. 2–23). Patients with impacted fractures of the femoral neck usually have no deformity, may be able to move the leg actively, and may show little on physical examination. One might suspect this diagnosis in a patient who has fallen and has residual pain in the hip area and tenderness over the anterior aspect of the hip joint. Fractures of the pubic rami have the same history and physical findings generally, although the location of tenderness is more medial.

Inflammatory Problems

In diagnosing inflammatory problems involving the hip joint, the history of onset and the presence of associated systemic signs are all important. The onset may be acute, and can be associated with severe systemic reactions in cases of acute septic arthritis or hematogenous osteomyelitis of the femoral neck. Conversely, the onset may be gradual, and can be associated with milder systemic reactions in cases of tuberculosis or rheumatoid arthritis. In any event, the systemic signs, such as elevation of temperature and general malaise, indicate the considerations of the inflammatory problems in the differential diagnosis. If a patient is acutely ill, the examination of the hip will consist of determining if hip motion is limited and painful. An accurate record of the motion is not important; it is enough to know that motion is limited and painful. Palpation is important to detect tenderness and increased warmth about the hip. It may be difficult to differentiate septic arthritis from osteomyelitis of the femoral neck in the early stages, although hip motion does not become as limited in uncomplicated osteomyelitis as it does in septic arthritis.

In the early stages of any condition associated with an effusion in the hip joint, the leg is maintained in the position of external rotation, moderate flexion, and abduction; this position allows the greatest relaxation of the hip capsule. In conditions which progress in severity and are associated with destruction of the joint, the hip later assumes a position of flexion and adduction.

Tuberculosis and monarticular arthritis have a less acute onset. In the early stages, limitation of motion and pain are not pronounced, and associated systemic reactions are mild to moderate.

Transient synovitis is seen in young children and may be of traumatic or inflammatory origin. It is characterized by an acute onset, varying degrees of pain, difficulty or inability to walk in the early stages, and moderate limitation of hip motion. Associated systemic signs are mild.

Summary

In attempting to diagnose hip problems, a good and accurate history is indispensable, as is familiarity with the common problems seen at specific age periods. The physician must be knowledgeable concerning the activities and mechanisms which produce specific types of injuries. A routine should be developed for examining a hip joint, and available methods for eliminating inaccuracies should be utilized.

Eponyms

1. Allis' sign: There is relaxation of the fascia between the crest of the ilium and the greater trochanter—a sign of fracture of the neck of the femur.
2. Allis' sign: When the hips and knees of a baby are flexed to 90°, with a dislocation of the hip, one thigh will appear shorter than the other.
3. Barlow's test: This is done in two parts. With the baby on its back and with the hips and knees flexed, the middle finger of each hand is placed over the greater trochanter and the thumb of each hand is placed on the medial thigh opposite the lesser trochanter. The thighs are carried into midabduction and forward pressure behind the greater trochanter is applied by the middle finger of one hand while the other hand holds the opposite femur and pelvis. If the femoral head slips forward into the acetabulum it is felt that the hip has been dislocated. If there is no noticeable movement of the femoral head, the hip is felt to be not dislocated. The second part of the test involves applying pressure backward and outward on the medial thigh with the thumb. If the head of the femur is felt to slip out over the rim of the acetabulum and slips back in again as soon as the pressure is released, the hip is felt to be unstable.[1]
4. Bryant's triangle: This is a triangle formed

by a perpendicular dropped from the anterior superior iliac spine when the patient is lying supine; the base of the triangle is a line extending from the tip of the trochanter to this perpendicular, while the hypotenuse is represented by the line joining the anterior superior iliac spine and the tip of the trochanter. The base of the triangle is shortened in any condition allowing upward displacement of the greater trochanter.

5. Desault's sign: This is a sign of intracapsular fracture of the femur and consists of alteration of the arc described by rotation of the greater trochanter, which normally describes the segment of the circle but in this fracture rotates only at the apex of the femur as it rotates about its own axis.
6. Dupuytren's sign: In congenital dislocation of the head of the femur there is a free up-and-down movement of the head of the bone (piston mobility).
7. Erichsen's sign: When the iliac bones are sharply pressed toward each other, pain is felt in sacroiliac disease but not in hip disease.
8. Fabere test: This means flexion, abduction, external rotation, and extension. See Patrick's test.
9. Frankel's sign: There is diminished tonicity of the muscles of the hip joint in tabes dorsalis.
10. Gill's sign: When the hip joint is swollen with fluid, the involved hip will feel thicker than the opposite one. Swelling of the joint is demonstrated by placing the thumb over the femoral artery where it crosses the inguinal ligament while the other four fingers are placed posteriorly over the buttock opposite the position of the thumb. In this way the joint with the soft tissues anterior and posterior to it is grasped between the thumb and the fingers.
11. Hart's sign: This is the limitation of abduction of the hips seen in congenital dislocation of the hip.
12. Jansen's test: This is indicative of osteoarthritis deformans of the hip. The patient is told to cross his legs with a point just above the ankle resting on the opposite knee. This motion is impossible when the disease exists.
13. Ludloff's sign: This is a sign of traumatic separation of the epiphysis of the lesser trochanter. Swelling and ecchymosis are found at the base of Scarpa's triangle and there is inability to raise the thigh when in a sitting position.
14. Nelaton's line: A line is drawn from the anterior superior iliac spine to the ischial tuberosity. Normally, the tip of the greater trochanter lies on or distal to this line.
15. Ober's test: With the patient lying on his side with the bottom thigh flexed to eliminate lordosis, the upper leg is abducted and extended while the knee is flexed 90°. This leg is then brought toward the examining table. If it stays in a position of abduction, it indicates contracture of the iliotibial band.
16. Ortolani's sign: A click is felt when a dislocated hip slips into the acetabulum as the thigh is abducted.
17. Patrick's test: The patient is supine. The thigh and knee are flexed and the external malleolus is placed over the patella of the opposite leg; the knee is depressed and, if pain is produced thereby, arthritis of the hip is indicated.
18. Putnam's sign: This is the lengthening of the leg in hysteric hip disease.
19. Schoemaker's line: A line is drawn from the tip of the greater trochanter through the anterior superior iliac spine and prolonged toward the midline. When the trochanter is displaced upward, the continuation of the line meets the midline of the body below the umbilicus, whereas normally the midline is reached above the umbilicus.
20. Thomas test: The good knee and hip are flexed on the abdomen; if the opposite leg cannot then be laid on the table, a flexion deformity is present and the test is positive.
21. Trendelenburg's sign: When the patient stands on the normal side, the buttock of the opposite side rises, for the gluteus medius contracts to raise the pelvis and bring the trunk more directly above the limb which is sustaining the body weight. When the patient stands on the side of the dislocated hip, the opposite buttock drops, for the gluteus medius is relatively inefficient and the pelvis cannot, therefore, be raised or even be kept horizontal. This test is not pathognomonic of congenital dislocation of the hip, but occurs with any interference with the action of the gluteus medius, e.g. paralysis or coxa vara.

Bibliography

1. Barlow, T. G.: Early diagnosis and treatment of congenital dislocation of the hip. J. Bone Joint Surg., 44B:292, 1962.
2. Ducroquet, R., et al.: *Walking and Limping, A Study of Normal and Pathological Walking.* Philadelphia, J. B. Lippincott, 1968.
3. *Measuring and Recording of Joint Motion.* American Academy of Orthopedic Surgeons, 1963.
4. Trendelenburg, F.: *Compte Rendu du Congress de la Societe Allem ande de Chirurgie* Hoffa, 1895.

CHAPTER 3

The Anatomy of the Hip Joint

MICHAEL HARTY

There is but little room for inexactness in the field of surgery; a deviation of even a centimeter or two from the correct approach may change success into disaster.
Lord Brock.[4]

The hip is a synovial joint of the ball-and-socket variety formed by the globular femoral head cupped into the acetabular or cotyloid cavity of the hip bone. It plays a major role in the static and dynamic physiology of the locomotor system and, although it is the most stable ball-and-socket joint in the body, it still maintains an extraordinary range of motion. Descriptively the hip joint is commonly discussed in the extended position. However, a clear mental picture of the anatomical changes which occur during the full range of joint motion forms an essential adjunct to an accurate evaluation of the functional and pathological problems encountered.

Osteology

Femur

The proximal end of the femur includes the head, the neck, and the trochanters. The neck, which is embryologically a continuation of the shaft, joins the latter at an angle which varies from 125 to 135° (Fig. 3–1). The angle between the plane of the femoral condyles and the axis of the femoral neck is the torsion or declination angle of the femur. It shows a wide degree of variation from anteversion to retroversion with an average figure of 14° anteversion [14] (Fig. 3–2). The head forms two-thirds of a sphere and joins the constricted neck at the subcapital sulcus. The joint face of the normal fully hydrated articular cartilage, which covers the femoral head, is perfectly spherical. The cartilage-covered area of the head is derived predominantly from the epiphysis, but inferiorly a tongue of diaphyseal bone extending medially also contributes to the lower articular surface (Fig. 3–3). As the neck is only three-fourths of the equatorial diameter of the head, a wide range of motion is possible before it impinges on the pliable labrum acetabulare.[27] The articular cartilage of the head thins toward the periphery and terminates at the subcapital sulcus. This sulcus is more pronounced at the superior and inferior aspects of the neck, where it may be occupied by a small subsynovial fat pad. In the absence of an anterior subcapital sulcus, a small articular facet encroaches onto the anterior aspect of the neck in 10% of specimens. It is in contact with the iliofemoral ligament during extension but slides under the anterior acetabular margin during flexion and internal rotation. The margins of the articular cartilage join the synovial membrane which covers the anterior aspect of the neck as far laterally as the intertrochanteric line, where the iliofemoral (Bigelow) [3] component of the capsule is firmly anchored. Only the medial half of the posterior surface of the neck is sheathed by synovium (Fig. 3–4). Schmorl [33] stated that the periosteum of the neck contained no cambium layer and so lacked osteogenic properties. Harris [13] and Banks [1] corroborated this observation and added that the neck did not exhibit the massive callus formation seen typically in extraarticular locations.

The greater trochanter, a typical traction

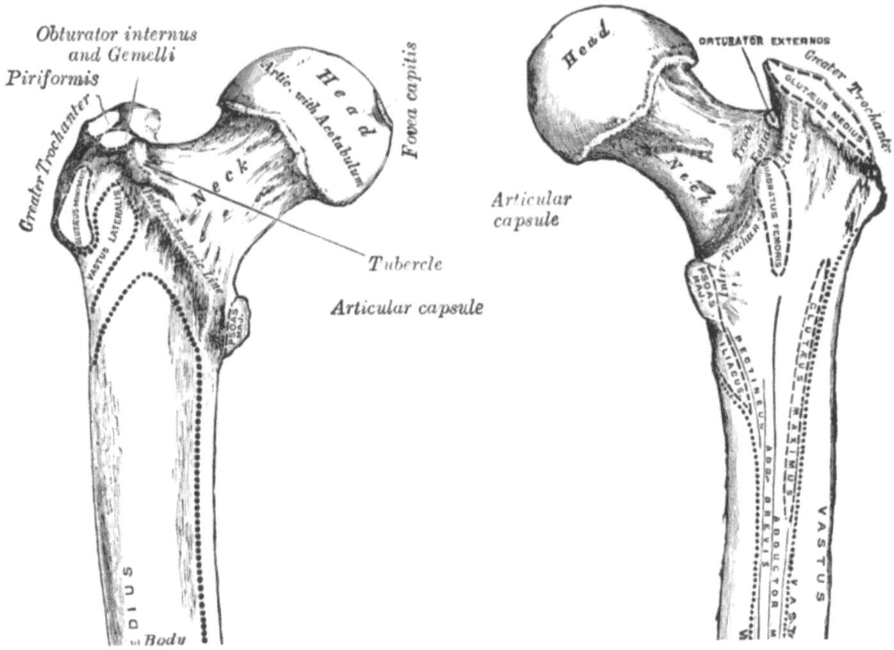

FIG. 3–1 Anterior (A) and posterior (P) aspects of right proximal femur. (Adapted from Fig. 4–178, from *Gray's Anatomy of the Human Body,* C. M. Goss, ed., 29th ed. Philadelphia, Lea & Febiger, 1973.)

epiphysis for insertion of the abductors, overhangs the expanded junction of neck and shaft. Posteriorly it is joined by the intertrochanteric crest to the lesser trochanter which projects from the posteromedial aspect of the proximal shaft (Fig. 3–1 B). The trochanteric line demarcates the anterior aspect of the neck from the shaft. The upper end forms the femoral tubercle and the inferior end continues distally as the spiral line giving origin to the vastus medialis. A muscle, although covering the medial surface of the femoral shaft, does not take origin from this aspect of the bone, but it protects the profunda femoris artery which may be traumatized by drills or screws protruding from the medial side of the shaft.[15] In the anatomy laboratories we see many examples of longitudinal or oblique splits in the cortex of the proximal femoral shaft following the insertion of screws or pins (Fig. 3–5). With correct and careful technical precautions this can and should be avoided, as it throws additional and unnecessary strains on the stability of the internal fixation.

Growth disturbances at the capital femoral epiphysis cause a coxa vara, while growth arrest of the growing greater trochanter produces a coxa valga.

Acetabular Fossa

The femoral head is cupped in the reciprocally curved acetabulum, made up of the iliac, ischial, and pubic components of the hip bone. The mouth of the acetabulum is directed laterally, distally, and anteriorly. It has a reinforcing prominent buttress of bone at its superior and posterior margins to counteract the strains and stresses exerted by the pressing femoral head, not alone in the erect attitude but also in the much more commonly utilized hip flexion position (Fig. 3–6). On the convex or male component of all joints, the articular cartilage is thickest centrally and thins toward the periphery. Precisely the opposite occurs on the concave or female component, where the thickest area of articular cartilage is found at the periphery, adjacent to the labrum acetabuli. In the acetabulum the weight-bearing cartilage-covered articular surface of horseshoe outline surrounds the nonarticular acetabular fossa (Fig. 3–7). This contains a fibroelastic fat pad (haversian * gland) [19] covered

---

* Clopton Havers (England, 1655–1702) described intraarticular fat pads and bone canals, although *pinguis pulvinus articuli* or "the fat cushion of the joint" was mentioned in classical Latin.

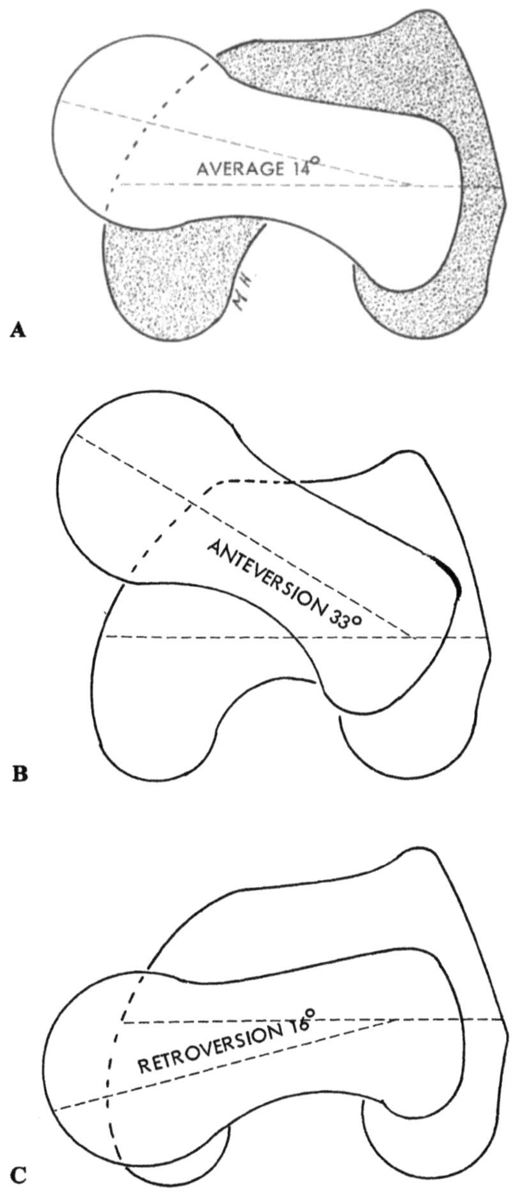

FIG. 3–2 **A** Average torsion angle of right femur. **B** Anteversion. **C** Retroversion.

on its lateral aspect by synovial membrane (Fig. 3–8). The round ligament (ligamentum teres) is neither round nor ligamentous. It is a flat fibrous band covered with synovium which extends from the acetabular notch and transverse ligament to the fovea capitis of the femoral head. It serves to transmit blood vessels to the femoral head.

The combination of a yielding fat pad and depressed acetabular fossa allows the ligament free

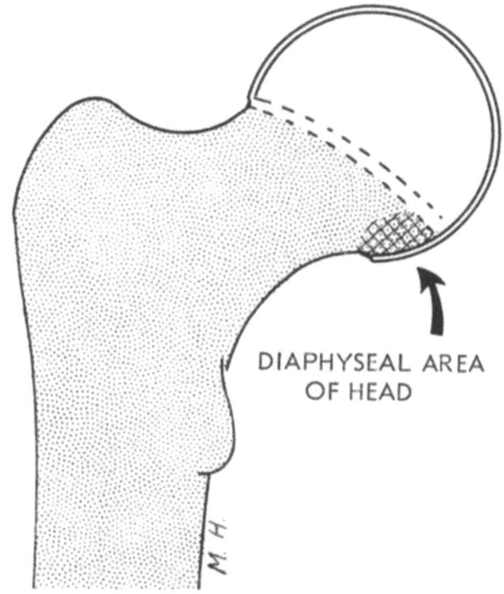

FIG. 3–3 Areas of the epiphysis and diaphysis covered by articular cartilage (double lines).

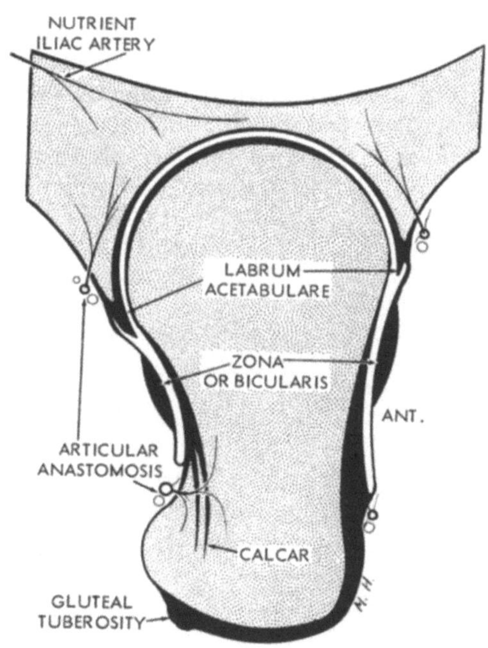

FIG. 3–4 Horizontal section of neck and joint, with capsule distended. Note zona orbicularis, extent of capsular reflection on neck, site of pericapsular anastomosis, and labrum acetabulare.

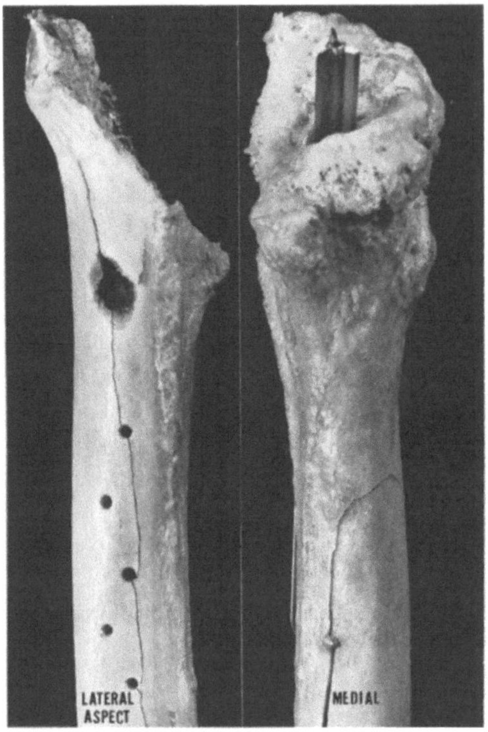

FIG. 3–5 Splits in femoral cortex following insertion of bone screw, lateral and medial aspects.

movement without exposing it to compression and friction forces between the facets of articular cartilage (Fig. 3–9). Although the articular surfaces are reciprocally and regularly curved, they are not coextensive. In any joint position only two-fifths of the head occupies the bony acetabulum. The bony acetabulum without its peripheral labrum is less than a true hemisphere, which is why such an excellent range of motion is possible at the hip joint.

A smaller femoral head with a corresponding smaller and shallower acetabulum is found in females.

Labrum

The acetabular notch is bridged by the fibrous transverse ligament, which continues as a tough but mobile fibrocartilaginous anulus (labrum acetabulare) attached to the bony margin. Because the labrum embraces the head tightly beyond its equator, it increases the depth of the acetabulum and enhances the stability of the hip joint. The labrum is most prominent at the posterosuperior region of the acetabulum, where it is covered by synovial membrane on both its superficial and deep aspects (Fig. 3–4). Thus, the superior margin or limbus (L. free edge) is mobile at the lateral margin and may rotate into the joint cavity of a congenitally dislocated hip.

The Capsule

The strong but sensitive fibrous capsule of the hip forms a closely fitting cuff which covers the lateral margins of the head of the femur and most of its neck. Anteriorly the capsule reaches to the intertrochanteric line, but posteriorly the lateral half

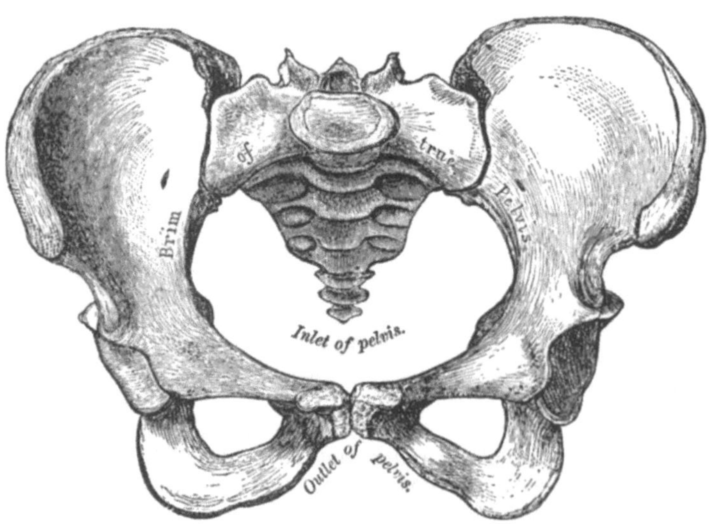

FIG. 3–6 Anterior view of pelvis to emphasize the prominent superior and posterior lip of acetabulum. (From *Gray's Anatomy,* 29th ed. Philadelphia, Lea & Febiger, 1973.)

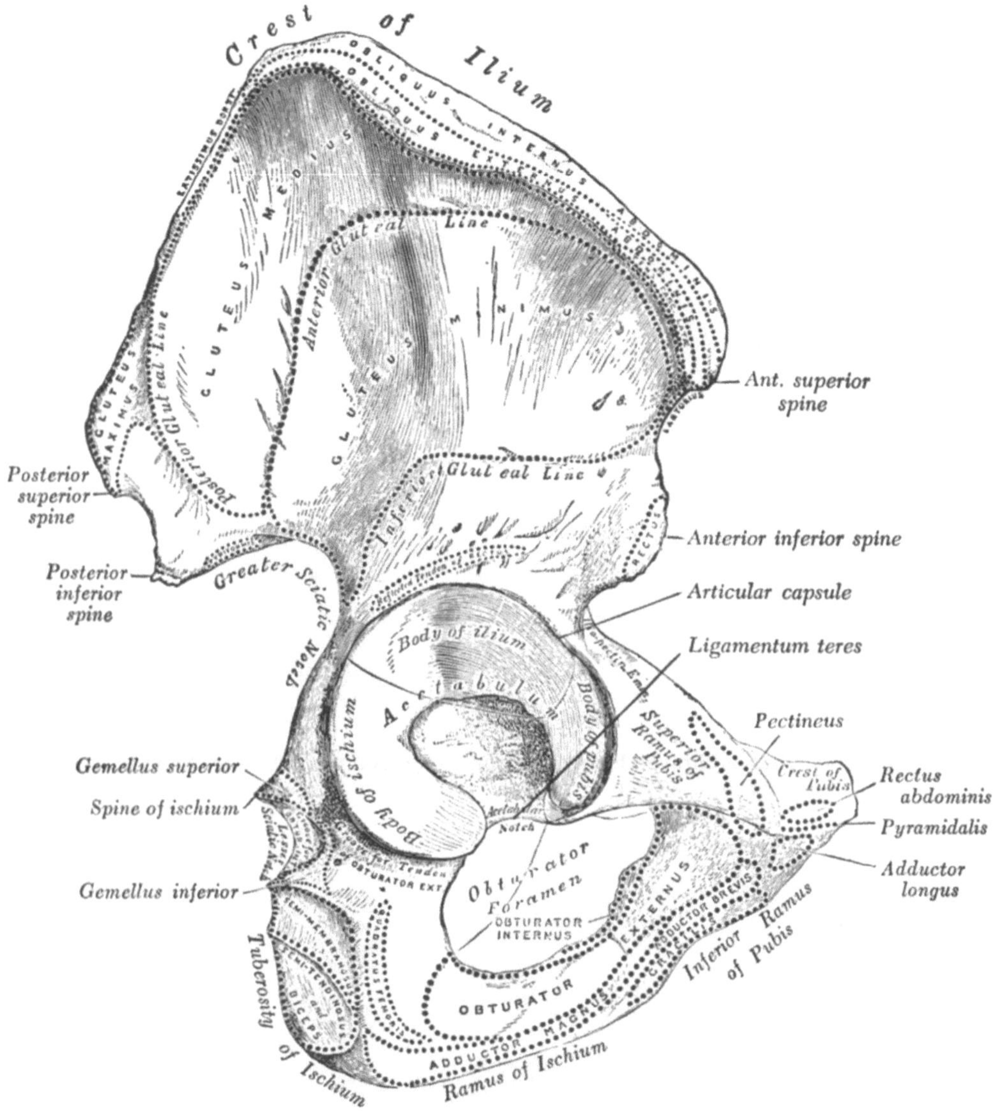

FIG. 3–7 **Right hip bone showing horseshoe-shaped articular facet. (From *Gray's Anatomy,* 29th ed. Philadelphia, Lea & Febiger, 1973.)**

of the neck is extracapsular (Fig. 3–4). The capsule is made up of dense, fibrous tissue reinforced anteriorly by the sturdy iliofemoral ligament of Bigelow, below by the pubofemoral condensation, and posteriorly by the thin ischiofemoral element. In the position of hip flexion and adduction, the femoral head may be easily forced through the attenuated posteroinferior capsule. The capsule is constricted around the narrowest area of the neck by the zona orbicularis—a condensed group of deeply placed circular fibers (Figs. 3–4 and 3–8) which reinforces the retaining action of the labrum acetabulare. The rest position at the hip joint is approximately 10° flexion, 10° abduction, and 10° external rotation. This position allows total capsular slackness and maximal joint capacity with complete muscular relaxation. It is the position classically assumed in the early stages of painless hip joint effusion or while the lower limb is supported by hydrostatic pressure.

The longitudinal fibers of the capsule are relaxed during hip flexion but become twisted and

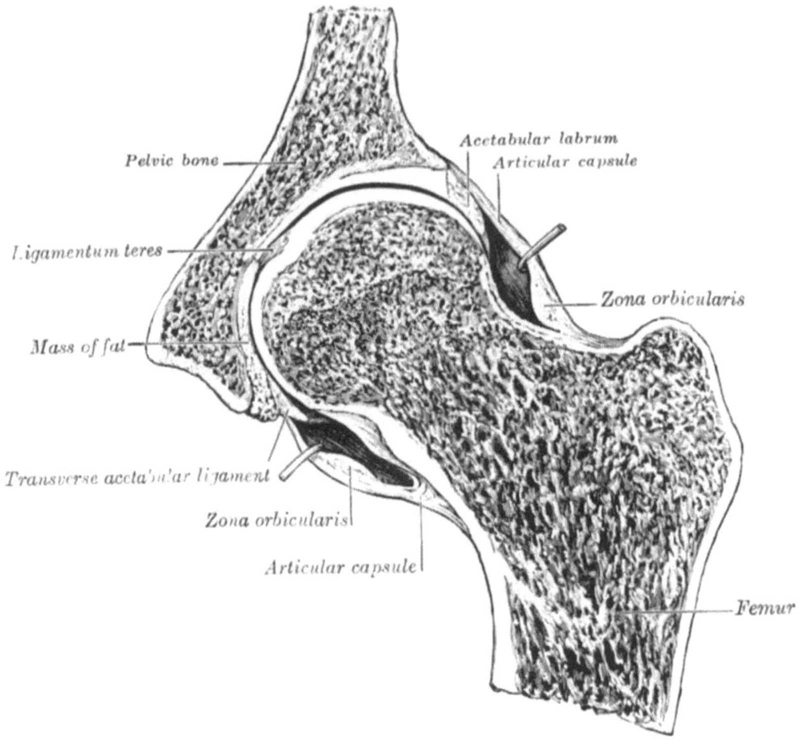

FIG. 3–8 Section through hip joint. (From *Gray's Anatomy,* 29th ed. Philadelphia, Lea & Febiger, 1973.)

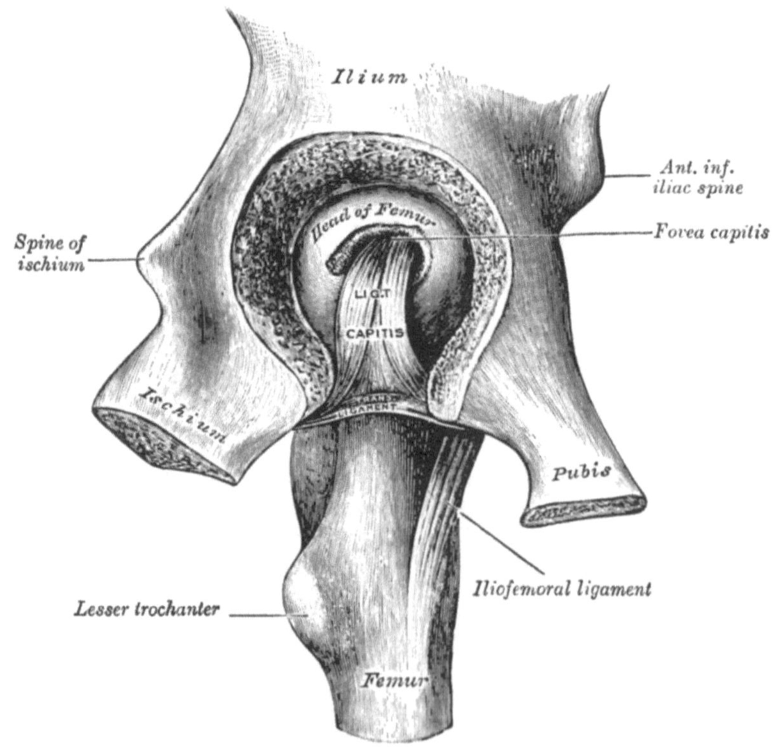

FIG. 3–9 Exposed left hip joint viewed from medial aspect. (From *Gray's Anatomy,* 29th ed. Philadelphia, Lea & Febiger, 1973.)

taut when the hip is in full extension, limiting that movement by torsional impaction of the femoral head into the acetabulum and producing the "close-packed position" (the terminal position commonly associated with tautening of ligaments and full congruity of articular surfaces [28]) (Fig. 3–10).

The femoral attachment of the capsule is reinforced by fibrous extensions into the many vascular foramina at the base of the neck. Some of the innermost fibers are reflected in a medial direction as retinacula onto the femoral neck, along which they pass to reach the subcapital articular sulcus. Covered by synovial membrane, these retinacula are concentrated superiorly, inferiorly, and occasionally anteriorly where they provide a relatively safe passage for the blood vessels to and from the femoral head in both children and adults [16] (Fig. 3–11). In the living the synovium is loosely attached to the neck and at the retinacular areas is lifted off into pliable folds.

Vascular Patterns

The human femoral head presents more vascular disorders, of both traumatic and nontraumatic origin, than any other skeletal element. This is partly attributable to the complete intraarticular position of the head and most of the neck, a feature which makes them dependent on the long vulnerable retinacular vessels for survival (Fig. 3–12). In all mammalian joints, the subsynovial tissues at the margins of the articular cartilage have a rich anastomosis described by William Hunter [24] in 1743 as the circulus articuli vasculosus, better known today as the subsynovial articular anastomosis. The sites of the capsular attachment to bone are also surrounded by a vascular circle, both of which contribute to the metabolic needs of the articular components.

Pericapsular

The capsular attachment to the acetabulum is surrounded by a vascular anastomosis fed by both femoral circumflex vessels, by the acetabular branches of the obturator, and by articular twigs from the superior gluteal (Fig. 3–4). It contributes capsular and osseous vessels to the acetabular margin and its deep ramifications anastomose with branches from the nutrient artery to the ilium on the deep aspect of the acetabular floor. This derivative of the internal iliac is the largest nutrient vessel to the hip bone, and when traumatized may occasionally bleed briskly. The acetabular anastomosis is united by pericapsular branches to a larger and more important corona of vessels which embraces the capsular attachment at the base of the neck—the *basal* or *trochanteric anastomosis.* It gets a rich blood supply inferiorly from the medial femoral circumflex artery, anteriorly from the ascending branch of the lateral circumflex, and superiorly from the superior gluteal tributaries [7] (Figs. 3–11 to 3–13). Deep to the quadratus femoris additional contributions come from the cruciate anastomosis at the confluence of the medial femoral circumflex, the inferior gluteal, the middle branches of the lateral femoral circumflex, and derivatives from the first perforator (Fig. 3–12). The terminal branches from this basal vascular plexus are capsular, muscular to the adjacent muscles, osseous via the many underlying bony foramina to the cancellous trochanteric bone, and retinacular piercing the capsule and entering the subsynovial retinacula to reach the subcapital anastomosis. This latter vascular circle supplies the epiphysis and metaphysis in the child and the head and the medial neck in the adult.

Subcapsular

The vessels in the superior retinacula deriving their blood supply from the upper end of the trochanteric anastomosis are always multiple and are distributed to the upper neck and approximately the upper two-thirds of the head (Figs. 3–12 and 3–13). At the superior subcapital sulcus, the vessels continue into the head on a smooth curved course parallel to the epiphyseal plate or scar. Smaller branches radiate to the subchondral cortex and the epiphyseal plate during the growth period (Figs. 3–13 and 3–40). The inferior retinaculum has a more mobile, pedunculated fold of synovial membrane enclosing a leash of blood vessels which pass directly to the subcapital anastomosis.[16] Having a double fold of synovial membrane on their deep aspects, they do not send branches to the neck as the deeper vessels do (Figs. 3–11 and 3–14). All articular arteries both pericapsular and subcapsular are accompanied by thin-walled venae comitantes which often assume plexiform dimen-

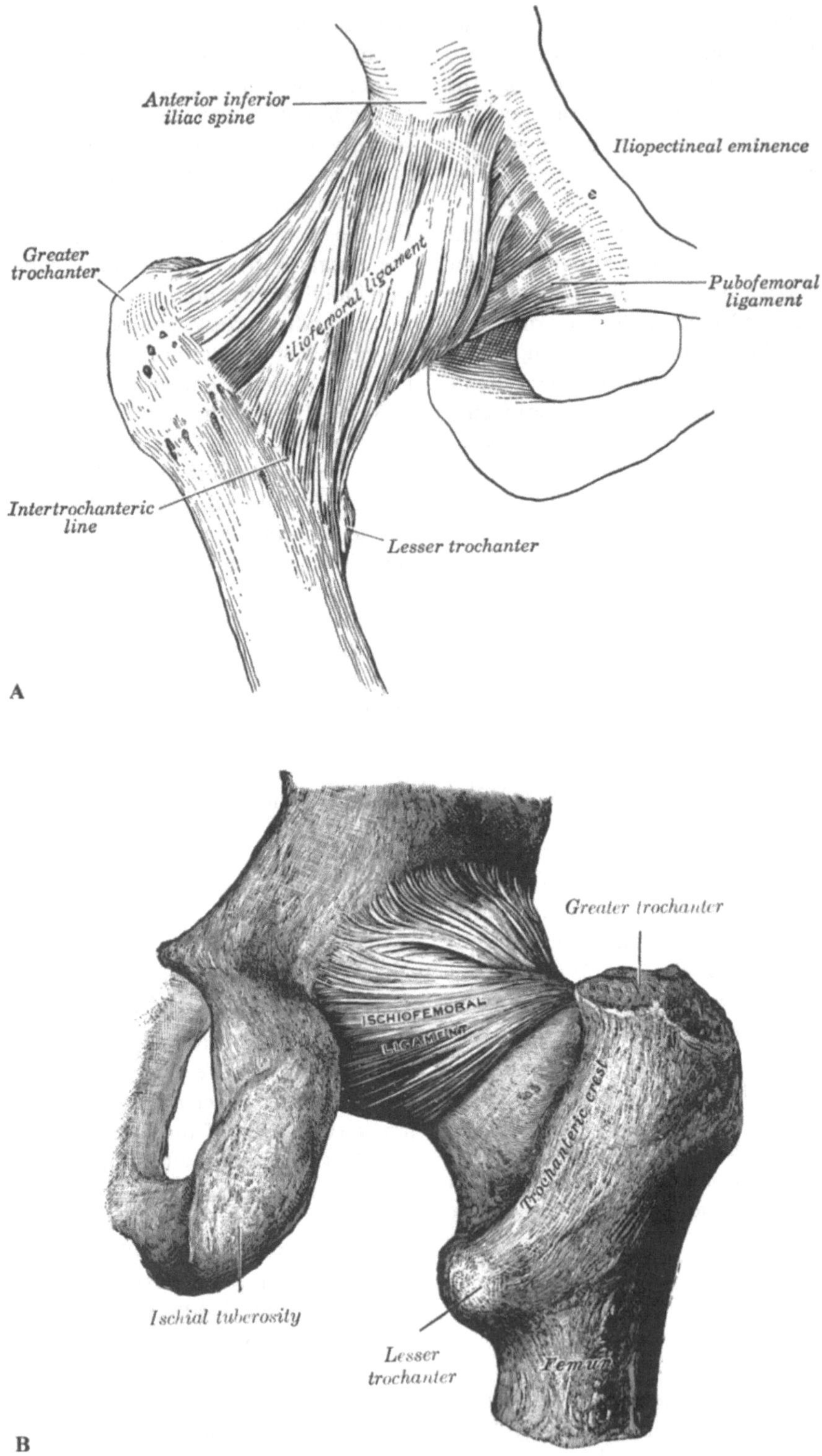

FIG. 3–10 Extended right hip joint to show twisting of capsule, anterior (**A**) and posterior (**B**). (From *Gray's Anatomy,* 29th ed. Philadelphia, Lea & Febiger, 1973.)

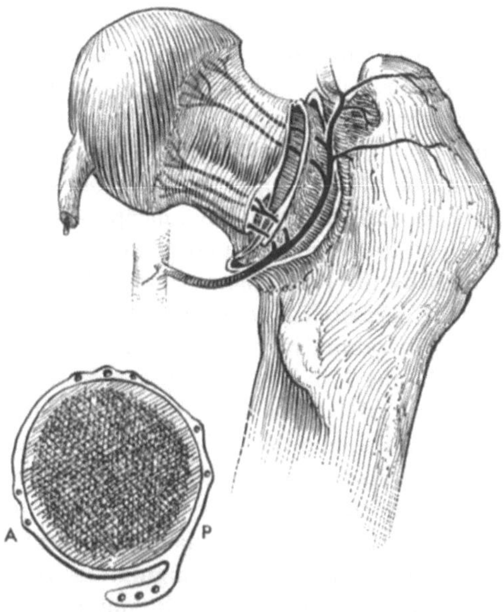

FIG. 3-11 Retinacula on femoral neck. Insert shows them concentrated superiorly and inferiorly.

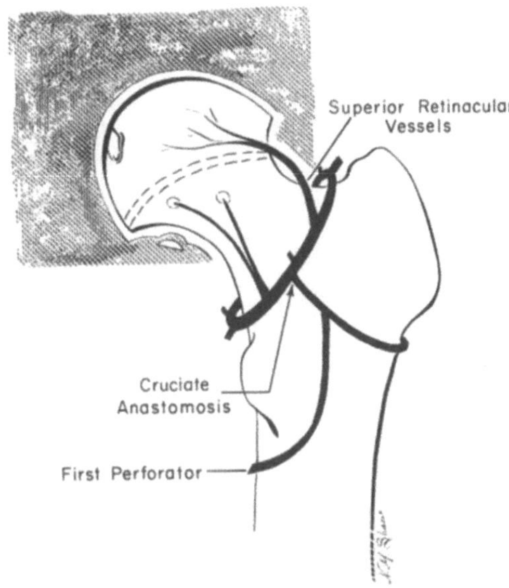

FIG. 3-12 The isolated femoral head at the end of the cervical pedicle. Basal anastomosis sending superior and inferior retinacular vessels to the head.

sions and are even more sensitive to extramural pressures than the arteries.

Variations of Blood Supply

The femoral head may possibly get a blood supply from the superior, the inferior, or the more inconstant anterior retinacular vessels, from the obturator artery via the ligamentum capitis femoris, or from the nutrient artery in the adult. As in all biological morphology, the vascular distribution shows considerable variations and the individual, partial, or total contributions of these vessels to the capital blood supply are equally variable. Savitt and Thompson's [32] elegant series of injected human specimens following total neck severance suggests that 70% or more of the heads depend on the retinacular vessels for survival. Only 5% showed a full head injection through the foveolar artery in the ligament. The remaining 25% exhibited a greater or lesser degree of total head injection. These authors also confirmed the findings of others that under normal average conditions the superior retinacular vessels contribute the major blood supply to the head in both children and adults.[16,32,35,36] The superior retinacular vessels enmeshed in a venous network may pass in the synovial folds, and may be partly or even fully embedded in the bone of the superior neck cortex. At

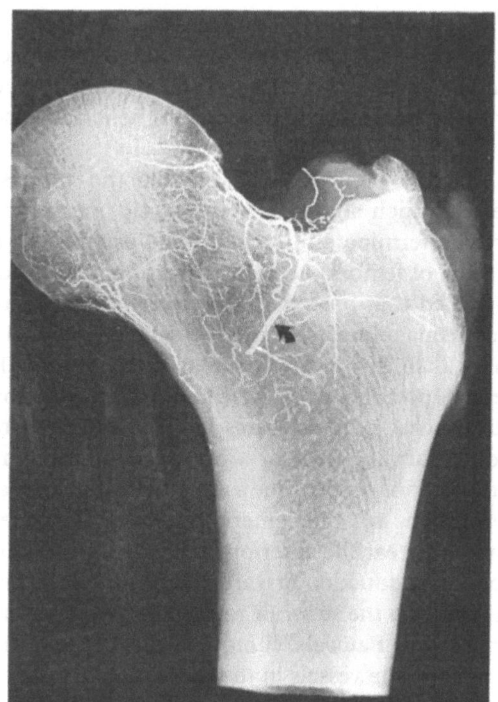

FIG. 3-13 Injected basal anastomosis supplying superior retinacular vessels to upper head and neck. (From Harty, M., and Joyce, J. J.: Surgical approaches to hip and femur. J. Bone Joint Surg., 45A:175, 1963. Used with permission of The Journal of Bone and Joint Surgery.)

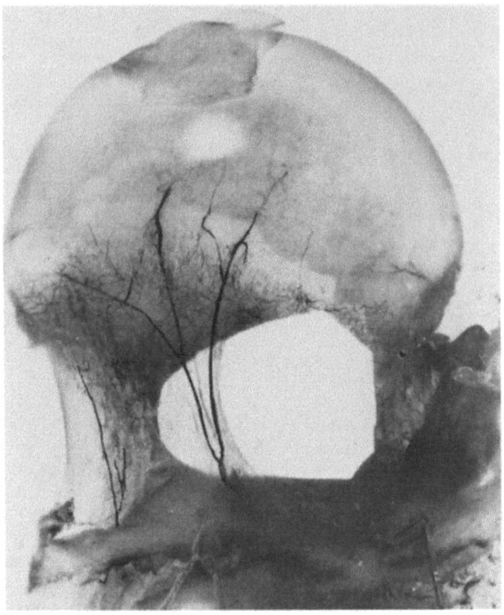

FIG. 3–14 Inferior retinacular vessels; white paper inserted between neck and pedunculated retinaculum.

the head–neck junction the intervascular bony ridges reinforce this area and afford protective covering to the underlying cancellous bone and vascular channels.

Harris [13] pointed out that, unlike the epiphyseal vessels which anastomose freely, the metaphyseal arteries terminate in loops as end-arteries. In the healing of femoral neck fractures, Bank's [1] studies indicated that open and intact vessels in the inferior retinaculum were more essential for head vitality than any other vascular contributors. The reasons postulated for these findings are as follows: All femoral neck fractures have an external rotation deformity with or without comminution of the posterior cortex. The associated angulation and separation of the anterior cortical fragments stretch or tear the anterior retinacular vessels. The common adduction or varus deformity has a similar effect on the superior retinacular vessel, as seen typically in Pauwels' [31] more vertical type of fracture line. The vessels in the more mobile pedunculated area of the inferior retinaculum, having no bony neck attachments, escape laceration except in the presence of more severe capital displacement or rotation. Undoubtedly the vessel may undergo torsional or angular deformity. White [39] and Hayes et al.[20] from their experimental and clinical investigations point out that faulty acetabulum–head relationship and alignment throw abnormal sheer stresses on the femoral neck. They maintain that this malalignment is sufficient to produce nonunion or later bearing failure complicated by head necrosis.

The major blood supply to the femoral head and neck is derived from the subcapital anastomoses united to the pericapsular plexus at the base of the neck by the retinacular vessels. The vessels lying in the pericervical retinacula are exposed to pressure and trauma in practically any abnormal condition of the hip joint. The presence of local hemorrhage and edema may further jeopardize the circulation to the head. In minor cervical or subcapital displacements associated with tearing or stretching of the attached synovium, the mobility and pliability of the retinacula allow some bony or cartilaginous distortion and angulation without vessel laceration. This alteration in alignment and lumen of the vessels may slow or obstruct either the arterial or venous circulation or both, leading eventually to restricted blood flow and subsequent avascularity of the head. Early reduction of displacement is advocated to reduce swelling, and nowhere is this dictum more essential than in acute hip joint injuries. *For cervical and capital survival, every effort must be made to preserve the retinacular vessels and the pericapsular arterial and venous anastomosis at the base of the neck.* Posteriorly this vascular ring is afforded some protection by the overhanging greater trochanter and trochanter crest, but anteriorly it is exposed and vulnerable on the prominence of the trochanteric line (Fig. 3–4). Extensive pericapsular stripping at the base of the neck should be avoided.

Muscles

The hip joint is surrounded by thick broad muscle groups which play a vital role in stability, support, and locomotion, but present difficulties in examination and palpation of the joint. Anteriorly the hip flexors are innervated by the lumbar nerve roots. Posterolaterally the extensors and abductors get their nerve supply from the lumbosacral plexus, and medially the joint is hidden by the adductors innervated by the obturator nerve (Fig. 3–15). Anteriorly the sartorius, the adductor longus, and the inguinal ligament outline the femoral triangle containing the femoral nerve, artery, and vein; they are separated from the hip joint by the

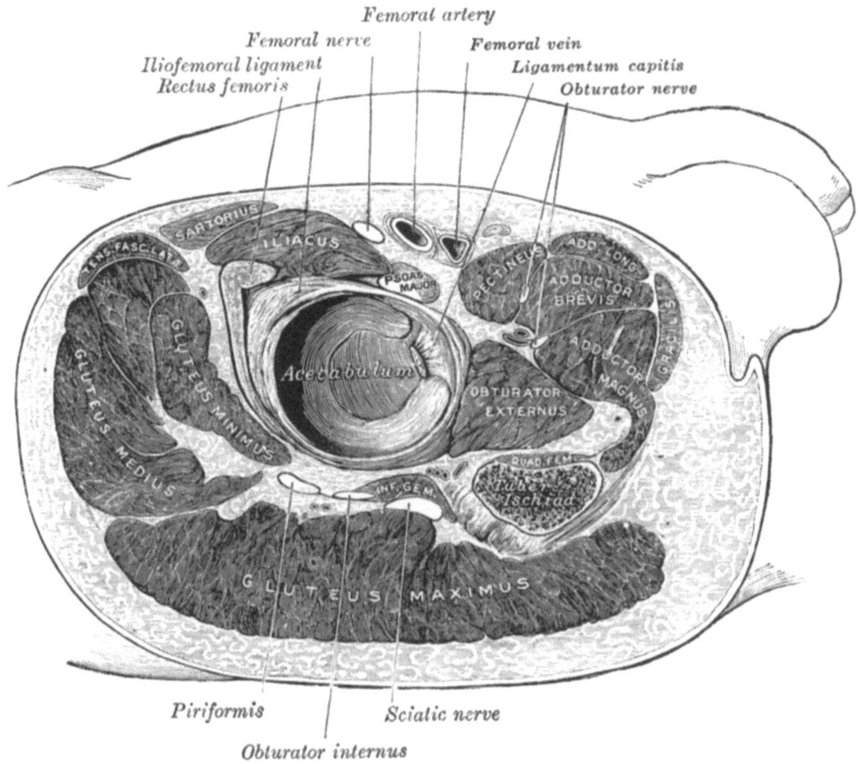

FIG. 3–15 Transverse section through hip joint to show the surrounding structures. (From *Gray's Anatomy,* 29th ed. Philadelphia, Lea & Febiger, 1973.)

combined tendon of the iliopsoas (Fig. 3–16). This hip flexor, par excellence, commonly overlies a bursa which in 10% of cases communicates with the hip joint and may appear as a swelling in the groin. The lateral margin of the tendon is often attached to the iliofemoral ligament (iliocapsularis) and may need sharp dissection to develop a line of cleavage during operative exposures. The floor of the femoral triangle is formed by the iliopsoas, the pectineus and adductor longus. The obturator nerve is not found in the triangle until the adductor longus is artificially separated from the pectineus; this exposes the anterior division of the nerve, crossing the adductor brevis which still hides the posterior division.

The prominence of the buttock and gluteus maximus, an exclusive human feature, provides a protective cover for the back of the hip joint (Fig. 3–17). The gluteal lid of Henry,[21] perhaps better known to the practicing surgeon as the gluteal barrier, is a thick, coarse-fiber muscle, firmly bound to the overlying fibrofatty layer and to an underlying rich but fragile vascular plexus. All of the superficial layer and the proximal part of the deeper layer of gluteus maximus insert on the iliotibial tract; the distal deeper portion joins the gluteal tuberosity of the femur (Fig. 3–4). The inferior gluteal nerve breaks up rapidly into smaller branches on entering the thick muscle mass and, for this reason, the upper and outer quadrant of the buttock is a favorite site for the administration of intramuscular injections. The posterior cutaneous nerve of the thigh adheres to the deep aspect of the muscle, but is separated by a layer of loose fatty tissue from the sciatic nerve and short lateral rotator muscles.

The neurovascular bundle and the piriformis muscle reach the buttock through the greater sciatic foramen (Fig. 3–17). Only the superior gluteal vessels and nerves pass out above the muscle, all other neurovascular structures leaving the pelvis below the piriformis (Fig. 3–18). In the buttock, the gluteus maximus and piriformis cover the sciatic nerve which overlies the short lateral rotator

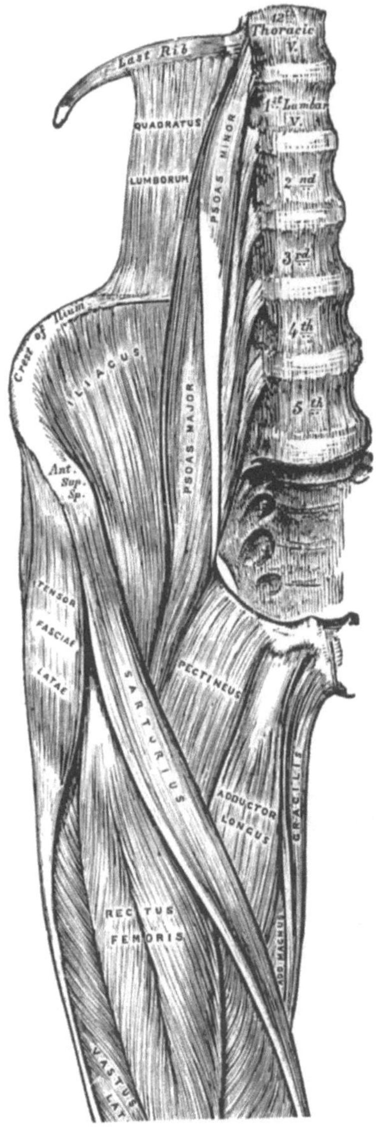

FIG. 3–16 Muscles on anterior aspect of right hip joint. (From *Gray's Anatomy,* 29th ed. Philadelphia, Lea & Febiger, 1973.)

muscles, but the capsule of the hip joint forms its most important anterior relationship because the nerve may be stretched tightly over the flexed joint (Fig. 3–19). During surgical exposures, the piriformis is sometimes confused with a lower detached segment of gluteus medius in this region, but the latter muscle does not come through the greater sciatic foramen.

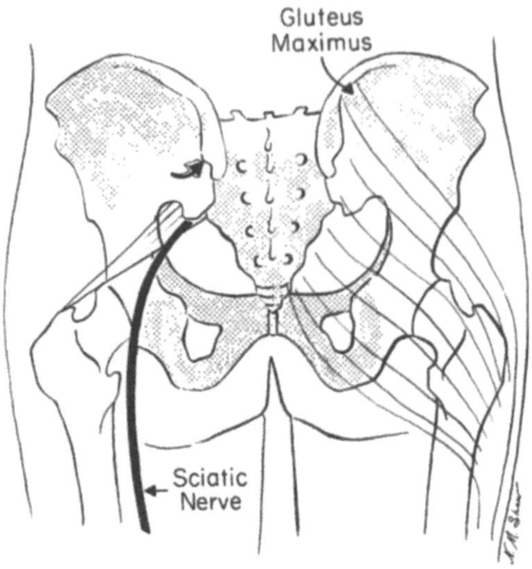

FIG. 3–17 Gluteus maximus overlying right hip joint. Left sciatic nerve and piriformis muscle indicated. Arrow points to left posterior superior iliac spine.

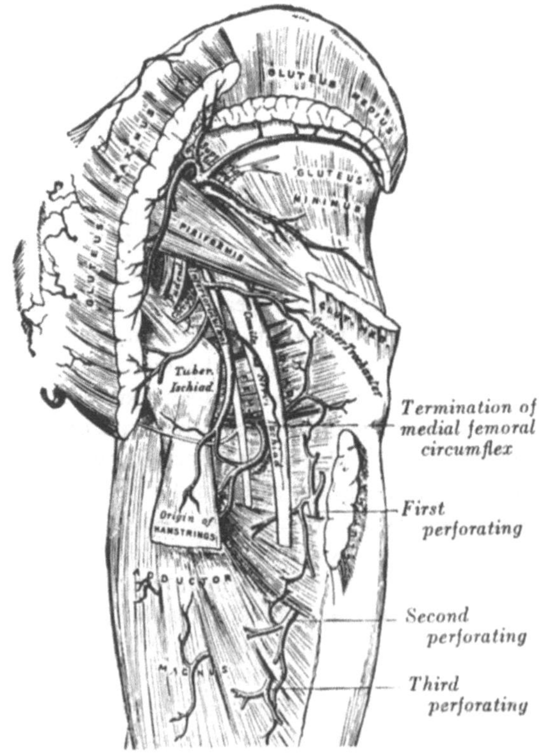

FIG. 3–18 Structures under gluteus maximus. (Adapted from Fig. 6–62, *Gray's Anatomy of the Human Body,* C. M. Goss, ed., 29th ed. Philadelphia, Lea & Febiger, 1973.)

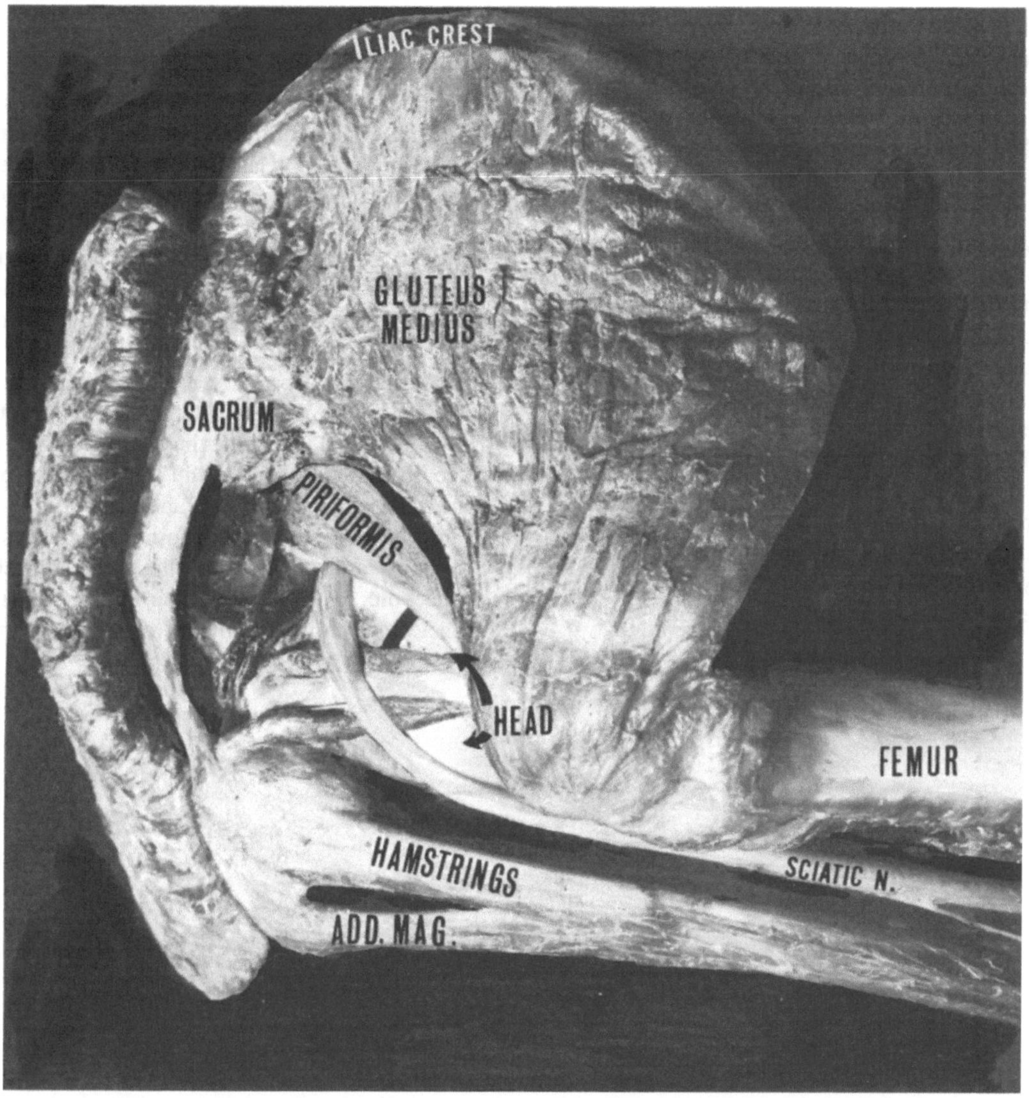

FIG. 3–19 Flexed right hip joint to show sciatic nerve tensed over the joint.

Abductor Stability

The glutei medius and minimus, passing from the dorsum ilii to the greater trochanter, cover the superior or lateral aspect of the joint. These two muscles together with the tensor fasciae latae are innervated by the superior gluteal nerve. This muscular trio is the major hip abductor, visualized by the beginner as abduction of the thigh. However, in the more common clinical interpretation, the thigh is fixed and abductor contraction prevents sagging of the pelvis to the opposite side. This smooth balanced action between the abductor and the adductors maintains the pelvis on a relatively level plane during locomotion. To prevent contralateral pelvic drop while weight bearing, e.g., walking, two factors are indispensable: (1) a stable hip joint which provides a painless fulcrum and (2) adequate and effective hip abductors. Loss of the fulcrum or incompetency of the abductors is characterized by contralateral pelvic sagging—Trendelenburg's sign. In maintaining a level pelvis during weight bearing, the hip abductors gain additional aid from contraction of the contralateral quadratus lumborum and sacrospinalis groups.

This fact is readily confirmed by palpation of the lumbar sacrospinalis muscles while walking, but still the importance and preservation of the gluteal abductors cannot be overemphasized.

The adductors clothe the inferior aspect of the hip joint and the medial aspect of the femur. Arising from the pubic bone, they are the adductor longus and brevis; with parts of the adductor magnus and obturator externus, all innervated by the obturator nerve, they adduct and flex the thigh. The ischial component of the adductor magnus reaches distally to the adductor tubercle; it is innervated by the sciatic nerve and adducts but also extends the thigh.

The iliopsoas anteriorly and inferolaterally and the obturator externus inferiorly and posteriorly (dependent area) have the most extensive intimate relationship to the capsule of the hip joint. Both may overlie a bursa which sometimes communicates with the joint cavity.

Muscle Action

Only in the eyeball and middle ear do we find muscles which act alone. Hip joint motions result from the contraction and controlled relaxation of muscle groups, and as such are these movements represented in the cerebral cortex. The initial position of the joint has a marked influence on the action of adjacent muscle. Starting from extension the glutei medius and minimus produce abduction of the hip joint, although the anterior fibers may aid in internal rotation and the posterior fibers in external rotation (Fig. 3–20*A*). The obturator internus is an external rotator. However, starting from the flexed position, the same glutei now produce internal rotation of the joint and the obturator internus has become an abductor (Fig. 3–20*B*). Similarly, at the flexed hip joint, the gluteus maximus slips anteriorly over the greater trochanter to become an abductor. The short pericapsular muscles are more important as postural muscles

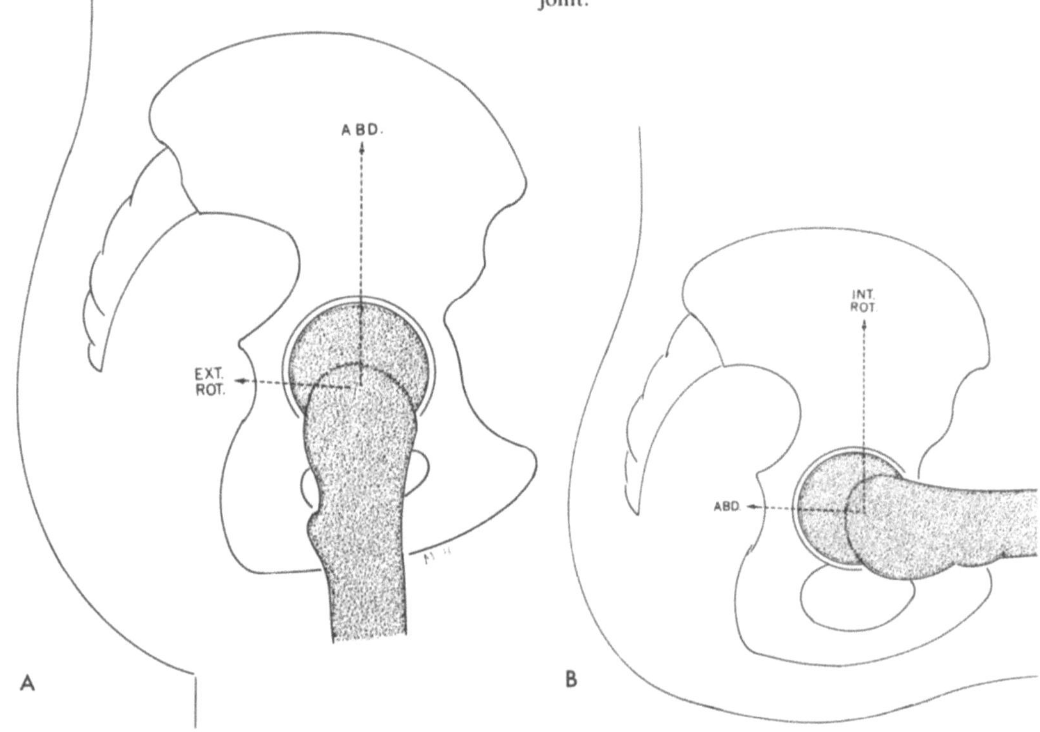

FIG. 3–20 **A** Muscle action on the extended hip joint (see text). **B** Action of same muscles on the flexed hip joint.

and stabilizers, reinforcing the capsule to which they are often attached, than as prime movers of the joint.

Summary of Hip Joint Movers

From the extended position with their innervation: *Flexion* (L. 3 and 4, more rarely L. 2 and 5): The iliopsoas is the principal hip flexor through the full range of motion. Flexion is also aided by the rectus femoris, the sartorius, the pectineus, and adductor longus. *Extension* (L. 4, 5 and S. 1, more rarely S. 2): The gluteus maximus, the long hamstrings, and the ischial part of the adductor magnus provide this motion. *Abduction* (L. 4, 5 and S. 1): The glutei medius, minimus, and tensor fasciae latae are the major hip abductors. *Adduction* (L. 2, 3, and 4): Adductor magnus, longus, brevis, pectineus, and gracilis adduct at the hip joint. *External rotation* (L. 5 with S. 1 and 2): Gluteus maximus, quadratus femoris, obturator externus with obturator internus and gemelli produce the motion. *Internal rotation* (L. 4, 5 and S. 1): Tensor fasciae latae with the anterior fibers of gluteus minimus produce this motion. Internal rotation is weak in full extension; for more effective medial rotation some hip flexion is always utilized (Fig. 3–20*B*).

Moment of force [11] between:	
Flexors and extensors	251:290
Adductors and abductors	210:347
External and internal rotation	146:54

The external rotators are practically three times more powerful than the internal rotators but, as mentioned above, internal rotation is reinforced by hip flexion. In patients with cerebral palsy hip flexion augments the action of the internal rotators, although the flexion may be apparently concealed by a lumbar lordosis. This is a basic breakdown of hip motion, but we must realize that under normal working conditions a single movement such as pure flexion is rarely executed. In parallel fibered muscles the major pull is always parallel to the direction of the muscle fasciculi. A glance at the orientation of gluteus maximus indicates that its primary action from the extended position is a combination of extension and external rotation.

Fascia

The deep fascia of the thigh ensheathes the muscles like a well-fitting lady's stocking. Distally it blends with the deep fascia of the leg and proximally it has an attachment in continuity to the iliac crest, the inguinal ligament, the ischiopubic ramus, and the sacrotuberous ligament. A thick condensation of fascia on the lateral side forms the iliotibial band, which splits into two layers at its proximal end to receive the insertion of the tensor fasciae latae and three-fourths of the gluteus maximus (the tensor gluteal internal intervening) (Fig. 3–21). The deep aspect gains an additional attachment to the linea aspera by a strong intermuscular septum between the vastus lateralis and biceps femoris. Another septum passes deeply at the anterior margins of the glutei medius, minimus, and tensor fasciae latae where it blends with the lateral edge of the iliofemoral ligament. This condensed layer, encountered during anterolateral surgical exposures of the joint, conceals the ascending branches of the lateral circumflex vessels [25] (Fig. 3–4). The iliotibial band, which joins the middle third of the iliac crest to the lateral tibial tubercle of Gerdy, provides an aponeurotic insertion for the tensor fasciae latae and the greater part of the gluteus maximus (Fig. 3–21). It slides freely over the greater trochanter as evidenced by the large bursa which covers that prominence both

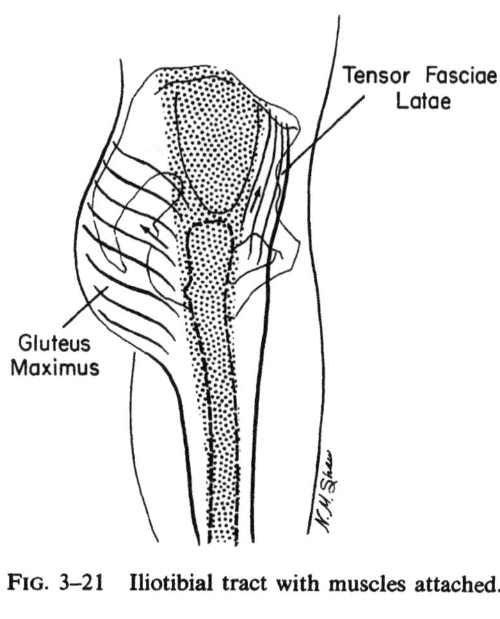

FIG. 3–21 Iliotibial tract with muscles attached.

laterally and posteriorly as well as the adjacent areas of gluteus medius and vastus lateralis. The deep aspect of the iliotibial tract is easily located at the bursal site and more distally, but proximally it gives origin to the superficial fibers of the gluteus medius which obscure the line of cleavage. The trochanteric or subgluteal bursa may be the site of acute or chronic (not uncommonly tuberculous) inflammatory changes. Sliding of a deep fibrous band across this bursa is one cause of snapping hip. Another bursa rarely seen today is located on the ischial tuberosity; it was commonly seen in the days of the hand loom and dignified by the august title of "weaver's bottom." Other smaller bursae are found deep to the muscles attached to the greater trochanter and between the lesser trochanter and adductor magnus muscle.

The inguinal ligament covers a vascular and neuromuscular lacuna in the groin. The psoas major, the iliacus, the femoral nerve, and the lateral cutaneous nerve of the thigh leave the abdomen through the lateral neuromuscular lacuna. They are enclosed in the psoas sheath which is attached to the brim of the true pelvis and more distally to the iliopectineal eminence (Fig. 3–22). The more medial vascular lacuna carries the femoral artery, vein, and canal, all three surrounded by the femoral sheath.

Innervation

The hip, like many other joints, has a rich distribution of nerve endings in the capsule, the ligaments, the intraarticular fat pads, and the articular blood vessels, but apparently none in the synovial membrane.[8] This innervation provides mechanoreceptors which exercise reflex, static, and dynamic influences on muscle control and aid in the appreciation of joint position, of motion, and of pain. The afferent articular nerves, which contain both myelinated and unmyelinated fibers, pass either directly to adjacent peripheral nerves (primary articular nerves) or to nerves in the pericapsular muscles (accessory articular nerves). The nerve to the quadratus femoris (immediately deep to the sciatic) innervates the posterior capsule. The anterior division of the obturator nerve carries impulses from the anterior capsule. Contributions from the posterior division of the obturator supply the ligamentum capitis femoris and haversian fat pad. At its origin the obturator externus is pierced by this nerve, which has an eventual distribution to the back of the knee joint and popliteal artery. The muscular branches to the pectineus, infrequently joined by recurrent twigs from the rectus femoris nerve, supplement the anterior and the inferior capsular sensory supply. The superior capsule also gets contributions from branches of the superior gluteal nerve in the gluteus minimus.[12] In addition to their afferent sensory branches, the subsynovial blood vessels also have an efferent autonomic (vasomotor) innervation.

Regardless of its severity or origin, joint pain is often diffuse, poorly localized, and may radiate to distal anatomical sites. John Hilton's statement (law) of 1863,[23] that "the same trunks of nerves whose branches supply the groups of muscles moving a joint furnish also a distribution of nerves to the skin over the insertion of the same muscles, and [what at this moment especially merits our attention] the interior of the joint receives its nerves from the same source," is as germane today as it was a century ago.

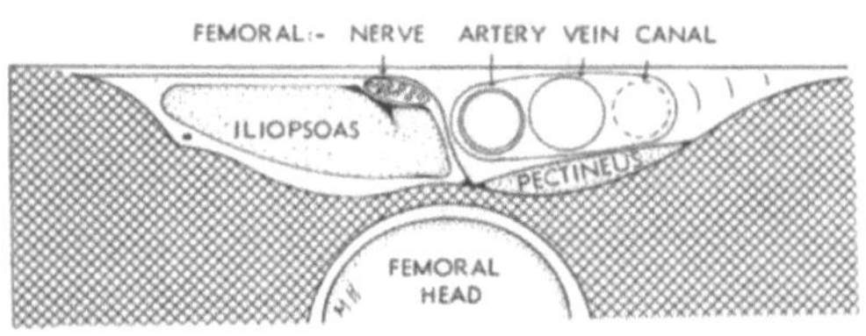

FIG. 3–22 Structures passing under inguinal ligament.

Normal Radiological Findings

The lesser trochanter is attached posteromedially to the femoral shaft; therefore a prominent lesser trochanter indicates an externally rotated hip joint confirmed by a foreshortened neck and overlap of the trochanteric and capital shadows. The lesser trochanter is overlapped by the femoral shaft during internal rotation. In either of these positions, the medial shaft, the lower margin of the neck and of the superior pubic ramus form the curved line of Shenton[34] (Fig. 3–23).

On tangential view, the subchondral bone in the roof (dome) of the acetabulum joins the cortical bone in the floor of the acetabular notch. From here it blends with the upper rim of the obturator foramen, where it recurves upward as the side wall of the true pelvis. The cortical shadow now curves

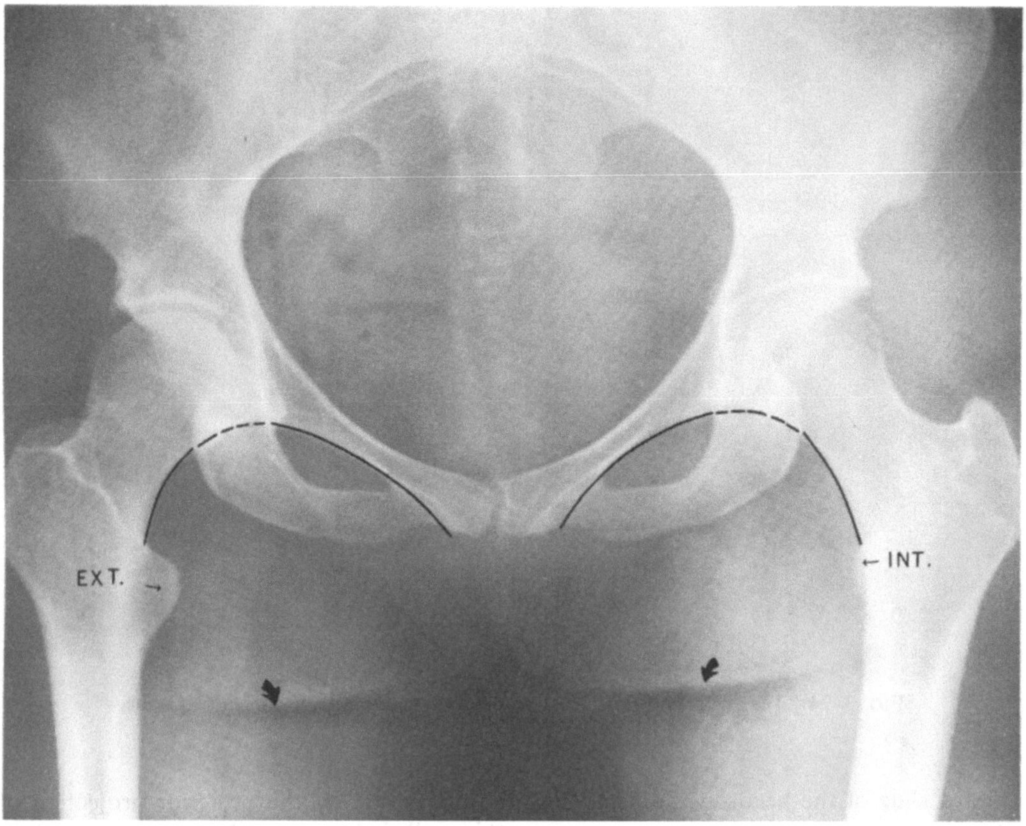

FIG. 3–23 Hips in external and internal rotation. Shenton's line indicated. Arrow points to gluteal fold.

laterally to form the floor of the greater sciatic notch and terminates at the lateral edge of the acetabular roof. The bottom of that outline forms the teardrop [17] (Fig. 3–24). A symmetrical right and left teardrop indicates a well-centered anteroposterior roentgenogram of the pelvis. A central displacement of the femoral head interrupts the characteristic outline of the teardrop and, when the femoral head fails to occupy the acetabulum, a wider teardrop shadow is expected and found. A crescent of perfectly normal trabeculated bone is outlined between the acetabular roof and the floor of the greater sciatic notch; this is not a region of demineralization (Fig. 3–24). The thin cortical bone of the greater trochanter also casts a faint shadow compared to the adjacent bony structure, both in children and the aged.

Koch [26] has shown by mathematical analysis that there is a remarkable adaptation of the inner structure of the femur to the mechanical requirements imposed by loading on the femoral head. Condensed pressure lamellae radiate from the thick cortex of the medial shaft to the superior subchondral aspect of the head. Less distinct lamellae curve from the cortex of the lateral shaft to the upper neck and continue in the direction of the epiphyseal scar. Ward (1838)[38] maintained that the former contributes by its rigidity and the latter by its tenacity to support the weight on the head—a valid supposition while considering vertical loading on an isolated and disarticulated femur. He also contrasted these lamellar condensations with the relatively alamellar triangles in the center of the neck and at the junction of head and neck (Fig. 3–25). Today the central cervical triangle still retains the eponym of Ward but the subcapital triangle is associated with the name of Babcock, who described it as the most common site for the early metaphyseal manifestations of bony tuberculosis of the hip joint in children. Normally the femoral head shadow overrides the superior margin of the neck; absence of this overriding indicates

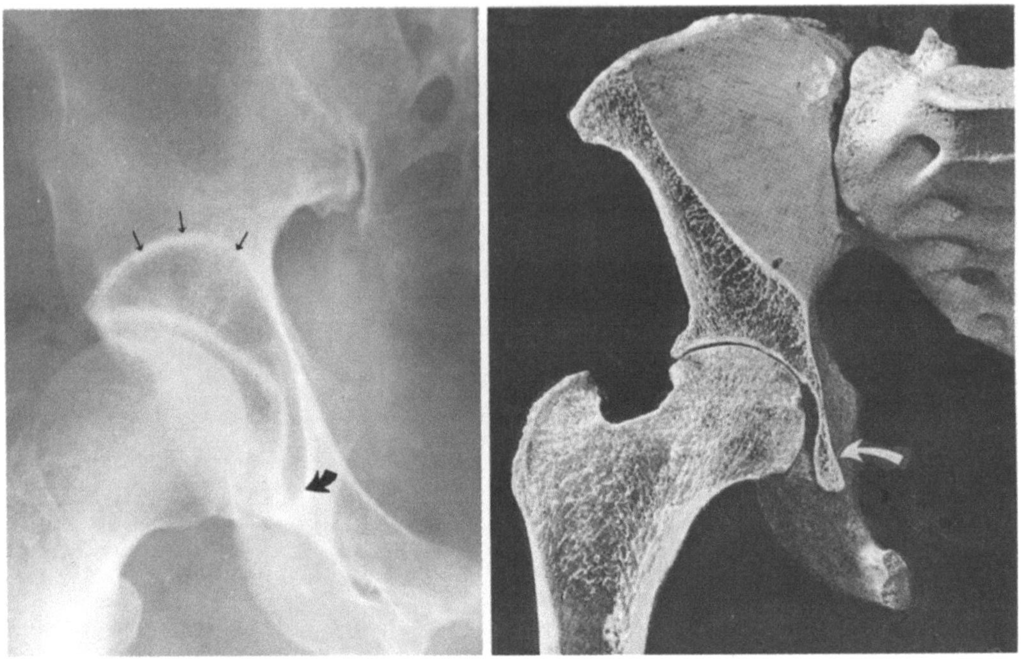

FIG. 3–24 Teardrop and normal supracetabular crescent of cancellous bone.

a downward slide of the head on the neck (Fig. 3–25).

The triangles at the head–neck junction are part of the subcapital tunnel that houses a circular venous and arterial anastomosis (Figs. 3–25 and 3–26B). Embryologically the superior triangle is of epiphyseal origin whereas the inferior one is a diaphyseal derivative. In surface replacement arthroplasty procedures the core of pressure lamellae is indispensable for adequate weight bearing and preservation of the superior retinacular blood supply is a prerequisite for its survival. Excessive reaming at the superior head–neck junction and/or low osteotomy of the greater trochanter may jeopardize these vital vessels.

Calcar

In orthopedic literature, the inferior cortex (beak) of the femoral neck is often incorrectly designated the calcar femorale.[18] The calcar femorale is a laminated vertical plate of condensed bone fanning laterally from the medial cortex toward the gluteal tubercle (Fig. 3–26). Proximally it blends with the posterior cortex of the neck, and distally beyond the lesser trochanter it fuses with the posteromedial shaft. The thick-walled tubular shaft pattern is interrupted by the posterior projection of the thin-walled lesser trochanter and trochanteric crest. The calcar femorale, representing the original cylindrical shaft, strives to maintain the tubular outline and counteract the posteroinferior compressive forces of the external rotators. In trochanteric fractures the wedge of the calcar femorale often forces the thin-walled trochanteric crest and lesser trochanter posteriorly off the thick-walled anterior parent shaft. The thick cortical bone of the shaft and neck contrasts sharply with the thin subchondral cortex of the head (Figs. 3–25 and 3–26*A*). The thickness change is also illustrated by the thin cortex on the lesser trochanter and quadrate tubercle posteriorly as compared to the thick-walled parent shaft anteriorly and laterally (Fig. 3–30). In the aged femur, the sparse lamellae in Ward's triangle are attenuated and occasionally completely absorbed. For this reason the so-called central or bull's-eye nail provides little resistance to vertical shearing forces in a fractured neck of femur.

The resultant forces passing across the joint cavity act at right angles to the articular surfaces at the area of contact.[2] This basic concept is well illustrated in primate weight-bearing joints, such as the ankle and knee, where the retention of the

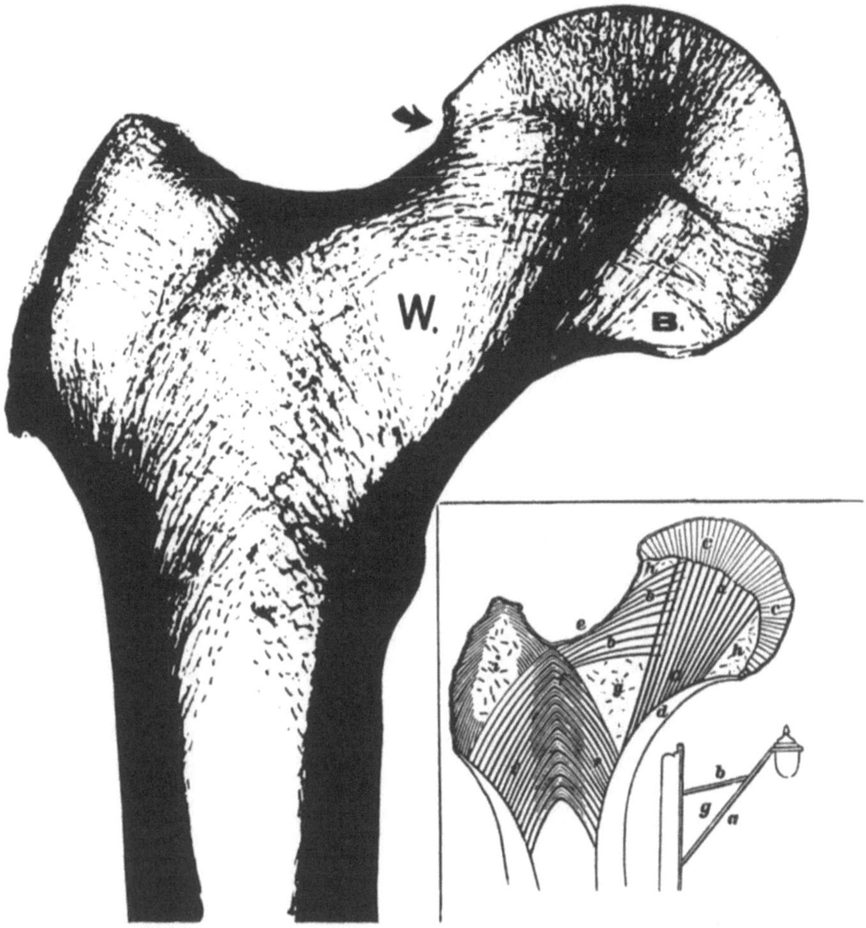

FIG. 3–25 Ward's (*W*) and Babcock's (*B*) triangles (insert of Ward's original illustration). Arrow indicates head projecting above cortex of neck. (Courtesy J. Bone Joint Surg.)

horizontal joint line enhances good painless function. The longitudinal rotary axis of the femur passes from the center of the head to the region of the intercondylar notch (Fig. 3–27). It is also called the mechanical axis and is 90° to the axis of the knee, which is an important relationship in the alignment of total knee replacement. While the proximal femur is intact, the course of this axis is outside the upper two-thirds of the shaft. Hence, internal rotation moves the greater trochanter anteriorly and external rotation moves it posteriorly (Fig. 3–28). Dissolution of the femoral neck (regardless of the cause) displaces the axis of rotation laterally into the marrow cavity of the shaft. This immediately converts all muscles passing from the pelvis to the linea aspera and lesser trochanter into uninhibited external rotators (Fig. 3–29). They unwind the femoral shaft into external rotation just as the biceps brachii unwinds the radius into supination. In a fractured femoral neck the normal anterior convexity of the neck is exaggerated (Fig. 3–30), a fact which must be recalled while inserting guidewires. Compression forces on this axis, whether due to muscle spasm, rotation, or direct contact, will collapse and comminute the posterior cortex at its two weak areas. These areas are found where the cortex is thinnest and exhibits a maximal angulation to longitudinal compression forces. They are located laterally where the neck joins the trochanteric crest and medially at the junction of the head and neck (arrow)—the classical site for femoral neck fractures. Needless to add, comminution of the posterior cortex cannot occur without a fracture of the thick anterior neck

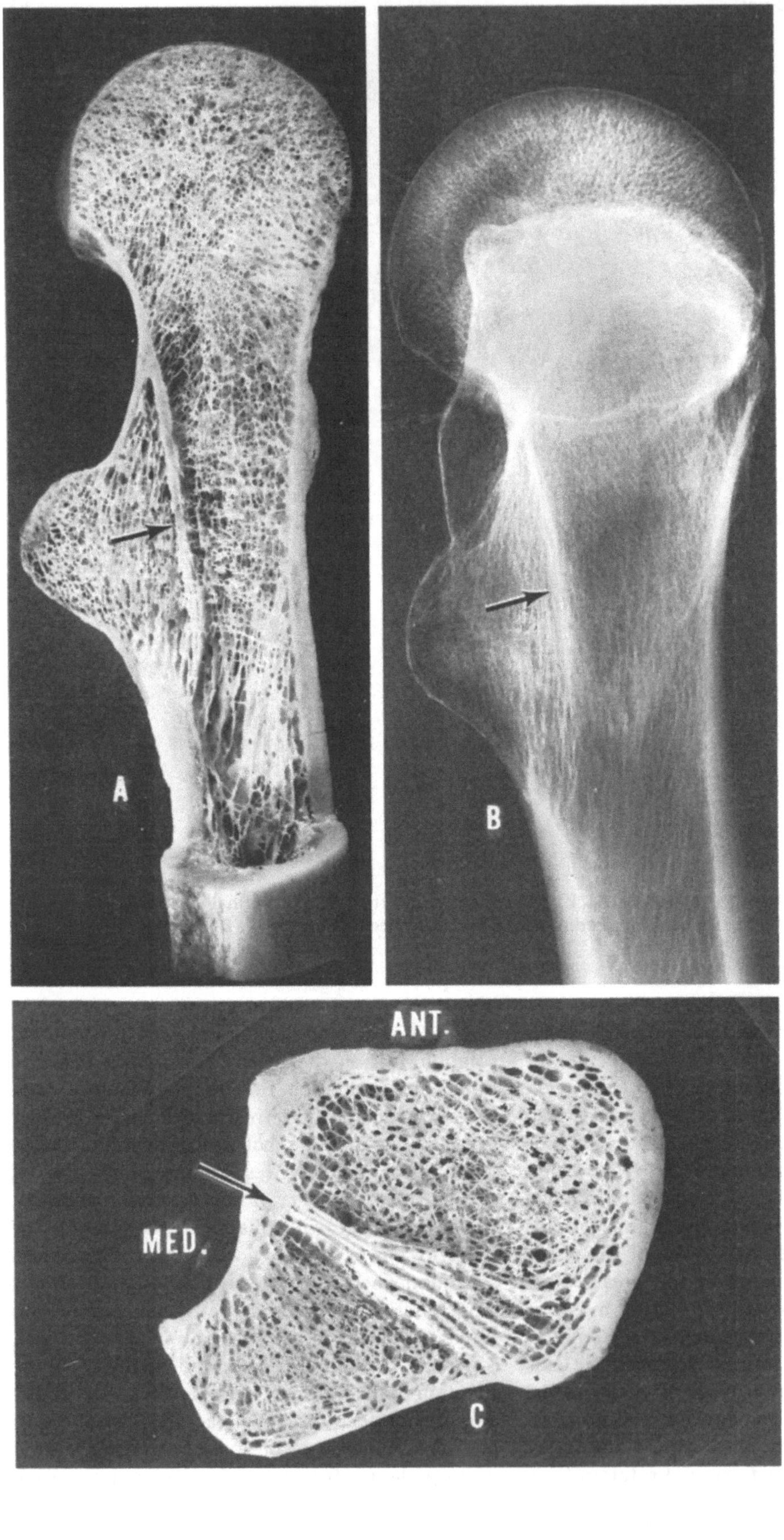

A B C

FIG. 3–26 Calcar femorale (*arrow*). **A** From lateral aspect. **B** On roentgenogram. **C** On transverse section through lesser trochanter. (From Harty M.: J. Bone Joint Surg. 39A:625, 1957. Used with permission of The Journal of Bone and Joint Surgery.)

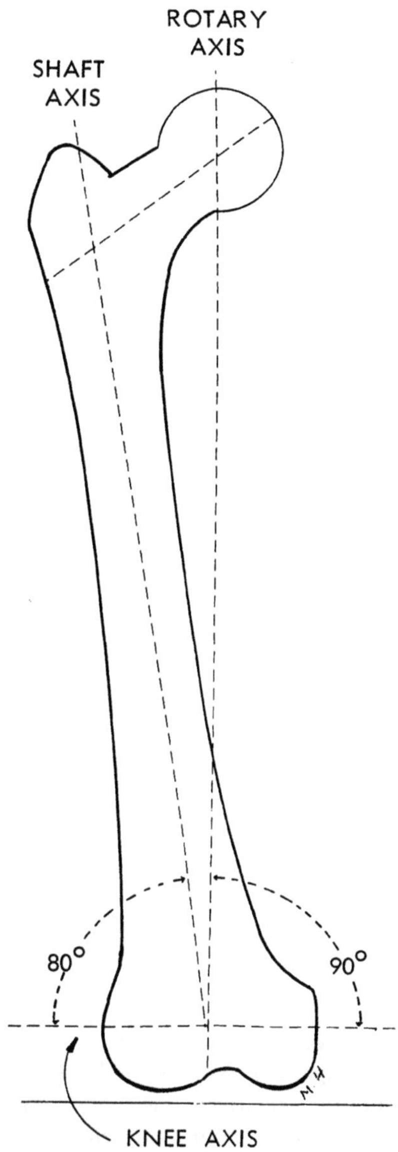

A

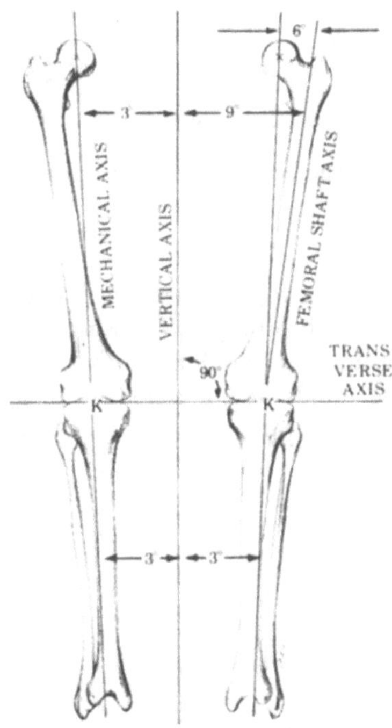

B

FIG. 3–27. **A** Longitudinal rotary axis of femur. **B** Relationship of rotary axis or mechanical axis to its companion femoral shaft axis and their interrelationship to the axis of tibial plateaus, or knee axis. (Courtesy of Howmedica.)

cortex. Incidentally, the subcapital site corresponds to the posterior margin of the subcapital epiphyseal plate where the head may slide backward on the neck.

Lubrication

Despite innumerable minor injuries and insults, the human hip joint operates as an efficient and comfortable bearing for our three score years and ten. This occurs in 65% of the population without the aid of maintenance, overhaul, or replacement of spare parts.

Articular Cartilage

This material forms a tough, springy, avascular, aneural, living layer on the bone ends. It supplies a yielding cover, which mitigates bone stresses, and a smooth gliding surface which reduces fric-

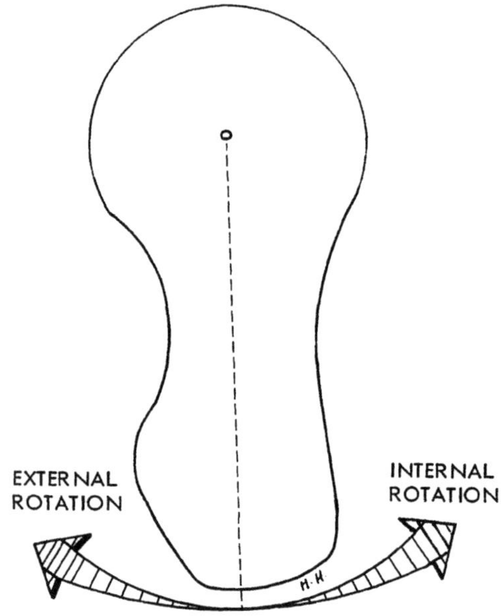

FIG. 3–28 Trochanteric displacement during femoral rotation.

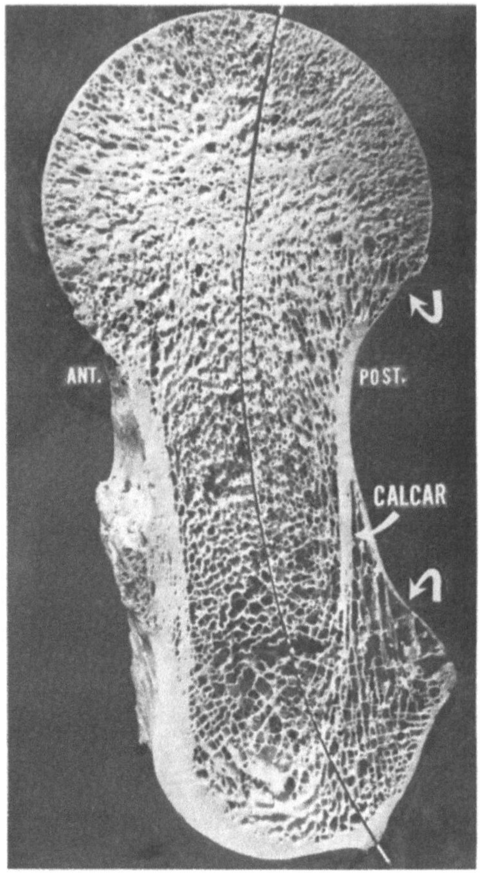

FIG. 3–30 Curved axis of femoral neck. Note tortuous outline of posterior cortex.

tion and facilitates free movements. Living cartilage, capable of absorbing and loosing fluids, displays a temporary swelling in response to exercise.[10] It molds and flattens under pressure but rapidly resumes its original dimensions, especially in the younger age groups. It is made up of a fibrocollagenous framework in a gelatinous matrix containing relatively few chondrocytes. The collagen fibers, by restricting the gelatinous matrix (fluid cushion), counteract the compression and tangential forces to which articular cartilage is exposed. Deeply, near the osteochondral level, the collagen fibers are irregularly oriented but form perilacunar baskets which enclose clusters of cartilage cells (chondrones). Superficially, very fine tangentially oriented collagen fibers of 50–100 Å diameter form the lamina splendens (MacConaill [29]) which is devoid of cells and almost devoid of the intervening ground substance. A transitional arrangement of cells and fibers is found at the intermediate level (Fig. 3–31). Walker et al.[37] have shown by scanning electron microscopy that the "smooth" articular cartilage has an undulating surface rather like beaten brass or silver. The crev-

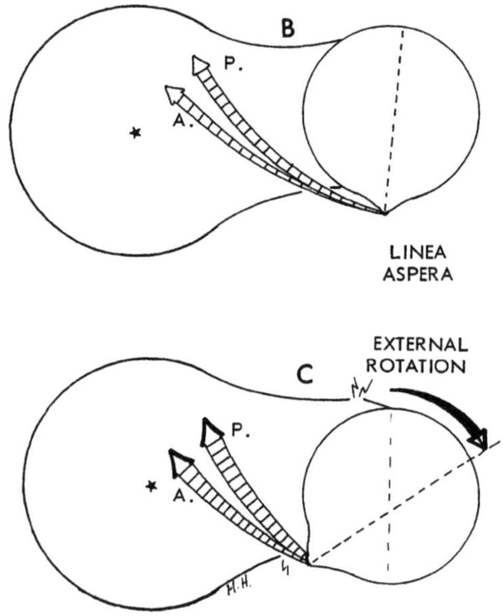

FIG. 3–29 Rotation of shaft by adductors (*A*) and pectineus (*P*). **B** Intact neck. **C** Fractured neck (see text).

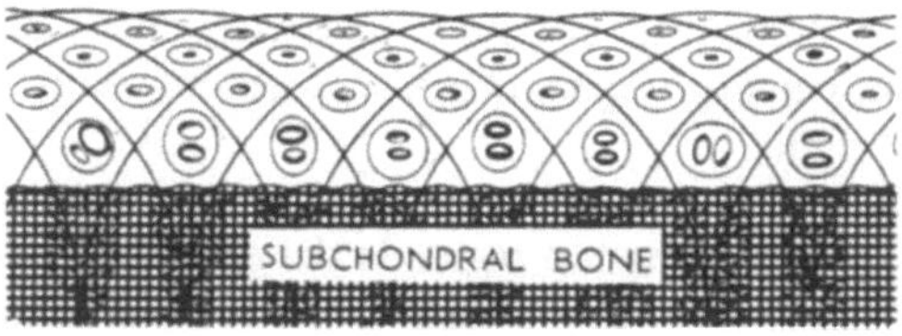

FIG. 3–31 Diagrammatic structure of articular cartilage.

ices which entrap the synovial fluid have a peak-to-valley height in the 2 to 5 mμ range, but as cartilage is elastic the number and size of these irregularities change repeatedly under pressure. The porosity of articular cartilage allows the low-molecular-weight components of synovial fluid, and possibly some fat molecules, to pass through its surface.

Synovial Fluid

This is a fibrinogen-free dialysate of blood plasma containing a high-molecular-weight long-chain polysaccharide—hyaluronic acid. This, probably in a protein complex, forms a tough, slippery film on articular cartilage which is highly resistant to rupture even under conditions of heavy loading. William Hunter[24] in 1743 stated that "synovial fluid was . . . a proper fluid for lubrication of the two contiguous surfaces . . ." Today we say that synovial fluid is an excellent lubricant but specifically and only for articular cartilage. We have also concluded that synovial fluid provides nutrition for the avascular articular cartilage, removes the end-products of metabolism, and aids in the dissipation of localized heat.

Lubrication in synovial joints is provided by the hyaluronic acid–protein complex in the fluid film (be it ever so thin) between the yielding surfaces of the articular cartilage. How this film is retained under conditions of static and dynamic loading has presented a problem to scientists and still awaits a unanimous answer. The more common current concepts on joint lubrication are classified as hydrodynamic, boundary, elastodynamic, squeeze-film, booster, weeping, hydrostatic, and mixed. The mechanical bearing of the engineer and the synovial joint have many features in common, but also have some pronounced differences. Movements in animal joints are a combination of sliding and rolling but not of continuous rotation. Speed of movements is slow as compared to current bearing speeds. Weights in the range of 200 kg/cm^2 are not excessive. The working temperature is in the moderate range of 98–100 F. The animal joint is not exposed to continuous action under severe pressure as occurs typically at the thrust block of ocean liners. During life the animal joint is never stationary except for short periods, and while healthy the articular surface is a compliant elastic and living structure.

Hydrodynamic Lubrication This proposes interlaminar slide in the synovial fluid wedged between two opposed, but not parallel, moving surfaces—a hydrodynamic wedge similar to that found in the Michels' thrust pads.[29]

Boundary Lubrication This refers to the adsorption of a molecular viscous coat of hyaluronic acid onto the articular cartilage.[6] This produces a physicochemical blend between the fluid and surfaces.

Elastohydrodynamic Lubrication A modified form of the hydrodynamic type introduces the deformation of the articular cartilage by hydrostatic and physical pressure.[9]

It has recently been reiterated that the surface of the cartilage covering the femoral head is perfectly spherical and that it exceeds the diameter of the acetabulum by about 1 μ. This incongruous proportion can occur only in the presence of pliant articular cartilage but the larger head provides "a more even distribution of contact stress" and spreads the load over the largest possible area—both well-accepted techniques for reducing surface pressure, attrition, and destruction.[22] Whatever the final answer may be, a compliant resilient bearing surface and an extremely low coefficient of friction characterize the animal joint—a combination which provides for the highly durable and trouble-free mechanism enjoyed by most of us. Any change in the harmonious reciprocity between the articular cartilage and the synovial fluid leads to a breakdown in joint lubrication and eventual degeneration.

Surface Anatomy

Unlike joints which provide palpable bony landmarks at the subcutaneous level, the hip joint is hidden on all aspects by thick muscle masses which are invariably covered by a layer of subcutaneous fat. Precise palpation of bony points is difficult, and for this reason many ingenious lines, measurements, and triangles have been devised to compare the relative positions of the available bony structures.

Bony Landmarks

The iliac crest terminating at the anterior and posterior iliac spines, the pubic symphysis, the ischiopubic ramus, and the well-covered ischial tuberosity provide the palpable bony features of the pelvis (Fig. 3–7). A constant dimple overlies the posterior superior iliac spine, which is the surface landmark for the sacroiliac joint; it is also at the level of the second sacral spinous process and the bottom of the subarachnoid space (Fig. 3–17). During hip extension the ischial tuberosity is covered by the fibrofatty layer of the buttock and the gluteus maximus, but in the flexed position the gluteus maximus slides laterally and allows a more precise palpation of the tuberosity. In the standing position a correctly oriented pelvis has both anterior superior iliac spines in the same perpendicular plane as the anterior margin of the pubis (Fig. 3–32). Classically in the female, the spines project 1 cm anterior to the pubic level. Needless to add, pelvic

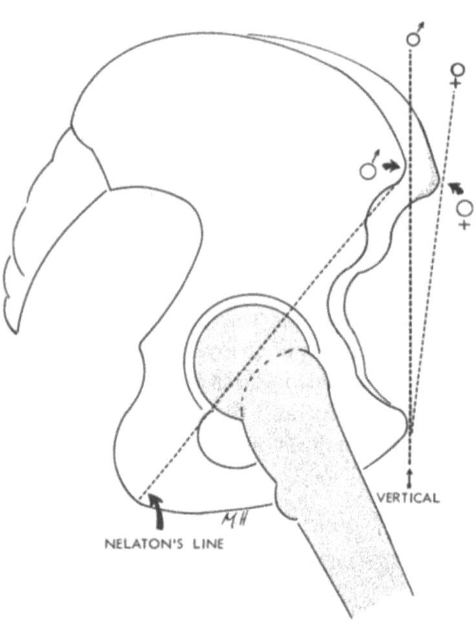

FIG. 3–32 Profile of male and female pelvis in standing position. Nelaton's line indicated.

tilt is influenced by other factors such as body build, poise or vogue, obesity, pregnancy, and ethnic origin.

The most prominent bony structure on the lateral aspect of the hip region is the greater trochanter; its tip normally indicates the level of the hip joint. The femoral shaft is well concealed by the quadriceps, hamstrings, and adductor muscle masses. Elevation of the greater trochanter is one of the more common manifestations of hip joint abnormality. Generations of medical students have demonstrated and confirmed this sign by the use of Nelaton's [30] line and Bryant's [5] triangle. Nelaton's line, which joins the anterior superior iliac spine to the ischial tuberosity, should pass proximal to the tip of the greater trochanter (Fig. 3–32). Bryant's triangle is illustrated in Fig. 3–33. Asymmetry in length of the basal (Bryant's) line is associated with dislocation of the hip joint, femoral neck dissolution, or alteration of the neck shaft angle. Elevation of the greater trochanter is also noticed by slackness at the proximal end of the iliotibial tract. The experienced clinician appreciates this sign, especially in children, simply by placing the thumbs on the patient's anterior superior iliac spines and palpating the tract and trochanters with the remaining fingers (Fig. 3–34).

The resistance offered by the femoral head which forces the iliopsoas anteriorly is located 5 cm distal to the center of the inguinal ligament. Femoral artery pulsations are also palpable on the tendon (Fig. 3–35). Even in the most obese patient, the tendinous origin of the adductor longus is not covered by subcutaneous fat. The fibrofatty subcutaneous layer covering the human gluteus maximus is limited distally by the horizontal gluteal fold. This fold is not produced by the lower edge of gluteus maximus but by the infolding of skin below the fibrofatty layer of the buttock (Figs. 3–17, 3–21, and 3–23). A similar shadow of infolded skin is often noticed at the proximal margin of the groin creases (Figs. 3–23 and 3–36). The comparative length of the lower limbs is utilized in the diagnosis and management of many hip disorders. However, measurements of limb length present two basic problems: (1) Exact bilateral symmetry is rarely encountered in the animal kingdom, e.g., right-handed persons may have a right humerus 5–10 mm longer than the left. (2) Precise palpation of bony points is difficult, especially in obese patients. True measurements are usually made from the anterior superior spine of the ilium

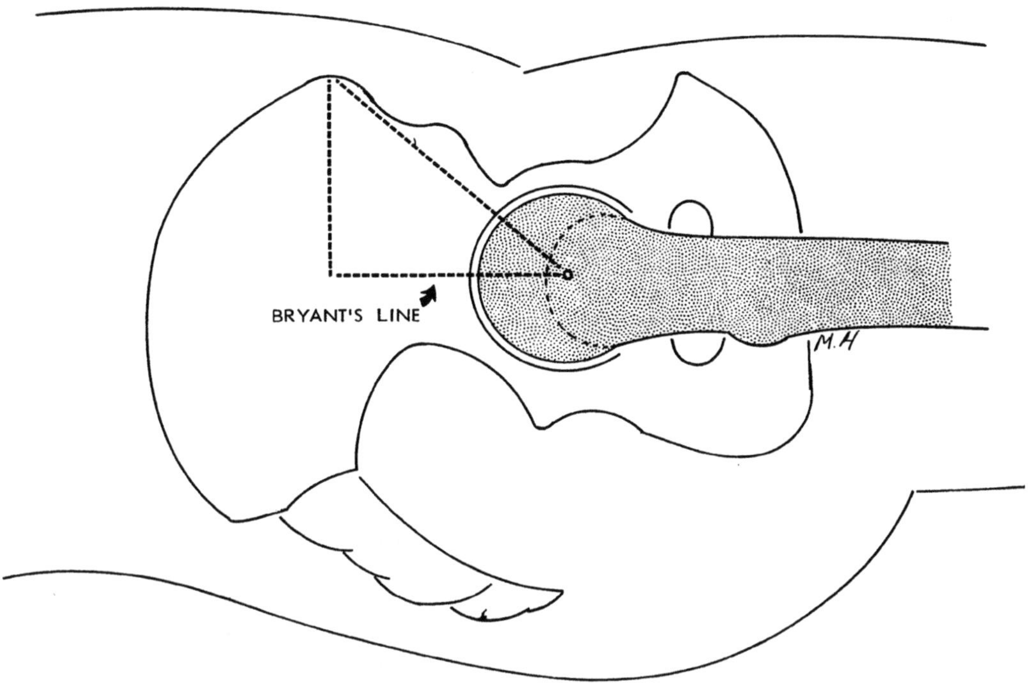

FIG. 3–33 Bryant's triangle and base line.

to the tip of the medial malleolus or the femoral adductor tubercle. If possible the limbs should be in corresponding positions and preferably perpendicular to the interspinal line (Fig. 3–34). As the line of measurement passes laterally to the axis of the hip joint (Fig. 3–36) moving from full abduction to full adduction increases limb length by 1 to 2 cm.

Joint Aspirations

The basic principles of joint aspiration follow: (1) Strict surgical asepsis is imperative. (2) Use position to get maximal relaxation of capsule and patient; this allows greatest joint capacity. (3) Avoid areas of major blood vessels and nerves. (4) Avoid injury to articular cartilage. (5) Utilize adjacent palpable bony landmarks for orientation.

The hip joint is commonly aspirated from the anterolateral aspect. The patient lies supine with the hip flexed to about 20° in slight abduction and internal rotation. This position relaxes the anterior capsule, and if an effusion is present it is forced on to the anterior aspect of the neck. The relevant bony landmarks are the anterior superior iliac spine and the greater trochanter. A 10-cm needle entered 6 cm anterior to the convexity of the greater trochanter is directed backward about 10° but in the general direction of the umbilicus. The needle point enters the joint cavity but not between the articular facets (Fig. 3–35).

Embryology and Ontogony

From the cradle to the grave the hip joint presents enigmas to the clinician. These range from congenital problems, adolescent displacements, and aged degeneration to the ever-recurring traumatic lesions. Congenital anomalies are found more frequently in the hip joint than in any other skeletal component. Because of restrictions imposed by the uterine wall during antenatal life, the hip joint develops and lives in the flexed position. Even in the first postnatal year, the infant still prefers to keep its hip flexed. Because the longitudinal fibers in the capsule were laid down in the flexed position, hip extension has a wringing and tautening effect which forces congruity of the articular facets and limits that motion (Fig. 3–10). This joint extension pulls the femoral artery, vein, and funnel-shaped collar of fascia transversalis distally into the thigh.

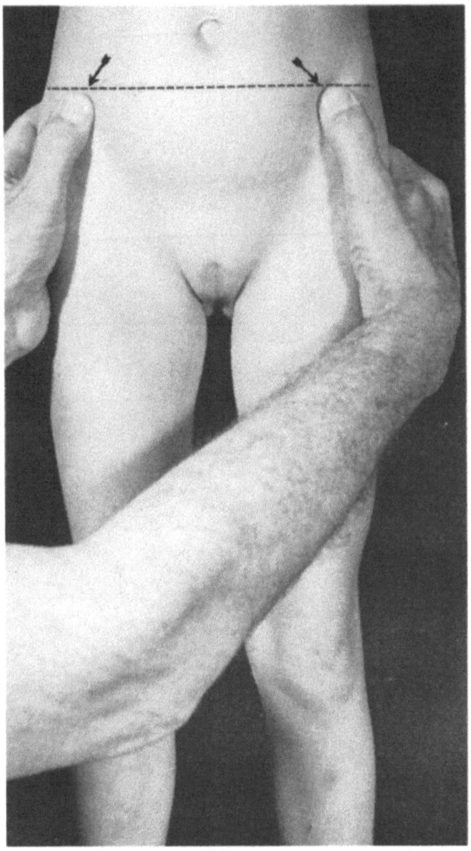

FIG. 3–34 Palpation of the iliotibial band and comparison of the greater trochanters in relation to the anterior superior iliac spines (*arrow*).

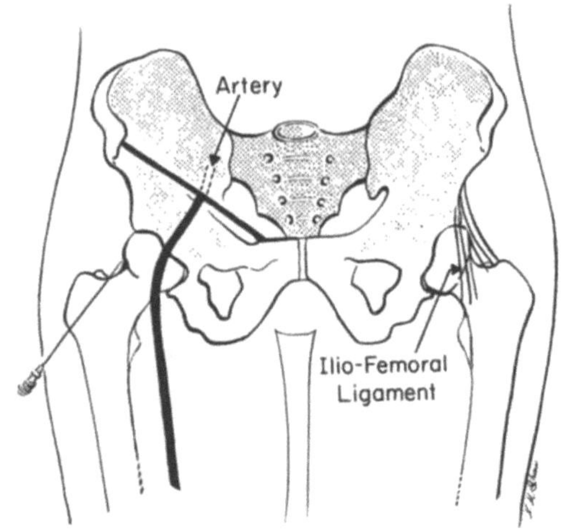

FIG. 3–35 Structures anterior to the hip joint. On right, femoral artery and needle indicate site of aspiration.

In the adult this collar, which also encloses the femoral canal, is known as the femoral sheath (Fig. 3–22).

Ossification

Although the chronological sequence rarely changes, the times of appearance of primary and secondary ossification centers are variable. Typically, secondary centers appear and fuse earlier in females than in males, but in both sexes the range may spread over a 1- to 3-year period. Primary ossification centers appear in long bones about the eighth week of intrauterine life, and contemporaneously cartilage cells at the site of future joints are compressed, soon liquefy, and form a joint cavity.

Figure 3–37 shows the ossification of the hip bone. The os acetabuli which appears about puberty in the triradiate cartilage may start as a single or multiple centers, and generally contributes the major part of the pubic component to the joint surface. Final union starts on the pelvic aspect and spreads laterally.

The shaft of the femur has ossified at birth, but the head, trochanter, and very short neck are still a cartilaginous mass (Figs. 3–38 and 3–39). During the first year a capital ossification center appears in the superior and lateral corner of the cartilaginous head. It is directly above the tongue of diaphyseal bone which forms the lower margin of the neck at this stage (Fig. 3–38). The combination of a short neck and an eccentric capital epiphyseal center produces a roentgenographic appearance of coxa valga with an almost horizontal epiphyseal plate. A growth spurt at about the seventh year gives an asymmetrical elongation of the neck which tilts the epiphyseal plate into a more vertical direction (Fig. 3–38). This tilt converts a stable compression stress into an unstable shearing (slipping) stress. During growth in the normal hip joint, the neck shaft angle of inclination changes from 160° to the 125° range, and the torsion angle moves from about 35° anteversion to about 15° anteversion (Figs. 3–2 and 3–38).

Changes in Vascular Patterns

In the growing child the retinacular vessels reach the epiphysis only by the fibrocartilaginous anulus (perichondrium) which surrounds the epiphyseal

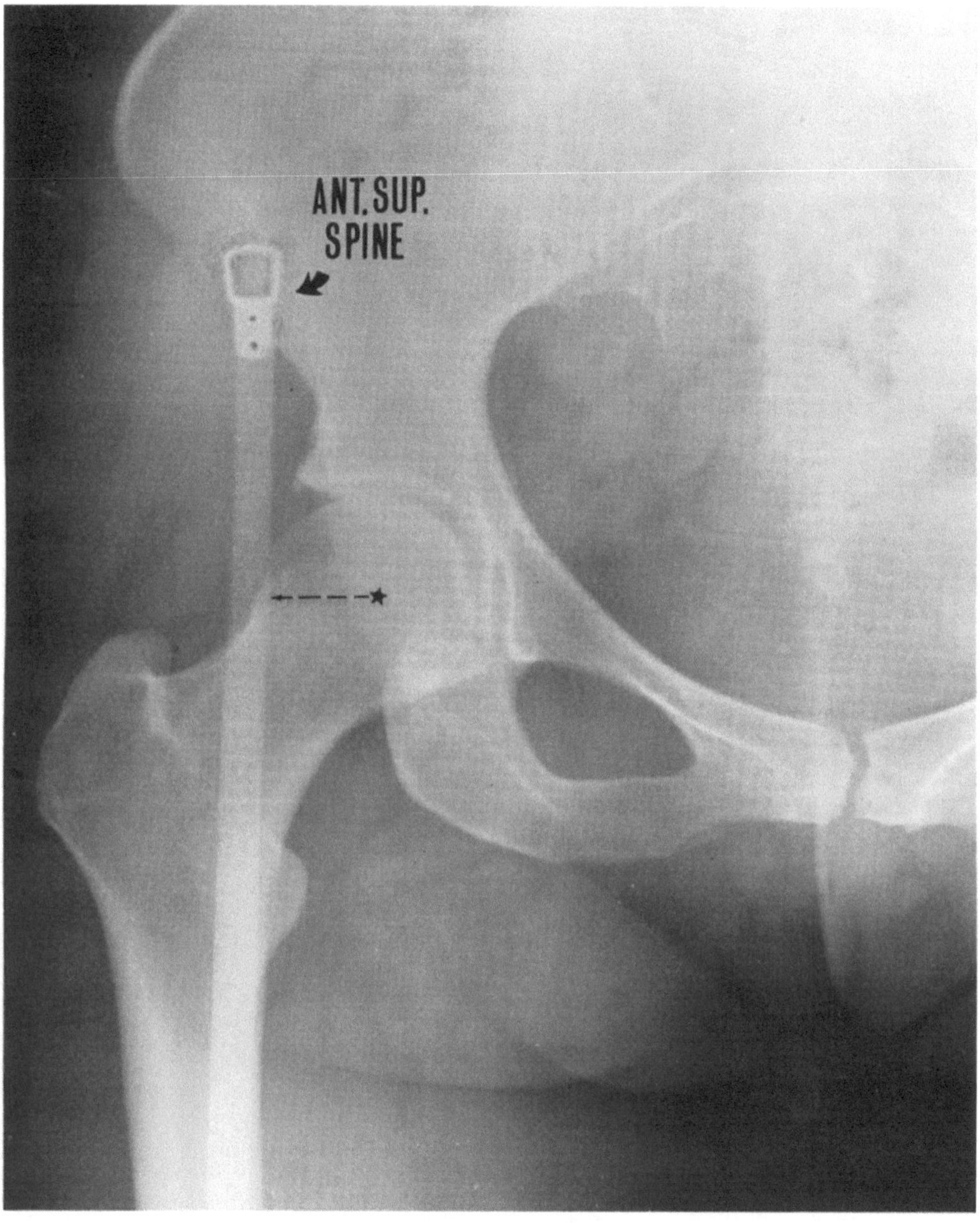

FIG. 3–36 Steel tape stretched from anterior superior iliac spine to medial malleolus. Note relationship to axis of hip joint.

plate. Following the disappearance of this plate at about the 18th year, the diaphyseal and epiphyseal vessels may communicate. In the child the retinacula, like the neck, are shorter and are attached more firmly to the neck by numerous pericervical vessels than are the retinacula in the adult. The epiphyseal plate derives its nourishment from the capital vessels only, so an avascular head is complicated by arrest of growth at the epiphyseal plate (Fig. 3–40). At all age groups the superior retinacular vessels contribute the major blood supply to the epiphysis and head. In the 8- to 16-year growth spurt the juxtaepiphyseal area shows intense cellular activity and an augmented blood

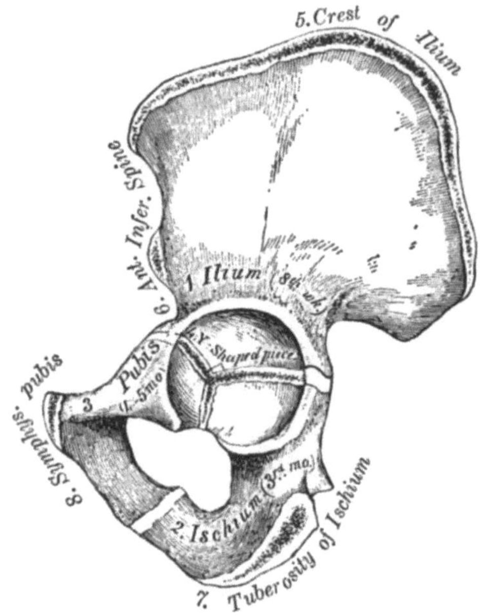

FIG. 3–37 Ossification of the hip bone by eight centers: three primary (ilium, ischium, and pubis), five secondary. (From *Gray's Anatomy*, 29th ed. Philadelphia, Lea & Febiger, 1973.)

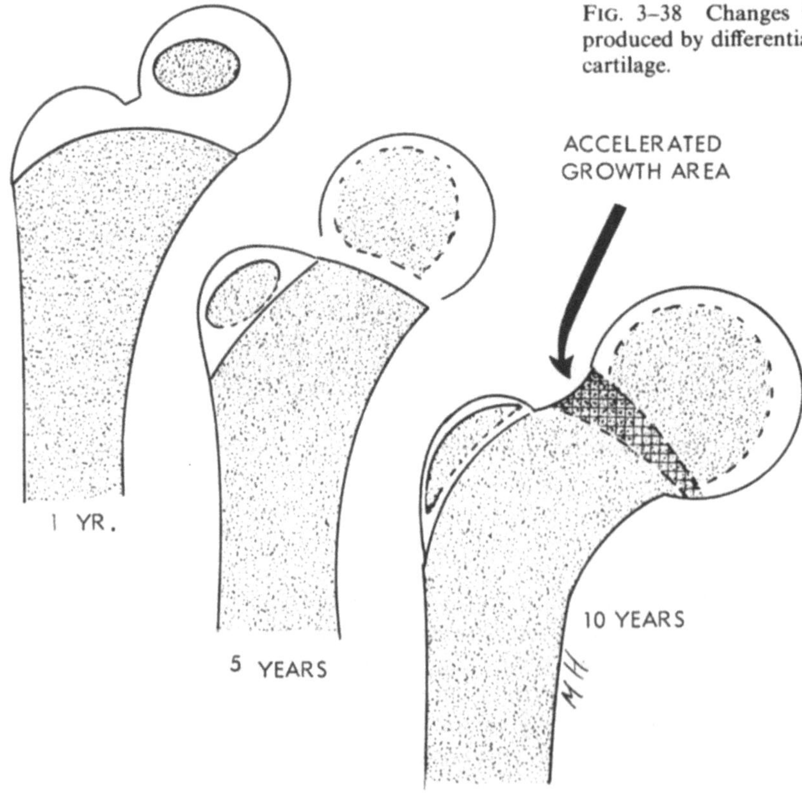

FIG. 3–38 Changes in direction of epiphyseal plate, produced by differential rates of growth in metaphyseal cartilage.

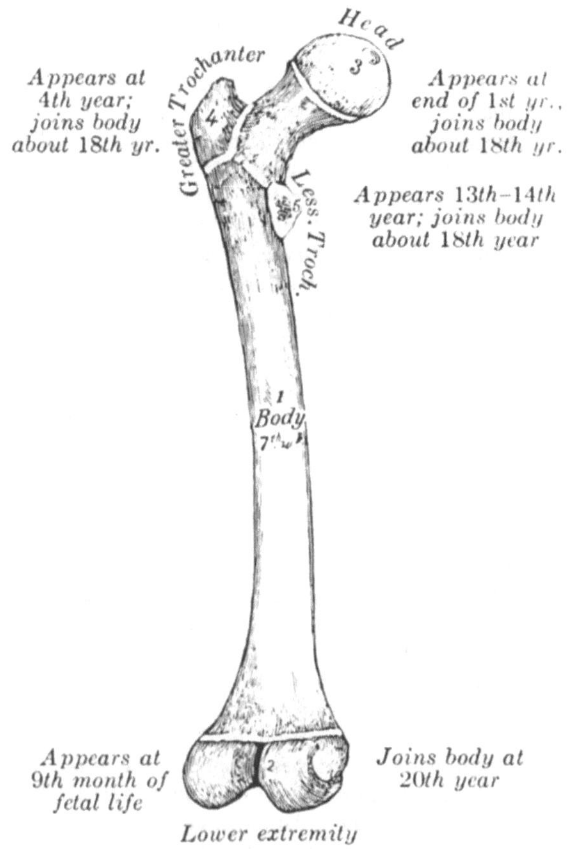

FIG. 3–39 Ossification of femur. (From *Gray's Anatomy,* 29th ed. Philadelphia, Lea & Febiger, 1973.)

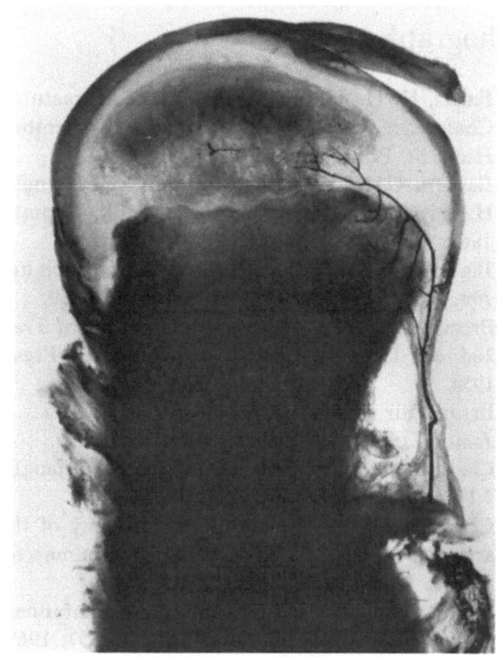

FIG. 3–40 Injected vessels in the pedunculated inferior retinaculum, passing on the peripheral margin of the growth plate to supply the epiphysis and its disc.

supply.[35] Both of these disappear after fusion at the epiphyseal plate and there is no evidence of a diminishing blood supply associated with advancing age. Capital displacement may stretch the retinacular vessels over the margin of the metaphysis, as seen typically in slipped epiphysis. Needless to add, there is a limit to which these vessels will stretch and kink before obstruction occurs. The femoral head gets a variable and minor blood supply through the capital ligament but the consensus is that without the retinacular contributions this supply would be insufficient to maintain capital vitality at any age in 95% of femoral heads.

The more commonly encountered dimensions and their variation of the femoral head, the neck, and the greater trochanter form an indispensible part of the orthopaedic surgeon's armamentarium (Fig. 3–41).

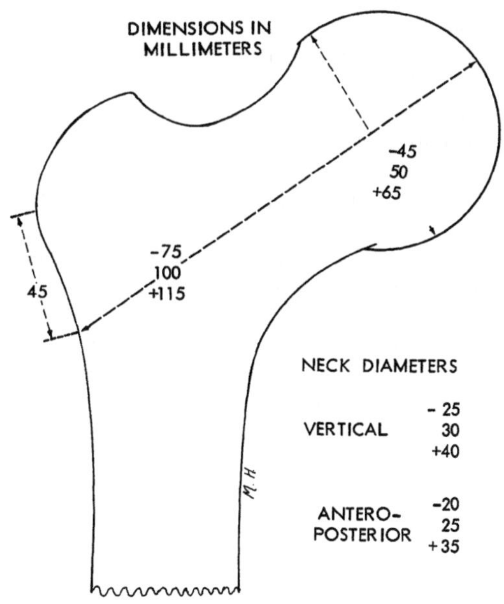

FIG. 3–41 Some dimensions of the proximal femur in millimeters.

Bibliography

1. Banks, H. H.: Healing of femoral neck fractures. Conference On Aseptic Necrosis Of Femoral Head, St. Louis, January 1964.
2. Barnett, C. H., Davies, D. V., and MacConnaill, H. A.: *Synovial Joints.* Springfield, Ill., Thomas, 1961.
3. Bigelow, H. J.: *The Mechanism of Dislocation and Fracture of the Hip.* Boston, Sampson, 1869.
4. Brock, Lord: *The Anatomy of the Bronchial Tree,* 2nd ed. London, Cambridge University Press, 1954.
5. Bryant, Sir Thomas: *The Diseases and Injuries of Joints.* London, Clinical Surgery, 1861.
6. Charnley, J.: How joints are lubricated. Triangle, 4:175, 1960.
7. Crock, H. V.: A revision of the anatomy of the arteries supplying the upper end of the human femur. J. Anat., 99:77, 1965.
8. Dee, R.: Structure and function of hip joint innervation. Ann. Roy. Coll. Surg. Eng., 45:357, 1969.
9. Dintenfass, L.: Rheology of complex fluids and some observations on joint lubrication. Fed. Proc., 25:1054, 1966.
10. Ekholm, R., and Norback, B.: Relationship between articular changes and function. Acta Orthop. Scand., 21:81, 1951.
11. Fick, R.: *Handbook der Anatomie und Mechanik der Gelenke,* Vols. 3, 9. Gena, Fischer, 1911.
12. Gardner, E.: The innervation of the hip joint. Anat. Rec., 101:353, 1948.
13. Harris, H. A.: *Bone Growth in Health and Disease.* London, Oxford University Press, 1933.
14. Harty, M.: Position of the foot in walking. Lancet, 2:275, 1953.
15. Harty, M., and Kostowiecki, M.: Vascular injuries in limb surgery. Surg. Gynec. Obstet., 121:339, 1965.
16. Harty, M.: Blood supply to the femoral head. Brit. Med. J., 2:1236, 1953.
17. Harty, M.: Some aspects of the surgical anatomy of the hip joint. J. Bone Joint Surg., 48A:197, 1966.
18. Harty, M.: The calcar femorale and the femoral neck. J. Bone Joint Surg., 39A:625, 1957.
19. Havers, C.: *Retrosynovial Pads or Fringes of Synovial Membrane Consisting Of Intra-articular Fat.* London, Osteologia Nova, 1691.
20. Hayes, A. G., and Groth, H. E.: The influence of rotational malposition on intracapsular fracture of the femoral neck. Surg. Gynec. Obstet., 124:40, 1967.
21. Henry, A. K.: *Extensile Exposures,* 2nd ed. Baltimore, Williams & Wilkins, 1957.
22. Hill, A. G. S., Ed.: *Modern Trends In Rheumatology 2.* New York, Appleton-Century-Croft, 1971.
23. Hilton, J.: *Rest and Pain.* London, Bell, 1863.
24. Hunter, W.: Of the structure and diseases of articulating cartilage. Philos. Trans. Roy. Soc., London, 42:470, 514, 1743.
25. Joyce, J. J., and Harty, M.: *Orthopaedic Approaches.* Baltimore, Williams & Wilkins, 1961.
26. Koch, J. C.: The laws of bone architecture. Amer. J. Anat., 21:177, 1917.
27. Last, R. J.: *Anatomy, Regional and Applied,* 2nd ed. Boston, Little, Brown, 1959.
28. MacConaill, M. A.: The movements of bones and joints. J. Bone Joint Surg., 328:244, 1950.
29. MacConaill, M. A.: J. Anat., 68:210, 1932.
30. Nelaton, A.: *Elements de Pathologie Chirurgicale.* Paris, 1844.
31. Pauwels, F.: *Der Schenkelhalsbruch ein mechanisches Problem.* Stuttgart, Enke, 1935.
32. Savitt, S., and Thompson, R. C.: Distribution and anastomoses of arteries supplying the head and neck of the femur. J. Bone Joint Surg., 47B:3, 1965.
33. Schmorl, G.: Die Pathologische Anatomie der Schenkelhalsbrekturen. Munchen Med. Wschr., 71:1381, 1924.
34. Shenton, E. W. A.: *Diseases of Bone.* London, Macmillan, 1911.
35. Trueta, J.: *Studies of the Development and Decay of the Human Frame.* Philadelphia, Saunders, 1968.
36. Tucker, F. R.: Arterial supply of the femoral head and its clinical importance. J. Bone Joint Surg., 31B:82, 1949.
37. Walker, P., et al.: Lubrication mechanism in human joints. Lubrication and Wear In Joints Symposium, Leich. Sector Co., London, 1969.
38. Ward, F. O.: *Human Anatomy.* London, Renshaw, 1838.
39. White, R. K.: The cause of non-union of femoral neck fractures. Conference On Aseptic Necrosis of the Femoral Head, St. Louis, January 1964.

CHAPTER 4

Surgical Approaches to the Hip

RAYMOND G. TRONZO *

Planning a surgical approach to the hip joint demands a thorough knowledge of the involved anatomy, not only in what is considered normal relationships but in possible or probable variants of normal. The outcroppings of bone around the hip which serve as attachments for muscles also provide convenient landmarks for dissection. They are the iliac crest, anterior superior and inferior iliac spines, the wing of the ilium, the symphysis pubis, and most importantly, the greater trochanter *with the foot held in as much neutral rotation as possible.*

Henry's *Extensile Exposure* should be read for its principles of how surgical incisions may be extended by following basic anatomy.[21]

Plans for the operation will have several components: the surgical anatomy, the instruments needed to aid in the procedure, and the specific surgical exposure. One should thoroughly know what can be expected from one surgical approach versus another. Surgical exposures can be baffling if there is pure reliance on eponyms alone: *surgical approaches* may be confused with *surgical procedures.* Modern orthopedic surgery has become even more complex by the number of instruments available for various named procedures. Using the same surgical approach, authors of different procedures may have specific instrumentation which facilitates their given operation. To be unprepared for lack of these instruments, e.g., Müller neck retractors, Smith-Petersen cobra retractors, Hohmann retractors, will cause difficulties. These special instruments can push bone up out of the way or stretch tissue to make a small opening larger during certain steps in any given procedure.

Options for Osteotomizing the Greater Trochanter

Many neophyte hip surgeons look upon the greater trochanter and its abductor muscles with great trepidation. Charnley contributed to this confusion by creating an aura around the abductor complex in developing his total hip arthroplasty. It was essential to his principles of total hip arthroplasty to transfer the abductors distally to improve gait, not to improve his exposure. In recent years, some workers in this field have added more mystique to the issue by insisting that one surgical approach is needed if the greater trochanter is left untouched and yet another if it is osteotomized. Such a rigid attitude is anatomically unfounded.

There is no anatomical basis to such recommendations: The trochanter can be osteotomized at any time during the course of any hip procedure if improved exposure is needed. Exposure to the hip joint can be increased and the surgical procedure can be facilitated by taking off the greater trochanter as a means of reflecting upwards the abductor muscles, but it is done at a price to be paid at the end of the operation and during the patient's rehabilitation. Undoubtedly, the morbidity is increased with the reattachment process and with non-unions, delayed unions, and chronic bursitis around wire knots.

Another option is to widen the exposure by cutting part of the abductor tendon and resuturing

* Parts have been freely borrowed from Chapter 4, by Rush Acton, of the first edition of this text.

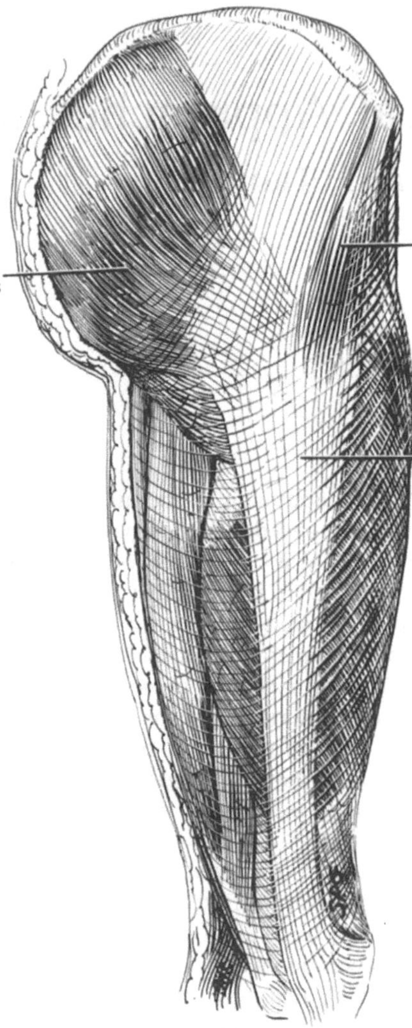

FIG. 4–1 The fascia lata is a very important structure around the hip joint. It is the deep fascia which is a strong envelope surrounding the entire thigh, but also completely encasing the gluteus maximus and the tensor fasciae latae. Both muscles have their attachments, or insertions, onto the central thickened portion of the fascia lata which is called the iliotibial band. Any entrance to the hip joint must deal with the fascia lata and the two superficial muscles.

it during closure of the wound. This author has seen Mittelmeier remove at least a third of it while inserting his Autophor hip prosthesis anterolaterally and resuturing it with double figure-of-eight stitch without any postoperative weakness. Müller does likewise anteriorly. This author cuts it posteriorly when inserting his Bio-Bond prosthesis.

Key Structures of Surgical Importance

Tensor Fascia Lata

The fascia lata (Fig. 4–1) is a very important sheet of fascial tissue which envelops the thigh with distinct boundaries. It extends from the wing of the ilium above to the knee below and the inguinal ligament medially, disappearing posteriorly at the sacroiliac joint and sacrum. It is thickest around the trochanteric area, becoming a distinct band from there to the lateral side of the knee. This part is called the iliotibial band. Figure 4–2 should be studied carefully for it shows the doorway to the hip joint. The anterolateral portion of the iliotibial band engulfs the tensor fascia femoris (tensor fasciae latae) muscle while its posterior segement engulfs the gluteus maximus muscle. An important extension of the tensor fascia lata attaches to the posterior femoral cortex. Here it is a thick, broad band which aids as a powerful tool for extending the hip joint. When contracted, it causes the typical external rotation deformity of the fractured hip. It therefore frequently must be severed to gain better exposure and to correct any contracture deformity. Beware of a large branch of the perforating artery which is immediately beneath the muscle. It is also a powerful deforming force in comminuted intertrochanteric fractures which must be cut in order to achieve proper reduction of the fracture.

Note that the gluteus medius is deep to the tensor fasciae latae. Often the anterior edge of the gluteus medius blends closely with the anterior edge of the overlying muscle. When entering the hip joint in any direction, one must always deal with the tensor fasciae latae. It can be cut in any direction for better exposure since it easily grows back together once sutured.

Gluteus Medius

The insertion of this important muscle is usually described as a single point which fans upward symmetrically (Fig. 4–3A). The actual arrangement is seen in Fig. 4–3B. The insertion on the greater

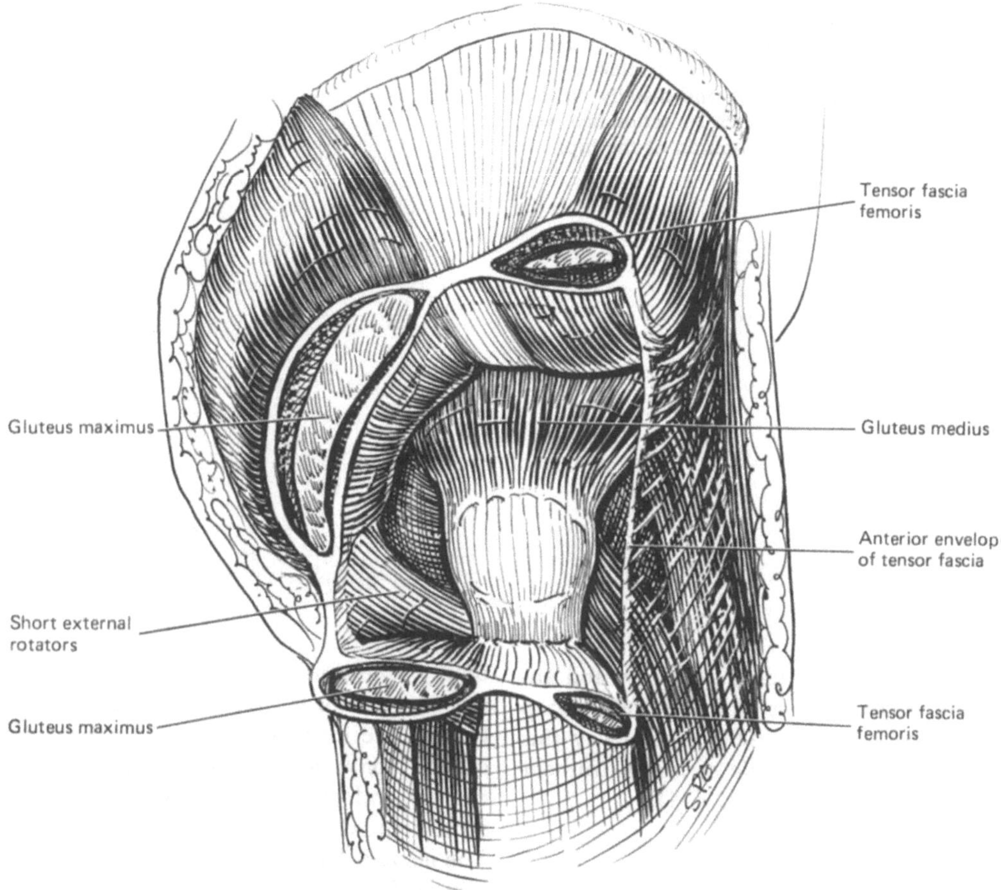

FIG. 4–2 The "doorway" to the hip joint is through the fascial envelope. The tensor fasciae latae and gluteus maximus are the covers to the hip joint; all other muscles are deep to the fascia and have no intimate relationship to it.

trochanter is more of an "L" shape because there are two distinct components to this powerful muscle: the anterior quarter attaches to the anterior segment of the trochanter, making the gluteus medius a flexor as well as an abductor and internal rotator; the back portion is also an abductor but externally rotates and aids in hip extension. The anterior portion lies immediately below the tensor fasciae latae and is often confused with this muscle, especially as the two are so intimate. However, there are distinct differences: The tensor's fibers are parallel and finer than those of the gluteus medius whose fibers are coarser and converge as they are traced down into the anterior edge of the trochanter. They end in bone, blending with the attachments of the vastus lateralis and intermedius, whereas the fibers of the tensor pass directly into the fascia lata and become the thick iliotibial band. These two muscles can be easily separated by blunt dissection once the plane between them is recognized by these anatomical characteristics.

Inferior Capsule

In disease states, especially in advanced osteoarthritis and in failed arthroplasties, the inferomedial portion of the capsule contracts and often becomes thickened like a steel cable. It acts as a tether on the upper end of the femur, keeping the neck pulled inward like an adduction contracture. It will resist dislocation or adequate mobilization even after the head is amputated. The best and safest method of severing it is as follows: First dissect the capsule away from the deeper tissue, especially keeping away from the inferomedial femoral circumflex artery. Then a large sponge

FIG. 4–3 **A** and **B** The gluteus medius is often mistakenly depicted as a fan-shaped muscle centered over the greater trochanter. Rather, it has a distinct anterior portion which attaches well anteriorly and distally on the trochanter in an "L"-shaped manner. Its action involves flexion, abduction, and internal rotation of the hip.

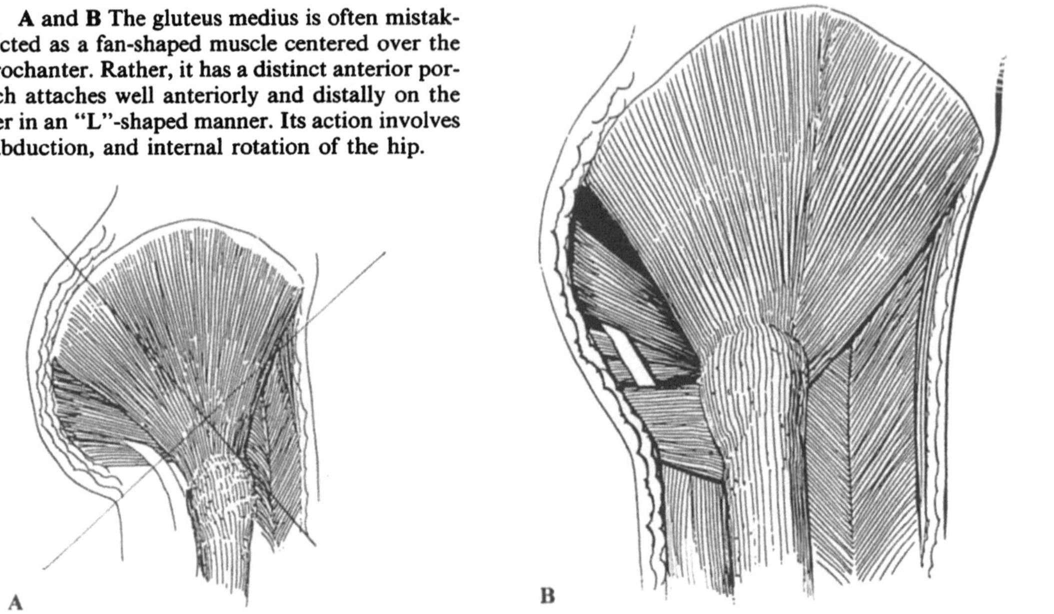

can be packed on either side, posteriorly and anteromedially. Once this is done, a very sharp periosteal elevator can be used to cut away this cablelike thickening of capsule as the instrument is able to cut against bone (Fig. 4–4).

Structures Covering the Inner Acetabulum

It is important to be aware of the structures covering the inner floor of the acetabulum since there is always a threat of violating this area during an arthroplasty. Where is the bladder, the periosteum, the internal iliac artery? The acetabular floor is covered with a thick layer of periosteum. Then one portion of the acetabulum is covered by the obturator internus muscle and the other by the piriformis muscle, both overlapping each other at the central area. Over these structures is the iliopsoas, then the bladder, well away from bone (Fig. 4–5). The internal iliac artery and vein are along the superior rim of inner pelvis as they lay on top of the iliacus, *but* they can be penetrated easily enough by a guide pin when nailing a fractured hip.

Contents of the Greater Sciatic Notch

The greater sciatic notch is becoming an increasingly important landmark, especially for innominate osteotomies and variations of the Chiari osteotomy. The contents are shown in Fig. 4–6. They are engulfed in a thin but strong fascial sheath, but yet are intimately related to the periosteum of the bony notch. The sciatic nerve quickly emerges independently, diverging from the other structures as it passes under the piriformis muscle. The nerve is large and surrounded by a protective tube of fatlike tissue. This whole complex can be eased away from the notch by dissection with a sharp periosteal elevator which peels away the periosteum, thereby protecting these structures as they are packed away with an intervening sponge.

Sites of Major Bleeders

Excessive bleeding can occur at the following sites if not carefully controlled. The major vessel to the hip joint is the *medial femoral cortex artery.* It supplies most of the hip capsule, i.e., the posterior, superior, and especially the inferior portions. The vessel enters the hip posteriorly and medially where it anastomoses with the inferior pudendal and inferior gluteal arteries. This area is thus luxuriously supplied with arterial branches; therefore when cutting away the capsule, significant bleeding will ensue. The main branch when cut will bleed profusely. It sends a large branch along the proximal inner edge of the quadratus femoris muscle (Fig. 4–24A). It is frequently cut along with the muscle for better exposure. Brisk bleeding can be

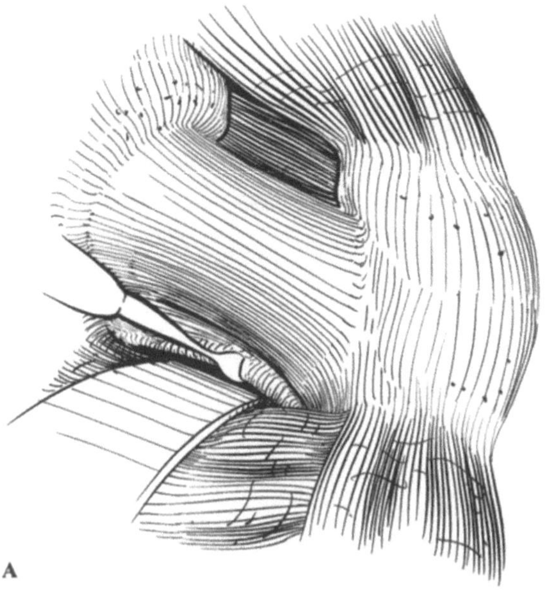

A

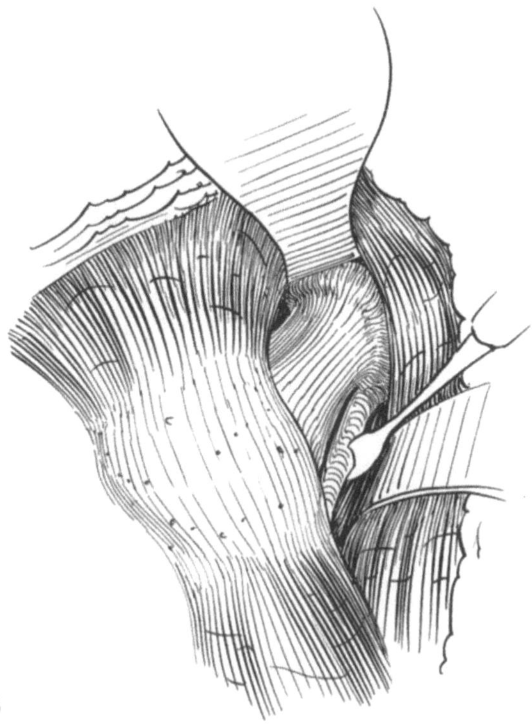

B

FIG. 4–4 The inferior (medial) capsule, when contracted in disease states, becomes a tether causing an adduction contracture. It can feel like a steel cable. Once dissected away from the medial femoral circumflex artery, it can be cut with a strong, sharp periosteal elevator. **A**, posterior view; **B**, anterior view.

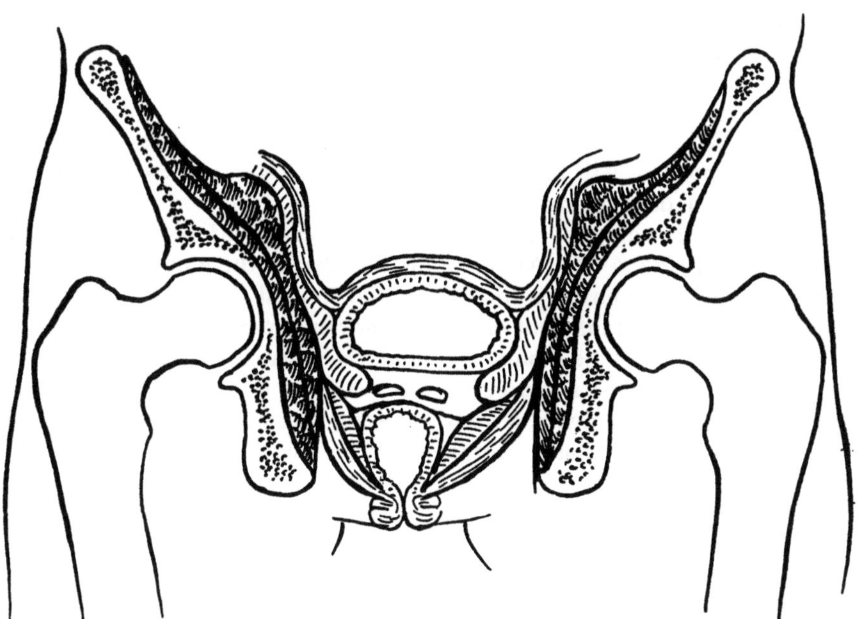

FIG. 4–5 The structures covering the floor of the acetabulum are the thick periosteum, the obturator internus, and the piriformis; the iliopsoas overlies there structures.

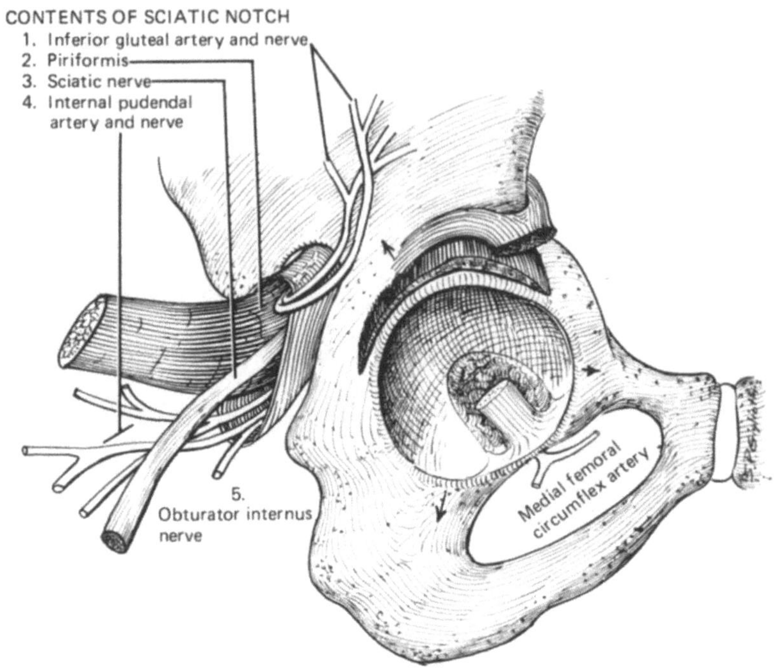

FIG. 4–6 Contents of the greater sciatic notch.

expected, which can be prevented if a heavy suture is first placed deep into the quadratus femoris muscle just distal to the proximal cut into the muscle before it is retracted away. From there, it sends retinacular branches along the posterior superior border of the femoral neck and then forms the important lateral epiphyseal vessels. In rheumatoid and hypertrophic arthritis, the capsule, especially the postero-medial portion, will bleed profusely when cut. Putting a deep figure-of-eight suture into the entire muscle edge will prevent postoperative hemorrhaging (Fig. 4–25). Another area for profuse bleeding to occur postoperatively is deep to the infero-medial area. It may not bleed much during surgery when all of these tissues are stretched, but they can certainly be a source of significant hemorrhaging later. Here again, a deep figure-of-eight suture should be placed as a routine step in one's protocol for hemostasis.

When utilizing one of the posterior approaches where the gluteus maximus is split, the *superior gluteal artery* and any of its branches may be ruptured or cut and cause more blood loss than is realized. A deep suture tie is recommended.

The *lateral femoral circumflex artery* enters the hip at the anterior corner of the greater trochanter where the gluteus medius meets the vastus intermedius. This vessel sends branches into the sulcus of the head–neck junction as well as into the head anastomosis (the vascular supply to the femoral neck is not relevant here), and a few others along the anteroinferior neck which anastomose with the medial femoral circumflex branches. One must be careful to coagulate these branches as they go into the capsule.

The fourth major site is just below the broad flat tendon of the gluteus maximus as it attaches to the femoral shaft. This is a branch of the *profunda femoris artery* which must be ligated or carefully coagulated; otherwise, when cut too close to the bone it will slip away deep to the thigh causing considerable frustration.

If the postoperative bleeding is excessive after the first 48 hours, embolization should be considered. At this writing, the most popular method employs the Granturco coil or Gelfoam. The procedure is called transcatheter arterial embolization and is very successful. The medial femoral circumflex artery is the most frequent cause of the bleeding.

Basic Principles of Surgical Exposure

Being a ball-and-socket joint, an enarthrosis, the hip is capable of movement around an infinite number of axes with a common center. Any combination of movement planes are possible within the limits of the restraining ligaments and muscular attachments. There are 21 muscles which span the hip joint (Fig. 4–7). Their attachments to the upper femur are seen in Fig. 4–8. Thirteen of these are one-joint muscles attaching to the ilium and femur, six attach to the ilium and tibia and/or fibula, one spans the lumbar spine to the femur, and one goes from the sacrum to the femur (Table 4–1). The groupings in Table 4–1 delineate their main motor functions. For example, every muscle in group A, supplied by the femoral nerve, spans the axis of flexion of the hip, making this group a team of flexors. Their relations to the other axes, i.e., abduction, adduction, internal and external rotation, and extension, determine whether another action is associated with this group, keeping in mind that rarely does one muscle have a single isolated action on the hip joint. Thus, any given muscle could be classified in more than one category. An external rotator spans the axis of rotation posteriorly, the internal rotators are situated ante-

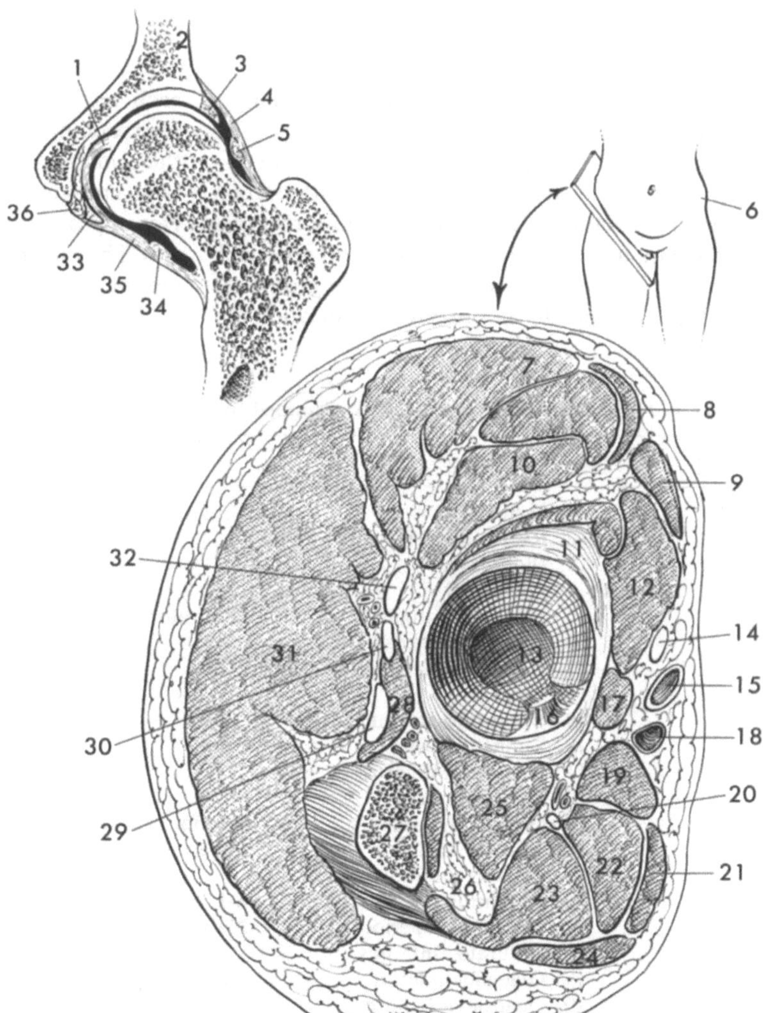

FIG. 4–7 Anatomy of the hip joint. *1,* ligamentum teres; *2,* innominate bone; *3,* acetabular labrum; *4,* articular capsule; *5,* zona orbicularis; *6,* iliac crest; *7,* gluteus medius; *8,* tensor fasciae latae; *9,* sartorius; *10,* gluteus minimus; *11,* rectus femoris, iliofemoral ligament of rectus femoris; *12,* iliacus; *13,* acetabulum; *14,* femoral nerve; *15,* femoral artery; *16,* ligamentum teres; *17,* psoas major; *18,* femoral vein; *19,* pectineus; *20,* obturator nerve; *21,* adductor longus; *22,* adductor brevis; *23,* adductor magnus; *24,* gracilis; *25,* obturator externus; *26,* quadratus femoris; *27,* tuberosity ischium; *28,* inferior gemellus; *29,* sciatic nerve; *30,* obturator internus; *31,* gluteus maximus; *32,* piriformis; *33,* transverse acetabular ligament; *34,* zona orbicularis; *35,* articular capsule; *36,* fat.

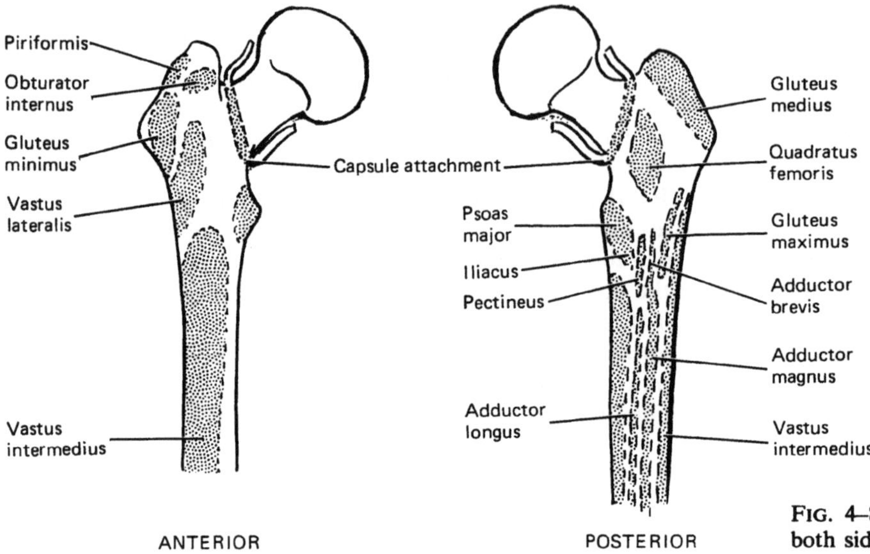

FIG. 4–8 Muscle attachments to both sides of the upper femur.

riorly, and so on (Fig. 4–9). Table 4–2 attempts to classify hip muscles by nerve distribution. The four main nerves to the hip musculature have distinct functional capabilities as listed, with certain exceptions. Figure 4–10 shows the major nerves to the hip musculature. Any surgical approach to the hip must take advantage of these groupings which in turn create an orderly classification for each territory being explored. Thus the *anterior* approach passes between muscle groups I and II, the *anterolateral* approach between tensor fasciae latae and gluteus medius (group I), and the *posterior* approach involves the last four nerve territories. The *medial* approach passes between the muscles of group III.

The *anterolateral* approach passes between the

TABLE 4–1 Muscles Spanning the Hip, Grouped by Function

Group	Muscle	Nerve	Principal Group Action
A	1. Sartorius	Femoral	Flexion
	2. Rectus femoris		
	3. Iliopsoas*		
	4. Pectineus†		
B	5. Adductor longus	Obturator	Adduction
	6. Adductor brevis		
	7. Adductor magnus		
	8. Gracilis		
	9. Obturator externus		
C	10. Semitendinosus	Sciatic	Extension
	11. Semimembranosus		
	12. Biceps femoris		
	13. Gluteus maximus	Inferior gluteal	
D	14. Gluteus medius	Superior gluteal	Abduction
	15. Gluteus minimus		
E	16. Piriformis	S-1, S-2	External rotation
	17. Gemellus superior	Nerve to obturator internus	
	18. Obturator internus		
	19. Gemellus inferior	Nerve to quadratus femoris	
	20. Quadratus femoris		

* The psoas major is innervated by L-2 and L-3 fibers.

† The pectineus is sometimes supplied by accessory obturator or obturator.

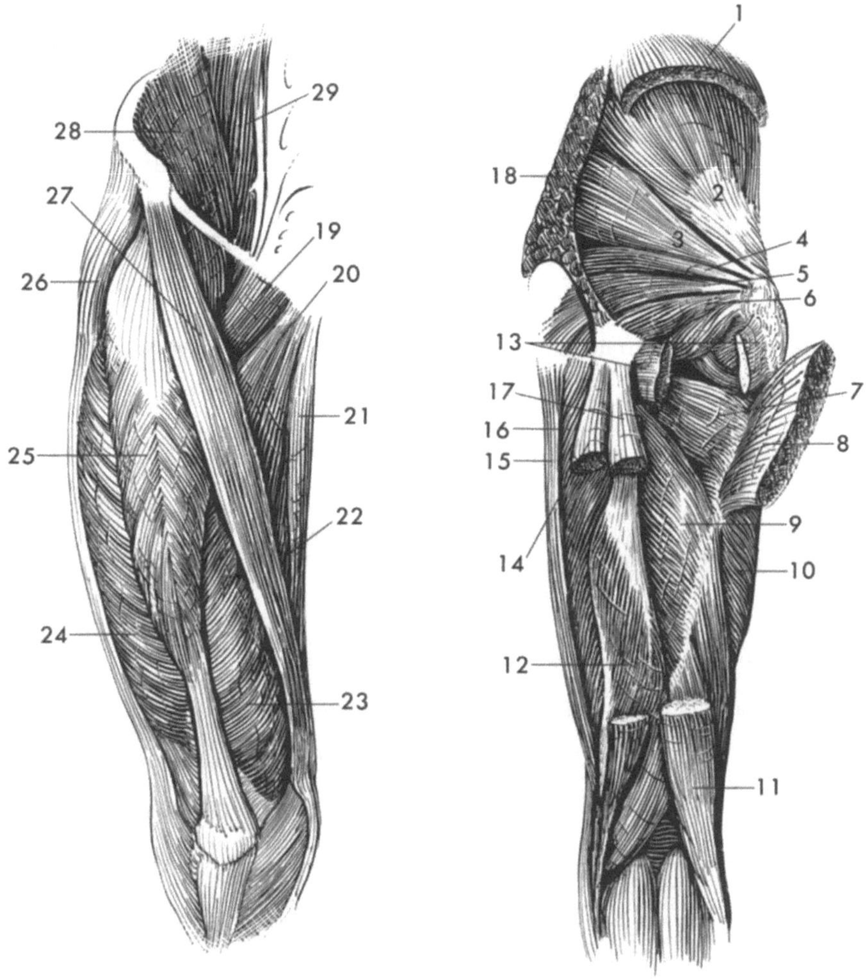

FIG. 4–9 Muscles of the hip joint. *1*, gluteus medius; *2*, gluteus minimus; *3*, piriformis; *4*, superior gemellus; *5*, obturator internus; *6*, inferior gemellus; *7*, adductor minimus; *8*, gluteus maximus; *9*, adductor magnus; *10*, vastus lateralis; *11*, biceps femoris; *12*, semimembranosus; *13*, quadratus femoris; *14*, semitendinosus; *15*, gracilis; *16*, adductor magnus; *17*, biceps femoris; *18*, gluteus maximus; *19*, pectineus; *20*, adductor longus; *21*, gracilis; *22*, adductor magnus; *23*, vastus medialis; *24*, vastus lateralis; *25*, rectus femoris; *26*, tensor fasciae latae; *27*, sartorius; *28*, iliopsoas; *29*, psoas major.

gluteus medius and tensor fasciae latae. Any dissection between these muscles is in a cephalad direction and must stop short of the inferior branch of the superior gluteal nerve as it passes from gluteus medius to tensor fasciae latae. The posterior approach generally involves splitting or retracting the gluteus maximus at an area well away from the inferior gluteal nerve.

Tables 4–3 to 4–6 provide technical considerations of the various surgical approaches to the hip. Appropriate references are provided.

The fascia lata is an important structure which must be fully appreciated before one can be knowledgeable about surgical anatomy of the hip joint (Fig. 4–1). Any extension of an incision must take into account the restraining dimensions of the fascia lata. To gain access to the deeper muscles and hip joint, this structure must be entered either anterior to the tensor fasciae latae or posterior to the muscle, or between it and the gluteus medius. The tensor fascia latae can be transected as it blends into the iliotibial tract as in the Calahan type of incision or it can be split in the middle of the iliotibial tract and divided transversely at

TABLE 4–2 Muscles Spanning the Hip by Nerve Distribution

Group	Nerve	Divisions of Lumbosacral Plexus	Muscles	Principal Action	Other Actions
I.	Superior gluteal	Dorsal L-4, 5 S-1	Gluteus medius Gluteus minimus Tensor fasciae latae	Abduction	Flexion, rotation (internal and external)
II.	Femoral	Dorsal L-2 L-3 L-4	Iliopsoas Pectineus Sartorius Rectus femoris	Flexion	Adduction, rotation (internal and external)
III.	Obturator	Ventral L-2 L-3 L-4	Adductor longus Adductor brevis Adductor magnus Gracilis Obturator externus	Adduction	Extension, flexion, rotation (internal and external)
IV.	Sciatic	Ventral L-4 L-5 S-1 S-2 S-3 Dorsal, same except S-3	Biceps femoris Semitendinosus Semimembranosus Adductor magnus	Extension	Adduction, rotation (internal)
V.	N. to obturator internus	L-5, S-1, S-2	Obturator internus Superior gemellus	External rotation	
VI.	N. to quadratus femoris	L-4, L-5, S-1	Quadratus femoris Inferior gemellus	External rotation	
VII.	Inferior gluteal	L-5, S-1, S-2	Gluteus maximus	Extension	External rotation
VIII.	N. to piriformis	S-1, S-2	Piriformis	Extension	

either end, as in Tronzo's lateral approach, all done to expand the opening either superiorly or inferiorly. Figure 4–2 shows transection at the greater trochanter to depict anatomic boundaries as the fascia engulfs the two muscles and overlays the trochanteric bursa.

Anterior Incisions

Anterior approaches are based on entering the hip by cutting through the fascia lata at the anterior border of the tensor fasciae latae. A plane is developed between the under surface of this muscle (with the gluteus medius deep to it) and the sartorius. The anatomy of the anterior thigh over the hip area is reviewed in Fig. 4–11.

All six incisions listed as anterior approaches (Table 4–3) pass between the muscles of group I and group II. The exception to this is the "simplified surgical approach to the hip" described by Sutherland and Rowe in 1944.[42] They felt that the Smith-Petersen incision had postoperative disadvantages such as scar adhering to the iliac crest, weakness of gluteal abductor muscles, hemorrhage, and delayed mobility. They tried to avoid these by removal of the sartorius attachment with its anterior superior spine, detaching the anterior inferior spine with the straight head of the rectus femoris, and retracting of the gluteus medius and minimus with osteotomy of the greater trochanter. In closing, the bony processes were then reattached by metal fixation, often transplanting the trochanter distally on the shaft of the femur to increase leverage of the abductors. In one sense, the anterior approach is the most physiological since, properly done, it is impossible to divide muscle groups without dividing their motor supply. The muscles to be reflected laterally are innervated by the superior gluteal nerve and those to be reflected medially by the femoral nerve.

A comprehensive and extensive anterior expo-

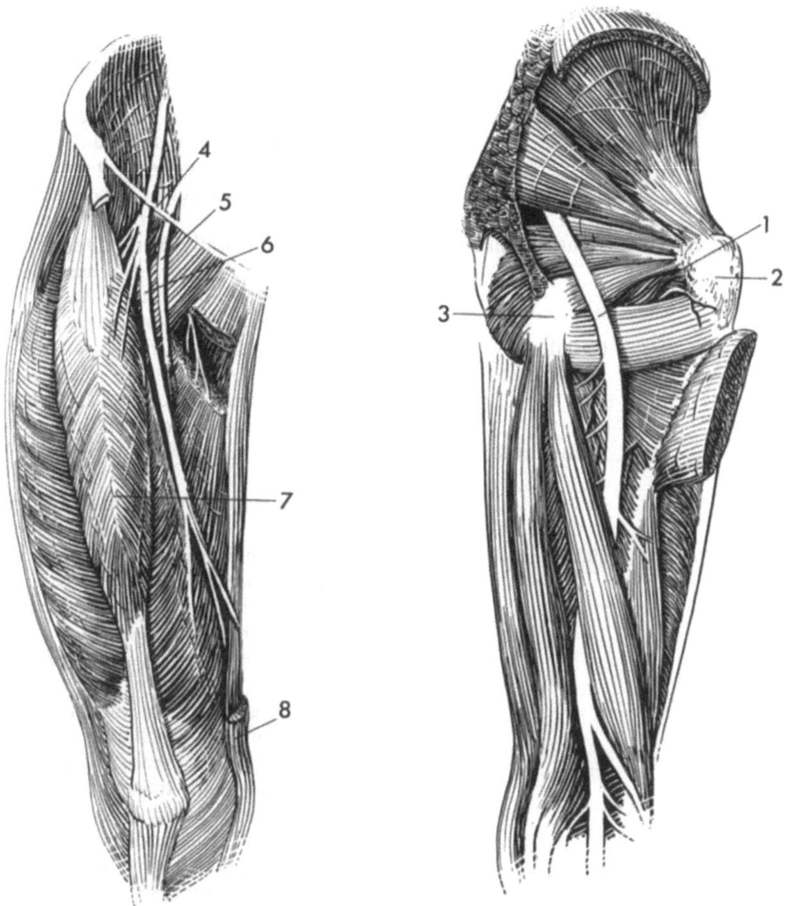

FIG. 4–10 Innervation of the hip joint. *1,* sciatic nerve; *2,* greater trochanter; *3,* ischial tuberosity; *4,* inguinal ligament; *5,* femoral artery; *6,* femoral nerve; *7,* rectus femoris; *8,* sartorius.

sure is the Smith-Petersen iliofemoral approach.[37] The original parameters are shown in Fig. 4–12. It is an extensive exposure as the wing of the ilium is scraped free of the gluteal muscle attachments and the tensor fasciae latae. The less radical version is depicted in Fig. 4–12A–C whereas the original version is shown in Fig. 4–12D–G.

The skin incision as described by Smith-Petersen passes over the anterior third or more of the iliac crest, curves distally along the anterior border of the tensor fasciae latae, then curves posteriorly across the insertion of the tensor into the iliotibial band about 3 or 4 inches below the base of the greater trochanter of the femur. The muscles innervated by the superior gluteal nerve. i.e., the tensor fasciae latae, gluteus medius, and gluteus minimus, are dissected subperiosteally in a single flap from the iliac crest as far posteriorly as necessary. The periosteal elevator follows the surface by the ilium and bleeding is controlled by packing. The dissection continues in a plane between the tensor laterally and the sartorius and rectus femoris medially. The ascending branch of the lateral femoral circumflex artery is ligated and the lateral femoral cutaneous nerve is retracted medially before capsulotomy of the hip is performed, or the nerve may be cut if it gets in the way rather than retracting it so severely as to cause incisional pain. The anterior spine may be osteotomized if necessary.

Smith-Petersen reported on this technique in 1917 [37] and again in 1931.[39] In 1931, Cave and Vangorder [39] reported a modification in which the fascial incision along the anterior border of the

TABLE 4–3 Anterior Approaches to the Hip

No.	Date	References	Eponym	Technique
1.	1917	4, 37, 38, 39	Smith-Petersen	1. Anterior half crest ilium to spine and distally 5″ 2. Strip medius, minimus, and tensor from ilium 3. Separate and pass between tensor and sartorius-rectus 4. Osteotomize anterior superior spine 5. Ligate ascending branch of lateral femoral circumflex
2.		4, 6, 40	Heuter Schede	1. Incise 7″ distally from anterior superior spine 2. Pass between tensor and sartorius-rectus 3. Ligate ascending branch lateral femoral circumflex 4. Cut reflected head of rectus
3.	1939	13	Callahan	1. Incise 8″ distally from spine with posterior hockey stick 2. Pass between tensor and sartorius-rectus 3. Ligate lateral femoral circumflex
4.	1944	42	Sutherland-Rowe	1. Incise from anterior spine to trochanter and distally along the femur 2. Cut spines and trochanter and reattach with metal fixation
5.	1949	15	Fahey	1. Straight incision spine to below trochanter 2. Between tensor and sartorius 3. Cut iliotibial band distal to tensor 4. Cut straight head rectus 5. Ligate ascending and lateral branch of lateral femoral circumflex 6. Retract psoas tendon medially 7. May transplant trochanter
6.	1955	25, 42	Luck	1. Incise in flexor crease from over head of femur to lateral to greater trochanter 2. Cut tensor in distal third 3. Retract sartorius and rectus medially 4. May transplant greater trochanter

tensor fasciae latae is curved posteriorly across the insertion of the tensor into the iliotibial tract 3 or 4 inches below the trochanteric region. This exposes the lateral portion of the rectus femoris and the vastus lateralis. In 1936, Smith-Petersen [38] further suggested reflecting not only the direct but the reflected head of the rectus femoris in the final capsular dissection. In addition, the abdominal oblique muscle, the sartorius, and the iliacus are dissected from the crest and inner surface of the ilium, respectively, exposing the inner surface of the ilium, the deep surface of the ilium, or iliac fossa as far down as the upper margin of the anterior acetabular wall.

Indications The Smith-Petersen approach is useful in arthroplasties of the hip joint, specifically a cup arthroplasty, arthrodesis of the hip joint, or osteotomies of the pelvis (e.g., Salter osteotomy, Pemberton osteotomy [12]) when combined with inner pelvic dissection. It can also be used for open reduction of congenital dysplasia of the hip when combined with or without a shelf procedure.

Callahan Modification In 1939 Callahan [13] reported an approach that he had developed in the anatomical laboratory which compares with the anterior femoral approach as modified by Smith-Petersen, Cave, and Vangorder. Callahan's skin incision is essentially the upper portion of the Smith-Petersen incision from the anterior spine distally, except that Callahan's drawing shows a sharper curve posteriorly over the iliotibial tract to make a "hockey-stick" incision (Fig. 4–13). The gluteus medius and minimus are mobilized by subperiosteal dissection and a transverse incision across the tensor fasciae latae. The entire flap is reflected laterally and direct access to the hip joint is thereby attained. This approach is good for open

TABLE 4–4 Lateral Approaches to the Hip

No.	Date	References	Eponym	Technique
7.	1881	4 36	Ollier Senegas	1. U incision from anterior spine to trochanter to midway between trochanter and posterior spine 2. Between gluteus medius and tensor to capsule
8.	1903	4	Murphy goblet	1. As above 2. Add 10 cm extension distally
9.	1912	6	Brackett	1. Anterior spine to trochanter and distally 2″ 2. Between tensor and gluteus medius 3. Cut femoral attachment of fascia lata and free vastus externus 4. Cut maximus fascia and osteotomize trochanter
10.	1935	10	Colonna	1. Backward C from 1″ below spine to 5″ below trochanter 2. Cut fascia and cut all muscles attached to trochanter 3. Remove head of femur, place stump in acetabulum, and reattach abductors distally
11.	1936	46	Watson-Jones	1. Incise from 1″ inferolateral to spine, curve posteriorly and distally to 2″ inferior to base of trochanter 2. Between gluteus medius and tensor to capsule
12.	1954	7	Burwell-Scott	1. Incise from 3″ anterior to posterior spine to upper 6″ of femur along anterior border 2. Cut gluteal aponeurosis and iliotibial tract under skin 3. Between glutei and tensor to 1″ below crest 4. Capsulotomy and dislocate head of femur
13.	1955	23	Jergensen-Abbott	1. Anterior spine to trochanter and distally between biceps and vastus lateralis to 5 cm below gluteal fold 2. Cut iliotibial band over trochanter 3. Between tensor and gluteus medius 4. Cut aponeurosis of maximus and reflected tendon of rectus 5. Between rectus and iliacus 6. Cut trochanter and short external rotators and retract 7. May cut lesser trochanter
14.	1969	44, 45	Tronzo	See text

reduction of femoral neck fractures and open biopsies of the femoral head and/or neck because it can be extended easily.

Fahey Approach In 1949, Fahey [15] discribed an approach to the hip which involves the same intermuscular planes of dissection but with a different skin incision. A straight-line incision extends obliquely inferoposteriorly from the anterior superior iliac spine to a point posterior and distal to the greater trochanter of the femur. One then develops a plane of dissection between the tensor fasciae latae and sartorius; the insertion of the tensor fasciae latae as it blends into the iliotibial band and the straight head of the rectus femoris just distal to the anterior inferior iliac spine are divided. The ascending and lateral branches of the lateral circumflex artery are ligated. The psoas major is separated from the capsule and retracted medially, and the capsule is opened. The vastus lateralis may then be retracted anteriorly from the lateral intermuscular septum with the trochanter osteotomized and transplanted if desired.

Luck Approach In 1954, Luck [25] reported a transverse anterior approach to the hip which utilizes a long transverse incision from just superficial to the femoral head along the flexor crease of the hip to the greater trochanter. Its lateral end can be extended proximally or distally as needed for certain modifications of the incision. The same intermuscular planes are developed as in the anterior iliofemoral incision; however, the tensor fasciae latae is divided transversely across the distal third of its belly rather than at its insertion into the iliotibial band. The sartorius, rectus femoris, and iliopsoas are retracted medially and the origin of the rectus from the anterior inferior spine may be divided. The glutei medius and minimus may be divided from the greater trochanter or the trochanter may be osteotomized with its tendinous insertions.

TABLE 4–5 Posterior Approaches to the Hip

No.	Date	References	Eponym	Technique
15.	1874 1887 1949	4	Langenbeck Kocher Gibson	1. 1.5″ inferior to trochanter, 4″ obliquely, between piriformis and gluteus medius 2. Anterior border maximus and 6″ distal from trochanter; divide maximus aponeurosis and retract maximus; cut and retract abductors forward and external rotators posteriorly
16.	1920	20, 41	Stookey	1. ? incision posterior spine, upper border maximus, curves medial to trochanter, and under gluteal fold to midpoint and distally 2. Split maximus to bony insertion, cut 2 cm from bone and reflect
17.	1924	34	Ober	1. Incise from posterolateral femur to sacrococcygeal 2. Separate maximus fibers, pass between rotators or incise them
18.	1930	35	Osborne	1. Incise 1.75″ inferior to posterior spine to trochanter and distally 2″ 2. Retract maximus fibers; cut piriformis, gemelli, and obturator internus
19.	1943	8	Caldwell	1. Grater trochanter distally for 8–10″ 2. Cut fascial insertion of maximus; separate biceps and vastus lateralis
20.	1945	21	Henry	1. ? incision posterior superior spine 2.5″ along crest obliquely to trochanter, to gluteal fold, medially and distally along mid-posterior thigh 2. Cut iliotibial tract along femur and along superior border of maximus and attachments of maximus to femur, and retract
21	1952	22	Horwitz	1. Incise from trochanter 3″ toward posterior spine and from trochanter distally for 6″ 2. Incise fascia lata and split downward (from trochanter); split maximus fibers upward 3. Elevate vastus lateralis and retract trochanteric crest fragment or detach quadratus femoris and obturator externus
22.	1954	27	Marcy-Fletcher	1. From trochanter 6″ distally and from trochanter 6″ obliquely to a point 2″ anterior to posterior spine 2. Cut superior border of maximus (fascia lata) 3. Cut aponeurotic insertion of maximus and all external rotators
23.	1954	29	McFarland-Osborne	1. Incise from trochanter distally and from trochanter proximally between tensor and maximus 2. Cut fascia lata; retract maximus and tensor in opposite directions 3. Gluteus medius and vastus lateralis elevated and retracted forward as one 4. Cut minimus and retract; do capsulotomy
24.	1956	43	Zahradnicek	1. T incision inferior to anterior spine, curve cover trochanter and up to ischial tuberosity; vertical limb over femur 2. Cut fascia lata and osteotomize trochanter with maximus, medius, and minimus
25.	1957	30, 31	Moore	1. Incise from 2″ below inferior spine along maximus fibers to greater trochanter and then 4–5″ below on posterolateral thigh 2. Spread maximus fibers and divide maximus insertion on femur and short external rotators

TABLE 4–6 Medial Approaches to the Hip

No.	Date	References	Eponym	Technique
26.	1913	4, 26	Ludloff	1. Incise 15 cm parallel to femur from Poupart's down (with hip abducted 90°) on lateral border of adductor longus 2. Bluntly spread adductors to capsule
27.	1946	14	Etienne, Lapeyrie, and Campo	1. Incise 7–10 cm on medial thigh two fingers breadth distally from a line drawn between the pubic spine and ischial spine (hip flexed, abducted, and externally rotated) 2. Pass between rectus femoris and adductor magnus and then between adductor magnus and brevis

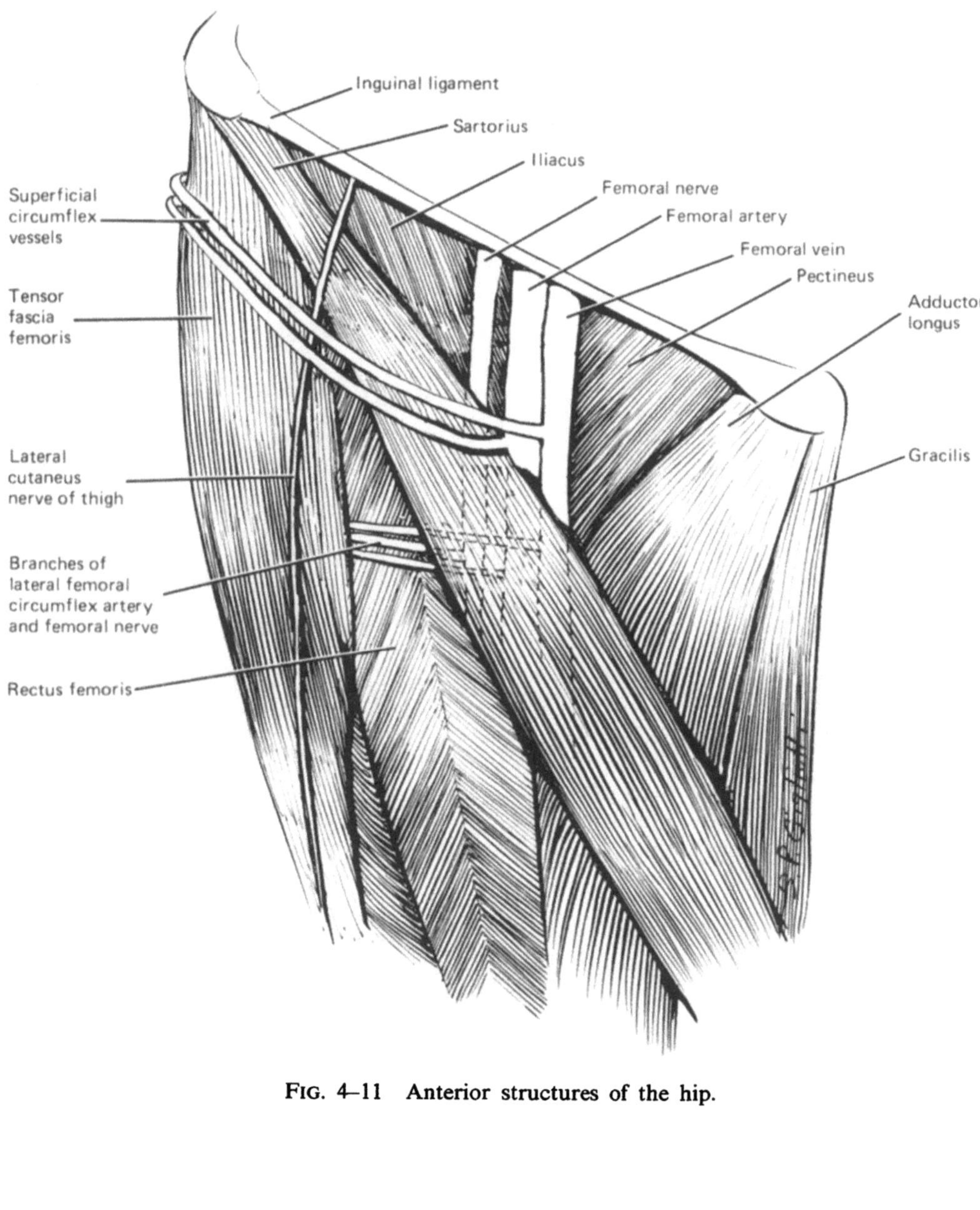

FIG. 4–11 Anterior structures of the hip.

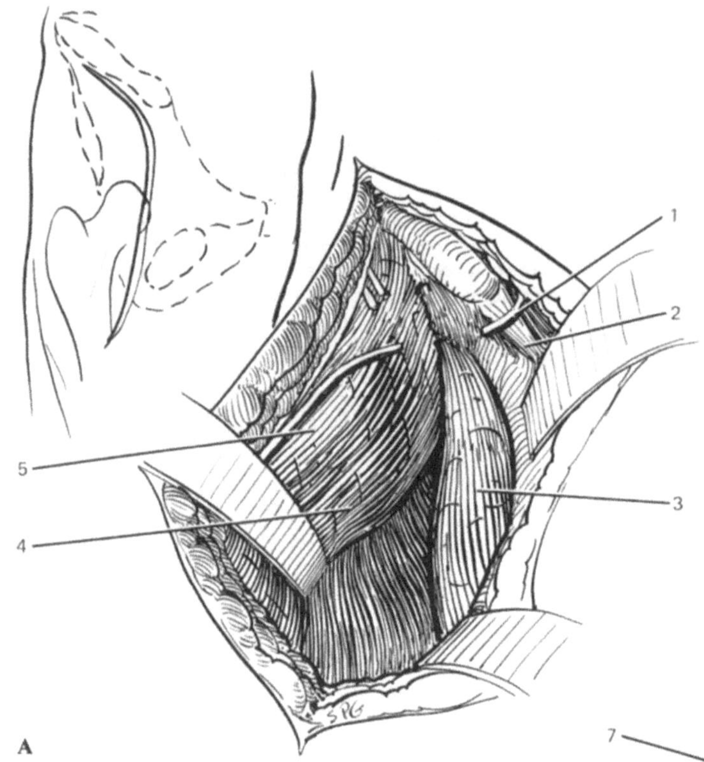

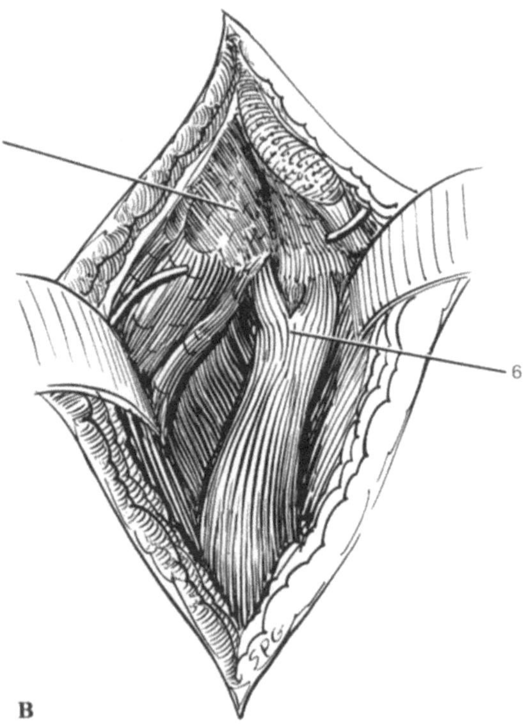

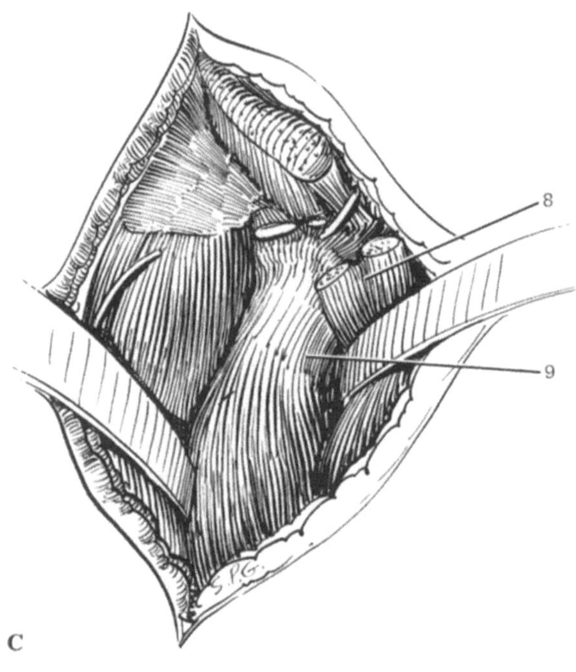

FIG. 4–12 **A** Anterior iliofemoral exposure of Smith-Petersen. 1, lateral cutaneous nerve of the thigh; 2, sartorius; 3, rectus femoris; 4, gluteus medius and minimus; 5, tensor fascia femoris; 6, short and reflected heads of rectus femoris overlying capsule; 7, tensor and gluteal muscles peeled from ilium; 8, tendons of rectus reflected; 9, joint capsule.

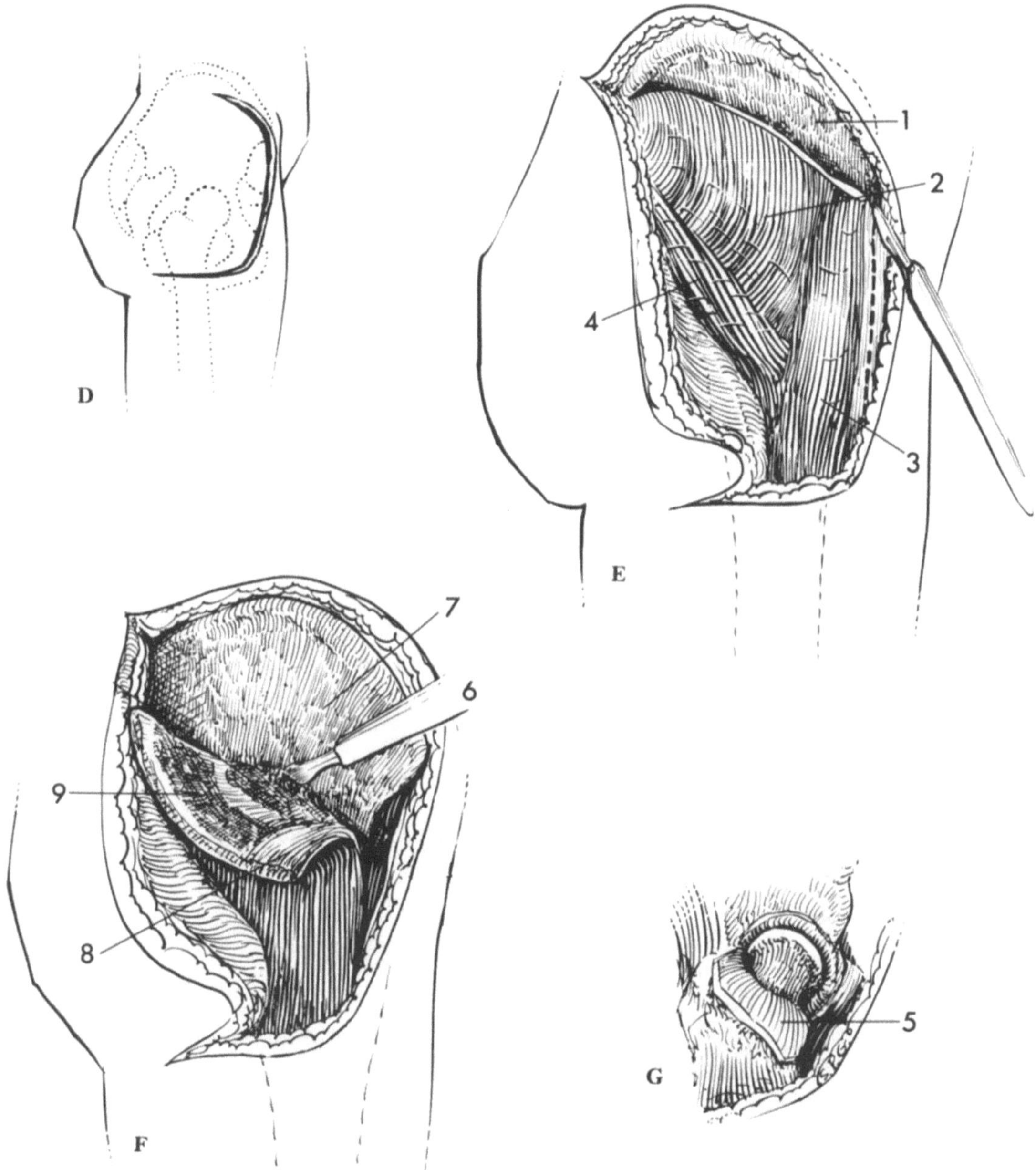

FIG. 4–12 **D-G** Lateral aspect of Smith-Petersen approach. *1,* scrape clear; *2,* gluteus medius; *3,* Tensor fasciae latae; *4,* gluteus maximus; *5,* capsule; *6,* periosteal elevator; *7,* lateral wall of ileum; *8,* tensor fasciae latae; *9,* gluteus minimus and medius.

Anteropelvic Approach

This approach was developed by Judet and Letournel [23a] (Fig. 4–14). The sartorius is detached from its insertion and the rectus femoris identified along its medial border and retracted laterally. Both the major and minor portions of the iliopsoas are identified as they traverse the corner of the hip and arise from the inner wall of the ilium. By sharp subperiosteal dissection, starting with the inner anterior iliac crest, this large muscle mass is dissected away from the inner wall and the pelvic

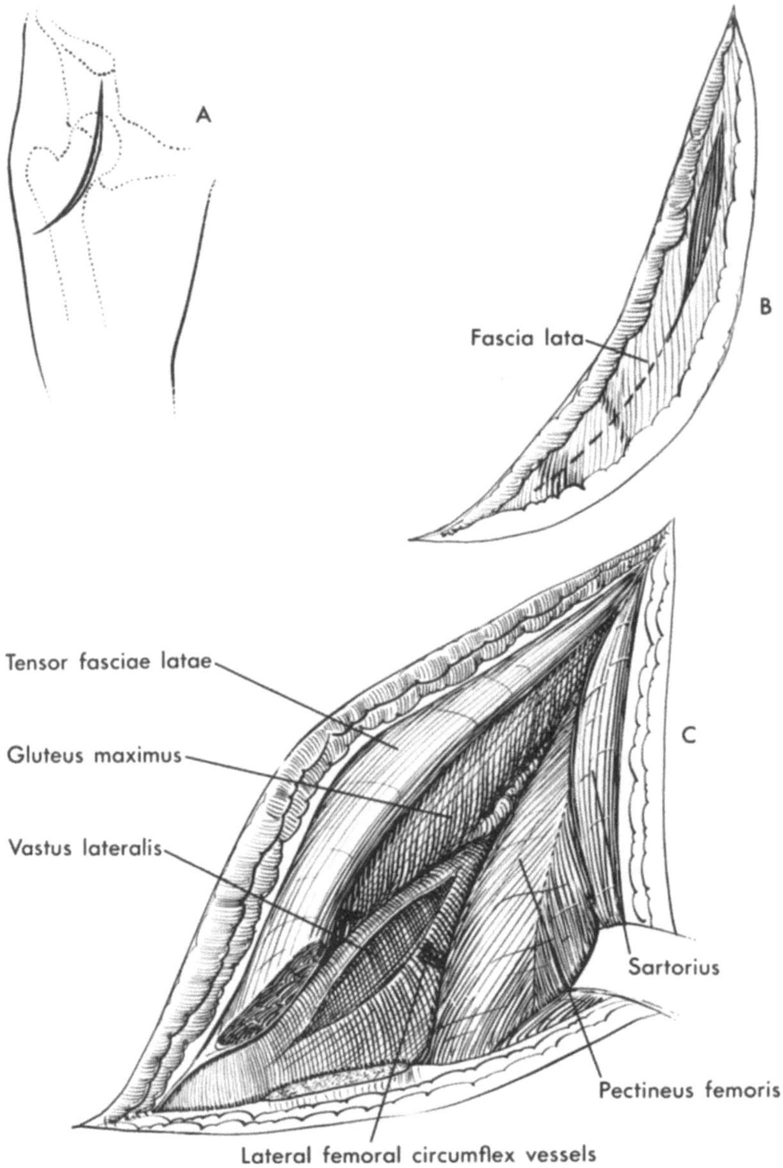

FIG. 4–13 Callahan anterior exposure.

portion of the acetabulum down to the iliac notch. The obliquus abdominis is left attached to the iliacus and the entire muscle mass is retracted medially with a large blunt Dever retractor.

Indications This approach is used primarily for reducing acetabular fractures of the inner wall. It can be used for hip flexor release in paralytic lesions of the hip joint.

Anterolateral Approaches

The anterolateral anatomy of the fascia lata must be reviewed (Figs. 4–1 and 4–2). The gluteus medius is closely adhered to the under surface of the tensor fasciae latae; the two can be mistaken for one muscle *if* they are approached at the very front edge of the tensor muscle. But by going just posterior to the tensor fasciae latae, a plane can be developed which keeps the tensor muscle anteri-

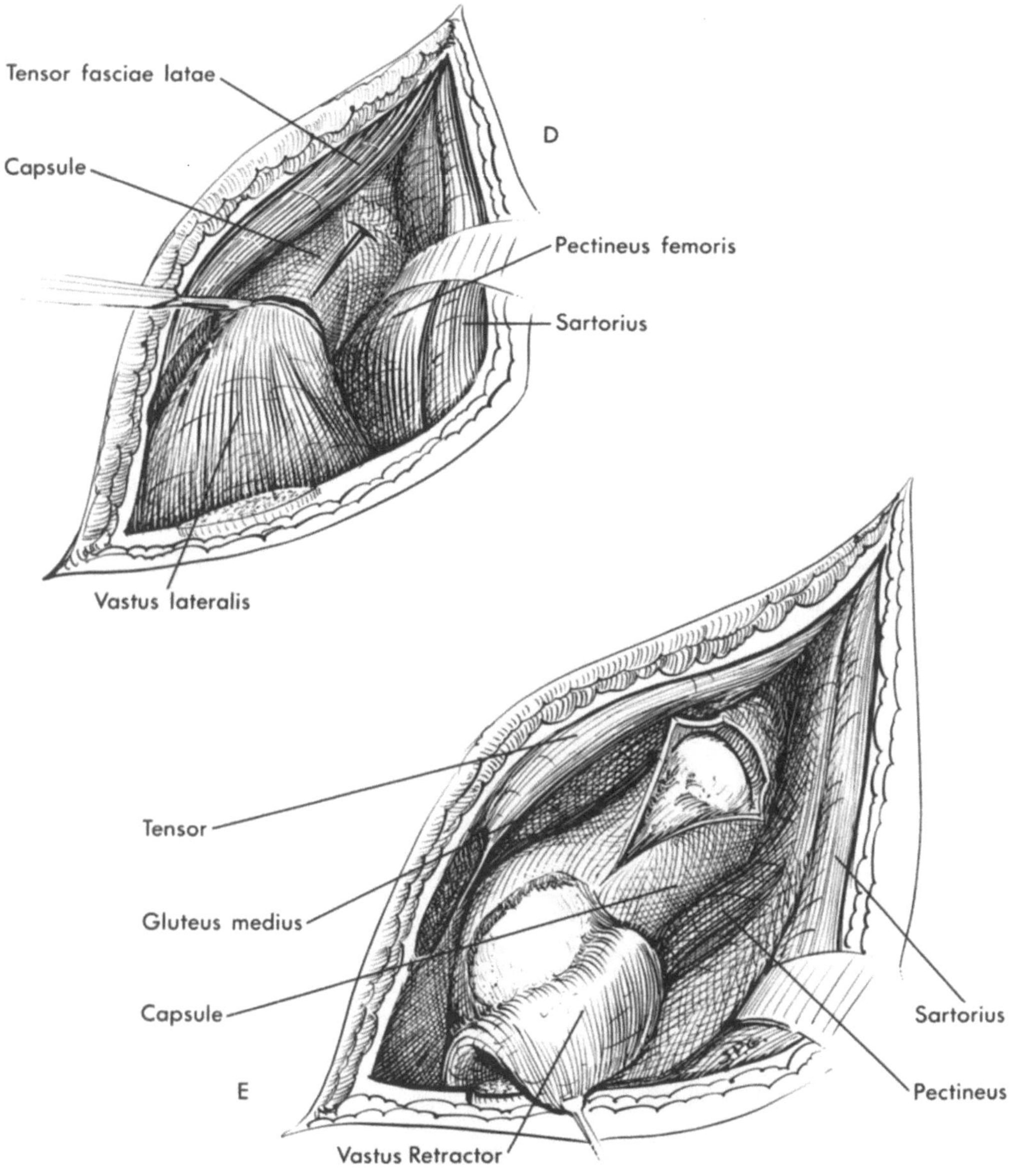

FIG. 4–13 (*Cont.*)

orly with the fascia lata, maintaining the gluteus medius posteriorly. This then is the basic plane of entry for anterolateral approaches.

Watson-Jones is credited with developing the anterolateral approach.[16] It has become a popular incision for total cup arthroplasties as modified as a *procedure* by Charnley and Müller. Figure 4–15 depicts the basic Watson-Jones approach.

The patient is placed supine with possibly a small sandbag under the hip for better draping. There are three landmarks to be connected which will help to outline the skin incision: The first point is approximately 1 inch below and 1 inch posterior to the anterior superior iliac crest. The second point is just posterior to the greater trochanter assuming that the foot lies straight up on the table. The third point is 3 inches distal to the greater trochanter parallel with the femoral shaft. Connecting these three points results in a long, lazy curve. Next, the plane between the glu-

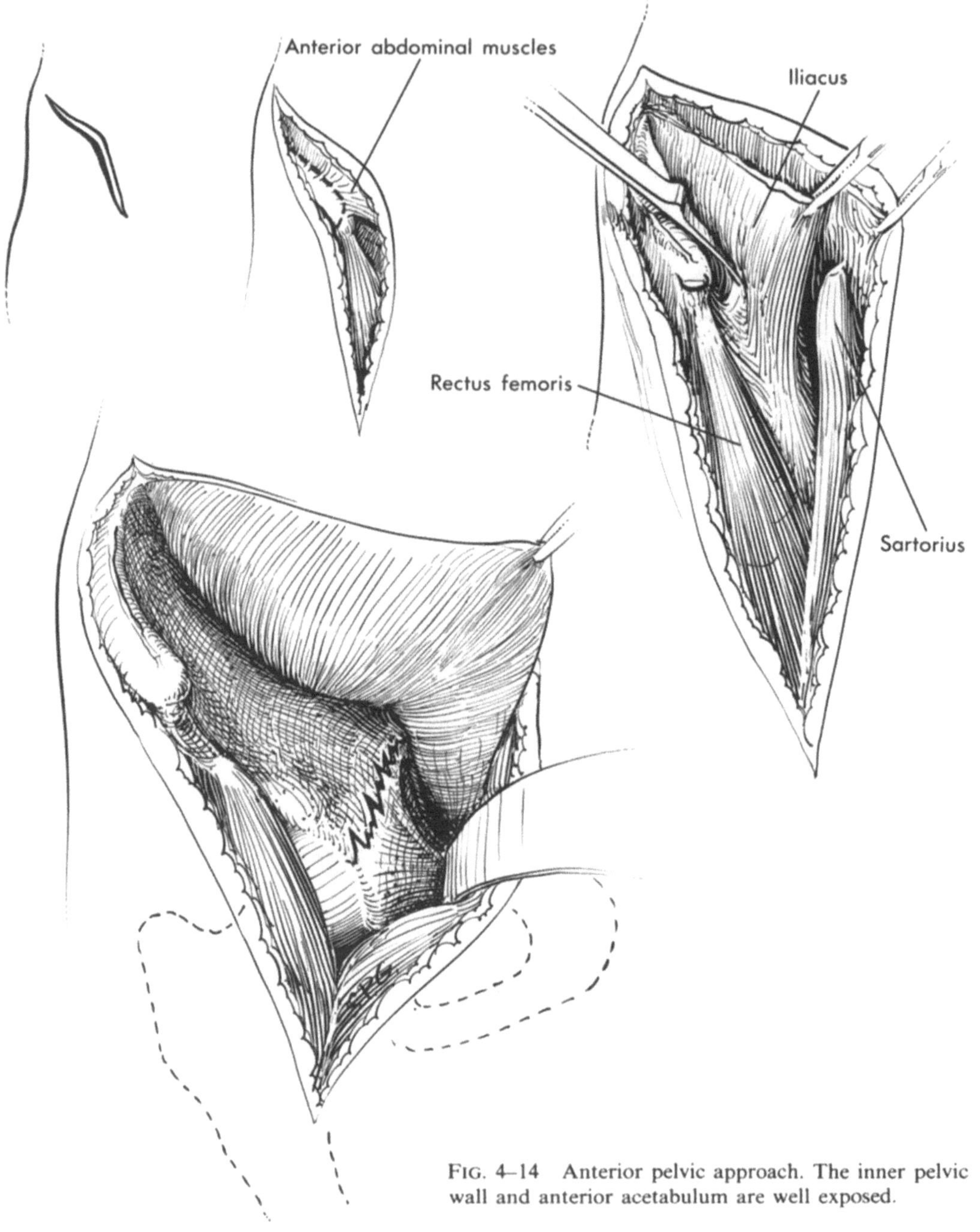

FIG. 4–14 Anterior pelvic approach. The inner pelvic wall and anterior acetabulum are well exposed.

teus medius and the tensor fasciae latae is identified.

Initially, the iliotibial band is split just *below* the greater trochanter; then, using a pair of Mayo scissors, the incision is curved upward to the point at which the inferior border of the tensor fasciae latae can be visualized. With blunt dissection using the surgeon's finger, the plane between the tensor fasciae latae and the gluteus medius is opened. From this point, using a periosteal elevator, the anterior aspect of the neck of the femur and the anterior portion of the trochanter can be identified. The thick tendon of the rectus femoris overlying the capsule may be peeled away as needed while the thick anterior capsule is incised or excised.

If the plane between the two muscles is not

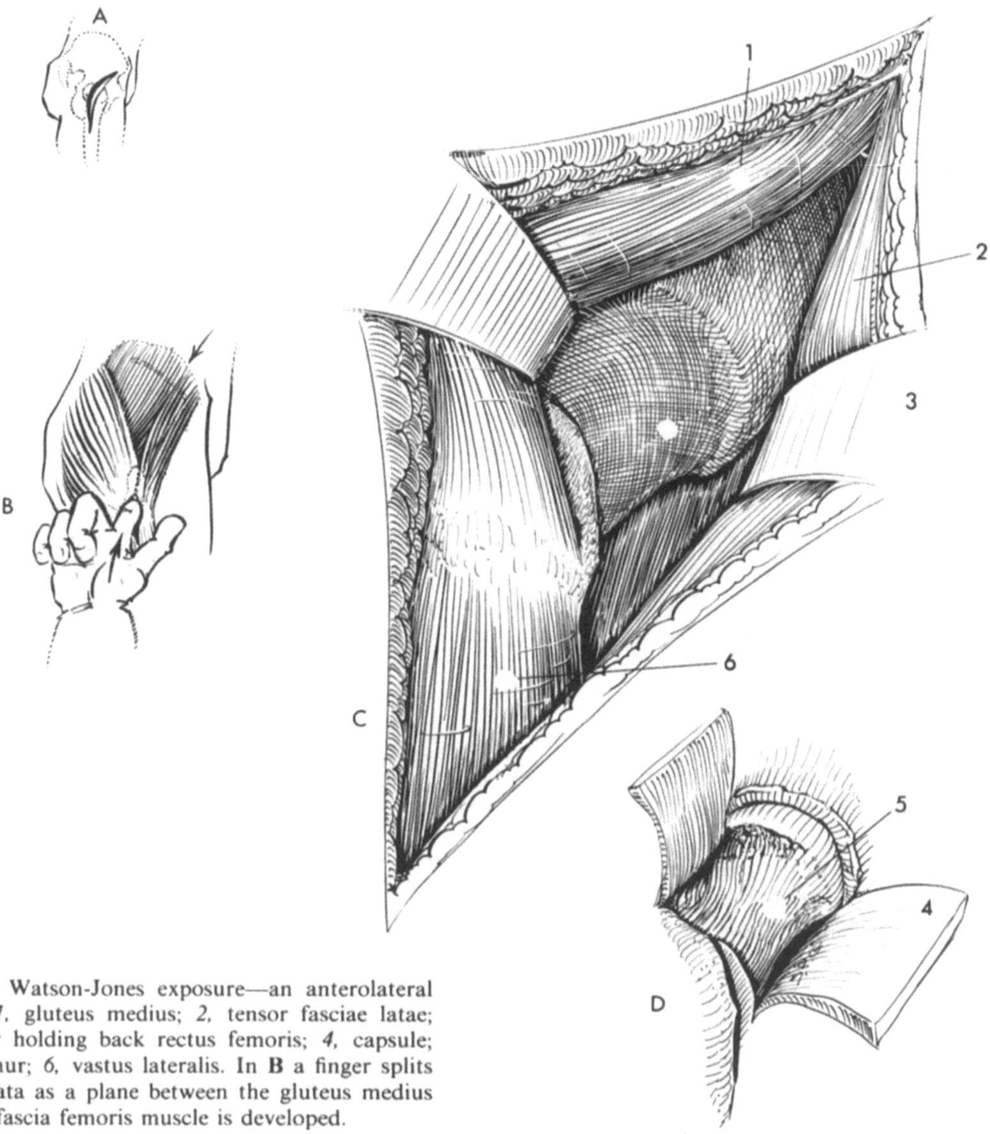

FIG. 4–15 Watson-Jones exposure—an anterolateral approach. *1*, gluteus medius; *2*, tensor fasciae latae; *3*, retractor holding back rectus femoris; *4*, capsule; *5*, neck femur; *6*, vastus lateralis. In **B** a finger splits the fascia lata as a plane between the gluteus medius and tensor fascia femoris muscle is developed.

found properly, the upper or superior portion of the incision may be tight; as a result, the incision may have to be extended to the anterior area of the acetabulum in order to facilitate retraction of these muscles. Flexing the hip with a sandbag will help relax these muscles. Extending the skin incision more distally enables one to split the tensor fasciae latae further which will also aid in relaxing tension on the retractor.

The biggest error in this incision lies in not properly identifying the posterior boundary of the greater trochanter. The incision must run just inferior to its posterior border and then headward parallel to the femoral shaft. If this is not done, the tight tensor fasciae latae and gluteus medius will interfere with further exposure of the lateral shaft of the femur.

Another way to help define the interval between the gluteus medius and tensor fasciae latae is to look at the grain of muscle fibers. The gluteus medius fibers are coarse and tend to curve upward and backward, in an almost vertical direction. The tensor fasciae latae fibers are finer and tend to curve upward entirely in a parallel fashion.

The vastus lateralis can be detached from its insertion on the lateral side of the greater trochanter as one large flap or the vastus lateralis can be split longitudinally, whichever is more efficient, or a flap of muscle containing the lateralis and intermedius can be peeled away at the base of the greater trochanter.

Historically, Brackett [6] in 1912 described an incision similar to that of Watson-Jones with the exception that Brackett made a plane by splitting the fascia of the gluteus maximus posterior to the greater trochanter in order to release this otherwise restricting structure in a procedure very similar to that described by Harris in 1967 and 1957 [19] as a "new lateral approach."

Colonna developed the "C" incision, useful for modern total hip joint replacement, and perfected his capsular arthroplasty procedure through this approach.[10] He severed all of the abductors from the greater trochanter rather than osteotomizing them. One must remember, however, that Colonna protected the resutured muscle tendons by placing the patient in a body spica, which became part of the Colonna arthroplasty.

Indications The Watson-Jones approach has wide application for open reduction of fractures of the upper end of the femur and is excellent for arthroplasties as performed by Müller. It has some limitations in the treatment of femoral neck fractures, because one cannot visualize the head and lip of the acetabulum well; but for intertrochanteric and subtrochanteric fractures it is ideal. If the Zickel nail is to be used for subtrochanteric fractures, the patient can be placed on the table in the lateral upright position. The surgeon should not hesitate to detach part of the anterior tendon of the gluteus medius from the greater trochanter for easier access to the upper portion for placement of a guide pin or even split the tendon vertically to make a hole in the trochanter–neck junction. The tendon can be easily reattached without any functional disability.

Müller's Total Hip Arthroplasty Using Watson-Jones Approach Arthroplasties can be done through this approach, as pointed out by Müller who advocated total hip replacement *without* detaching the greater trochanter,[18] whereas Charnley cut the trochanter away but basically used the same surgical planes. Muller's technique is depicted in Fig. 4–16A. His incision is a lazy "C" curve whose distal half is parallel to the line of the upper femur and shaft. This point is important, because the incision can be extended as needed for any dissection at the upper end of the femur. He does not hesitate *to cut the insertion of the gluteus medius* for better exposure of the femoral neck. Here is an example where special Hohmann retractors greatly facilitate the exposure (Fig. 4–16C). This approach has no limitations when one wants to extend the incision down the femoral shaft. Muller cuts just below the greater trochanter and the fascia lata; extending into the gluteus maximus in order to release this tight band.

Müller gains easy access to the hip by not dislocating it, as is so commonly done in the United States, but rather the capsule is first exposed and then the neck amputated for its complete removal and dislocation as a second step. The leg can then be manipulated in various positions. The posterior capsule can be entered for release of the external rotators as needed. (Fig. 4–16D). However, this approach does not afford much access to the posterior portion of the hip where significant contractures may be present.

All such surgical approaches for total hip replacement are done with the patient in the supine position with the hip flat on the table for orientation when the acetabular cup is inserted. The main pathway to the hip is primarily through the anterior side of the joint; thus all instrumentation and surgical techniques are done from this angle. Such approaches do not afford very easy access to the posterior aspect of the hip joint to release tight, short rotators or, frequently, a tight gluteus maximus attachment to the femur. All of these structures can be scarred and shortened, especially when a revision operation becomes necessary. The anterolateral approach is fairly easy in the so-called virgin hip. But here again, if the surgeon knows his anatomy well and has become adept in this approach, he can tailor it for any problem that arises in the course of the procedure and may reach the posterior structures by removing the greater trochanter. Müller's technique of reattachment is excellent and depicted in Fig. 4–16F.

The leg must be held in extreme external rotation with the severely flexed knee placed over the abdomen. *Cases of vascular compression have been reported when the leg is held in such a distorted posture during the step of preparing the femoral canal.* Anyone with tenuous vascularity to the lower extremity should not be subjected to this approach, for if the disease is ignored a below-

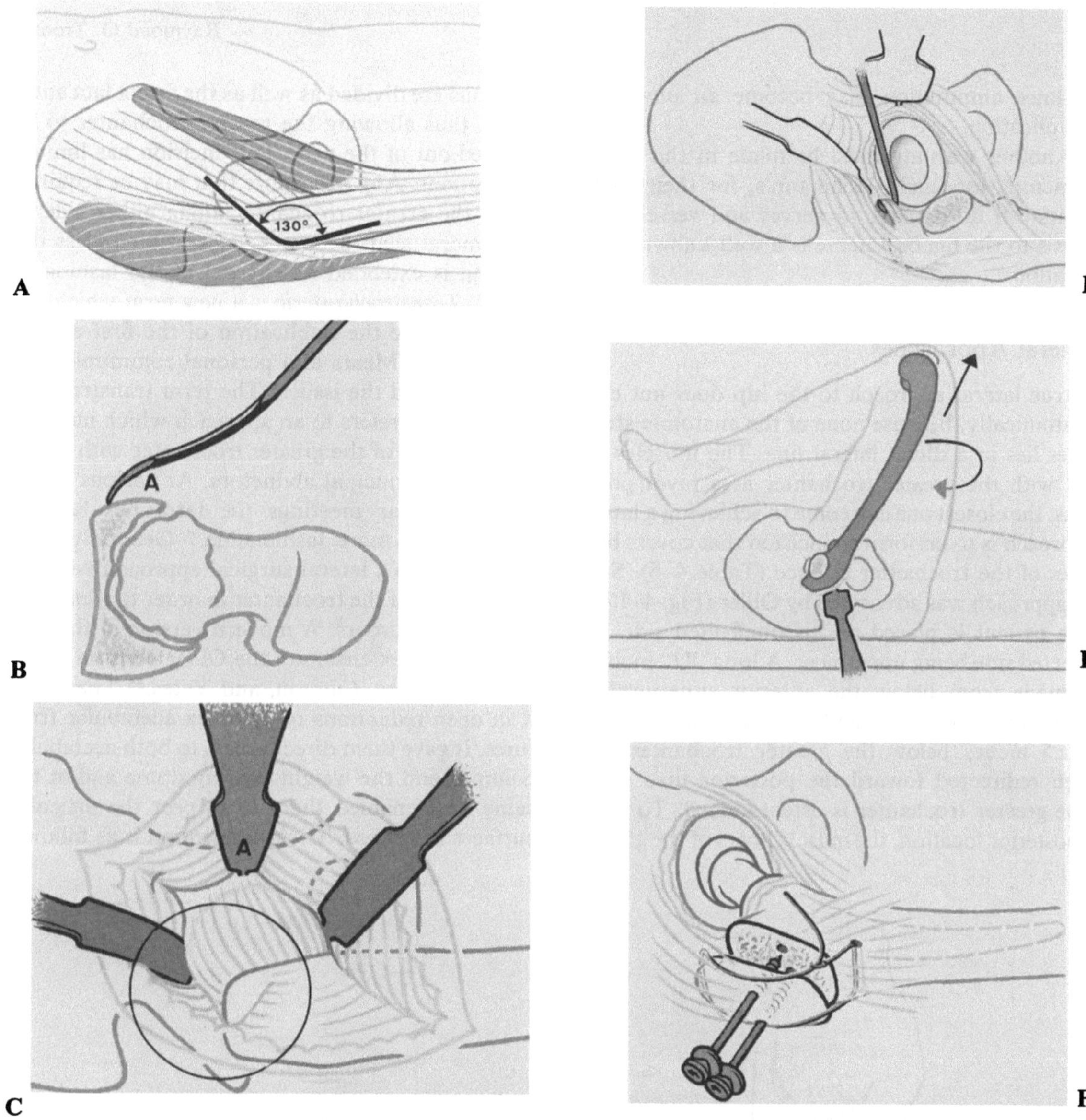

FIG. 4–16 Müller application of the Watson-Jones approach for total hip arthroplasty. **A** Patient supine. Curved incision 12 to 15 cm long starting from the midpoint of a line joining the anterosuperior iliac spine and the tip of the greater trochanter. The distal part of the incision is parallel to the femoral shaft. The angle between the two arms of the incision is about 130°. The point of the angle is just behind the greater trochanter. Curved incision of the underlying iliotibial band. In obese patients the incision should be straight and longer. **B–C** Approach to the interval between tensor fasciae latae and glutei, sparing the nerve to tensor fasciae latae. Transverse incision of the distal gluteal attachment until the bursa between the gluteus minimus and greater trochanter is opened. Exposure of the joint capsule. Placement of the three narrow, long, pointed retractors: two are found on the capsule on each side of the neck; the point of the third has a grip on the pelvis behind the anterior lip of the acetabulum (**C**). Note that the anterior tendon of the gluteus medius has been severed. **D–E** Division of the short external rotators is required, especially if the limb was in external rotation before the operation. Place the limb in internal rotation, and if the short external rotators, especially the piriformis, are under great tension, they should be pulled forward on a bone hook and cut with a knife. Never cut the quadratus femoris since its artery can cause serious postoperative hematomas. **F** Technique of the attachment of the greater trochanter. A 3.2-mm hole is drilled in the diaphysis, 1 cm distal to the osteotomy of the greater trochanter. A metallic wire, 1.5 mm in diameter, is passed above the trochanter through the glutei to return in front. Two malleolar screws with a washer are passed through the greater trochanter and two holes are made on both sides of the prosthesis in the cement through the base of the greater trochanter. At first the two malleolar screws are introduced into the holes and the compression plane of section of the greater trochanter to prevent rotation. Then the wire is put under tension and made fast.

the-knee amputation may become an unwanted complication.

Another warning must be made in the use of retractors, especially Hohmann's, for their sharp points can do damage to nerves and vessels. Paralysis to the femoral nerve is a well-known complication.

Lateral Approaches

A true lateral approach to the hip does not exist anatomically, because none of the anatomic structures lies in a direct lateral line. The muscles fan out with the greater trochanter as a pivot point; thus, the closest one can come to achieving a lateral approach is to perform an incision that covers both sides of the trochanter at once (Table 4–6). Such an approach was advocated by Ollier (Fig. 4–17).[21] The patient is placed on his unaffected side, the affected side being uppermost. A long "U" incision is made from below the anterior superior iliac spine, directed down and around a point about 1–1.5 inches below the greater trochanter, and then redirected toward the posterior iliac spine. The greater trochanter is osteotomized. To reach a posterior location, the muscle fibers of the gluteus maximus are divided as well as the fascia lata anteriorly, thus allowing the greater trochanter to be elevated out of the way. This incision has limited applications. Any procedure that may be required below the greater trochanter along either side of the femoral shaft becomes inaccessible unless the incision is extended downward in the fashion of a "Y." *Transtrochanteric* is a new term which has emerged since the publication of the first edition of this book. Mears in a personal communication has elucidated the issue: "The term transtrochanteric incision refers to an approach which includes an osteotomy of the greater trochanter with elevation of the principal abductors. At various pelvic and acetabular meetings the term has become progressively more fashionable." Generally, it is a reference to a lateral surgical approach with osteotomizing of the trochanter in order to transcend anatomical borders. A modern version of that approach is an extension of the Ollier incision modified by Senegas, Liorzou, and Yates.[36] They used it in open reductions of complex acetabular fractures. It gave them direct access to both acetabular columns and the weight bearing dome and at the same time enabled them to inspect the articular surfaces as needed. Their description is as follows:

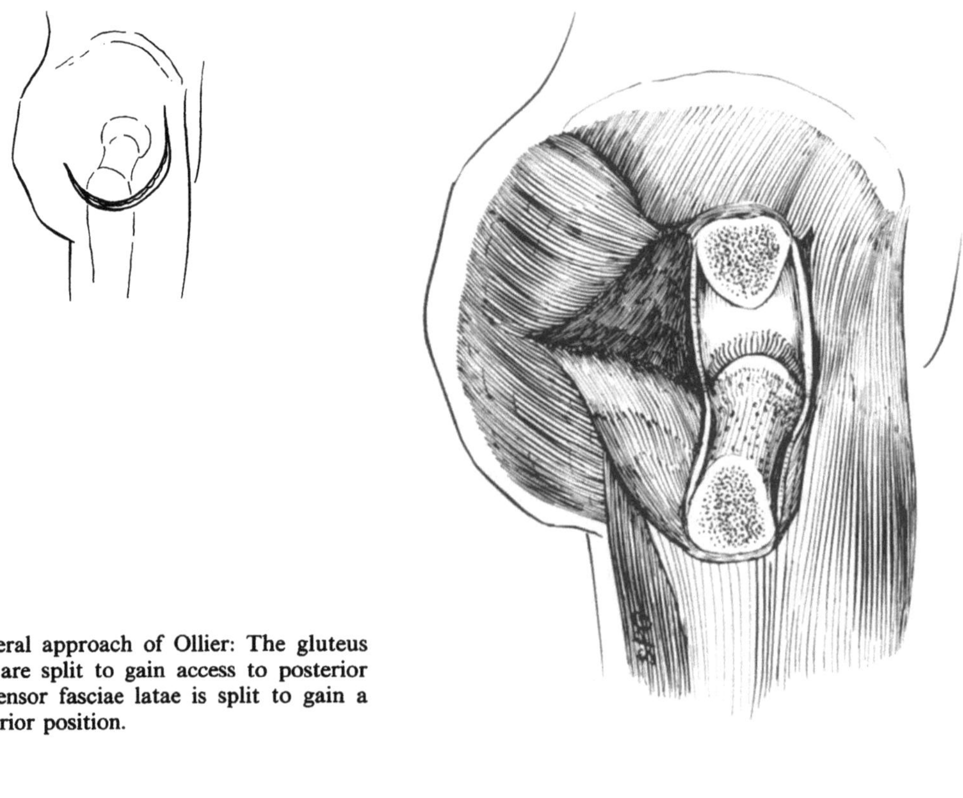

FIG. 4–17 Lateral approach of Ollier: The gluteus maximus fibers are split to gain access to posterior areas and the tensor fasciae latae is split to gain a view of the anterior position.

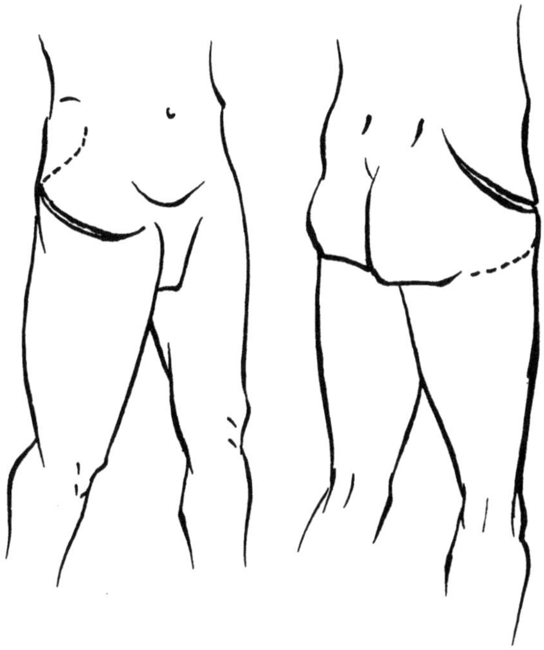

FIG. 4–18 Senegas Approach: Cutaneous incision for the proposed lateral surgical approach in complex acetabular fractures.

The patient is placed in the lateral decubitus position, then tilted 60° in order to expose the anterolateral hip surface. The lower limb on the fracture side is left free, permitting intraoperative manipulation. The skin incision corresponds to that of Ollier's posteriorly, while anteriorly, instead of going to the anterior superior iliac spine, we proceed horizontally to the lateral border of the femoral triangle (Fig. 4–18). The gluteus maximus is separated along its fiber direction and the tensor fascia lata is sectioned horizontally. The greater trochanter is then osteotomized taking only a thin portion of bone along with the glutei. The articular capsule with its vessels is left untouched. The external rotators of the hip are sectioned adjacent to their distal insertion. This allows for excellent access to the posterior acetabular column (Fig. 4–19).

Access to the anterior column is facilitated by detaching the rectus femoris from the anterior inferior iliac spine. The psoas tendon is retracted medially and maintained in place with a Steinmann pin. The articular capsule is opened by an incision above the acetabulum permitting access to the joint. Visualization of the articular surface is necessary in order to verify reduction, and more specifically to avoid leaving any loose bone fragments in the joint. Acetabular surface continuity is reestablished piece by piece as if it were a puzzle. An

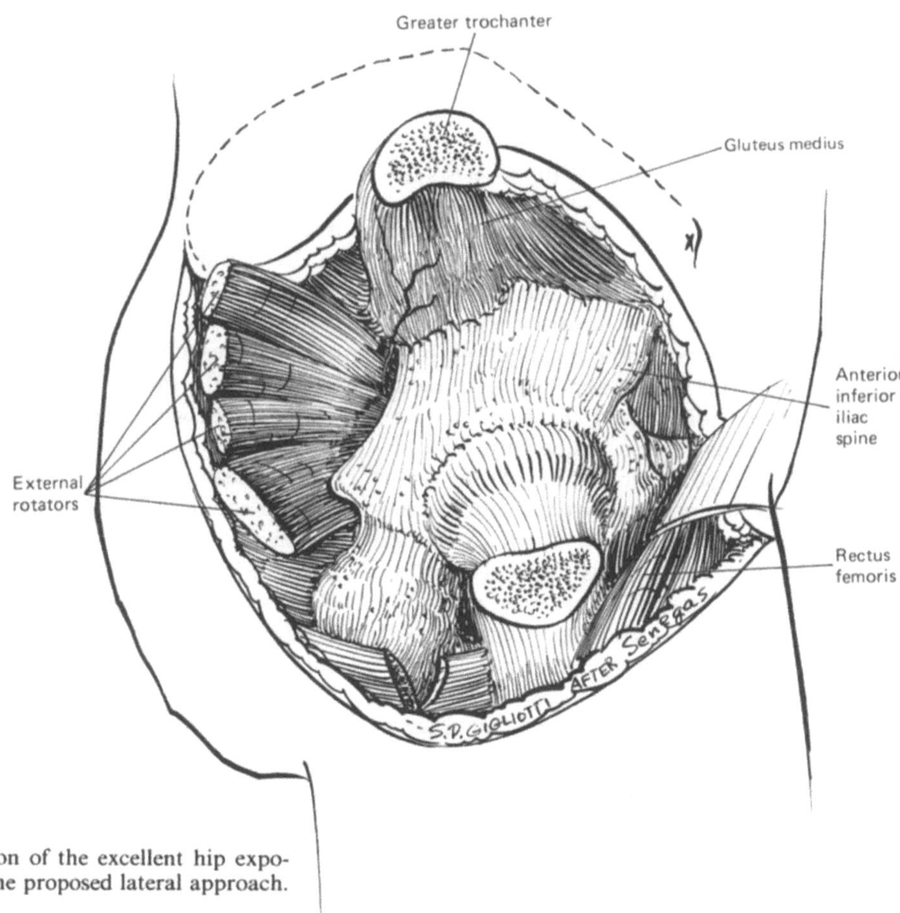

FIG. 4–19 Illustration of the excellent hip exposure obtained using the proposed lateral approach.

eye bolt is inserted temporarily into each major bone fragment and maintained in place by self-retaining bone holders. Fixation is only undertaken after all displacements are reduced. Usually, fixation is performed using a plate fastened to the posterior acetabular column and an oblique screw inserted into the anterior column. This provides accurate impaction of the fragments.

Another similar, more comprehensive lateral exposure is that of Mears, which he calls the "Y lateral exposure." It is shown in detail in Volume II, "Fractures of the Acetabulum."

The most recent transtrochanteric approach has been advocated by McLaughlin.[28] He calls it the "Strocathro Approach." It is a true lateral incision whereby a straight vertical split is made with an osteotome into the greater trochanter in an oblique enough direction as to preserve the neck. The bony slices of trochanter remain attached to the gluteus medius and minimus above and the vastus lateralis below. The author claims he has used such a surgical incision on over two thousand total hip arthroplasties without complications, except for a mild self-limiting bursitis.

Approach of Jergensen and Abbott A fairly comprehensive lateral incision was developed by Jergensen and Abbott [23] (Fig. 4–20). It begins as a long, lazy "S" incision that traverses from front to back. It also depends on osteotomy of the greater trochanter for a more comprehensive exposure of either side of the femoral neck. It is more physiological because it opens up the restricting iliotibial fascia.

The incision runs obliquely inferior to posterior starting with the anterior superior iliac spine, across the greater trochanter at about its lower level, and then curving to about 2 to 3 inches below the gluteal fold. Flaps are developed and the iliotibial band is divided in line with the junction between the posterior border of the rectus femoris and the anterior border of the gluteus medius; the incision then extends down to a point at which the gluteus maximus fascia blends into the tensor fasciae latae. The anterior capsule is exposed by retracting the gluteus medius and pulling aside the rectus femoris anteriorly, and for even deeper exposure, the iliopsoas. Any of the quadratus femoris fibers may be cut in order to obtain more exposure to the back of the femoral neck. For further exposure to the posterior aspect of the hip, the femoral attachment of the gluteus maximus is incised. A capsulectomy is performed as needed.

Tronzo Lateral Exposure This surgical approach was developed originally in 1969 when the author first began work with total hip arthroplasties.[44,45] At that time, most surgeons were following the procedure as taught by Charnley and Müller: with the patient supine they adopted a Watson-Jones incision for total hip arthroplasties.

Gradually it seemed easier for the author to place the patient in a straight lateral posture and move the initial incision in a straight lateral fashion *and* anterior to the front edge of the gluteus maximus (Fig. 4–21). This allowed a convenient view of the *anterior* aspect of the hip joint as well as the *posterior* structures. The approach avoids splitting the gluteus maximus and ripping open the superior gluteal arteries by staying in the avascular tensor fasciae latae. *Maneuvering the femur is essential for facilitating the anterior exposure* (Fig. 4–24D, 4–26A). The distinguishing feature of this method is that the hip is opened widely by traversing the avascular central portion of the tensor fascia lata (Fig. 4–22). The short external rotator tendons are severed and folded over the sciatic nerve.

In this approach, the sciatic nerve is left protected in its enveloping tube of fat and not specifically exposed because the general area is kept covered by the tendons of the external rotators (Fig. 4–23). Remembering that the tensor fasciae latae forms a thickened core around the gluteus maximus so as to form an attachment for the muscle to the femur (Fig. 4–24C), the opening through the tensor fasciae latae is facilitated by severing the tendinous extension of the gluteus maximus as it attaches to the posterolateral area of the upper femoral shaft; this is an essential feature of such a lateral approach because it allows the lower half of the fascial envelope to fall away with retraction. In hip disease, the joint is often contracted in flexion and rotation. The incision is centered directly lateral to the thigh which places the cut in the center of the iliotibial tract over the greater trochanter (about an inch anterior to the gluteus maximus edge), thus entering the hip through the avascular tensor fasciae latae. For wider exposure in tight situations, the tensor fascial envelope is opened by extending the incision upward or downward.

Advantages of this approach include the following: (1) the sciatic nerve is not exposed but protected by staying superior to it; (2) skin, fat, and muscles fold away naturally on either side of the

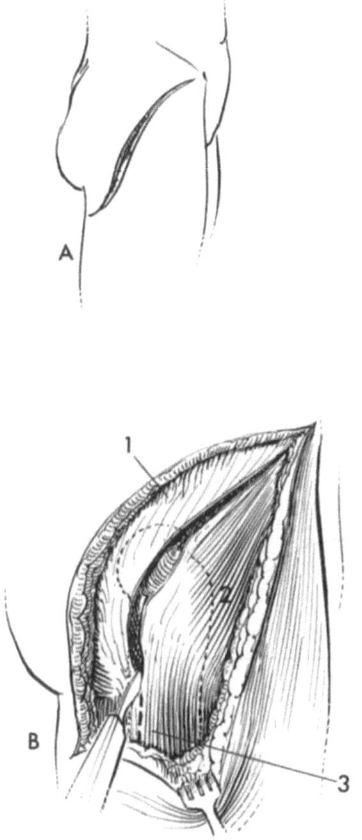

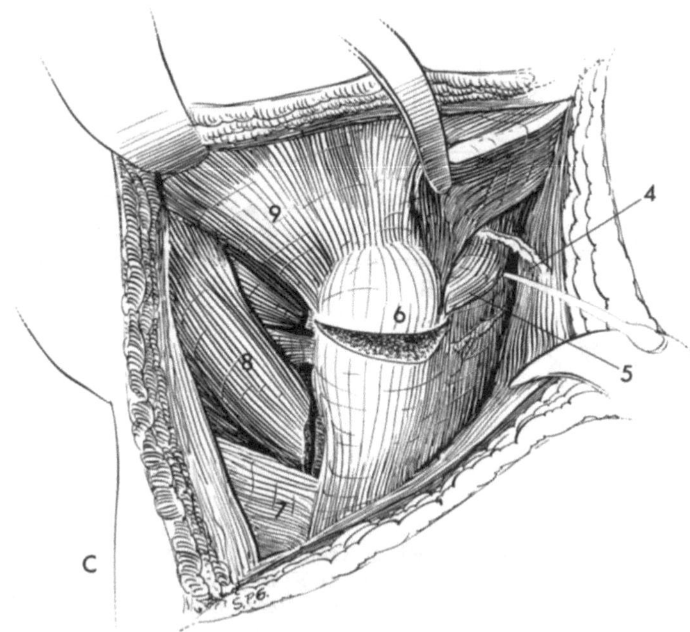

FIG. 4–20 Jergensen–Abbott approach—lazy "S" incision. **A–C** *1*, gluteus medius; *2*, tensor fasciae latae; *3*, iliotibial band split; *4*, rectus femoris; *5*, iliopsoas; *6*, trochanter divided; *7*, quadratus femoris; *8*, gluteus maximus; *9*, gluteus medius. **D** and **E** *1*, obturator internus; *2*, greater trochanter; *3*, capsule; *4*, vastus lateralis; *5*, quadratus femoris; *6*, iliopsoas and insertion.

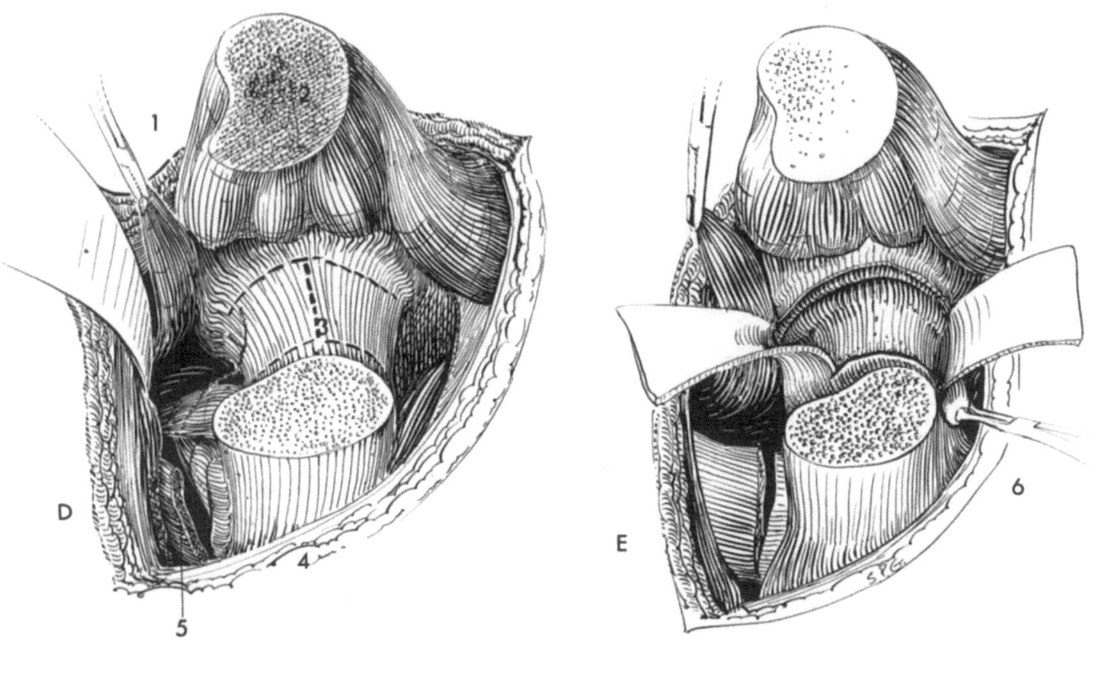

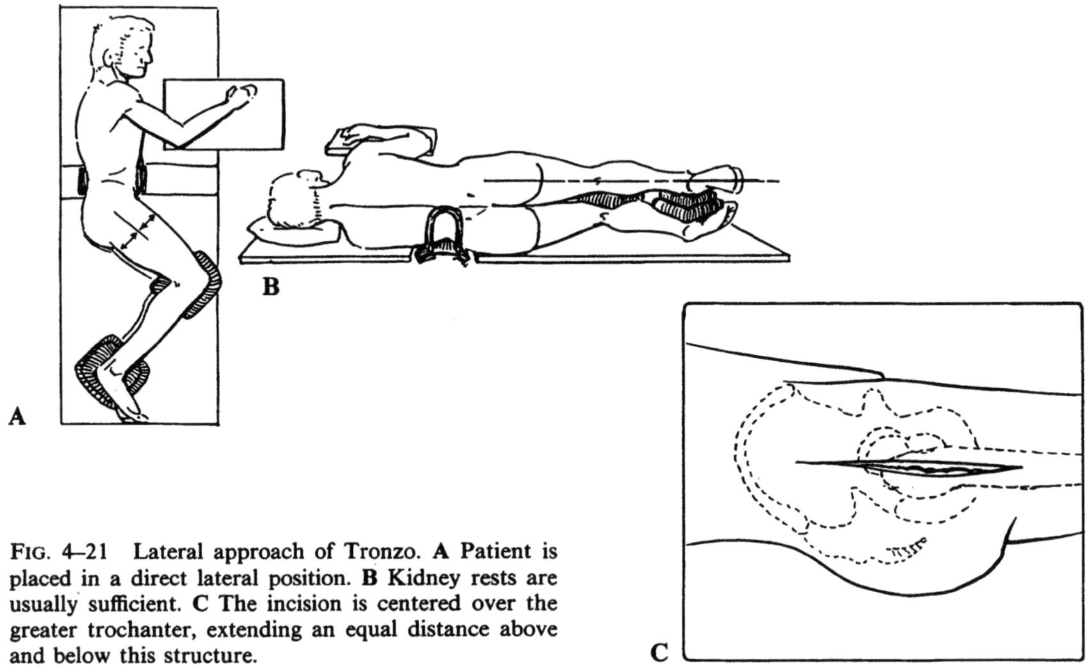

FIG. 4–21 Lateral approach of Tronzo. **A** Patient is placed in a direct lateral position. **B** Kidney rests are usually sufficient. **C** The incision is centered over the greater trochanter, extending an equal distance above and below this structure.

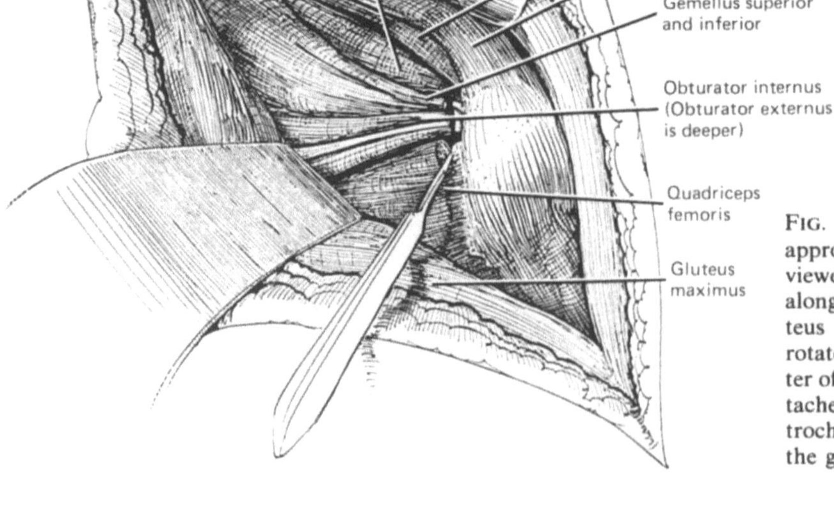

FIG. 4–22 In the Tronzo lateral approach, the posterior side is viewed by cutting the fascia lata along the leading edge of the gluteus maximus. The short external rotators as well as the upper quarter of the quadratus femoris are detached from the back of the greater trochanter. The cut is done *under* the gluteus minimus.

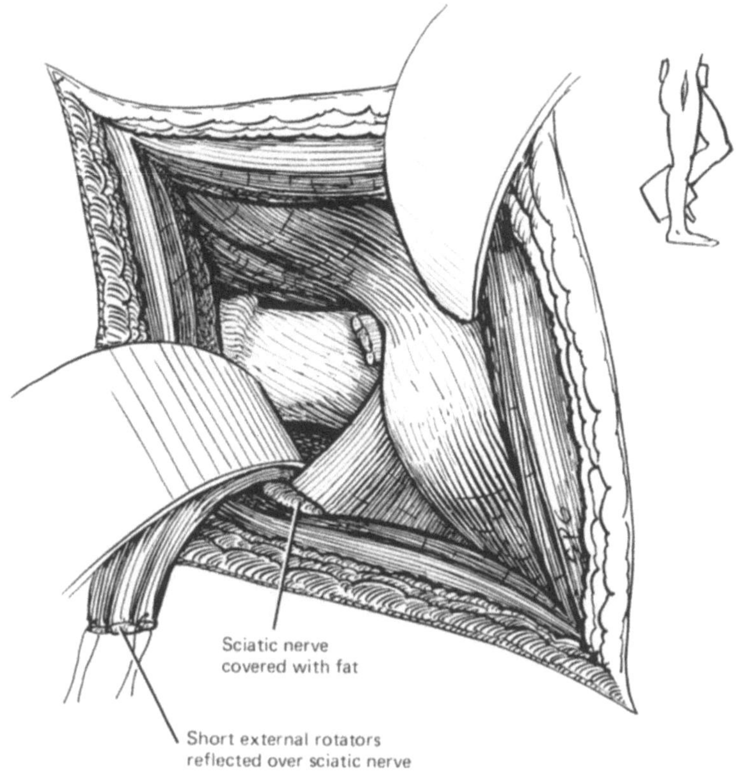

FIG. 4–23 The sciatic nerve is not visualized per se because the short rotators are pulled over the area of its usual location. This maneuver protects it at all times.

incision for easier retraction because the patient is positioned straight up on his side rather than being prone as in the classic Gibson approach; (3) the leg can be maneuvered easily in any position for appropriate access to the hip joint; (4) the approach is comprehensive since both the anterior and posterior regions of the hip joint can be exposed simultaneously; and (5) the entire femoral shaft can be easily exposed on either side, especially the posterior region where most restricting tissues must be freed. The patient is held in place by standard kidney rests with rolled drapes placed between the abdomen and the rest as needed. "Bean bags" should be avoided: they are so bulky they block the leg in adduction when such a position is needed to look down the shaft of the femur.

Depending on the patient's size, an incision is made usually about 3 inches above and 3 inches below the greater trochanter. To keep the incision truly lateral, the leg and foot are positioned in neutral rotation and abduction-adduction. The incision is centered over the lateral femoral shaft. Gradually, *internally rotate* the leg for better exposure of the external rotator tendons (Fig. 4–24D).

Once through the tensor fasciae latae, the short external rotators are cleared of fatty tissue and the small branches of the medial femoral circumflex arteries electrocoagulated. They are cut deep under the trochanter. Part of the quadratus femoris may be resected, but first the large branch of the medial femoral circumflex artery must be tied (Fig. 4–25). The gluteus minimus is closely adherent to the capsule and can be inadvertently cut if not carefully dissected away. It is retracted superiorly with the gluteus medius. The posterior or anterior edge of the abductor tendon may be partially transected whenever indicated for improving exposure. Resuturing is simple enough and no postoperative weakness will occur.

A generous capsulectomy is performed with attention given to cutting well into both the inferior and superior capsule (Fig. 4–25). When the hip has been scarred from previous surgery (e.g., open reduction for hip nailing, reconstructive procedures such as cup arthroplasties or total hip replacement), the femoral attachment of the gluteus maximus will be shortened and very tight. This should be cut, thus freeing the shaft for rotation and easier dislocation. A large arterial branch from the profundus femoris lies immediately below this

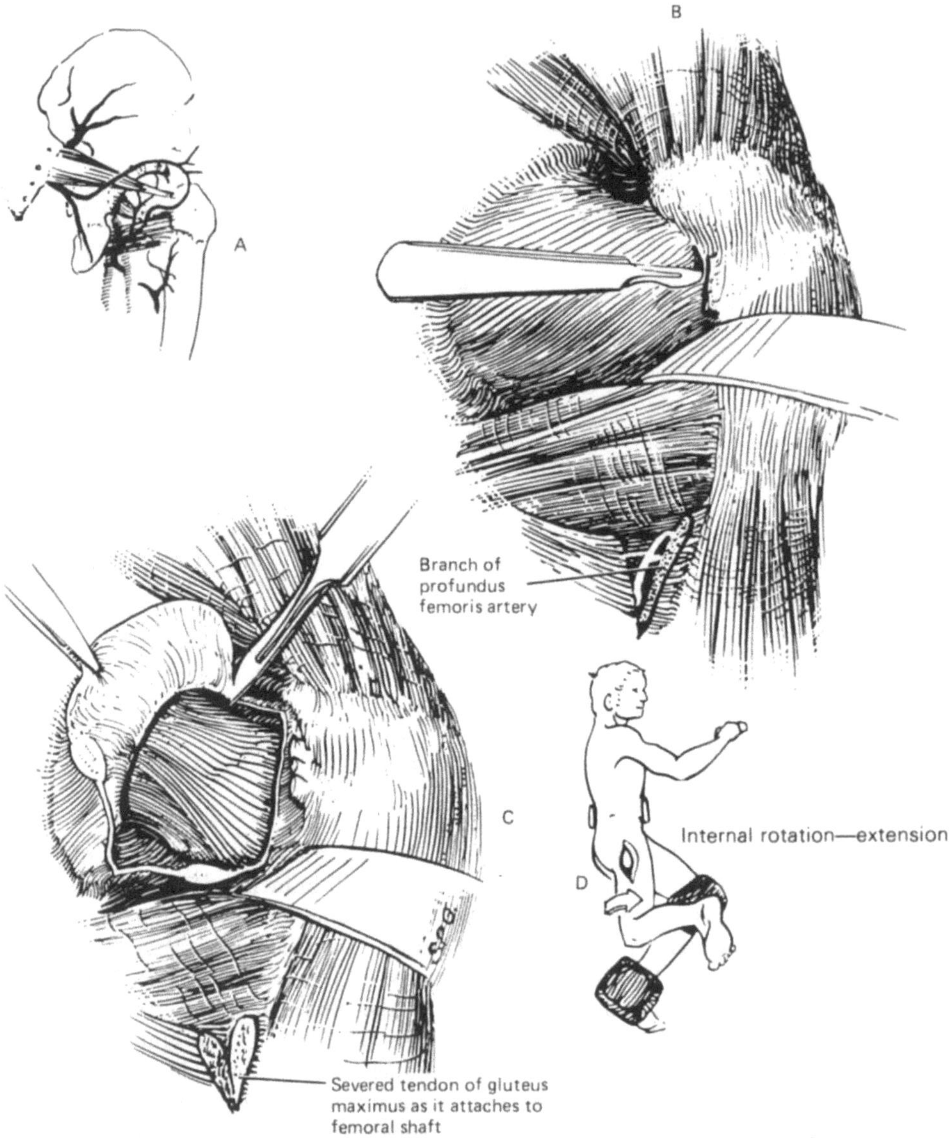

FIG. 4–24 For under exposure the gluteus maximus is retracted downward, after cutting its tendon as it enters the femur. One must be alert for the large branch of deep perforator artery. The leg is kept *internally* rotated and extended, which takes tension off the gluteus maximus flap. A generous capsulectomy is done.

tendon. It bleeds briskly when cut, so the surgeon must be prepared to ligate this artery with large Kelly clamps.

The femoral head is dislocated by marked adduction and internal rotation (Fig. 4–25). At this point, osteophytes on the head can be trimmed away; the remaining capsular structures are cut away in order to identify the neck. One may have to dissect some of the quadratus femoris *and the inferior capsule* in order to reach the inferior edge of the neck. Once these structures are cleared, the head may be amputated. Any anteriorly placed synovial tissue which may be pedunculated or hypertrophied can also be removed after the head is removed.

The anterior portion of the hip can be readily viewed by appropriate maneuvers (Fig. 4–26). If the hip is flexed, *abducted,* and externally rotated

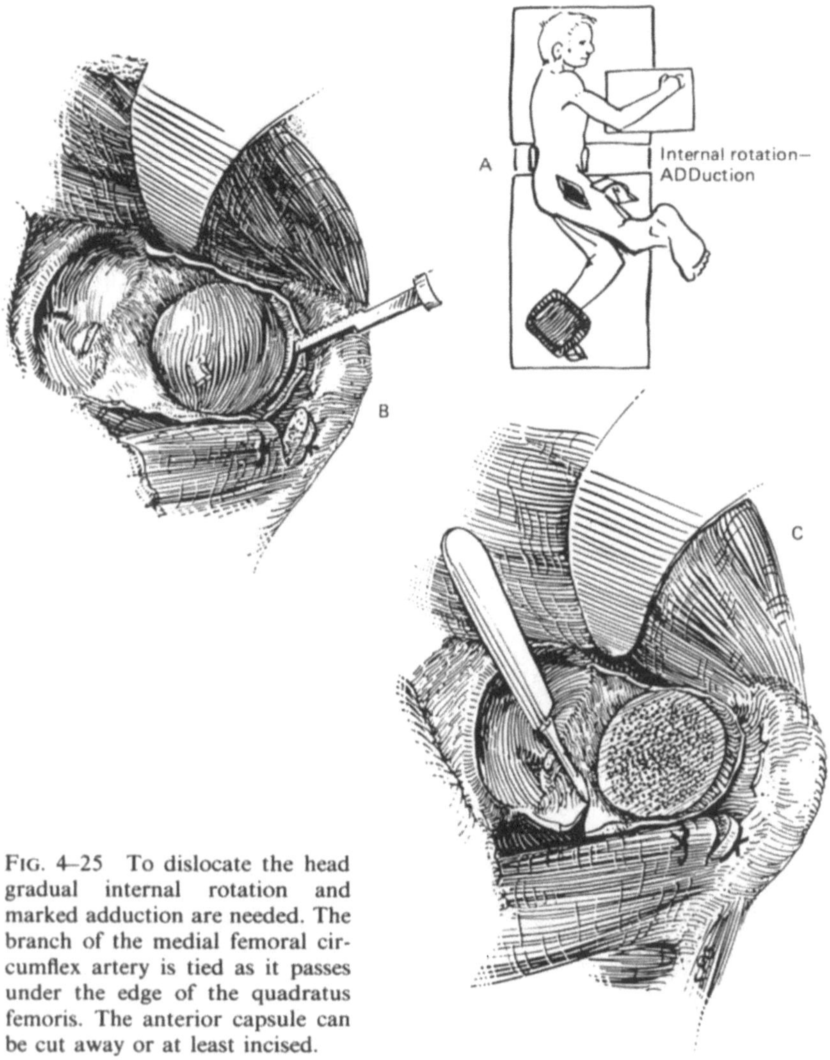

FIG. 4–25 To dislocate the head gradual internal rotation and marked adduction are needed. The branch of the medial femoral circumflex artery is tied as it passes under the edge of the quadratus femoris. The anterior capsule can be cut away or at least incised.

the anterior femoral neck and capsule come into view; with appropriate retractors, a capsulotomy can be performed and the anterior lip of the acetabulum visualized. Such a procedure allows access to the anterior portion of the acetabulum for any further reconstruction or release of a tight rectus femoris tendon.

In double-cup arthroplasties, this incision is valuable because the greater trochanter need not be removed. Here again, the hip can be dislocated initially and, by bringing the head around posteriorly, the appropriate sculpturing is done or preparation of the femoral neck carried out before capping of the femoral shaft. Once this is accomplished the maneuver of flexion, abduction, and external rotation is carried out and any contracted anterior capsule removed, thus exposing the acetabulum from an anterior pathway for its preparation. Should this not be possible, the anterior third of the gluteus medius tendon can be severed. After the head is prepared and the anterior capsule excised, the head and neck can be held down and pointed posteriorly out of the way of the acetabulum by use of the femoral neck retractor. The acetabulum is then prepared from the anterior pathway.

Osteotomy of the greater trochanter, if necessary, can be done easily through this approach (Fig. 4–27). By doing so, a better global view of the acetabulum may be achieved, particularly needed for revision surgery. Before sawing off the trochanter, it is best to first detach the external

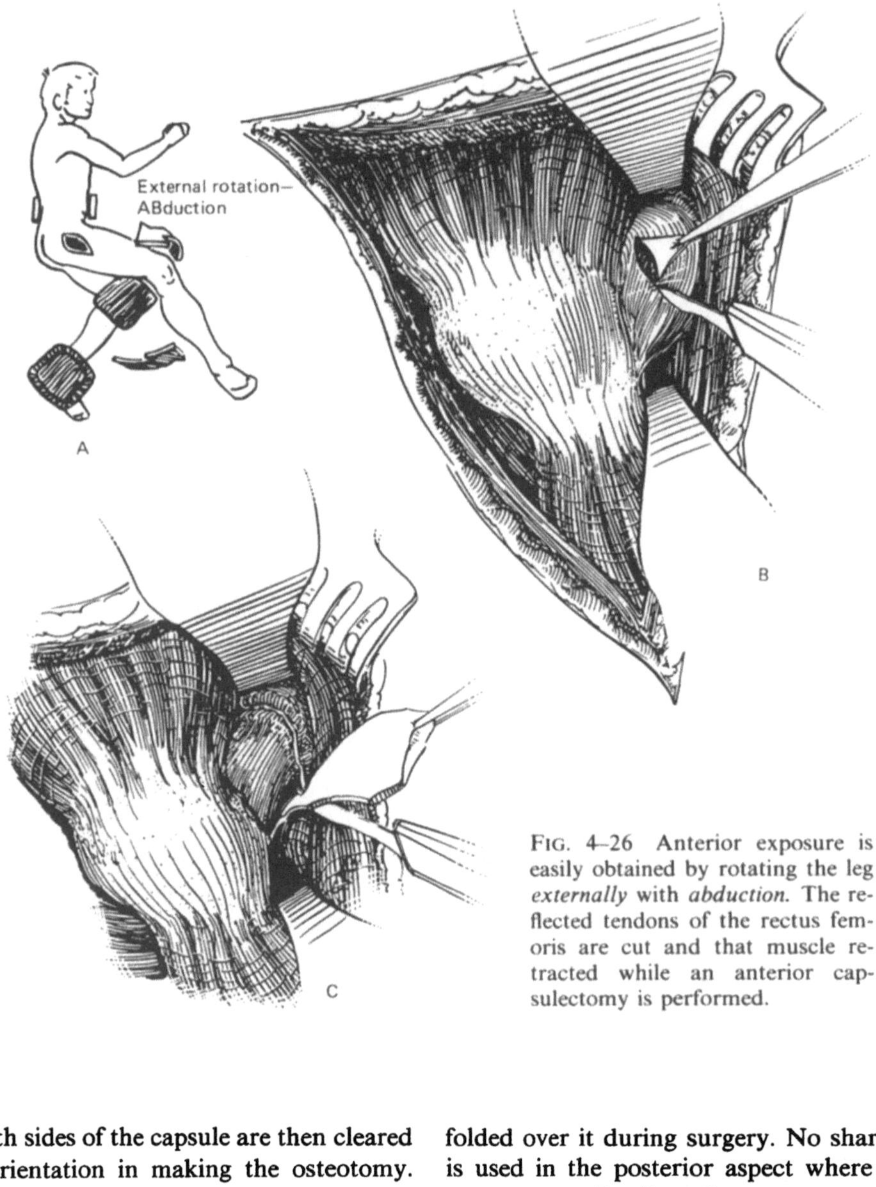

FIG. 4–26 Anterior exposure is easily obtained by rotating the leg *externally* with *abduction*. The reflected tendons of the rectus femoris are cut and that muscle retracted while an anterior capsulectomy is performed.

rotators. Both sides of the capsule are then cleared for better orientation in making the osteotomy.

INDICATIONS This particular comprehensive lateral incision appears to be a most useful surgical approach, especially for total hip replacement, arthroplasties of all types, and hip fusion. It is the author's preferred incision for open reduction of femoral neck fractures because it clearly exposes the posterior comminution of the neck when a posterior graft is indicated. The lateral shaft is also easily accessible for insertion of pins for fixing the head. In using this incision, the author constantly packs large sponges into the wound as retraction is carried out, so that the sciatic nerve is always protected by keeping the rotator muscles folded over it during surgery. No sharp retractor is used in the posterior aspect where the sciatic nerve generally lies. Sponges must always be placed over the fatty tissue which engulfs the nerve before any retraction is done.

Approach of Burwell and Scott In 1954, Burwell and Scott [7] reported a lateral intermuscular approach to the hip which was essentially the same as that of Watson-Jones, except that the proximal end of the incision began 3 inches anterior to the posterior superior iliac spine and curved backward to the trochanter instead of forward from the anterior spine (Fig. 4–28). The gluteal aponeurosis is incised over the superior border of the gluteus

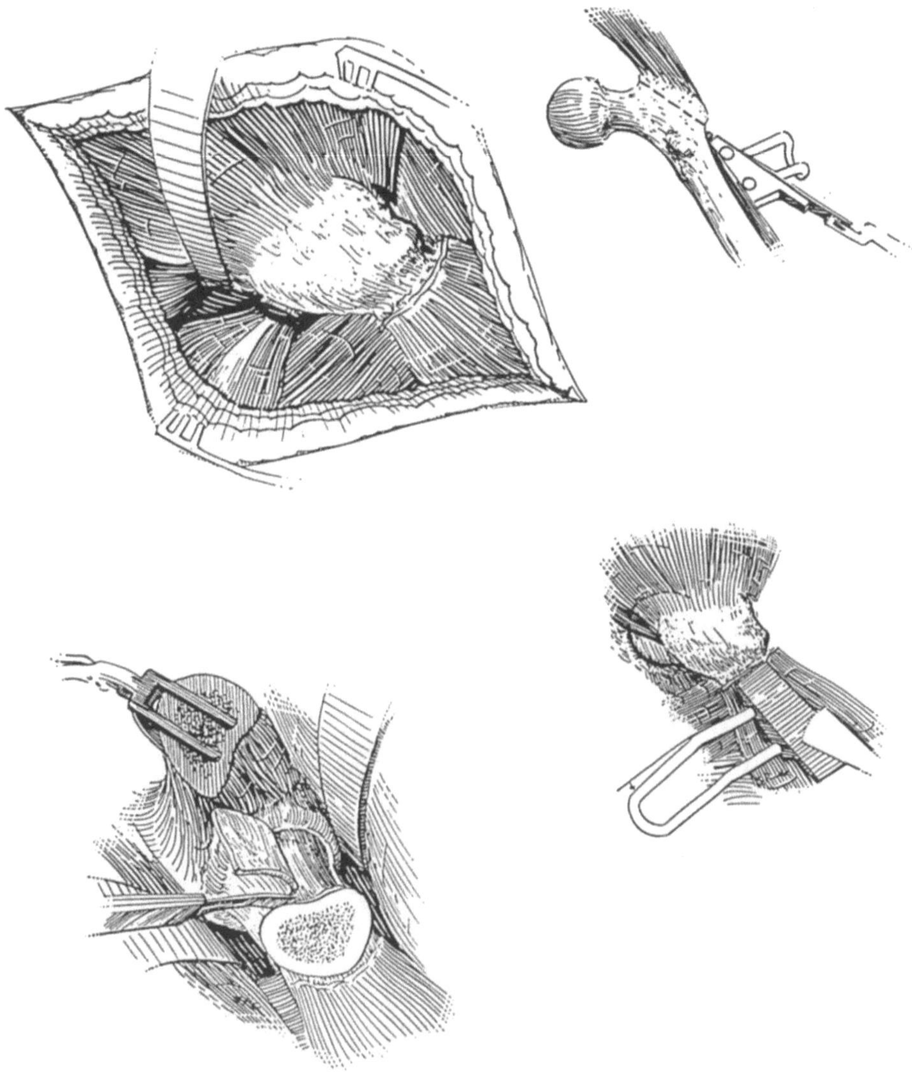

FIG. 4–27 If the greater trochanter is to be divided, first the external rotators are detached and a small portion of the gluteus medius tendon is cut to clear away the anterior capsule. *It is best to develop a plane between the glutei and the capsule* before osteotomizing it, because a neater capsulectomy can be performed without damaging the glutei. (The guide shown is used with the author's method to obtain a generous block of bone which is easier to reattach than is a small one.)

maximus and the iliotibial tract is incised over the femur deep to the distal limb of the incision, which passes 6 inches distally along the shaft of the femur. The thigh is laterally rotated and the interval between the gluteus medius and tensor fasciae latae is developed almost to the iliac crest. Since this incision is described for prosthetic arthroplasty, the head is dislocated after capsulotomy.

Posterior Approaches

History The first description of a posterior incision was recorded by von Langenbeck (Table 4–5) in 1874.[27] Dumont described in detail Kocher's modification of the von Langenbeck procedure, and thus it is commonly referred to as the Kocher-Langenbeck incision.[27] The most common posterior incision is that of Gibson, who first described

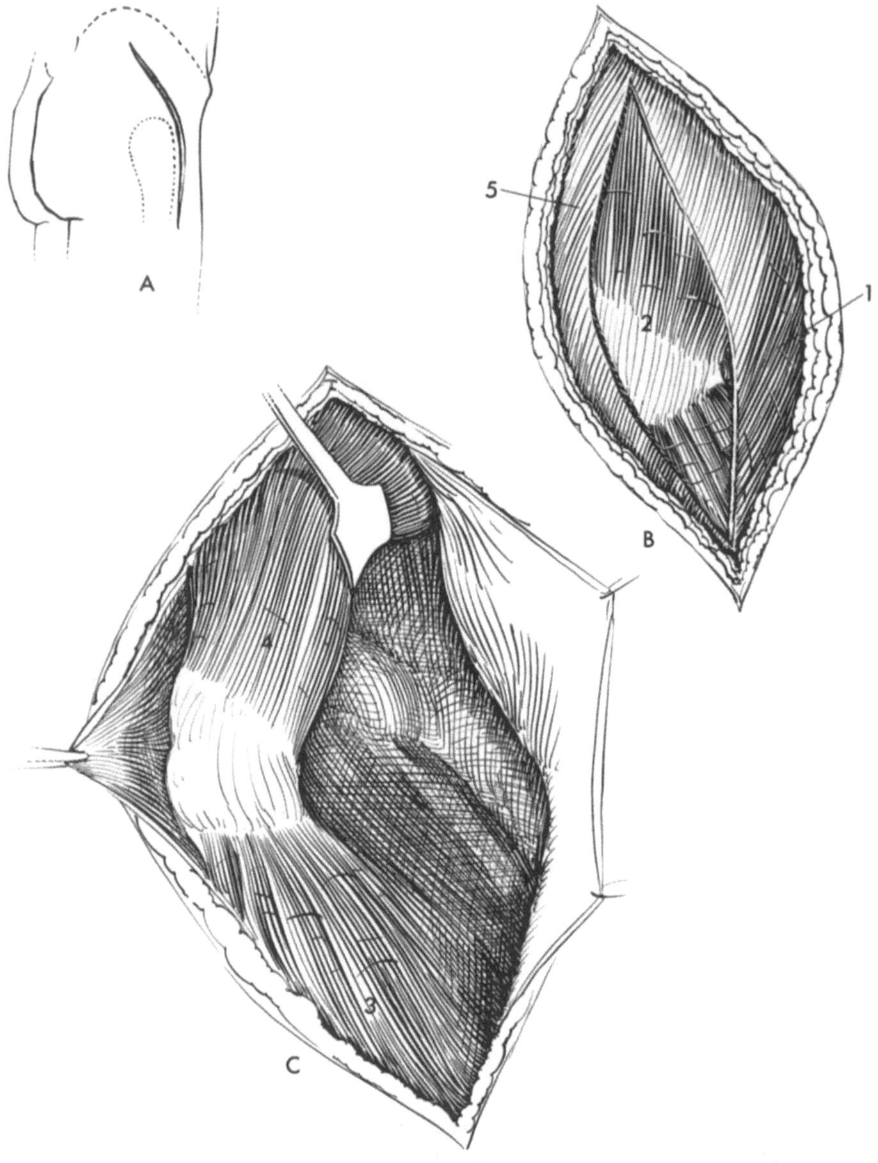

FIG. 4–28 Burwell-Scott lateral approach which gives a more generous exposure to the anterior hip than it does posteriorly. *1*, tensor fasciae latae; *2*, gluteus medius; *3*, vastus lateralis; *4*, gluteus medius; *5*, gluteus maximus.

his posterolateral approach in 1950.[16] With the introduction of the Austin-Moore endoprosthesis, Moore simplified the technique by what he called the "Southern approach" reported in 1957[31] (Fig. 4–29).

Gibson [17] relates the history of von Langenbeck and Kocher's subsequent use of this approach dating from 1874 and 1907, respectively. *Gibson depended on detaching the entire gluteal musculature and short rotators from the greater trochanter!* Bôst listed 11 posterior approaches to the hip joint described over a period of 83 years.[4] All three above mentioned approaches involve splitting incisions into the gluteus maximus (Fig. 4–29). The incisions are essentially alike, varying only in their position with relation to splitting the gluteus maximus. The most popular method is that of Kocher-Langenbeck (Fig. 4–29B). A more comprehensive poste-

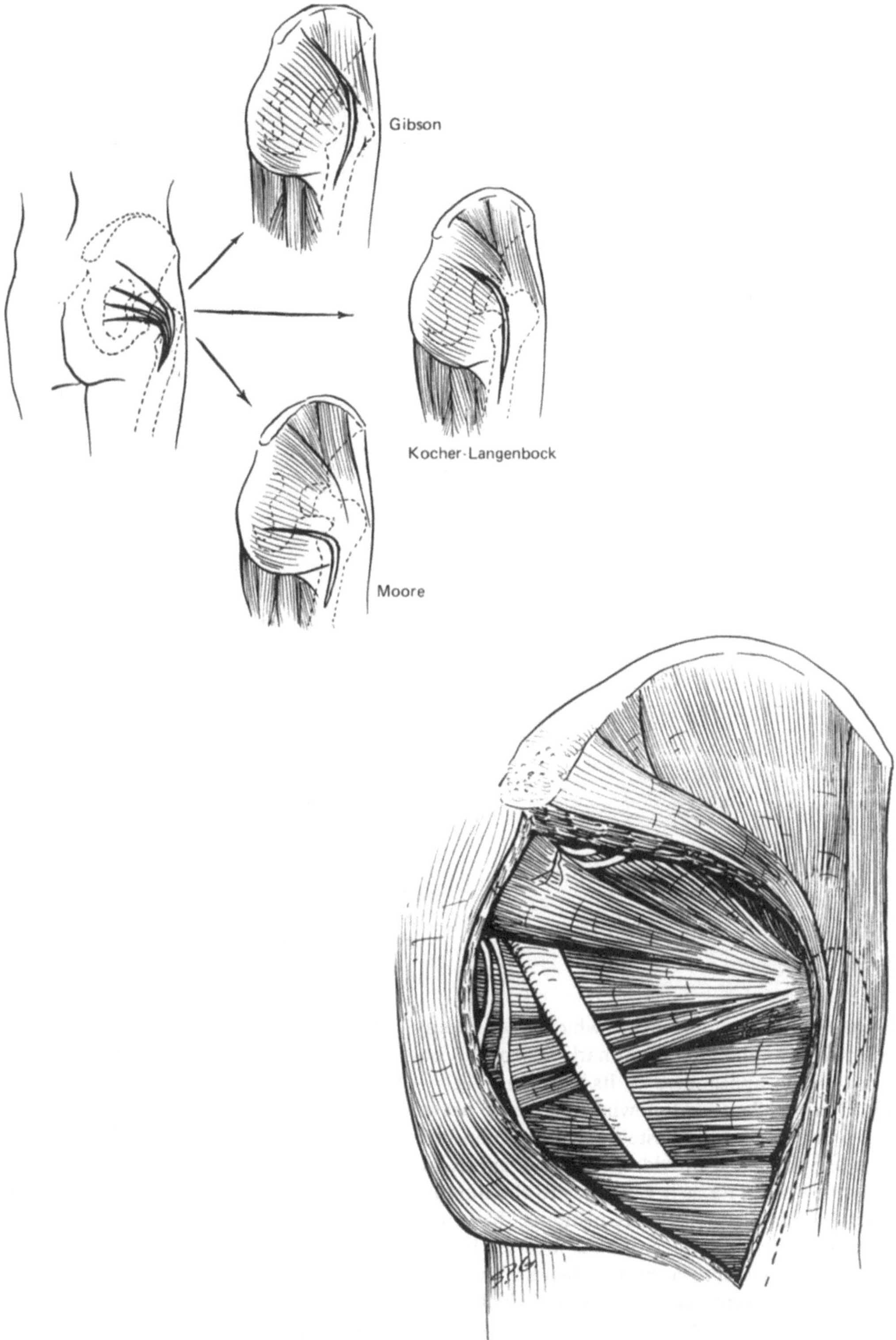

FIG. 4–29 All posterior exposures generally divide the gluteus maximus into three general levels: Gibson, Kocher-Langenbeck, Moore, *with the patient prone on the table.*

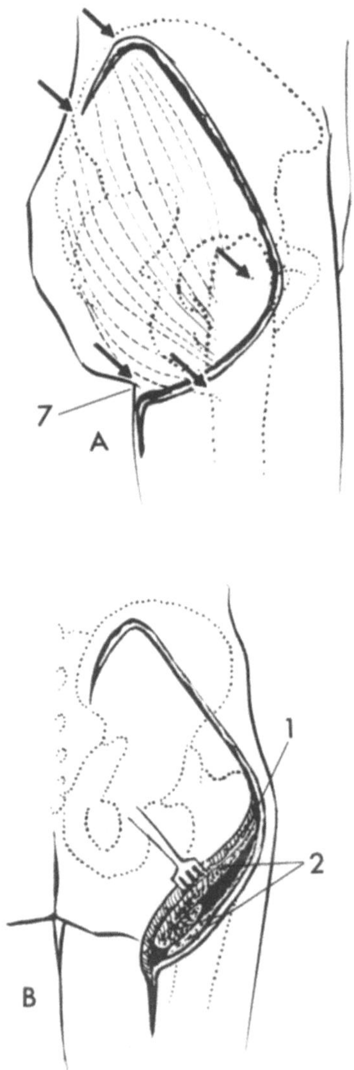

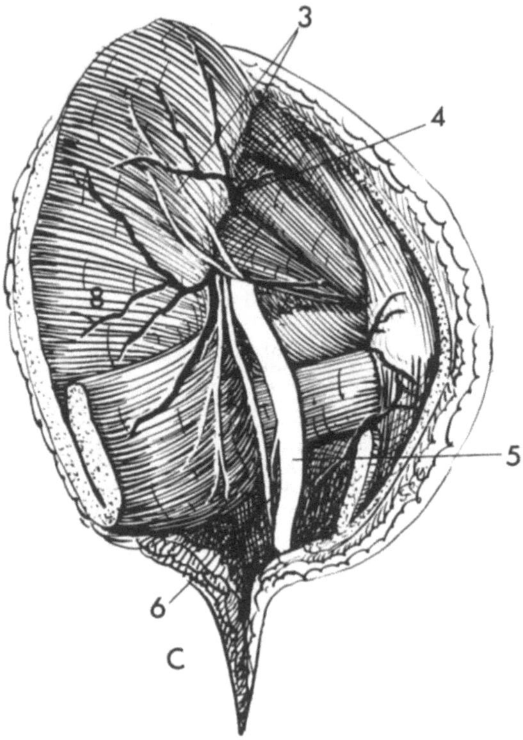

FIG. 4–30 The Henry "question-mark" approach is a radical exposure to the posterior aspect of the hip and is excellent for following the sciatic nerve. *1,* iliotibial tract cut; *2,* gluteus maximus; *3,* inferior gluteal artery and nerve; *4,* superior gluteal artery; *5,* sciatic nerve and arterial comitans; *6,* posterior cutaneous nerve; *7,* gluteal fold; *8,* gluteus maximus.

rior incision is that of Henry [21] which is commonly referred to as the "question-mark approach" because of the appearance of its incision (Fig. 4–30). It is excellent for following the sciatic nerve.

To understand the posterior approach and the type of exposure it provides, one must appreciate fully the fascia lata as it extends into the iliotibial tract. It folds over the gluteus maximus, thickening over the anterior border of that muscle. It then further thickens into a discrete band of tissue as it covers the deeper gluteus medius (which is not adherent to it), splitting again as it engulfs the more superficial tensor fasciae latae just as it had engulfed the gluteus maximus posteriorly. Acton has stated in the first edition of this text:

We have thus looked at more than a dozen accounts of a posterior approach to the hip joint which are essentially one and the same technique with certain modifications. In many instances, the modifications are so slight as to question the existence of a truly new technique. Furthermore, as previously mentioned, surgeons often use eponyms for their favorite technique without a full knowledge of the alternate variations available.[4]

The patient is placed prone with a sand bag under the anterior iliac crest so the hip is raised slightly from the table. The gluteus maximus is split and the hip readily entered, immediately revealing all the posterior structures. The sciatic nerve is especially vulnerable because it lays naked in the wound, most apparent in the Moore incision.

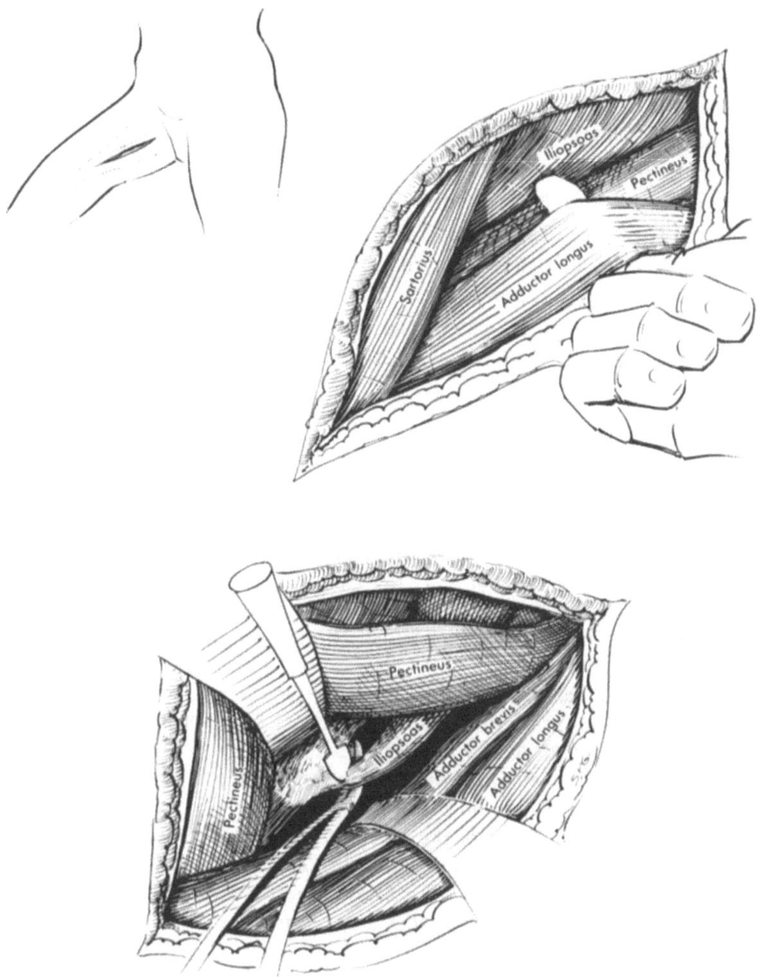

FIG. 4–31 Medial exposure. Technique of releasing the iliopsoas tendon with or without resection of the adductor tendons (adapted from Keats and Morgese[7]). The key to this anteromedial approach is proper positioning of the thigh to bring the lesser trochanter into prominence anteriorly—flexed, abducted, and externally rotated. The incision is made from the pubis and follows the lateral margin of the bulging adductor longus for about 6 inches. By blunt dissection the adductor longus is separated from the adductor brevis, taking care not to harm the anterior obturator nerve or the branches of the greater saphenous vein. The adductor brevis, upper fibers of the adductor magnus, and the adductor longus are retracted medially while the pectineus is pulled laterally. The taut tendon of the iliopsoas is exposed and isolated as it attaches to the lesser trochanter. A Kelly hemostat is pushed under the tendon as a guard against which it is severed. The incision may be extended well into the groin for selective release of any adductor muscle tight enough to be a deforming force, with a neurectomy of the anterior obturator nerve if so indicated.

Indications The posterior approach is especially valuable in open reduction of fractures of the posterior acetabulum. It is excellent for arthroplasties, with or without removal of the greater trochanter, and essential in exploring the sciatic nerve for damage and repair. It can be used for open reduction of fractures of the femoral neck when posterior comminution of the femoral neck must be exposed and treated with bone grafting.

The Medial Approach

The first medial approach was described by Ludloff in 1913 [14] and later in greater detail by Etienne et al.[15] It is depicted in Fig. 4–31. The technique involves releasing the iliopsoas tendon with or without resection of the adductor tendons (adapted from Keats and Morgese [10]). The key to this anteromedial approach is proper positioning of the thigh, bringing the lesser trochanter into prominence with anterior flexion, abduction, and external rotation. The incision is made from the pubis and follows the lateral margin of the bulging adductor longus for about 6 inches. By blunt dissection the adductor longus is separated from the adductor brevis, with care being taken not to harm the anterior obturator nerve or the branches of the greater saphenous vein. The adductor brevis, upper fibers of the adductor magnus, and adductor longus are retracted medially while the pectineus is pulled laterally. The taut tendon of the iliopsoas is exposed and isolated as it attaches to the lesser trochanter. A Kelly hemostat is pushed under the tendon as a support against which it is severed. The incision may be extended well into the groin for selective release of any adductor muscle tight enough to be a deforming force, with neurectomy of the anterior obturator nerve if so indicated.

Indications This is an excellent procedure for treatment of adductor spasm in cerebral palsy. It allows complete release of the iliopsoas muscle which in these conditions may have a broad insertion into the lesser trochanter, requiring complete osteotomy of the lesser trochanter before the iliopsoas is fully released. Biopsy of the lesser trochanter can be done through this exposure.

Bibliography

1. Allison, N.: Arthrotomy of the hip. Surg. Gynec. Obstet., 47:375, 1928.
2. Aufranc, O. E.: *Constructive Surgery of the Hip.* St. Louis, Mosby, 1962.
3. Banks, S. W., and Laufman, H.: *An Atlas of Surgical Exposures of the Extremities.* Philadelphia, Saunders, 1968.
4. Bost, F. C., Schottstaedt, E. R., and Larsen, L. J.: Surgical approaches to the hip joint. Instructional Course Lectures, AAOS, 11:131, 1954.
5. Boyd, H. B.: Anatomic disarticulation of the hip. Surg. Gynec. Obstet., 84:346, 1947.
6. Brackett, E. G.: Study of the different approaches to the hip joint. Boston Med. Surg., 166:235, 1912.
7. Burwell, H. N., and Scott, D.: A lateral intermuscular approach to the hip joint. J. Bone Joint Surg., 36B:104, 1954.
8. Caldwell, J. A.: Subtrochanteric fractures of the femur. Amer. J. Surg., 59:370, 1943.
9. Capener, N.: The approach to the hip joint. J. Bone Joint Surg., 32B:147, 1950.
10. Colonna, P. C.: The trochanteric reconstruction operation for ununited fractures of the upper end of the femur. J. Bone Joint Surg., 42B:5, 1960.
11. Cox, H. T.: The cleavage lines of the skin. Brit. J. Surg., 24:234, 1942.
12. Crenshaw, A. M.: *Campbell's Operative Orthopaedics.* St. Louis, Mosby, 1963.
13. Cubbins, W. R., Callahan, J. J., and Scuderi, C. S.: Fractures of the neck of the femur. Surg. Gynec. Obstet., 68:87, 1939.
14. Etienne, E., Lapeyrie, M., and Campo, A.: The route of internal access to the hip joint. Int. Abstr. Surg., 84:276, 1947.
15. Fahey, J. J.: Surgical approaches to bones and joints. Surg. Clin. N. Amer., 29:65, 1949.
16. Gibson, A.: Posterior exposure of the hip joint. J. Bone Joint Surg., 32B:183, 1950.
17. Gibson, A.: The posterolateral approach to the hip joint. Instructional Course Lectures, AAOS, 10:175, 1953.
18. Gibson, A.: Vitallium-cup arthroplasty of the hip joint. J. Bone Joint Surg., 31A:861, 1949.
19. Harris, W. H.: A new lateral approach to the hip joint., J. Bone Joint Surg., 49A:891, 1957.
20. Harty, M., and Joyce, J. J.: Surgical approaches to hip and femur. J. Bone Joint Surg., 45A:175, 1963.
21. Henry, A. K.: *Extensile Exposure.* Edinburgh, Livingstone, 1966.
22. Horwitz, T.: The posterolateral approach in the surgical management of basilar neck, intertrochanteric and sub-trochanteric fractures of the femur. Surg. Gynec. Obstet., 95:45, 1952.
23. Jergensen, F., and Abbott, L. C.: A comprehensive exposure of the hip joint. J. Bone Joint Surg., 37A:798, 1955.

23a. Letournel, E., and Judet, R.: Fractures of the Acetabulum. New York, Springer-Verlag, 1981, pp. 242–243.

24. Lipscomb, P. R.: A comparison of the Gibson posterolateral and Smith-Petersen iliofemoral approaches to the hip for Vitallium mold arthroplasty. Amer. J. Surg., 87:4, 1954.
25. Luck, V. C.: A transverse anterior approach to the hip. J. Bone Joint Surg., 37A:534, 1955.
26. Ludloff, K.: The open reduction of the congenital hip dislocation and anterior incision. Amer. J. Orthop. Surg., 10:438, 1913.
27. Marcy, G. H., and Fletcher, R. S.: Modification of the posterolateral approach to the hip for insertion of femoral-head prosthesis. J. Bone Joint Surg., 36A:142, 1954.
28. McLaughlin, J.: The strocathro approach to the hip. J. Bone Joint Surg. 66B:30–31, 1984.
29. McFarland, B., and Osborne, G.: Approach to the hip. J. Bone Joint Surg., 36B:364, 1954.
30. Moore, A. T.: The Moore self-locking Vitallium prosthesis in fresh femoral neck fractures. Instructional Course Lectures, AAOS, 16:309, 1959.
31. Moore, A. T.: The self-locking metal hip prosthesis. J. Bone Joint Surg., 39A:811, 1957.
32. Mosely, H. F.: *An Atlas of Musculoskeletal Exposures.* Phildelphia, Lippincott, 1955.
33. Nicola, T.: *Atlas of Orthopaedic Exposures.* Baltimore, Williams & Wilkins, 1966.
34. Ober, F. R.: Posterior arthrotomy of the hip joint. J.A.M.A., 83:1500, 1924.
35. Osborne, R. P.: Brit. J. Surg., 18:49, 1930.
36. Senegas, Liorzou, Yates: Clin. Orthop., 151:107, 1980.
37. Smith-Petersen, M. N.: A new supra-articular subperiosteal approach to the hip joint. Amer. J. Orthop. Surg., 15:592, 1917.
38. Smith-Petersen, M. N.: Treatment of malum coxae

senilis by means of acetabuloplasty. J. Bone Joint Surg., 18:869, 1936.

39. Smith-Petersen, M. N., Cave, E. F., and Vangorder, G. W.: Intracapsular fractures of the neck of the femur. Arch. Surg., 23:715, 1931.
40. Stein, A. H., and Costen, W. S.: Hip arthroplasty with the metallic prosthesis. J. Bone Joint Surg., 44A:1158, 1962.
41. Stookey, B.: Technique of nerve suture. J.A.M.A., 74:1380, 1920.
42. Sutherland, R., and Rowe, J., Jr.: Simplified surgical approach to the hip. Arch. Surg., 48:144, 1944.
43. Thompson, J. E. M.: The Jan Zahradnicek surgical approach to the problem of congenital hip dislocation. Clin. Orthop., 8:237, 1956.
44. Tronzo, R. G.: Comprehensive Lateral Exposure to the Hip. Technical Publication, Richards Mfg. Co., 1970.
45. Tronzo, R. G.: Surgical approaches to the hip joint. J. C. E. Orthop., 0:17, 1978.
46. Watson-Jones, R.: Fractures of the neck of the femur. Brit. J. Surg., 23:787, 1936.
47. Wilson, P. D.: Trochanteric arthroplasty in the treatment of ununited fractures of the neck of the femur. J. Bone Joint Surg., 29:313, 1947.

CHAPTER 5

Biomechanics of the Hip *

VICTOR H. FRANKEL AND JAMES W. PUGH

Biomechanics is the science which combines principles of engineering, basic laws of physics, and orthopaedic surgery. Biomechanics research enables the surgeon to achieve a greater understanding of the variety of mechanical derangements of the body, to formulate a precise surgical correction of a problem, and to design an effective rehabilitation program.

Through biomechanics the medical scientist can attain a clear picture of the mechanical characteristics of joint structure, the key relationship between internal and externally imposed loads, and the direction of such joint and muscle forces. In the following chapter basic biomechanical concepts and methods will be applied to the study of the hip joint. The chapter will examine the roles that muscular, joint, and gravitational forces play in motion, the bioenergetics of fracture mechanisms, the loading behavior of the hip joint in normal and pathological situations, and the basic characteristics of prostheses and fixation devices.

The Hip

The hip is one of the largest joints of the body; its intrinsic stability is due to its ball-and-socket configuration. The hip joint, however, bears large forces and a derangement of the ball-and-socket configuration can produce abnormal stresses throughout the joint cartilage and bone. Stresses and strains in the hip joint can also lead to degenerative arthritis which when coupled with the already large forces borne by the joint may produce further damage to the hip.[2]

The normal hip joint allows for a wide range of motion required for such diverse activities as walking, sitting, bending, and squatting. To accomplish such everyday activities without difficulty requires, however, that the acetabulum remain precisely aligned with the femoral head.

The Mechanical Properties of Bone

Strength and stiffness, measured as a function of stress and strain, are the key mechanical properties of bone. Stress–strain curves are used to determine the relative loading behavior of cancellous and cortical bone and of other different materials, such as steel, used in prosthesis design. Stress can be described as the load per unit area on a plane surface, as a result of an externally imposed load. Strain is the percentage of deformation—the lengthening or shortening—of a material at a point under active loading. Furthermore, specific materials are classified as brittle or ductile, depending on the degree of stretching they can withstand before failure is reached.

Cortical bone, being stiffer than cancellous bone, can withstand greater stresses but only comparable strains before failure. When the strain in vivo exceeds 2% of the original length cortical bone fractures, but cancellous bone can withstand somewhat greater strains before fracturing. This greater strain is due to cancellous bone's porosity—from 30 to 90%—which in cortical bone is only from 5 to 30% in comparison.[5]

Muscle contraction also plays a vital role in

* The authors would like to thank Peter L. Ferrara for his editorial assistance in preparing this chapter.

the supportive functions of the hip joint. During propulsion, bending moments are applied at the femoral neck, and tensile stress and strain are produced on the superior cortex. The contraction of the gluteus medius, however, generates a compressive stress and strain that, acting as a counterbalance, neutralize the tensile stress and strain. The overall result is that neither the compressive nor the tensile stress and strain act significantly on the superior cortex, which enables the femoral neck to sustain higher loads than would otherwise be possible (Fig. 5–1).

The testing of bone in vitro demonstrates that bone fatigues rapidly when the load or deformation approximates the yield strength of the bone and the number of repetitions needed to produce a fracture decreases.[5] In repetitive loading the frequency of loading as well as the magnitude of the load and the number of repetitions affect the fatiguing process. Fatigue fractures are usually sustained as a result of continuous, strenuous physical activity which causes the muscles to gradually fatigue. When the fatigue point is reached the muscles' ability to contract and thus store energy and neutralize the stress on the bone is seriously diminished. The energy storage capacity of bone also varies directly according to the speed at which it is loaded.

Failure may occur on the tensile side, the compressive side, or on both sides of the bone. In the case of a backpacker who continues to hike strenuously with a heavy pack on his back, abductor muscle fatigue may produce the loading configuration shown in Fig. 5–1. The high tensile strains on the superior surface may lead to an overload fracture of the femoral neck; or as pointed out by Chamay,[6] fatigue fracture results at the site of compression in a bending bone due to a "slip line" formation in the collagen fibers of the bone.

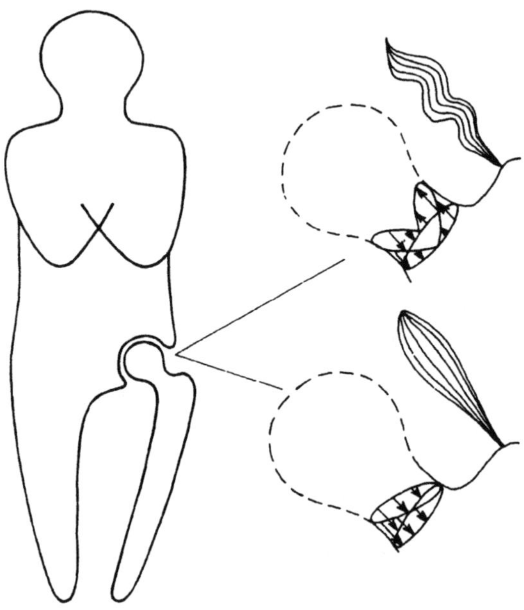

FIG. 5–1 The distribution of tensile and compressive stresses in a femoral neck subjected to bending. **Top** When the gluteus medius muscle is relaxed the femoral neck is loaded in a nonphysiological, more vertical, manner such as in the case of severe muscle fatigue. Large tensile stresses are found in the superior cortex while higher compressive stresses act on the inferior cortex. **Bottom** Contraction of the gluteus medius neutralizes the tensile stresses in the superior cortex while increasing compressive stresses act on the inferior cortex, thus loading the shaft in a physiological manner.

The Mechanical Properties of Tissue

The collagenous tissues—the ligaments (including the joint capsule) and tendons—are very different from common engineering materials. Collagenous tissues exhibit viscoelastic and anisotropic behavior, demonstrating different loading behavior when loaded in different directions. The most important mechanical properties of collagenous tissues are strength and stiffness.[12] Tendons, for instance, 80% of whose dry weight may be composed of collagen fibers, have a tensile stiffness of 1×10^3 megapascals (the pressure produced by a force of 1 newton over 1 mm^2) and a tensile strength of 50 megapascals. Comparatively, steel has a tensile stiffness of 200×10^3 megapascals and a strength of about 700 megapascals, whereas aluminum has a stiffness of 70×10^3 megapascals and a strength of 150 pascals.[5]

Several theories and techniques of measuring tissue behavior have been reported.[8,16,18,31] Adequate testing, however, should describe the strain or load rate since the ultimate stress, strain, and energy absorption depend directly on the strain rate.

In bone the relation of the orientation of collagen fibers to the mechanical properties of the bony tissue is all important.[11,12] A rough approximation of the relative modulus of elasticity of stainless steel to cortical bone to cancellous bone to articular cartilage under compressive loading is 1000:100:10:1.

Bone demonstrates anisotropy: its structure, which is different in the transverse and longitudinal directions, varies in strength depending on the direction in which it is loaded. Strength and stiffness are greatest in the direction in which loads are most commonly applied to the bone. Variations in strength and stiffness for cortical bone samples from a human femoral shaft, tested in four directions, were demonstrated by Frankel and Burstein in 1970.[16] The highest values for both parameters were obtained for the samples when loaded in the longitudinal direction (Fig. 5–2).

The direction of the joint reaction force imposed on the head of the femur may also be correlated with the anatomy of the upper end of the femur.[19,25] The interior of the femoral neck is composed of cancellous bone which is divided into the medial and lateral trabecular systems. The joint reaction force on the femoral head parallels the trabeculae of the medial trabecular system (Frankel),[13] indicating that this system is important in supporting the joint reaction force. It is probable that the lateral trabecular system resists the compressive force produced by the contraction of the abductor muscles. The epiphyseal plate is at right angles to the trabeculae of the medial trabecular system, and is considered to be perpendicular to the joint reaction force on the femoral head.[19] The thin shell of cortical bone around the

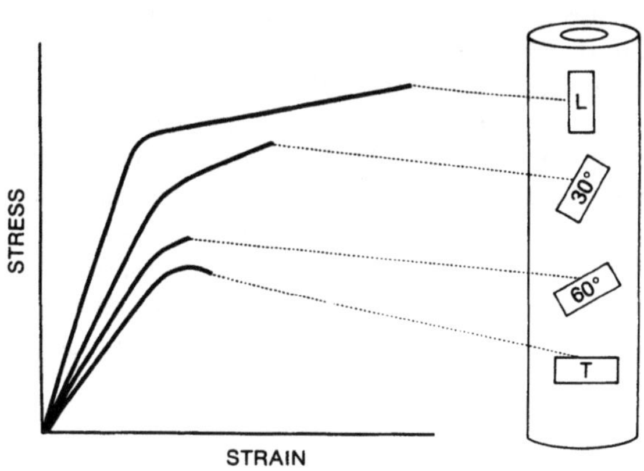

FIG. 5–2 Anisotropic behavior of cortical bone specimens from a human femoral shaft tested in four directions: longitudinal (*L*), tilted 30° with respect to the neutral axis of the bone, tilted 60°, and transverse (*T*). (From Frankel and Burstein.[16] Used with permission from Lea and Febiger.)

superior femoral neck gradually thickens in the inferior region. With the aging process the femoral neck gradually undergoes degenerative modifications wherein the cortical bone is thinned and cancellated and the trabeculae are gradually resorbed. These degenerative modifications may predispose the femoral neck to fracture.

Moreover, experimental studies have also indicated that fracture characteristics depend on the final resultant direction of the joint reaction force on the femoral neck, and not on the total exerted force.[13] Typical subcapital fractures resulted from high axial-to-bending load ratios. Intermediate ratios produced subcapital fractures with a "spike of neck." McLaughlin and Frankel[22] also analyzed the data from the earlier experimental study by classifying the bones according to osteoporosis.[33] Figure 5–3 shows a regression line for the strength of the bone, expressed as fracture force/square of the diameter of the neck. The chart indicates a steady decrease with age; older bones absorbed about 25% less energy to failure than did younger bones. A regression line indicating osteoporosis versus age is also shown in Fig. 5–3. The energy absorption failure point averaged 60 kg_f-cm for female bones which is highly significant in investigating the cause of fractures during falls.

The average female femoral neck required 600 kg_f for failure whereas the average male neck required 900 kg_f. An investigation into the biomechanical energetics of fractures of the femoral neck showed that two distinct mechanisms of fracture were operable.[15] In one type, where a person slips but does not fall, sufficient muscle force must be exerted to fracture the femoral neck. If the average femoral neck of an elderly female requires 600 kg_f to produce a fracture, then the amount of muscle tissue that must contract simultaneously to produce sufficient fracture force is available in the muscle which spans the hip joint (120–300 cm^2 at a ratio of 2–5 kg of force per cm^2). Indeed, weakness of the neck and osteoporosis are not necessarily contributing factors because fractures have been known to occur due to muscle forces during electric shock, in the "stiffman syndrome,"[34] and during seizures. Instead of deficient bone strength, such fractures may be caused by aging of the neuromuscular apparatus—the overloading of the bone occurring due to a lack of inhibitory impulses to the muscles during a slip.

Similarly, femoral neck fractures sustained during actual falls do not require weak bone tissue

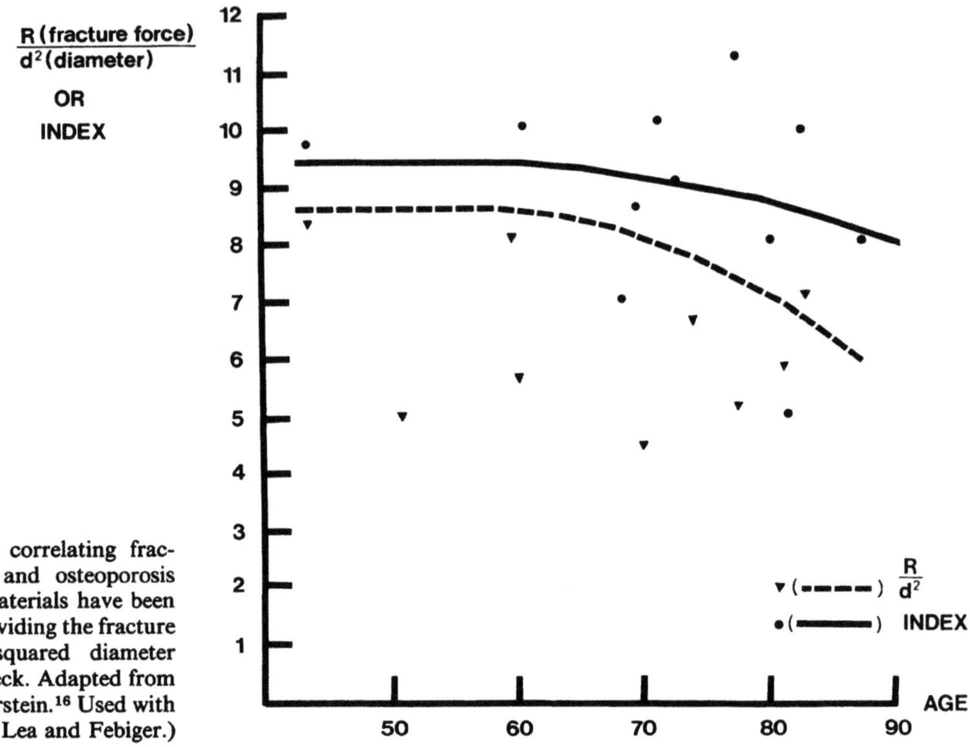

FIG. 5–3 Data correlating fracture force (R) and osteoporosis with age. The materials have been normalized by dividing the fracture force by the squared diameter of the femoral neck. Adapted from (Frankel and Burstein.[16] Used with permission from Lea and Febiger.)

as the primary causal factor. The mechanism by which an elderly female who falls dissipates the potential energy stored by her body is depicted in Fig. 5–4. In the illustrated example 3700 kg_f-cm must be dissipated, but since the femoral neck can absorb only 60 kg_f-cm of energy before failure other absorption and dissipation systems are active. Most of the energy in a fall is absorbed by active muscle contractions: the quadriceps alone can absorb ten times more energy than can the femur during a fall. In this situation, however, about 40 times as much energy than is necessary to fracture the femoral neck is available and this energy cannot be dissipated quickly enough through muscle contractions or through the conversion of strain to kinetic energy. Consequently, when the level of stored energy in the neck of the femur rises above its threshold level a fracture will occur.

Similar relationships between stored energy and the ability of the musculoskeletal system to absorb that energy also exist for a younger person. A typical subcapital fracture was observed in a healthy, vigorous skier who attempted to negotiate a 360° turn on an icy slope. Although the skier was accustomed to falling in snow, the event occurred so suddenly that his neuromuscular mechanisms for energy dissipation could not respond in time.

Energy absorption–dissipation studies for femoral neck fractures, dislocations of the hip joint, intertrochanteric fractures, and acetabular fractures should account for the role played by muscle forces as well as ground reaction forces and externally applied loads. Neuromuscular control data and the effect of aging on the neuromuscular system should also be taken into account. It was found in one study [1] that patients with diabetes, hemiplegia, and rheumatoid arthritis—all conditions associated with possible neuromuscular pathologies—sustained a greater incidence of fracture of the femoral neck than normal. A great deal of biomechanical research remains to be done in the area of hip joint trauma, so that bioengineers and other medical scientists can work with accurate bone failure data, such data being essential to the design of sports equipment, vehicles, workplace situations, and prostheses.

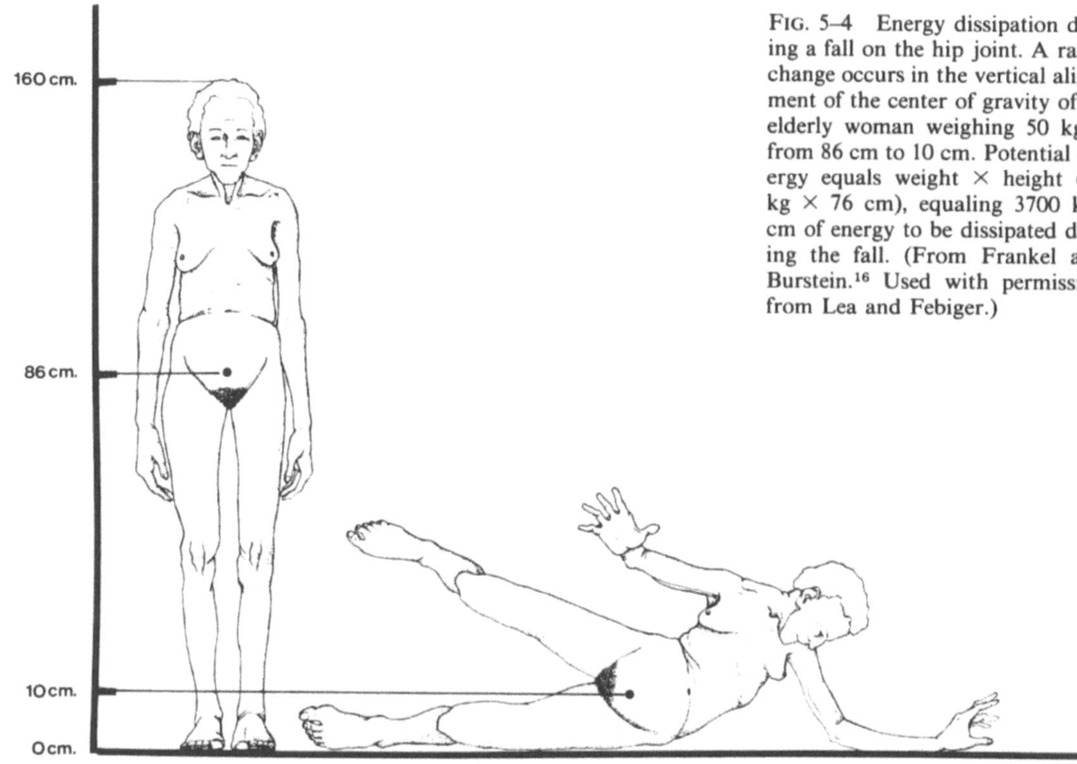

FIG. 5–4 Energy dissipation during a fall on the hip joint. A rapid change occurs in the vertical alignment of the center of gravity of an elderly woman weighing 50 kg—from 86 cm to 10 cm. Potential energy equals weight × height (50 kg × 76 cm), equaling 3700 kg/cm of energy to be dissipated during the fall. (From Frankel and Burstein.[16] Used with permission from Lea and Febiger.)

Kinematics

Kinematics is the branch of biomechanics that describes the motion of a body without reference to either mass or force. Kinematic studies define the range of motion and the surface joint motion along three planes: the coronal (frontal), the sagittal, and the transverse (or horizontal).

Gross measurements can be made by goniometry but more accurate measurements must be achieved with such methods as electrogoniometry, roentgenographs, special photographic techniques, or through computerized video motion analysis using light reflective spots, special cameras, and a variety of specially designed hardware.

Hip joint motion occurs in all three planes but is greatest in the sagittal plane where flexion ranges from 0 to 140° and extension from 0 to 15°.[23] In the frontal plane abduction ranges from 0 to 30° whereas adduction is slightly less, from 0 to 25°. In the transverse plane external rotation ranges from 0 to 90°, whereas internal rotation ranges from 0 to 70° when the hip joint is flexed. Less rotation occurs, however, during extension as a result of the restrictive function of the soft tissues.

The dynamic range of motion in the hip joint in the sagittal plane during level walking was studied with a computerized video motion analysis system.* In the normal gait pattern the hip is maximally flexed during the late swing phase as the leg moves forward for heel strike. The hip joint is then extended as the body is propelled forward at the beginning of the stance phase (Fig. 5–5A). Maximum extension is reached just prior to toe off. The hip shifts into flexion during the swing phase, reaching maximum flexion prior to heel strike. In marked contrast is the angle-angle plot for the patient with a Trendelenburg gait (Fig. 5–5B). The Trendelenburg pattern indicates that sufficient abductor muscle force is not available, leading to pelvis sag over the affected hip. The stance phase is significantly reduced and the overall gait cycle is also shortened, providing greater

* Research performed at the Bioengineering Lab, the Orthopaedic Institute, Hospital for Joint Diseases, New York, New York.

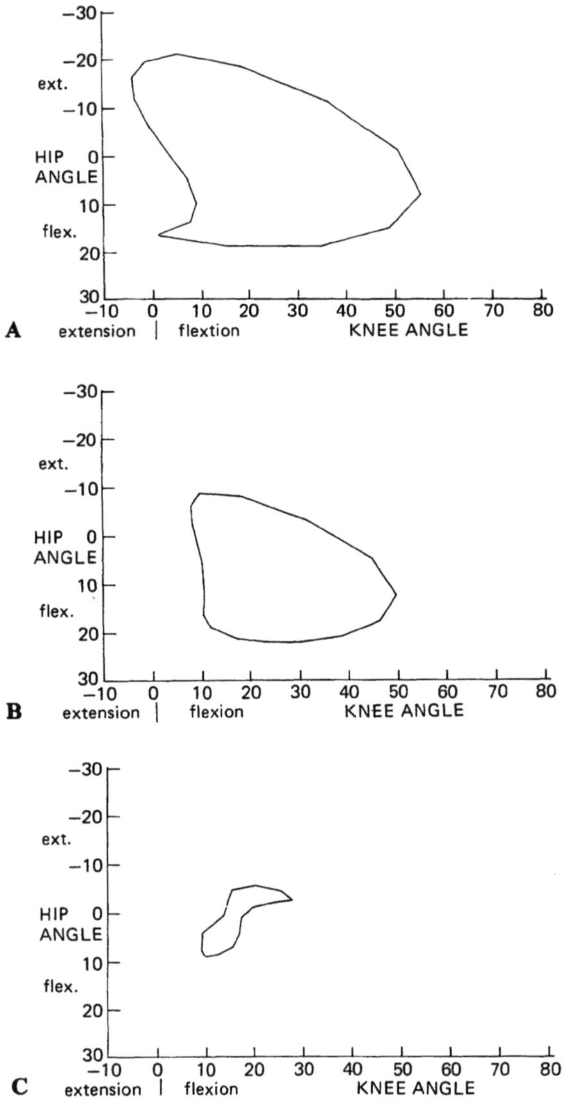

FIG. 5–5 Angle-angle plots showing dynamic range of motion of hip and knee joints during the gait cycle, as produced by computerized video motion analysis system. Progression of motion is clockwise, heel strike occurring at lower left. **A** Normal pattern. **B** Trendelenburg pattern. **C** Antalgic pattern. (From Pugh et al.[28])

frequency of joint motion and thus more stress on the hip joint.

Furthermore, in the severely restricted antalgic gait pattern (Fig. 5–5C) both the stance and swing phases are drastically shortened. Due to severe pain from degenerative arthritis the hip is lifted up and over the affected limb, almost exactly the reverse of the characteristic sag of the Trendelenburg pattern. Neither flexion nor extension at any point in the gait cycle exceeds 10°, less than half the range of motion in the normal gait pattern. Throwing the hip over the affected joint deranges the body's center of gravity and produces joint forces that are only slightly larger than 1 × body weight.

Once the motion of the hip joint has been recorded with computerized video motion analysis or other special photographic methods the angular accelerations about the joint can be calculated with simple formulas. The resultant information is particularly useful, when correlated with phasic muscle activity, in demonstrating the function of muscle in gait. Figure 5–6 illustrates the actions of the muscles which produce accelerations about the hip joint. Variations in the accelerations displayed in the charts, or aberrations in the stance phase of the angle-angle plot, may signal a pathological condition. The angle-angle plot of the Trendelenburg gait, for example, indicates that the shortened stance phase results in greater and more frequent eccentric and concentric contractions of the hip and knee extensors. This pathological gait pattern, due to weakness of the abductor muscles, causes the trunk to be accelerated over the affected hip joint. For orthopedic surgeons the acceleration rate data are all important in calculating the forces and moments acting on the hip joint.

Johnston and Smidt,[20] using an electrogoniometer, studied hip joint motion in the frontal and transverse planes during the gait cycle (Fig. 5–7). It was found that in the frontal plane abduction occurs during the swing phase, and reaches a peak just after toe off. The hip joint then reverses into adduction at heel strike, and continues until late stance phase.

As age advances the gait pattern changes considerably, demonstrating a diminished range of motion in the joints of the lower limb. One particular study [24] examined the walking patterns of 67 normal men of similar height and weight, ranging in age from 20 to 87 years. When the gait patterns of the younger and older men were compared the differences in the sagittal position at heel strike of the two groups were dramatic (Fig. 5–8). The older men displayed shorter leg lengths, limited range of hip flexion and extension, decreased plantarflexion of the ankle, and a decreased heel-floor angle of elevation of the toe of the forward limb.

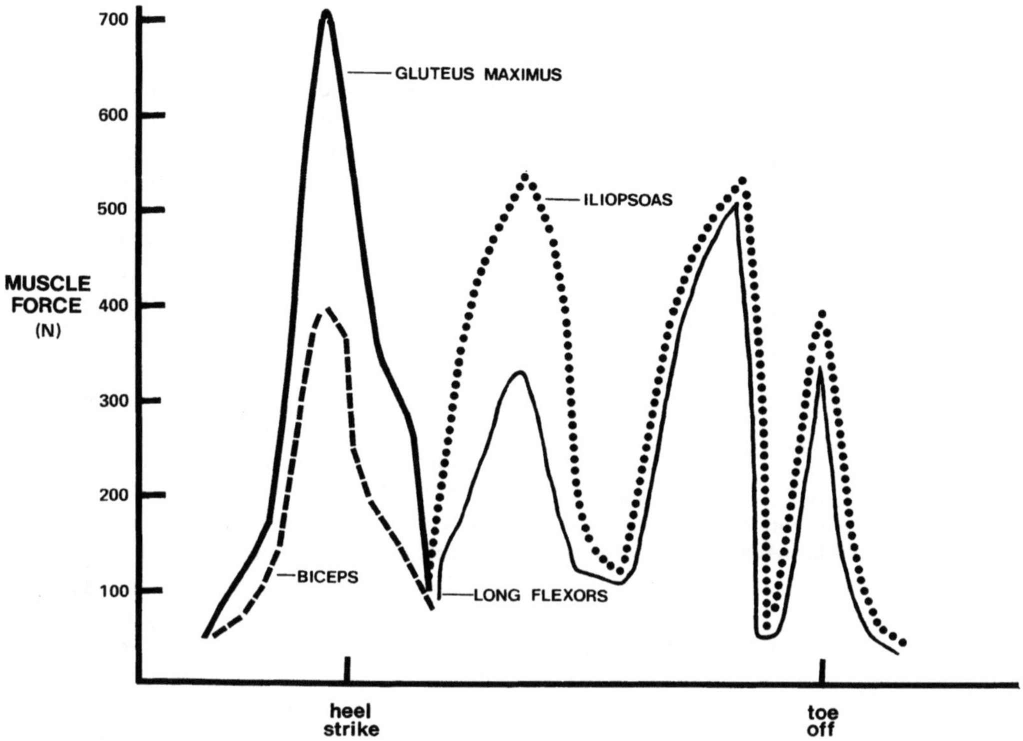

A

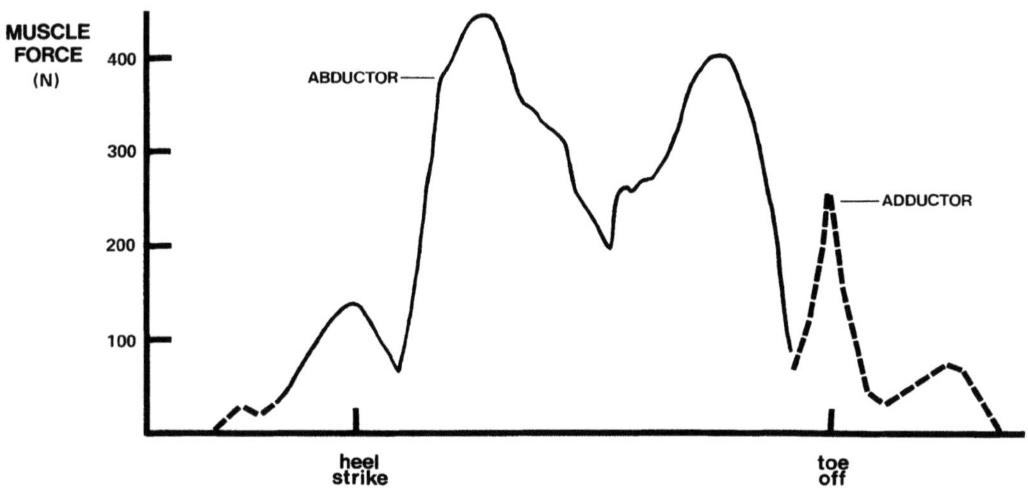

B

FIG. 5–6 **A** Variations in muscle tension about the hip joint during the gait cycle. Note the heel strike and toe off. **B** Tension in the abductor and adductor muscles during walking, one gait cycle. (From Paul.[25])

Surface Joint Motion

Surface motion in the hip joint may be viewed as the sliding of the femoral head on the acetabulum. This sliding of the joint surfaces is produced by the pivoting action of the ball-and-socket configuration in three planes around the center of rotation of the femoral head.[3] If incongruity occurs, for instance, in the femoral head—with a displaced center of rotation—sliding may not be parallel or

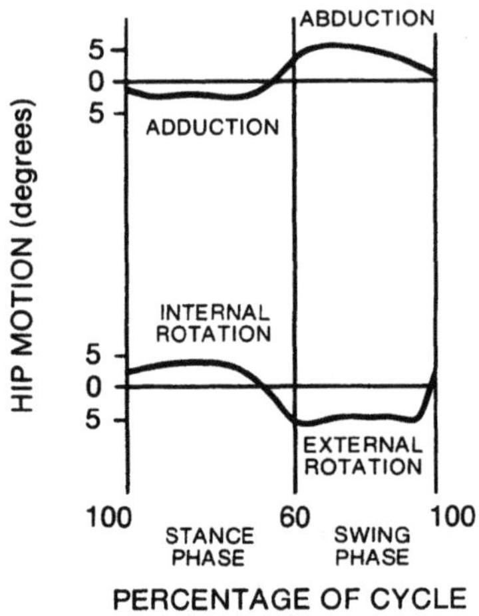

FIG. 5–7 A typical pattern for range of motion in the frontal (**top**) and transverse (**bottom**) planes during level walking for one gait cycle. (Adapted from Johnston and Smidt.[20])

tangential to the surface, and the joint cartilage may be abnormally compressed or distracted, creating a plowlike action. An instant center analysis which would detect derangements in a joint such as the knee is not possible in the hip since motion occurs in all three planes simultaneously.

Kinetics

A thorough understanding of the loads imposed on the hip joint is essential in the management of patients with hip disorders. Large forces are imposed on the hip during simple, everyday activities and the balanced distribution of these forces acting on the body depends on a rational neutralization of the forces of gravity by physiological counterforces. The diverse factors and circumstances which produce these considerable forces must be first fully determined if a rational and effective rehabilitation program is to be developed for pathological conditions of the hip.

Kinetics, which involves the application of Newton's laws to the motion of a body that is under the action of specific forces, can be used to analyze the forces acting on the hip joint. Statics, the study of forces acting on a body in equilibrium, and dynamics, the study of forces acting on a body which do not sum to zero, are the two chief analytic methods of kinetics. Kinetic analysis allows the scientist to determine the magnitude and direction of the forces imposed on the hip joint—produced by the muscles, body weight, the connective tissues, and externally applied loads.

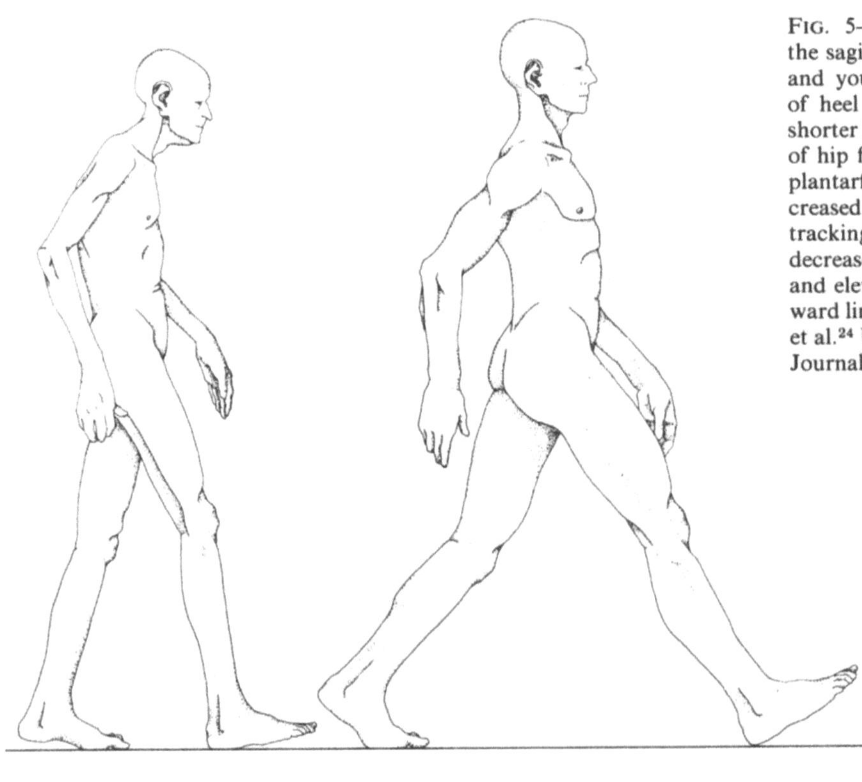

FIG. 5–8 Marked differences in the sagittal body positions of older and younger men at the moment of heel strike. Older men exhibit shorter leg lengths, restricted range of hip flexion-extension, decreased plantarflexion of the ankle, and decreased heel-floor angle of the tracking limb. Older men also show decreased dorsiflexion of the ankle and elevation of the toe of the forward limb. (Adapted from Murray, et al.[24] Used with permission of the Journal of Gerontology.)

More importantly, kinetic analysis can help to identify those loading situations which may produce excessively high, damaging forces.

The two main methods for determining joint reaction force imposed on the head of the femur are the free body technique for coplanar forces and the moment method with the use of equilibrium equations.

Statics: Free Body Technique

Static analysis may be performed for the hip joint under any loading configuration. A simplified technique—the free body analysis—allows the three principal coplanar forces to be determined by considering one portion of the body as discrete and distinct from the entire body.[17] A free body diagram of the upper body and lower supporting limb is drawn (Fig. 5–9) and, through the use of vectors, leads to the identification and determination of the three principal coplanar forces acting on the free body. The forces are designated as vectors since specific characteristics are known: magnitude, sense, and direction—or line of application and point of application. By using the lines of application a triangle of forces can be drawn, and since in a static or equilibrium situation the coplanar forces are concurrent and intersect at a common point, the magnitude of all three coplanar forces can be scaled from this construction. To estimate the joint reaction force in the frontal plane on the femoral head during a single-leg stance with the pelvis in neutral position, the three main forces would be identified as the force of gravity (W = ground reaction force) against the foot which is transmitted through the tibia to the femoral condyles, the force produced by the contraction of the abductor muscles (M), and the joint reaction force on the head of the femur (J). Scaling the triangle of forces determines that the muscle force is approximately 2 × body weight and the joint force is 2.75 × body weight.

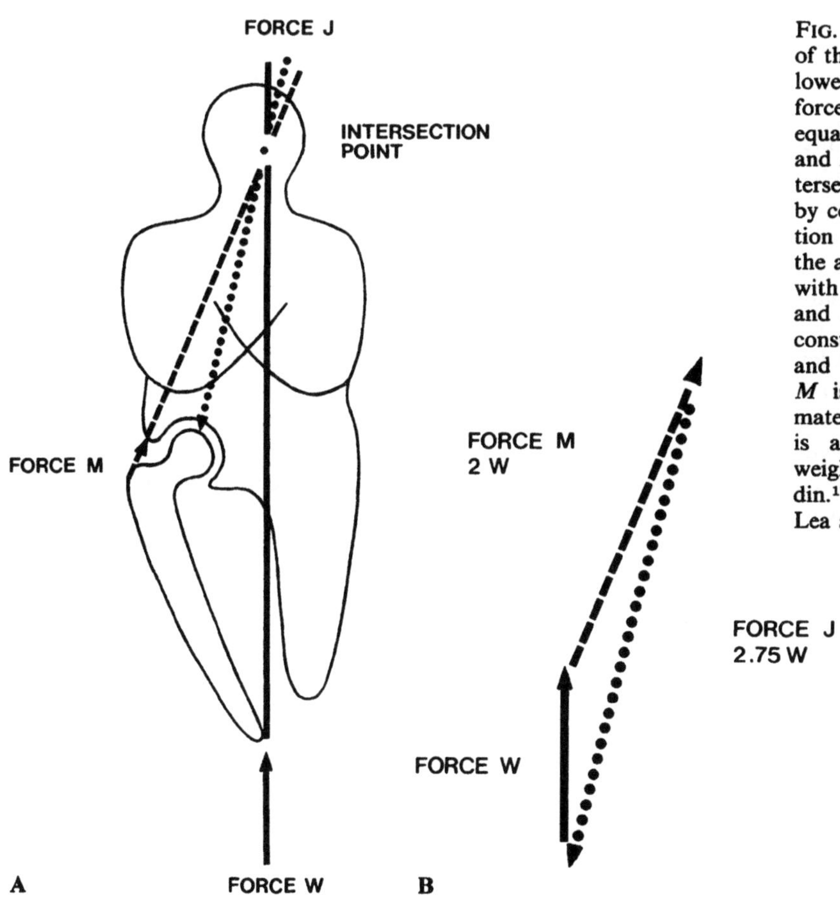

Fig. 5–9 **A** A free body diagram of the upper body and supporting lower limb. Lines of application for forces W (ground reaction force, equal to five-sixths body weight) and M (abductor muscle force) intersect, and force J is determined by connecting its point of application (the point of contact between the acetabulum and femoral head) with the intersection of lines for W and M. **B** A triangle of forces is constructed. The magnitudes of M and J are scaled from W. Force M is determined to be approximately 2 × body weight, while J is approximately 2.75 × body weight. (From Frankel and Nordin.[17] Used with permission from Lea and Febiger.)

Statics: Moment Method Analysis

A method of calculating the internal joint forces which is related to the free body technique is the moment method analysis. The moment method calculates the moments (the quantity required to angularly accelerate a body, in newton meters) acting on the hip during a single-leg stance by using an equilibrium equation. The derived knowledge of the moments then enables the investigator to determine the joint reaction force on the head of the femur. In a moment method analysis of the hip, the body is separated into distinct upper and lower free bodies. Roentgenograms are used to derive the gravitational force lever arm with intersecting plumb lines from the heel, the femoral head, and the gluteus medius. The direction of the muscle force of the gluteus medius is found, for example, to be 30° to the vertical. Then, from vector analysis and simple mathematical calculations,[10] the vertical and horizontal components of all forces acting on both free bodies are identified and determined. The joint reaction force on the femoral head in a single-leg stance with pelvis level is finally identified, for example, to be 2.75 × body weight while its direction is 69° from the horizontal.

Another essential factor influencing the magnitude of the joint reaction force on the femoral head is the ratio of the abductor muscle force lever arm to the gravitational force lever arm. The relationship of this ratio to the joint reaction force is shown in Fig. 5–10. Smaller ratios produce higher joint reaction forces on the femoral head than do large ratios. A short lever arm—as found in coxa valga—will result in a small ratio, and consequently a higher joint reaction force. Conversely, manipulating the greater trochanter laterally during total hip replacement will increase the lever arm ratio and thus lower the overall joint reaction force. Finally, setting a prosthetic cup deeper into the acetabulum will reduce the gravitational lever arm, thereby increasing the ratio and decreasing the joint reaction force. It is, however, very difficult to significantly reduce the joint reaction force on the femoral head by altering the lever arm ratio, as the curve becomes asymptotic when the ratio of c to b nears 0.8.

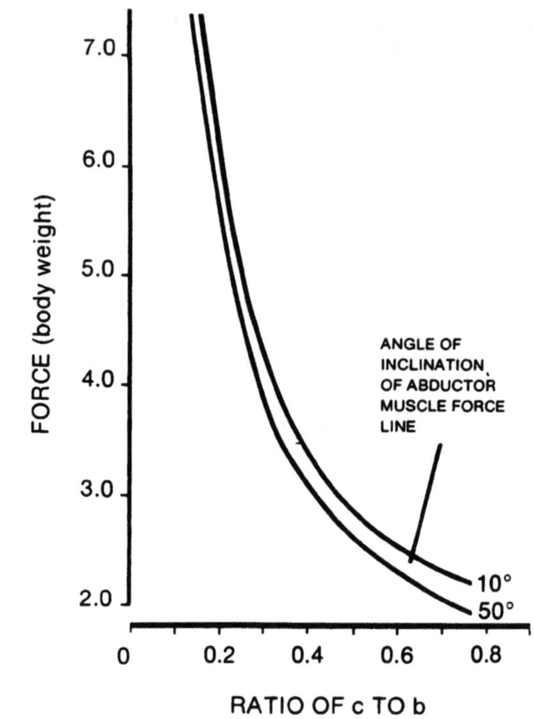

FIG. 5–10 The value of the ratio of the abductor muscle force lever arm (c) to the gravitational force lever arm (b) plotted against the joint reaction force on the femoral head in multiples of body weight. The force curve is plotted since it is known that the direction of the abductor muscle force has finite upper and lower limits of 10–50°. The curve can be used to determine the minimal force imposed on the femoral head during a one-leg stance if the ratio of c to b is known. (Adapted from Frankel.[13])

The ratio of the abductor muscle force lever arm (c) to the gravitational force lever arm (b) can also be determined with the use of roentgenograms and a plumbline. The ratio of c to b in a patient with degenerative arthritis in a single-leg stance is significantly altered after total hip surgery. After total hip replacement the line of gravity for a superincumbent body shifts laterally away from the affected hip joint as the patient assumes a more normal body alignment, having been relieved of the previous hip joint pain by the prosthetic replacement. The shift in the line of gravity increases the gravitational force lever arm and thus reduces the ratio of c to b. In one patient, where the direction of the muscle force was 15° to the vertical, the ratio of c to b before prosthetic replacement was 7.0 and the joint reaction force about 2.2 × body weight. After surgery, the ratio was reduced to 6.0 and the joint reaction force was approximately 2.5 × body weight.

Dynamics

The loads on the femoral head have been studied in static situations and were demonstrated to be considerably higher than body weight—up to 2.75 × body weight in a single-leg stance. Since large forces exist in static situations, the forces required to produce the accelerations during dynamic activities will impose even higher loads on the femoral head.

Several investigators have studied the forces imposed on the femoral head during dynamic activities.[25,28-30,32] Using a force plate system and kinematic data for the normal hip Paul [25] studied the joint reaction force on the femoral head during gait in normal men and women and correlated the peak magnitudes with specific muscle activities that were recorded electromyographically. In the group of men two peak forces were generated during the stance phase when the abductor muscles contracted to stabilize the pelvis. A peak of approximately 4.0 × body weight occurred just after heel strike and another, greater magnitude of about 7.0 × body weight was attained just before toe off (Fig. 5–11A). When the foot was flat the joint reaction force decreased to less than body weight due to the rapid lowering of the body's center of gravity. In the swing phase the joint reaction force was produced by contraction of the extensor muscles which were engaged in decelerating the thigh mass; the magnitude here was low, about equal to body weight.

In the group of women studied the force pattern was similar but the magnitudes were significantly lower, attaining a maximum of only 4.0 × body weight in the late stance phase (Fig. 5–11B). This lower magnitude of joint force may be attributed to several factors: a wider pelvis in females, a difference in the inclination of the neck–shaft angle, a difference in foot wear, and general differences in the gait pattern.

In an earlier study by Rydell [29] intravital measurements recorded through an instrumented prosthesis also demonstrated that a large joint reaction force acts on the femoral head during the late stance phase of a gait cycle. More importantly, the study indicated that at a faster pace the forces imposed on the prosthesis were greatly increased due to a proportional increase in muscle activity (Fig. 5–12). The forces recorded in the swing phase were about half the magnitude of the forces during the late stance phase.

In a more recent study [28] the angular and linear accelerations recorded through a computerized video motion analysis system were correlated with such data as mass characteristics of the body segments. Joint reaction forces derived through simple algorithms were plotted by the computer throughout the cycle of gait motion for the hip and the knee. Forces imposed on the hip joint—joint force plots—were depicted as multiples of body weight (Fig. 5–13). It was found that the joint reaction force imposed on the hip during the cycle for a patient with a Trendelenburg gait was about 5.0 × body weight. The antalgic gait pattern indicated forces that were below 2.0 × body weight, while the joint force for a normal gait pattern was recorded as approximately 4.0 × body weight. The greater forces in the Trendelenburg condition are accounted for by the pelvic sag over the affected hip, which displaces the center of gravity while simultaneously increasing the abductor muscle force. For further investigation, the kinematic data from the angular and linear accelerations are coupled with the mass characteristics of the body segments, and simple calculations yield an accurate description of the muscle forces required to produce propulsion. The muscle forces are then used to determine the joint forces throughout the cycle of motion, and the resultant data are consistent with data recorded by instrumented endoprostheses and by force plates.

In yet another study, an instrumented nail plate was used to measure the forces acting on a radiotelemeterized internal fixation device during common everyday activities following osteotomy or fracture of the femoral neck (Fig. 5–14).[14,21] The instrumented device measured forces on the nail plate but not on the hip joint itself. Through static analysis, however, it was possible to calculate the proportion of the load imposed on the implant and also to determine the total load imposed on the hip joint. In the case depicted in Fig. 5–14 the instrumented device transmitted one-fourth of the total load.[17]

Such diverse activities as raising onto a bedpan, transferral to a wheelchair, and walking imposed very large forces on the appliance. The magnitude of these forces was markedly modified by the skillful handling of the nurse or therapist, and by the patient's deliberate control. By far the largest forces encountered were those produced when the patient used his elbows and heels to lift himself onto a bedpan—imposing a force of about 47.5

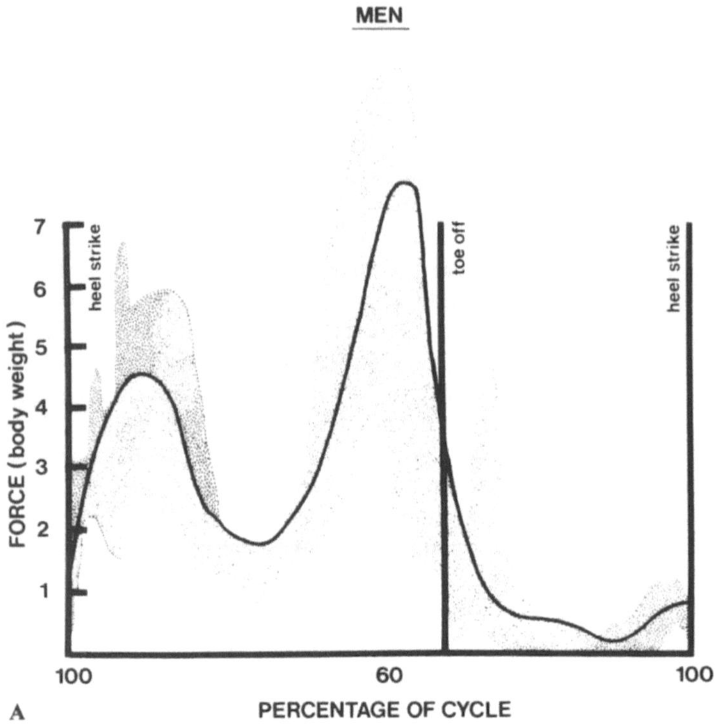

A

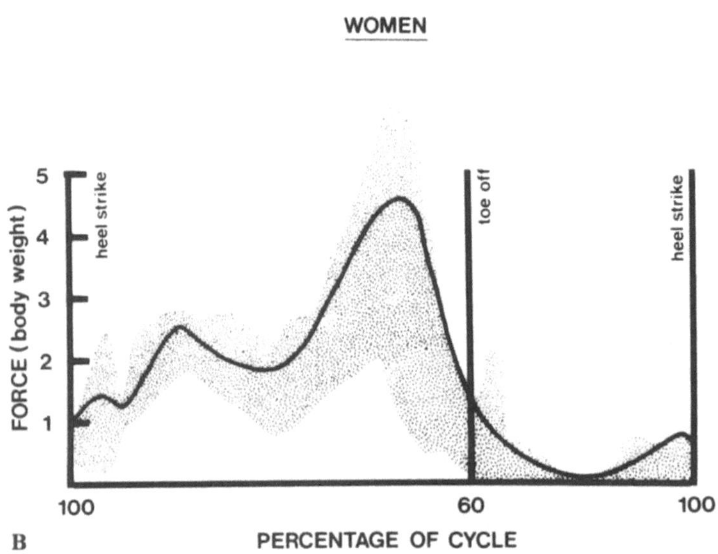

B

FIG. 5–11 Hip joint reaction force measured in multiples of body weight during walking for one gait cycle. Shaded portions indicate variations among subjects. **A** Joint force pattern for men. **B** Joint force pattern for women. (Adapted from Paul.[25])

kg_f on the device. Forces of up to 4.0 × body weight were imposed on the hip joint during the activity. Large forces were also encountered when the patient transferred himself from the bed to a wheelchair. Indeed, these abnormally high forces were greatly mitigated when a trapeze and an attendant were used to assist the patient onto the bedpan, and during the transfer.[21] Exercises of the hip—straight leg raising and hip flexion—on the operative leg in the fourth postoperative week produced high loads on the implant and great forces on the hip joint. It was found that foot and ankle exercises also imposed increased forces on the head of the femur. Overall, the use of a hip spica cast

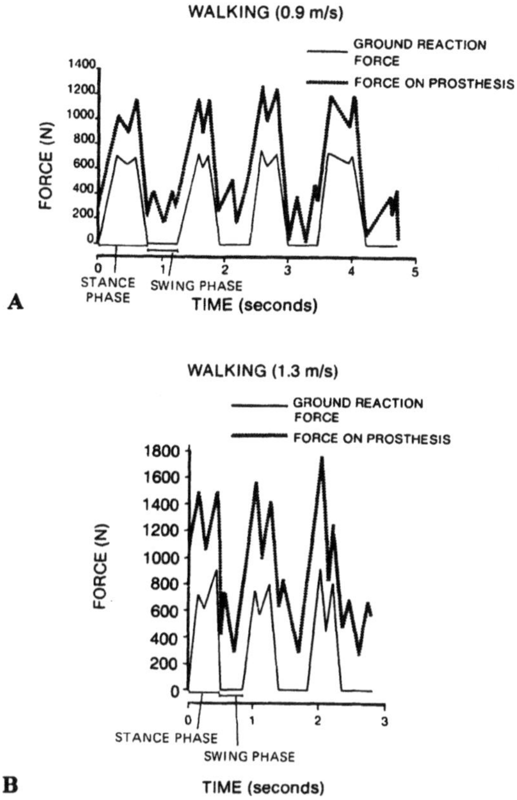

FIG. 5–12 Forces on an instrumented prosthesis during level walking. The solid line represents the ground reaction force and the broken line represents the force imposed on the prosthesis. **A** The walking speed is 0.9 m/s. **B** The walking speed is 1.3 m/s. (Adapted from Rydell.[29])

reduced the forces acting on the hip joint by two-thirds for all activities, but forces generated by muscle contraction were still present on a relatively low scale.

The instrumented nail plate study demonstrated that for a bedridden patient with a fractured femoral neck or an osteotomy, the forces acting on the femoral head during common daily activities were almost similar in magnitude to the forces acting on the implanted device during walking with external supports. Moreover, it was found that the magnitude of the moments acting on the nail plate junction in the horizontal plane was approximately one-half the magnitude of the moments acting on the vertical plane during various activities (Fig. 5–15).

Effects of External Support on the Hip Joint Reaction Force

Several studies [4,9,26] found through static analysis of the joint reaction force that when a cane is used it should be used on the opposite side of the painful or operated hip. More recently, using kinematic data from stroboscopic studies and torque calculations, it was demonstrated [17] that when a brace is used on the leg it does not necessarily reduce the joint reaction force on the femoral head. It was determined that, for an 8-year-old boy weighing 24 kg and wearing a long-leg brace, the joint reaction force on the femoral head in the braced limb was over 50% higher than the force produced by the nonbraced limb. The joint reaction force on the femoral head is equal to the muscle force (the extensor muscle force) minus the gravitational force. The muscle forces were 338 newtons for the nonbraced limb and 600 newtons for the braced limb, while the gravitational force was 40 newtons, thus making the joint reaction force on the nonbraced limb 298 newtons and on the braced limb 560 newtons.

Failure Criteria for Implant Materials

If one wishes to match or simulate properties of implant materials with those of the existing collagenous structures, precise data concerning the stress-strain-energy relationships under physiological strain and load rates are required. Three types of failure characteristics for internal fixation devices and prostheses are usually considered: brittle, plastic, and fatigue. Figure 5–16 depicts the load deformation curves for different types of materials. Brittle failure occurs when an implant behaves as if it were a material such as glass, instead of a material exhibiting plasticity. The nail plate in Fig. 5–17 broke when the patient was dropped 2 inches onto an x-ray table. A nail plate, however, may also deform plastically; it absorbs energy by yielding without fracturing. Fatigue failure of an implant occurs when a material is cyclically loaded and a minute crack is produced. Multiple small cracks form and coalesce, finally breaking the device as a result of increased fatigue.

Recent experimental tests of the mechanical failure of bone cement have been performed.[27] The

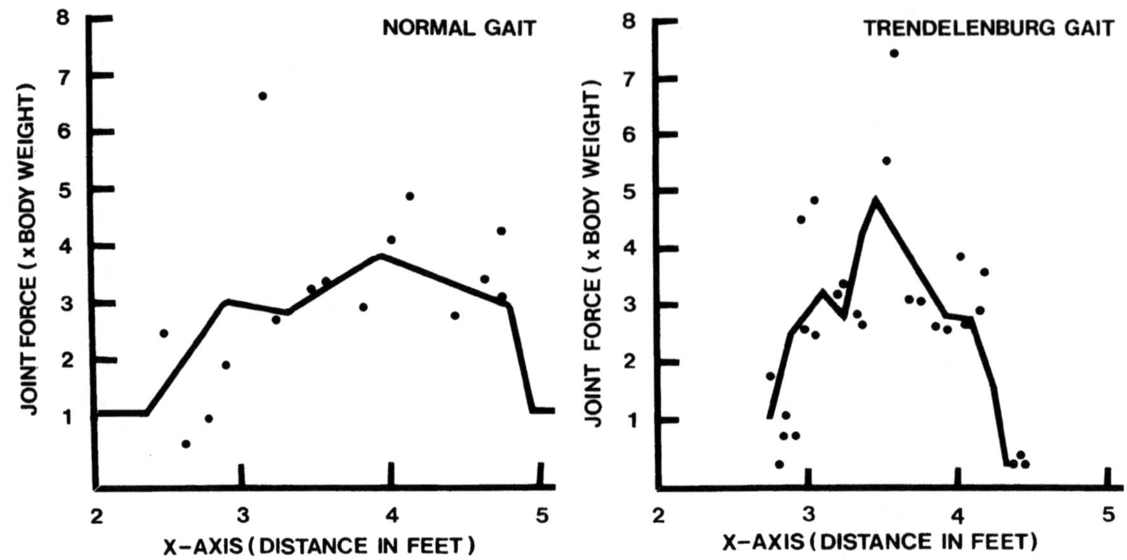

A B

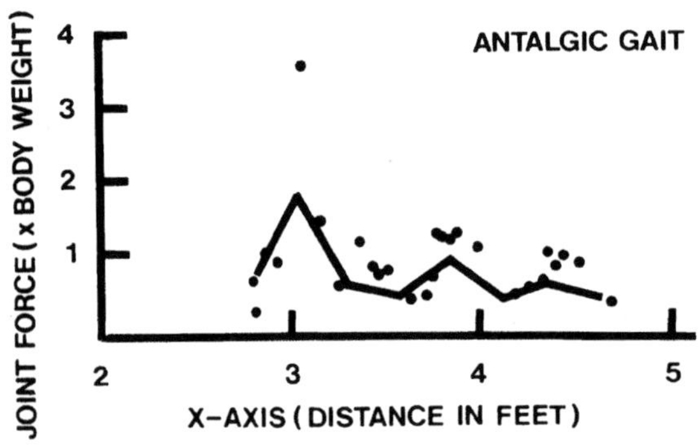

C

FIG. 5–13 Hip joint force plots depicted as multiples of body weight, produced by computerized video motion analysis. The forces acting on the hip joint are shown for a normal gait pattern (**A**), a Trendelenburg gait pattern (**B**), and an antalgic gait pattern (**C**). (From Pugh et al.[28])

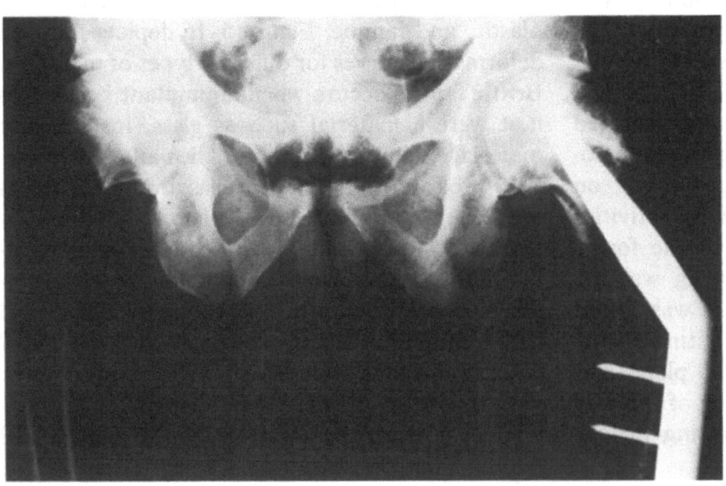

FIG. 5–14 An instrumented nail plate in the upper end of the femur, used to determine the forces imposed on the implant during common everyday activities following fracture of the femoral neck. In this case the nail plate was found to transmit one-fourth of the total load on the hip joint. (Adapted from Frankel and Nordin.[17])

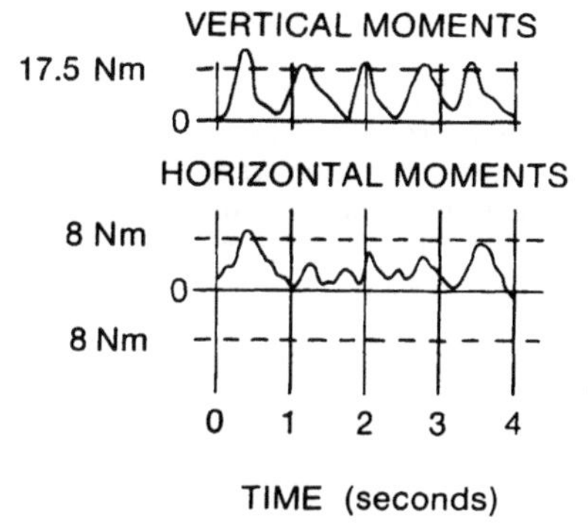

FIG. 5–15 Moments acting on the nail plate junction in the vertical and horizontal planes during unassisted walking. (Adapted from Frankel and Nordin.[17])

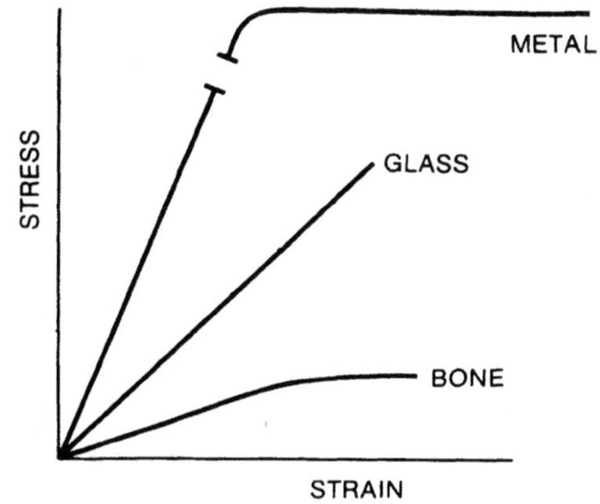

FIG. 5–16 Stress–strain curves for metal, glass, and bone. Stiffness is depicted by the slope of the curve in the elastic regions. For bone, the elastic region is slightly curved, indicating that bone is not linearly elastic in its behavior. Soft metal, which is ductile, has a long elastic region, whereas glass, a brittle material, has no elastic region.

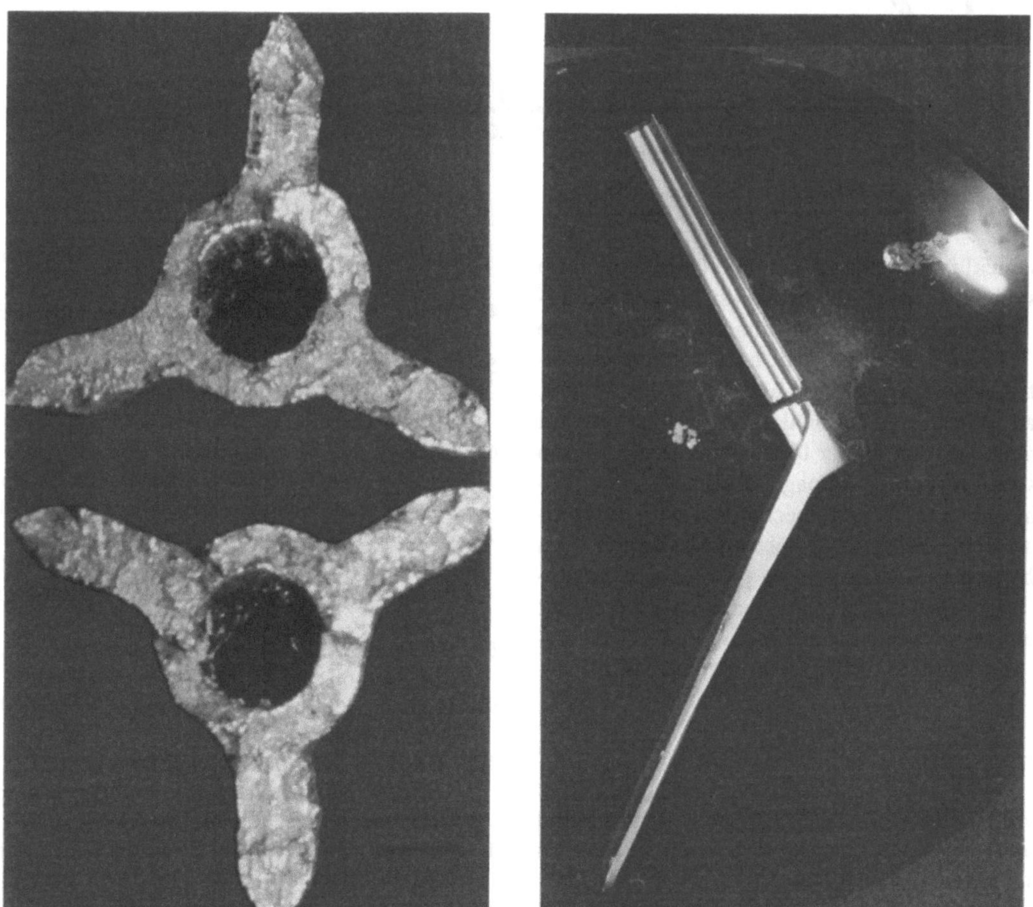

FIG. 5–17 Fracture of the nail plate followed dropping the patient 2 inches onto an x-ray table.

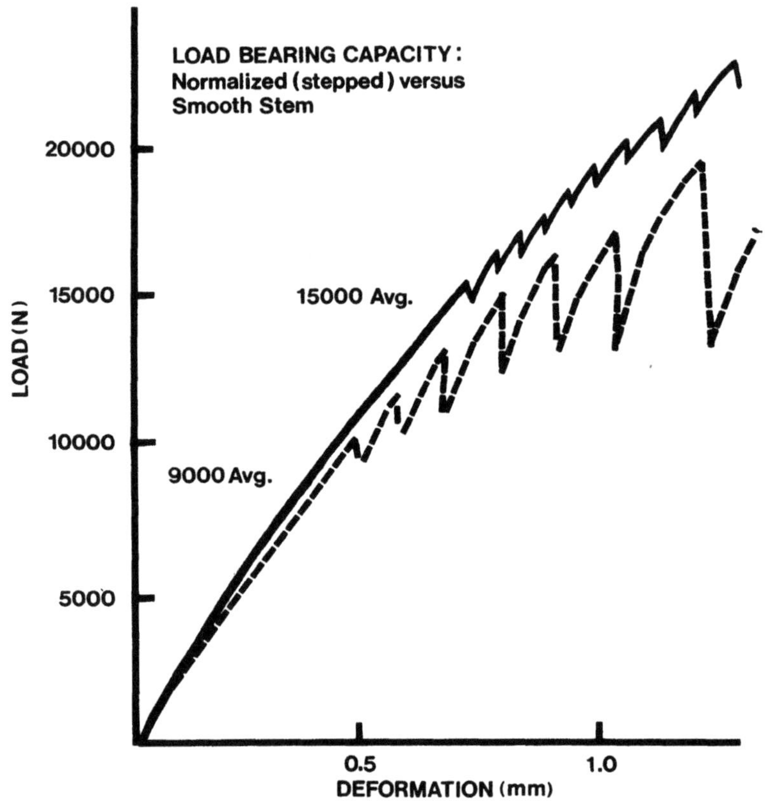

FIG. 5–18 The increased load-bearing potential of a stepped stem prosthesis vs. the conventional smooth stem prosthesis. The solid line represents the stepped stem, and the broken line the smooth stem. (From Pugh, et al.[27] Used with permission from Osteonics Corp.)

mechanical failure of bone cement, caused by hoop stress on the stem of the prosthesis, produced adverse bony reactions and ultimately failure of the stem. Through finite element analysis and modeling it was determined that a stepped taper stem, instead of the conventional taper system, would accommodate the higher loads generated by hoop stress by preventing slippage (Fig. 5–18).

The application of biomechanical data, in addition to being essential in prosthesis design, can also be useful in such diverse problems as pathogenesis of degenerative joint disease, management of the postfracture patient, bracing in Perthes' disease, and in many other pathological conditions.

Bibliography

1. Alffram, P. A.: An epidemiologic study of cervical and trochanteric fractures of the femur in an urban projection. Acta Orthop. Scand., Suppl. 65, 1964.
2. Backman, S.: The proximal end of the femur. Acta Radiol., Suppl. 146, 1957.
3. Bartel, D. L., and Johnston, R. C.: Mechanical analysis and optimization of a cup arthroplasty. J. Biomech., 2:97, 1969.
4. Blount, W. P.: Don't throw away the cane. J. Bone Joint Surg., 38A:695, 1956.
5. Carter, D. R., and Hayes, W. C.: The compressive behavior of bone as a two-phase porous structure. J. Bone Joint Surg., 59A:954, 1977.
6. Chamay, A.: Mechanical and Morphological Aspects of Experimental Overload and Fatigue in Bone, Vol. 3. London, Pergamon Press, 1970.
7. Contini, R., Gage, H. N., and Drillis, R.: Human gait characteristics. In: Biomechanics and Related Bioengineering Topics. London, Pergamon Press, 1965.
8. Currey, J. D.: The mechanical properties of bone. Clin. Orthop., 24:72, 1970.
9. Denham, R. A.: Hip mechanics. J. Bone Joint Surg., 41B:550, 1959.
10. Drillis, R., Contini, R., and Bluestein, M.: Body segment parameters. A survey of measurement techniques. Artif. Limbs, 8:44, 1964.
11. Evans, F. G.: Stress and Strain in Bones. Springfield, Ill., Thomas, 1957.
12. Evans, F. G., and Vincentelli, R.: Relation of collagen fiber orientation to some mechanical properties of human cortical bone. J. Biomech., 2:63, 1969.

13. Frankel, V. H.: The Femoral Neck: Function, Fracture Mechanisms, Internal Fixation. Springfield, Ill., Thomas, 1960.
14. Frankel, V. H.: Mechanical fixation of unstable fractures about the proximal end of the femur. Bull. Hosp. Joint Dis., 24:1, 1963.
15. Frankel, V. H., and Burstein, A. H.: Force and energetics of femoral neck fractures. Proceedings Dixieme Congres International de Chirurgie Orthopedique et de Traumatologie, Paris, 1966.
16. Frankel, V. H., and Burstein, A. H.: Orthopaedic Biomechanics. Philadelphia, Lea & Febiger, 1970.
17. Frankel, V. H., and Nordin, M.: Basic Biomechanics of the Skeletal System. Philadelphia, Lea & Febiger, 1980.
18. Frisen, M., Magi, M., Sonnerup, L., and Viidik, A.: Rheological analysis of soft collagenous tissues. J. Biomech., 2:13, 1969.
19. Inman, V. T.: Functional aspects of the abductor muscles of the hip. J. Bone Joint Surg., 29:607, 1947.
20. Johnston, R. C., and Smidt, G. L.: Measurement of hip joint motion during walking. Evaluation of an electrogoniometric method. J. Bone Joint Surg., 51A:1083, 1969.
21. Lygre, L.: The loads produced on the hip joint by nursing procedures: A telemeterization study. M.S. thesis (nursing), Case Western Reserve University, 1970.
22. McLaughlin, T., and Frankel, V. H.: A parametric study of the strength of the upper end of the femur. Unpublished data, 1970.
23. Murray, M. P.: Gait as a total pattern of movement. Amer. J. Phys. Med., 46:290, 1967.
24. Murray, M. P., Kory, R. C., and Clarkson, B. H.: Walking patterns in healthy old men. J. Gerontol., 24:169, 1969.
25. Paul, J. P.: Forces at the human hip joint. Thesis, University of Chicago, 1967.
26. Pauwels, F.: Der Schenkelhalsbruch, ein mechanisches Problem. Stuttgart, Enke, 1936.
27. Pugh, J., Averill, R., Pachtman, N., Bartel, D., and Jaffe, W.: Prothesis surface design to resist loosening; stress normalization. Technical Info. Bulletin, Osteonics Corp., New Jersey, 1982.
28. Pugh, J. P., Miller A., Tauber, C., and Au, J.: Static and dynamic analysis of forces acting on the hip joint during the gait cycle. A computerized video motion evaluation. Division of Bioengineering internal report, 1982. Available from authors.
29. Rydell, N. W.: Forces acting on the femoral head prosthesis. Acta Orthop. Scand., Suppl. 88, 1966.
30. Rydell, N. W.: Forces in the hip joint. In: Biomechanics and Related Bioengineering Topics. London, Pergamon Press, 1965, pp. 351–357.
31. Sedlin, E. D.: A rheological model for cortical bone. Acta Orthop. Scand., Suppl. 83, 1965.
32. Seirig, A., and Arvikar, R. J.: The prediction of muscular load sharing and joint forces in the lower extremities during walking. J. Biomech., 8:89, 1975.
33. Singh, M., Nagrath, A. R., and Naini, P. S.: Changes in trabecular pattern of the upper end of the femur as an index of osteoporosis. J. Bone Joint Surg., 52A:457, 1970.
34. Smith, L. D.: Hip fractures: A role of muscle contraction or intrinsic forces in the causation of fractures in the femoral neck. J. Bone Joint Surg., 35A:367, 1953.

CHAPTER 6

The Blood Supply of the Upper End of the Human Femur, Including Observations on the Venous Drainage of the Femoral Head

HENRY VERNON CROCK AND D. ROBERT V. DICKENS

The practical importance of the blood supply of some bones and their related soft tissues has led, in recent years, to the spectacular successes of microsurgical operations for the viable transpositioning of tissues from one part of the body to another. Although anatomists and orthopedic surgeons have continued to study the blood supply of the human hip joint since 1950, their efforts have been directed almost exclusively at the arterial side of this circulatory system. Meanwhile, radiological investigations designed to demonstrate the veins of the hip joint have failed to provide anatomically conclusive information.

The blood supply of the hip joint has consequently failed to attract the attention of practicing surgeons, nor is any significant attention paid to the teaching of this subject in most orthopedic training programs. The ultimate proof of its neglect and relegation to academic insignificance can be seen in the scant reference made to the arterial supply of the hip in many papers dealing with such important clinical problems as Perthes' disease, slipped upper femoral epiphysis, and intracapsular fractures of the neck of the femur—in which the authors usually refer to Trueta's work,[11] citing nomenclature long since shown to be incorrect by Lagrange and Dunoyer,[10] Crock,[4] and Chung.[1] On the contrary this anatomy is crucial to better appreciating the pathophysiology of these disease entities.

In this chapter the arterial supply of the head and neck of the femur in man will be described in detail, using terminology which supersedes that described previously by the Oxford school.[12,13] Observations on the venous drainage of the adult femoral head will be presented from previously unpublished work of Crock and Dickens, carried out in the Department of Surgery, St. Vincent's Hospital, within the University of Melbourne.

Origins of the Arteries Supplying the Upper End of the Femur

The medial and lateral femoral circumflex arteries are large branches of either the femoral or profunda femoris arteries. They are destined to supply most of the neck and head of the femur, with supplementary vessels in the ligament of the femoral head, usually derived from the obturator arteries. The importance of the macroscopic anatomy of these vessels has been stressed in the excellent paper by Howe and associates.[10]

The base of the femoral neck, at the level of the capsular attachments of the hip joint, is surrounded by a ring of arteries. The posterior circumference of the extracapsular arterial ring of the femoral neck is usually formed by a large, well-defined branch of the medial femoral circumflex artery, while anteriorly it is completed by branches of the lateral femoral circumflex artery (Fig. 6–1). Branches arise from this extracapsular arterial ring at regular intervals around its circumference, to enter the hip joint by passing through apertures in the capsule close to its insertion into bone. These ascending cervical branches pass upward along the femoral neck or downward and laterally from it, to supply the trochanters at the base of the neck.

The ascending cervical branches of the extracapsular arterial ring of the femoral neck penetrate

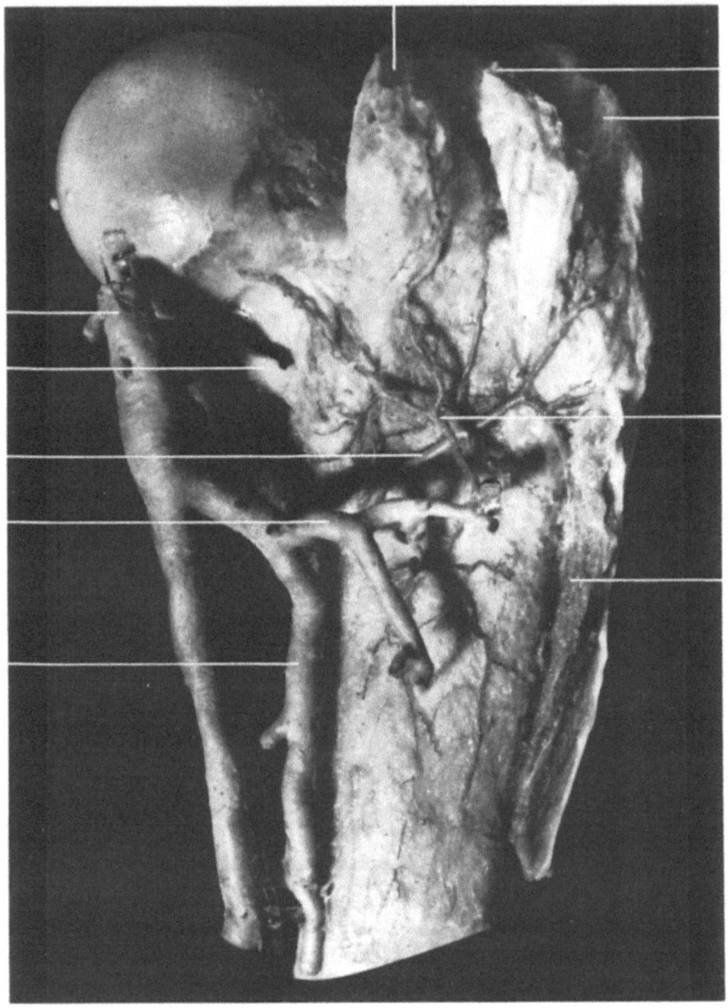

A

FIG. 6–1 **A** The anterior aspect of the upper end of the femur of a 50-year-old man. Arteries injected with red latex rubber. Dissected by Dr. S. Schofield. Reprinted with permission from Crock, H. V.: J. Anat. (Lond.), 99:86, 1965; and Crock, H. V.: The Blood Supply of the Lower Limb Bones in Man. Edinburgh, Livingstone, 1967. Iliofemoral ligament; gluteus medius; ascending branch of arterial ring of femoral neck; vastus lateralis; profunda femoris artery; lateral femoral circumflex artery; arterial ring of the femoral neck; capsule of the hip joint; femoral artery. **B** Posterior aspect of the specimen illustrated in **A.** Reprinted with permission from Crock, H. V.: J. Anat. (London.), 99:86, 1965; and Crock, H. V.: The Blood Supply of the Lower Limb Bones in Man. Edinburgh, Livingstone, 1967. Iliofemoral ligament; ligament of the head; ascending cervical branches of the arterial ring of the femoral neck; arterial ring of the femoral neck; medial femoral circumflex artery; lesser trochanter; profunda femoris artery; adductor brevis; perforating artery; superior nutrient artery; adductor magnus; gluteus maximus; vastus lateralis; obturator externus; orbicular zone; obturator internus and gemelli; gluteus medius; piriformis.

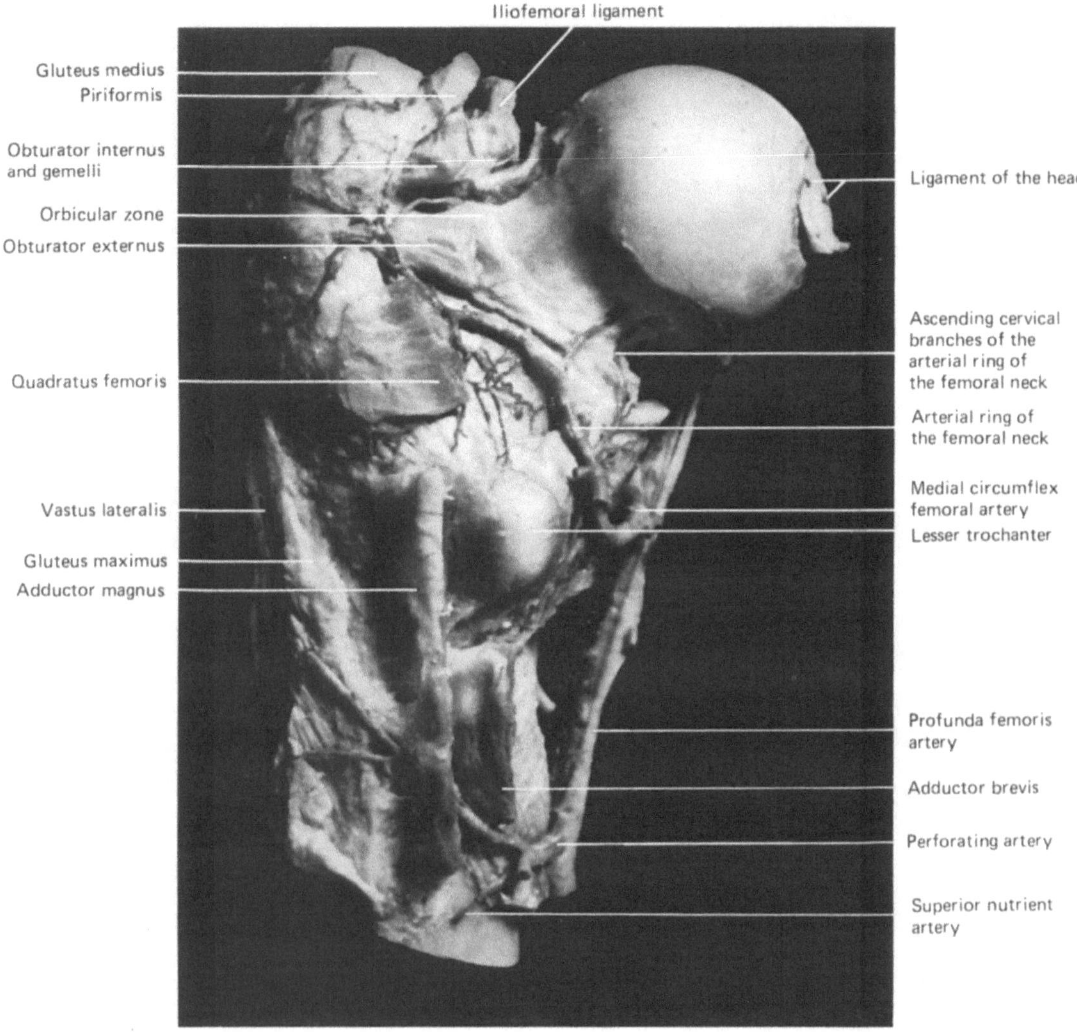

B

the capsule of the hip joint along the intertrochanteric line anteriorly, and on the posterior aspect they pass beneath the orbicular fibers of the capsule to run upward under the synovial reflection toward the articular cartilage rim which demarcates the femoral head from its neck. From these vessels arise the metaphyseal and epiphyseal arteries of the upper end of the femur.

In the most recent significant contribution to the study of the arterial supply of the upper end of the femur, Chung [1] has added an important dimension to the description of the anastomotic rings of arteries which are found in this area. He describes an extracapsular arterial ring formed by the medial and lateral femoral circumflex arteries, in accordance with Crock's [4,5,6] descriptions of the arterial ring of the femoral neck. There is also a subsynovial intraarticular arterial ring at the hyaline cartilage neck junction to which Chung has drawn attention for the first time. Disruption of this arterial ring may have particular significance in hip diseases, such as slipped upper femoral epiphysis in children, in high intracapsular fractures of the neck of the femur, and in the adult, hitherto unrecognized importance in the applied anatomy of femoral head blood supply in operations for surface replacement of the femoral head (Figs. 6–2 and 6–8).

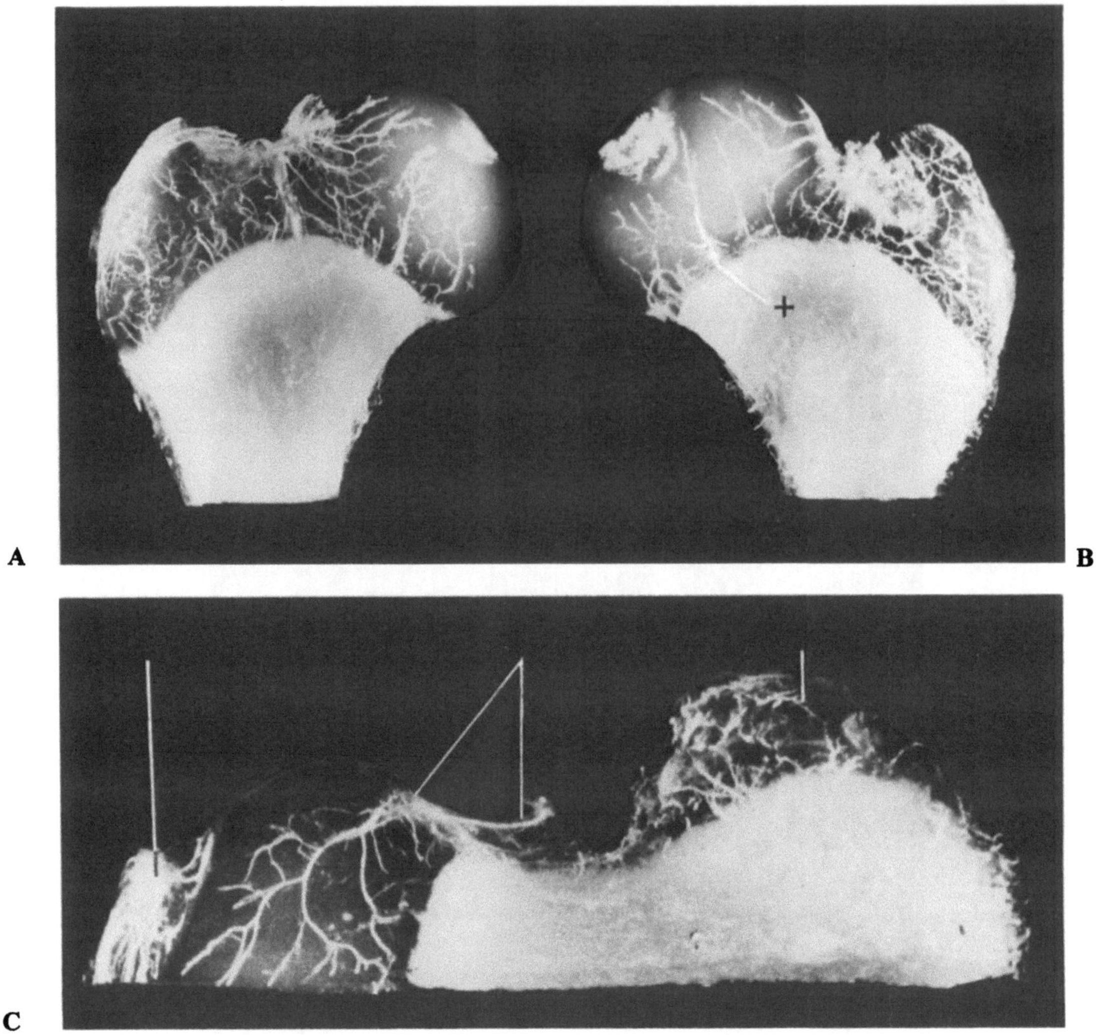

FIG. 6–2 The anterior (**A**) and posterior (**B**) halves of the upper end of the femur of a five-day-old girl. Coronal section. Arterial injection. Spalteholz cleared specimen, (× 2). The upper end of the femoral shaft with its dense injection is clearly demarcated from the femoral head and the greater trochanter. The sinusoidal terminations of the vessels within the epiphyses can be seen. The vessel marked with a cross in **B** is an epiphyseal artery lying on the surface of the femoral neck. Formerly it was described as a metaphyseal artery. Reprinted with permission from Crock, H. V.: J. Anat. (Lond.), 99:86, 1965; and Crock, H. V.: The Blood Supply of the Lower Limb Bones in Man. Edinburgh, Livingstone, 1967. **C** Horizontal section cut from the same specimen (× 3). Note the stem of the epiphyseal artery superficial to the femoral neck and its entry into the epiphysis. The arteries in the round ligament of the head of the femur are also marked. Reprinted with permission from Crock, H. V.: J. Anat. (Lond.), 99:87, 1965; and Crock, H. V.: The Blood Supply of the Lower Limb Bones in Man. Edinburgh, Livingstone, 1967.

The Arterial Supply at Birth

At birth, ossification of the shaft of the femur has extended to a clear-cut expanded upper end with a curved margin which is capped by the cartilaginous epiphyses of the femoral head and greater trochanter. The base of the femoral neck is surrounded by an extracapsular arterial ring from which, as in the adult, ascending cervical branches pass along the neck around its circumference. They penetrate the cartilage of the head, each branch terminating in sinusoidal expansions. All these ascending cervical branches of the extracapsular arterial ring of the femoral neck give rise to epiphyseal and metaphyseal branches. Within epiphyses,

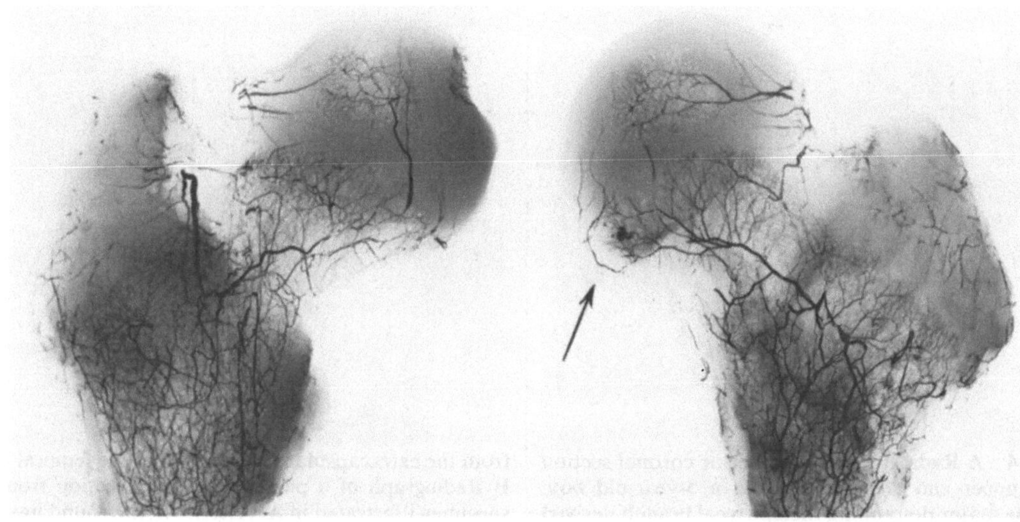

A B

FIG. 6–3 **A** Radiograph of the posterior half of the femoral head of a child, aged approximately 18 months, showing the pattern of arterial circulation in the neck of the femur based on an inferior metaphyseal artery. Epiphyseal vessels entering the femoral head have formed a plexiform pattern of anastomosing vessels in the small center of ossification, while at the margins of the cartilage of the head some of the epiphyseal vessels still terminate independently in cartilage. **B** Radiograph of the anterior half of the same femoral head. Note the epiphyseal arteries entering the inferomedial segment of the head (*arrow*). On the upper aspect of the neck note the well-defined metaphyseal artery derived from the subsynovial intraarticular arterial ring.

no anastomoses between sinusoidal terminations of epiphyseal arteries are found before the secondary centers of ossification appear. The gross vascular patterns which are established at birth remain unchanged throughout life. From birth until closure of the epiphyseal lines, vessels within the bone do not cross between the metaphysis and epiphysis, a major consideration in understanding why an infection in bone remains confined to the metaphysis in children.

The important details of the distribution and termination of arteries within the epiphysis and metaphysis of the femoral head during growth are illustrated in Figs. 6–2 to 6–7.

In the past, most authors have focused more attention on the blood supply of the capital femoral epiphysis and head of the femur than on the neck of the femur. In the present text, it seems appropriate to draw particular attention to the origins and distribution of metaphyseal arteries in the neck of the femur. Notice that some metaphyseal arteries arise from the extracapsular arterial ring of the femoral neck, passing vertically downward toward the center of the femoral shaft where branches anastomose with ascending branches of the superior nutrient artery system (Fig. 6–7B). Other metaphyseal branches spring from the subsynovial intraarticular arterial ring described by Chung. These vessels are well seen in Figs. 6–3B, 6–6, and 6–7B.

The greater trochanter is covered with an arterial plexus based on branches of the medial and lateral femoral circumflex vessels, and inferiorly contributed to by ascending branches of the perforating artery system and superiorly by descending branches of the gluteal system of arteries. In standard anatomical works, considerable attention is paid to the so-called cruciate anastomosis around the hip joint. Study of the material illustrated in this chapter shows that as a concept, this cruciate anastomosis is of little practical significance in the blood supply of the hip joint.

The Arterial Supply in the Adult

During growth, there is an effective anastomosis between epiphyseal and metaphyseal vessels on the surface of the femoral neck. Within the bone the epiphyseal plate constitutes a barrier to anastomoses between vessels supplying the epiphysis and metaphysis until maturity, when the two vascular systems blend (Figs. 6–8 and 6–9). The arterial supply of the upper end of the femur is derived

A 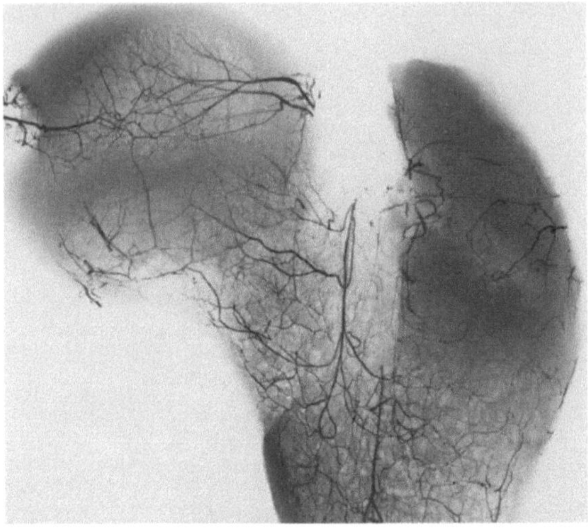 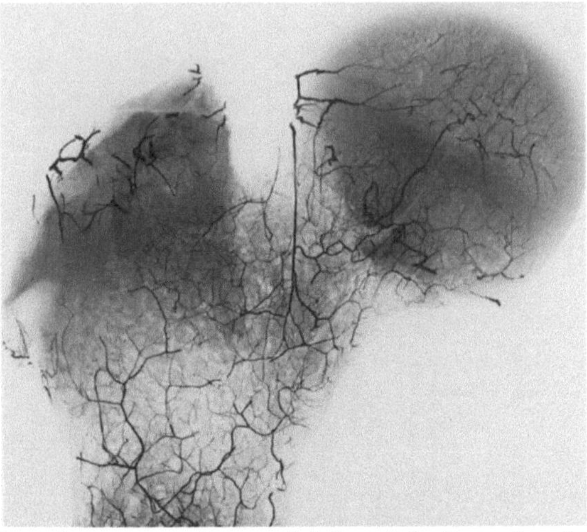 B

FIG. 6–4 **A** Radiograph of an anterior coronal section of the upper end of a femur from a 5-year-old boy. Note the major descending metaphyseal branch derived from the subsynovial intraarticular arterial ring of the femoral neck just below the inferolateral edge of the growth plate. The large artery in the center of the growth plate is an anterior ascending cervical branch derived from the extracapsular arterial ring of the femoral neck. **B** Radiograph of a posterior coronal section from the specimen illustrated in **A.** Arteries in the round ligament have already penetrated the bony nucleus of the femoral head. Note the large descending metaphyseal artery springing from the region of the extracapsular arterial ring of the femoral neck on its superolateral aspect.

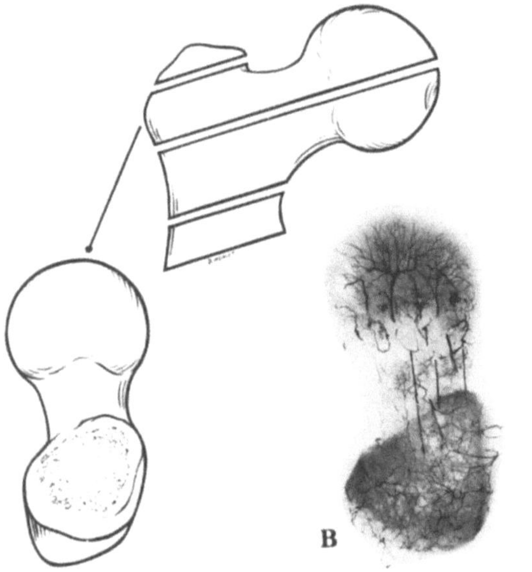

A B

FIG. 6–5 **A** Drawings to illustrate the appearance of of specimens cut horizontally, in the long axis of the neck, from the upper end of the femur, with the sections viewed from above. **B** Radiograph of a superior horizontal section of the head and neck of the femur from a male aged 13 years. The superior tip of the greater trochanter has been removed. The large stems of the four superolateral epiphyseal arteries are clearly seen. Just lateral to these, a row of shorter-stemmed arteries penetrates the superior metaphysis of the femoral neck. These are metaphyseal arteries originating from the subsynovial intraarticular ring of the femoral neck.

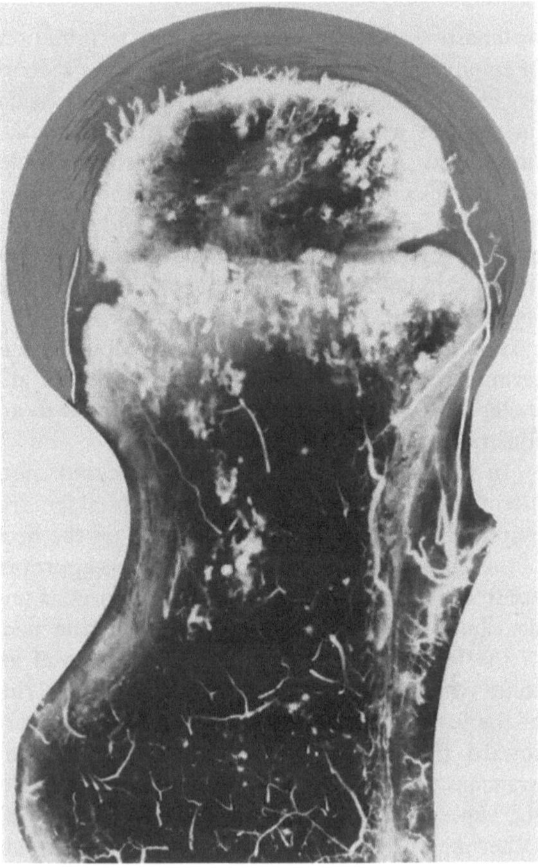

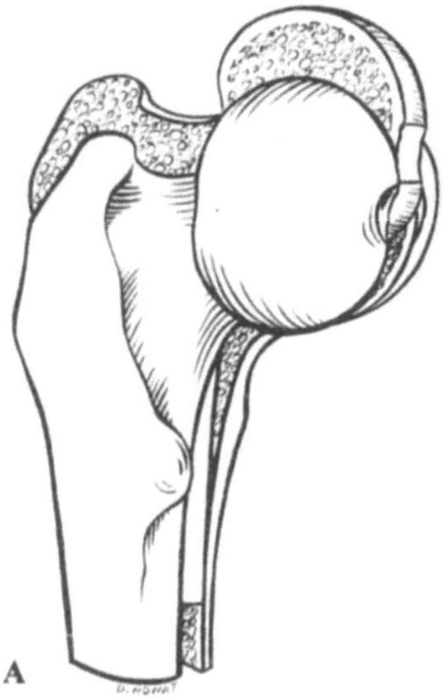

A

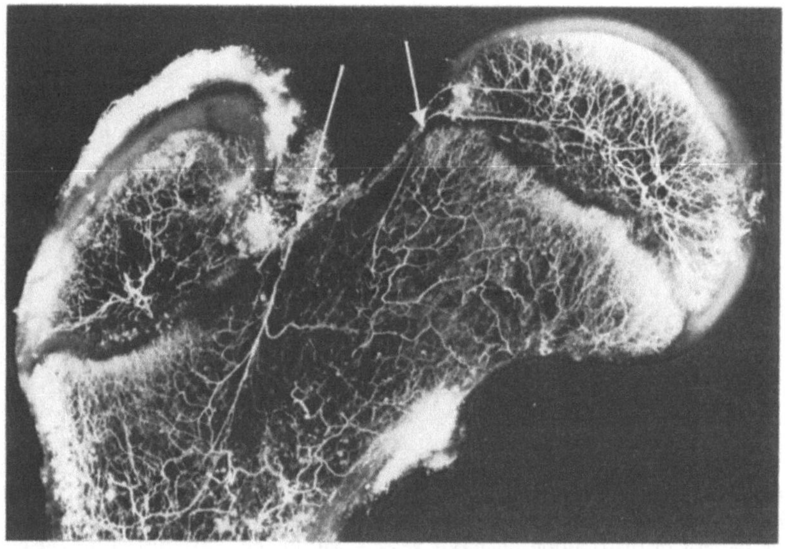

B

FIG. 6–7 **A** A drawing showing the site of removal of a coronal section from the upper end of the femur. Reprinted with permission from Crock, H.V.: J. Anat. (Lond.), 99:80, 1965; and Crock, H.V.: The Blood Supply of the Lower Limb Bones in Man. Edinburgh, Livingstone, 1967. **B** A coronal section (1 cm thick) cut from the upper end of the femur of a 13-year-old boy. Note the anastomosis between the epiphyseal arteries and those of the ligament of the femoral head. The origins of two descending metaphyseal arteries which have arisen respectively from the extracapsular and subsynovial intraarticular rings of the femoral neck are marked by arrows. Reprinted with permission from Crock, H.V.: J. Anat. (Lond.), 99:87, 1965; and Crock, H. V.: The Blood Supply of the Lower Limb Bones in Man. Edinburgh, Livingstone, 1967.

principally from branches of the extracapsular arterial ring of the femoral neck, and from branches of the subsynovial intraarticular ring described by Chung (Fig. 6–10). Arteries running in the ligament of the head of the femur supplement the blood supply of the head.

Branches from the nutrient artery system of the femoral shaft form a loose anastomosis with descending metaphyseal arteries, but they cannot be traced upward into the femoral neck as discrete trunks.

The relationship of the subchondral arterioles in the head of the femur to the main stems of the epiphyseal arteries is clearly shown in coronal and transverse sections (Figs. 6–8 and 6–11).

◀ FIG. 6–6 Horizontal section cut from the upper end of the femur of a 2.5-year-old boy. Note the secondary vascular sprouts from the bony nucleus of the capital epiphysis. New bone will form around these as growth of this secondary center of ossification proceeds. Reprinted with permission from Crock, H.V.: J. Anat. (Lond.), 99:88, 1965; and Crock, H.V.: The Blood Supply of the Lower Limb Bones in Man. Edinburgh, Livingstone, 1967.

Observations on the Venous Drainage of the Adult Human Femoral Head

Complex *subarticular collecting veins* have been described in many of the bones in the human skeleton by Crock,[3,5] Crock and Yoshizawa,[9] and Crock et al.[7,8] A similar system of veins exists in the head of the femur in adult man. These veins are oriented parallel to the subchondral bone plate of the femoral head (Fig. 6–12B). Subchondral capillaries run into venules which drain into this system, the subarticular collecting veins draining off at the fovea and at the articular margin of the head with the femoral neck. In that latter area, a complex aggregation of veins forms in a subsynovial position, corresponding to the subsynovial intraarticular arterial ring of Chung. From this subsynovial intraarticular venous plexus, individual veins of large caliber course down the femoral neck to run through the thick fibers of the capsule of the hip joint at the base of the femoral neck (Fig. 6–12A). Within the femoral head there are some direct connections between the subarticular collecting vein system and the principal veins in the head itself (Fig. 6–12B).

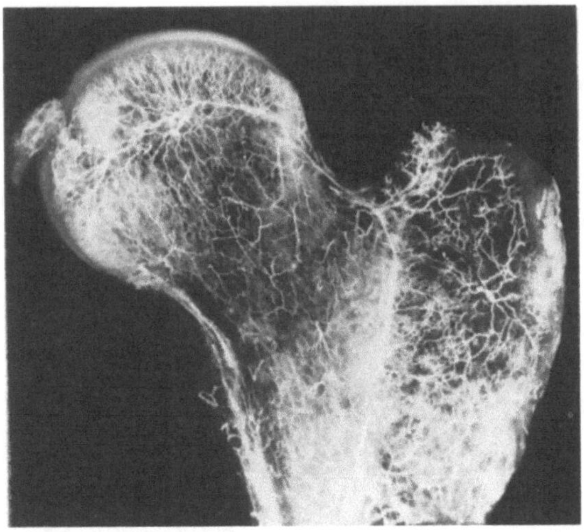

FIG. 6–8 Photograph of a coronal section (1.5 cm thick) cut from the upper end of the right femur of a 59-year-old female. Spalteholz cleared specimen. Note the pattern of distribution of major vessels within the head and neck of the femur. This corresponds precisely with the pattern already established at birth. The anastomosis between vessels across the site of the former growth plate, within the bone, is shown (× 1/3).

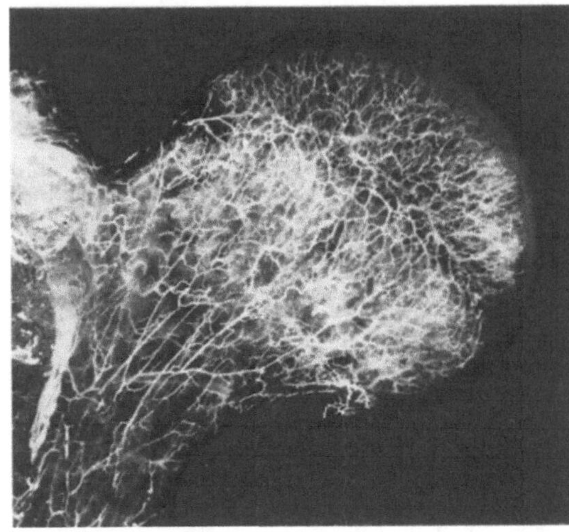

FIG. 6–9 Photograph of the posterior half of an adult femoral head showing the delicate plexiform anastomoses that exist between metaphyseal and epiphyseal arteries within the bone across the area of the obliterated growth plate. This complex system of vessels is nonetheless vulnerable, being based on the slender branches of the ascending cervical arteries which take origin from the extracapsular arterial ring at the base of the femoral neck.

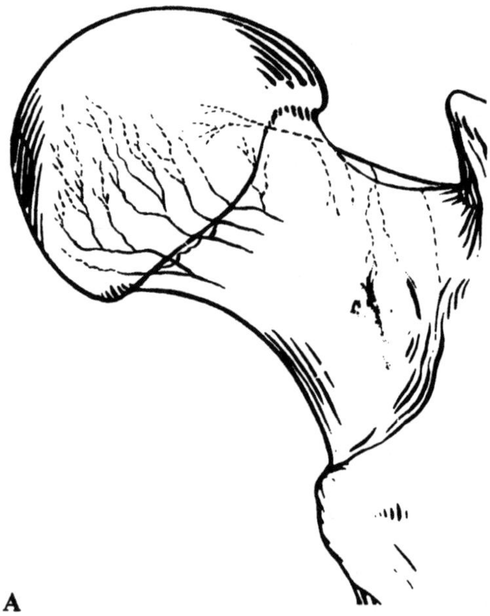

A

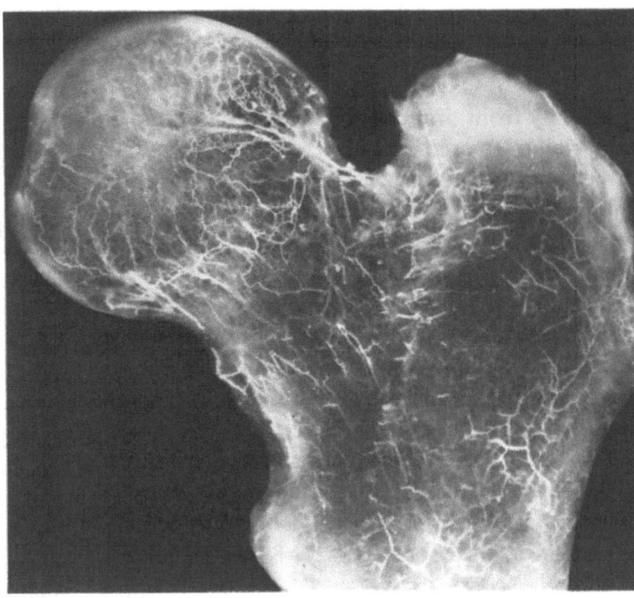

B

FIG. 6–10. **A** A drawing of the posterior half of the upper end of the femur, corresponding to **B.** Shading represents the outline of the articular cartilage–femoral neck junction. The terminations of posterior ascending cervical arteries are outlined; these vessels form a subsynovial intraarticular arterial ring with their epiphyseal branches passing upward into the head. Reprinted with permission from Crock, H. V.: The Blood Supply of the Lower Limb Bones in Man. Edinburgh, Livingstone, 1967. **B** The posterior surface of the upper end of the femur from a 27-year-old man. The terminal portions of the posterior ascending cervical branches of the extracapsular arterial ring of the femoral neck are shown forming the subsynovial intraarticular arterial ring, from which fine epiphyseal branches penetrate the femoral head to disappear out of focus at about its center. Reprinted with permission from Crock, H. V.: J. Anat. (Lond.), 99:86, 1965; and Crock, H. V.: The Blood Supply of the Lower Limb Bones in Man. Edinburgh, Livingstone, 1967.

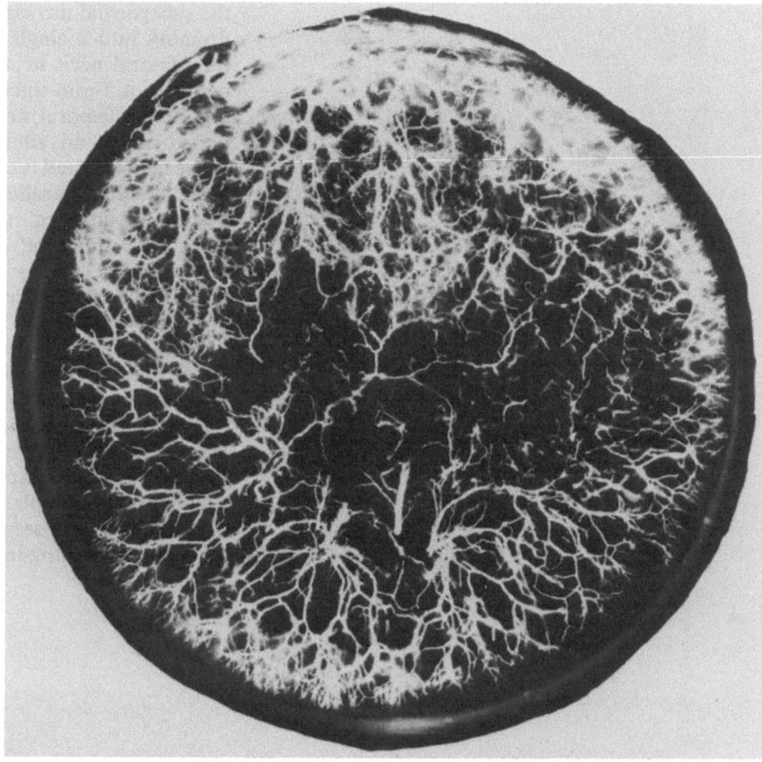

FIG. 6–11 Radiograph of a transverse section of the femoral head of an adult (1 cm thick) cut just proximal to the junction of the head with the neck of the femur. Arterial injection, showing the relationships of subchondral arterioles to the main stems of the epiphyseal arteries.

The clinical significance of these fascinating, complex subarticular collecting vein systems remains largely unknown, except for the observation of the development of subarticular osteoporosis which appears in the territory of these vessels in a variety of conditions, but most noticeably after trauma. An example of this pattern of localized osteoporosis is shown in the region of the knee joint (Fig. 6–13). Such a pattern of osteoporosis has been observed also in radiographs of the hip following traumatic dislocation.

Far from being academically sterile and clinically irrelevant, we believe that any future significant progress in the management of hip disorders awaits the practical acceptance of anatomical knowledge of the blood supply of the hip by surgeons and pathologists. Surgeons must devise new approaches to preserve this delicate and vulnerable blood supply, while pathologists should recommence the study of these vessels in thick and thin sections.

Perhaps some of the secrets of avascular necrosis of the femoral head and of the mechanisms leading to its segmental collapse are to be found in the pathology of these subarticular collecting veins.

Acknowledgements

H. V. Crock acknowledges with gratitude the permission of the editor of the *Journal of Anatomy,* London, and of the publishers, Churchill Livingstone, Edinburgh, and J. B. Lippincott & Co., Philadelphia, to reproduce his works previously published by them.

H. V. Crock and D. R. V. Dickens wish to express their appreciation for the financial support given to their work on the Venous Drainage of the Hip by the William Angliss Trust, the William Buckland Foundation, and the National Trustees and Executors Agency Limited, Melbourne.

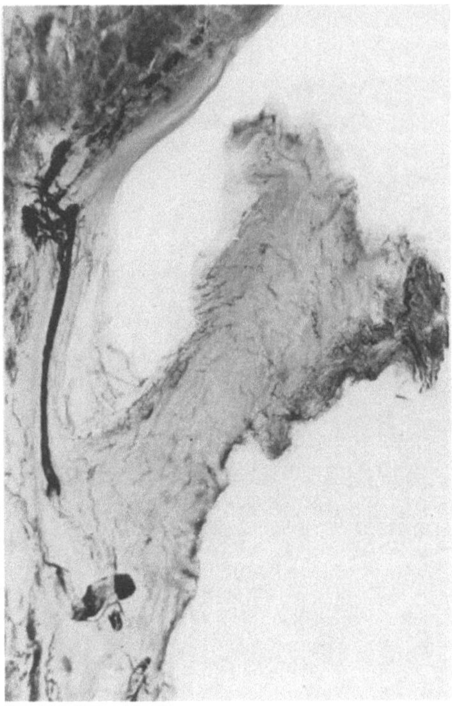

A

FIG. 6–12 **A** A detailed view of the anterior aspect of the femoral head and neck showing the confluence of veins in plexiform arrangement—corresponding to the subsynovial intraarticular arterial ring of Chung [1]—draining into a single large vein which courses down the femoral neck in a subsynovial position. **B** Photograph of a 5-mm-thick section cut horizontally in the line of the femoral neck from the anterior half of the upper end of an adult femur. The articular cartilage of the femoral head is clearly defined. Within the femoral head, oriented parallel to the subchondral bone plate, a large, blood-filled *subarticular collecting vein* can be seen. This drains off at the articular margin with the femoral neck into a subsynovial vein which courses down the femoral neck and joins veins in the capsule of the hip joint at the level of the anterior intertrochanteric line. Near the top of the specimen, the subarticular collecting vein drains also into one of the principal veins at the fovea capitis. **C** A microphotograph (× 80) taken from the middle section of the specimen illustrated in **B** showing the relationship of the subarticular collecting vein to the marrow spaces immediately adjacent to the subchondral bone plate. The calcified zone of articular cartilage is clearly seen near the top of the picture. Note the venules draining into the subarticular collecting vein along its course.

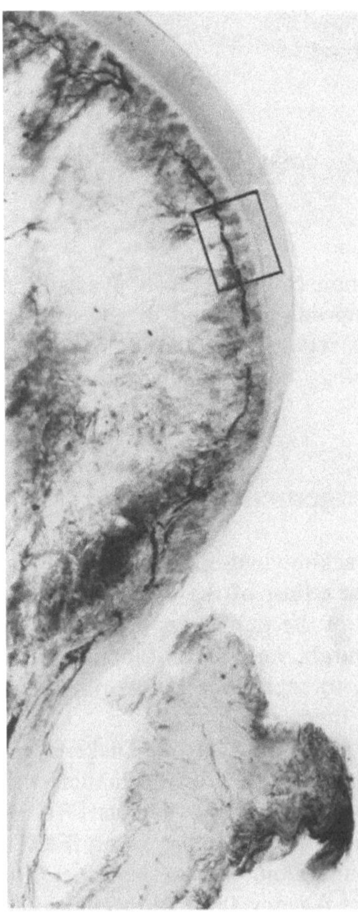

B

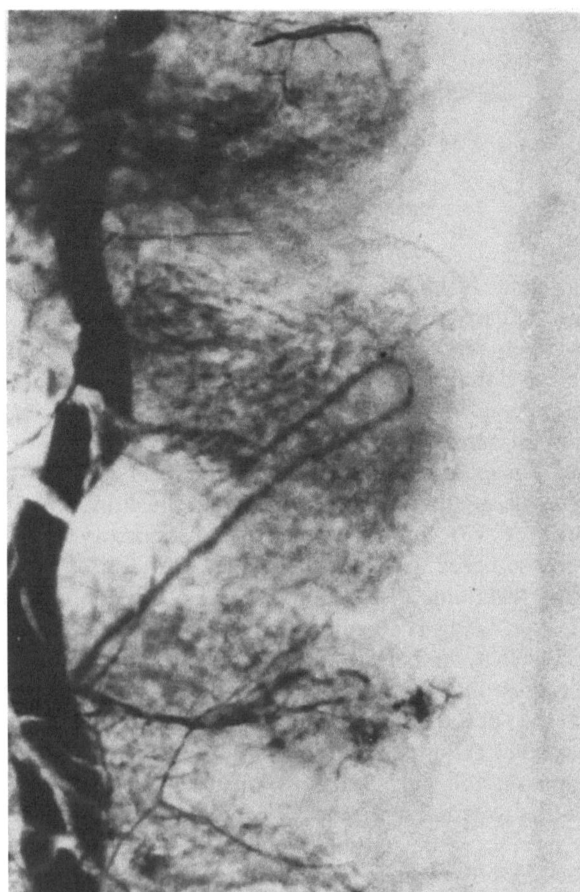

C

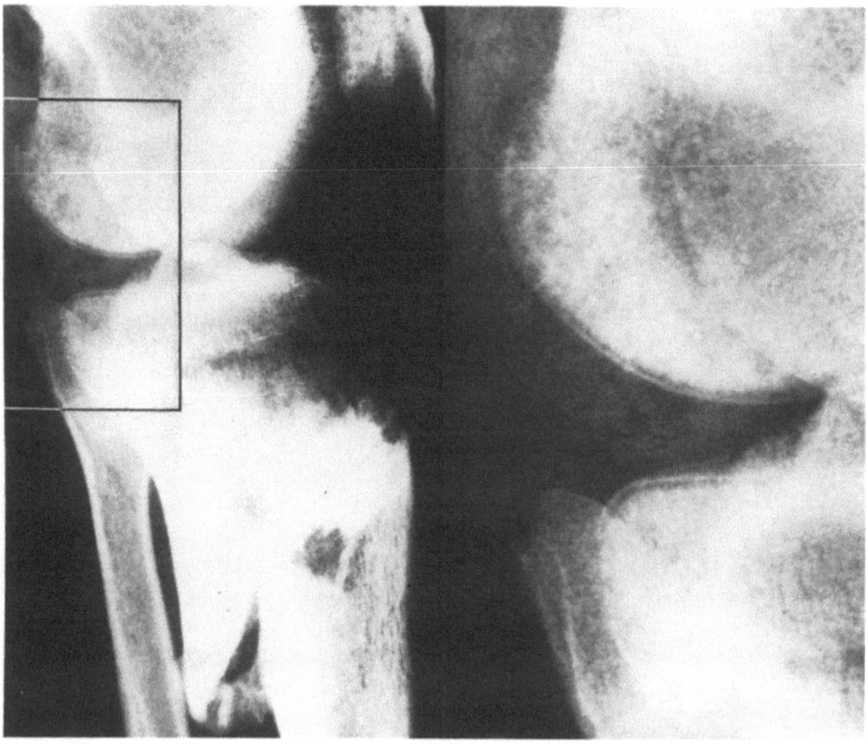

FIG. 6–13 Radiographs of the knee joint of a young adult showing the subarticular osteoporosis which has developed in adjacent joints following fractures of the tibia and fibula. This osteoporosis occurs in the region of the subarticular collecting vein systems.

Bibliography

1. Chung, S. M. K.: The arterial supply of the developing proximal end of the human femur. J. Bone Joint Surg., 58A:961, 1976.
2. Crock, H. V.: The arterial supply and venous drainage of the vertebral column of the dog. J. Anat., 94:88, 1960.
3. Crock, H. V.: The arterial supply and venous drainage of the bones of the human knee joint. Anat. Rec., 144:199, 1962.
4. Crock, H. V.: A revision of the anatomy of the arteries supplying the upper end of the human femur. J. Anat. (Lond.): 99:77, 1965.
5. Crock, H. V.: The Blood Supply of the Lower Limb Bones in Man. Edinburgh, Livingstone, 1967.
6. Crock, H. V.: An atlas of the arterial supply of the head and neck of the femur in man. Clin. Orthop., 152:17, 1980.
7. Crock, H. V., Chari, P. R., and Crock, M. C.: La vascularization des os du poignet et de la main chez l'homme. In Tubiana, R. (ed.): Traité de Chirurgie de la Main. Paris, Masson, 1980, pp. 361–371.
8. Crock, H. V., Chari, P. R., and Crock, M. C.: The blood supply of the wrist and hand bones in man. In Tubiana, R. (ed.): The Hand. Philadelphia, Saunders, 1981, pp. 335–347.
9. Crock, H. V., and Yoshizawa, H.: The Blood Supply of the Vertebral Column and Spinal Cord in Man. New York, Springer-Verlag, 1977.
10. Howe, W. W., Lacey, T., and Schwartz, R. P.: A Study of the gross anatomy of the arteries supplying the proximal portion of the femur and acetobulum. J. Bone Joint Surg. 32A:856, 1950.
11. Lagrange, J., and Dunoyer, J.: La vascularization de la tête femorale de l'enfant. Rev. Chir. Orthop., 48:123, 1962.
12. Trueta, J.: The normal vascular anatomy of the human femoral head during growth. J. Bone Joint Surg., 39:358, 1957.
13. Trueta, J., and Harrison, M. H. M.: The normal vascular anatomy of the femoral head in an adult man. J. Bone Joint Surg., 35:442, 1953.

Disorders of the Hip in Children

CHAPTER 7

Trauma, Hip Development, and Vascularity *

JOHN A. OGDEN

When considering both acute damage as well as the chronic sequelae of trauma to the skeletally immature hip region in the infant, child, or adolescent, it is important to remember there are significant, constantly changing anatomical, physiological, and biomechanical differences compared to the adult.[34,39,41,43,44-46] Such changes result in different fracture patterns, modalities of therapy, and predispositions to complications in each age group. The areas of major significance include (1) the complex cartilaginous components of the acetabulum, and development of secondary ossification centers within the triradiate cartilage and along the acetabular margin; (2) the progressive development of the proximal femur into functionally separate lesser trochanteric, greater trochanteric, and capital femoral epiphyses and physes; (3) cartilaginous posterosuperior physeal and epiphyseal anatomical continuities that may be fractured (but are not often considered a part of the injury since they are radiolucent); (4) the progressive changes in the blood supply, particularly the changing intracapsular course of the capital femoral blood vessels; and (5) the different patterns of susceptibility to vascular compromise that relate to age and anatomy.

The development of the proximal femoral chondro-osseous epiphysis and physis is probably the most complex of all longitudinal-latitudinal growth regions.[37,38] Similarly, the integrated development of the acetabular chondro-osseous components among themselves and relative to the proximal femur is equally complex. Fortunately, significant growth mechanism injuries secondary to either direct chondro-osseous trauma or selective vascular damage are infrequent. However, when such complications do occur, they assume great importance for subsequent limb development as well as hip and leg biomechanics.

Understanding the effects of traumatic injury to the acetabulum and proximal femur requires an appreciation of the complex anatomical changes occurring in both regions over time, as well as the changes in the dependence on differing patterns of blood supply.

The acetabulum develops a triradiate cartilage which eventually forms a secondary ossification center within its cartilage. Injury causing premature closure of one or more of the arms of this cartilage may lead to a shallow, significantly deformed acetabulum. Ossification which occurs secondarily within the triradiate cartilage is intimately related to the formation of the os acetabuli along the posterior margin, an area which should not be confused with a marginal hip fracture when the proximal femur is traumatically dislocated.

Similarly, the proximal femur undergoes major structural changes in transforming from a composite mass of cartilage which includes the greater trochanter and capital femur in the newborn, to one in which these two regions progressively separate. However, the two regions are connected throughout development by a bridge of cartilage along the superior and posterior regions (but not the anterior region) of the developing neck. The blood vessels to the femoral head have an intimate relationship to this bridging cartilage. It must be remembered that when a fracture is seen roent-

* Supported in part by grants from the Crippled Children's Aid Society, the National Institutes of Health (HD-10854 and AM-00300), and Skeletal Educational Associates, Inc.

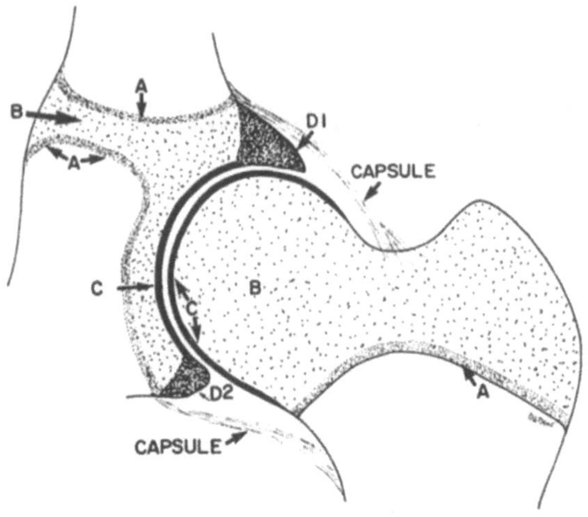

A

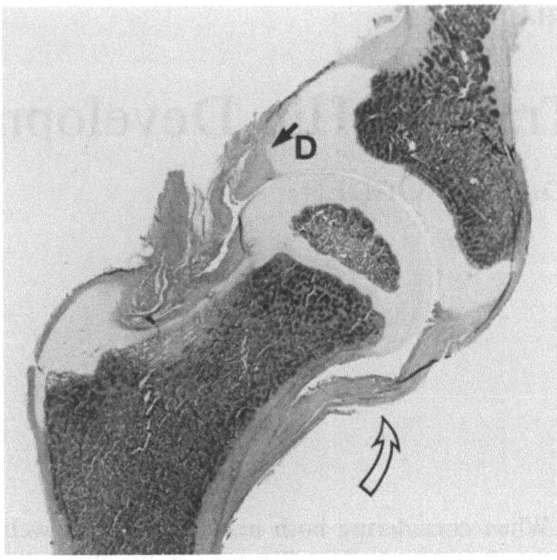

B

FIG. 7–1 **A** Schematic of the cartilaginous regions in a neonate. *A*, physeal cartilage; *B*, epiphyseal cartilage; *C*, articular cartilage; *D*, marginal fibrocartilage of the acetabular labrum (*D1*) and inferior transverse acetabular ligament (*D2*). **B** Histological section of hip from a 3-year-old shows the aforementioned regions, including labrum cartilage (*D, arrow*) and capsule (*open arrow*). (All artwork reproduced with permission of Skeletal Educational Associates, Inc.)

genographically across the osseous femoral neck, damage may occur to the cartilaginous portion and may result in maldevelopment of the femoral neck. Because of the close relationship of the blood vessels, direct vascular damage may occur.

The blood supply to the femoral head and the acetabulum is extremely dynamic and constantly changing, although there is a basic pattern of two major vessels (the posterosuperior and the posteroinferior vessels) originating from the medial circumflex artery. These vessels are susceptible to injury with a fracture of the femoral neck. The posterosuperior vessel is probably more susceptible, inasmuch as it tends to be intimately related to the cartilage along the neck, whereas the posteroinferior vessel tends to be in a retinacular fold and more mobile. In hip dislocation, these vessels may be severely attenuated. No matter what the underlying trauma, patterns of ischemic necrosis may occur when there is damage to these vessels. The patterns will be contingent upon the extent of vascular damage, the extent of potential for revascularization, and the stage of chondro-osseous maturation at the time of injury. The effect may manifest primarily in the secondary ossification center of the capital femur, the physis, or the metaphyseal neck, involving all regions or in any combination.

Acetabulum

Morphology

The acetabulum is comprised of four types of cartilage (Fig. 7–1). The first type, articular cartilage, is variably thick and merges imperceptibly with the second type, the epiphyseal cartilage, which has a discrete vascular system of cartilage canals and contributes cells to the third type, the physeal cartilage. The fourth type is the fibrocartilage of the labrum; grossly, histologically, and biomechanically this tissue is well demarcated from the adjacent epiphyseal cartilage.

The three pelvic growth sectors—iliac, pubic, and ischial—become confluent within the acetabulum, apposing each other through common epiphyses and physes that combine to form the triradiate cartilage (Fig. 7–2). The bone adjacent to each physis along this triradiate cartilage is analogous to a metaphysis, and thus represents bone capable of considerable remodeling, especially in the segment of ilium above the acetabulum. Further, these regions do not elaborate a secondary ossification center and distinct subchondral bone plate (cribriform plate) until late in adolescence, so interstitial expansion of the physis and epiphysis may occur. Functionally this intricate

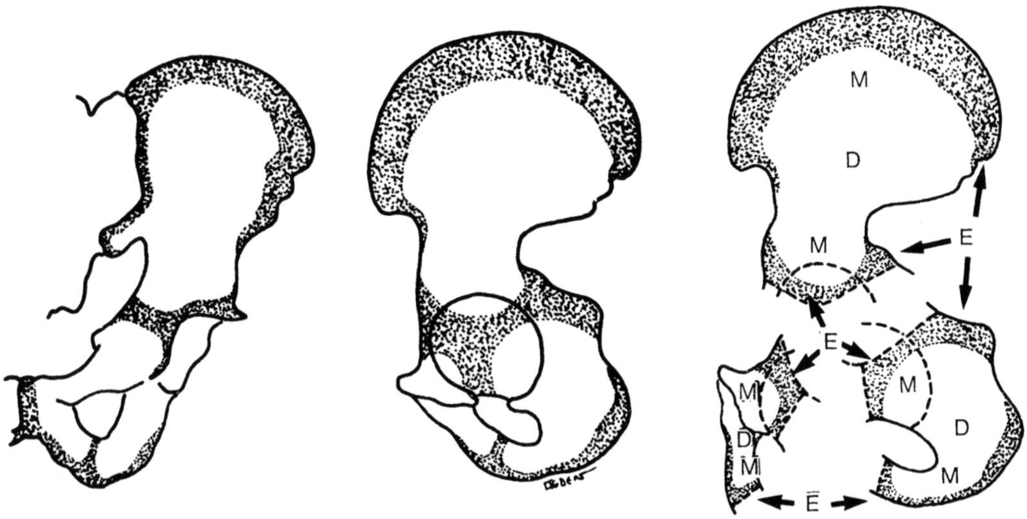

FIG. 7–2 Schematic of development of the pelvic or innominate bone. Stippled areas in the anterior view (*left*) and lateral view (*center*) represent regions of epiphyseal and physeal cartilage. The "exploded" view (right) shows how the three component bones—ilium, ischium, and pubis—come together at the triradiate cartilage. *E*, epiphysis; *M*, metaphysis; *D*, diaphysis. Note that each component pelvic bone has regions analogous to those in the long bones.

interrelationship between the acetabulum and the triradiate cartilage allows progressive expansion of the acetabular concavity to accommodate the proximal femoral convexity. Thus, the major function of the triradiate-acetabular cartilage unit is to allow an increase in absolute size of the hemispheric acetabulum, while maintaining congruency between acetabulum and femoral head. Deformation of the femoral head, damage to the triradiate cartilage, sustained alteration of biomechanical forces, or major neurological damage (e.g., sciatic nerve) consequent to pelvic injury will variably affect this acetabular/femoral head developmental congruence.

The triradiate cartilage in the newborn is wide. As the hip progressively develops throughout childhood and adolescence, the width of each arm progressively narrows until it is approximately 5 to 6 mm wide (Fig. 7–3). Because of the obliquity of roentgenograms used in the evaluation of pelvic trauma in children, it is not always easy to interpret the entire triradiate cartilage. During adolescence, secondary ossification centers, analogous to those seen in longitudinal bones, develop within the triradiate cartilage (Fig. 7–3B and C). Concomitantly, the acetabular rim develops a secondary ossification center (Fig. 7–4), which must not be misinterpreted as a discrete injury. This peripheral ossification, sometimes referred to as the os acetabuli, is usually continuous with portions of the triradiate secondary ossification in the anterior and posterior arms.

Injury Patterns

Fractures involving the triradiate cartilage are usually type 1, 2, or 5 growth mechanism injuries (Fig. 7–5), and often difficult to diagnose.[6,39] When fractures occur and lead to premature fusion of the growth plate, this process occurs extremely rapidly, and, depending on the age of the child, may result in significant growth deformity (Fig. 7–5). Resection of an osseous bridge early in its formation is probably not realistic, as many of these children seem to have extensive crushing injuries involving most of the anterior and/or posterior arms. They must be followed closely and due consideration given to appropriate means of augmenting the acetabulum (e.g., shelf procedure, pelvic osteotomy).

Fractures involving the acetabular rim (Fig. 7–6) are not always easy to diagnose, particularly when accompanying traumatic dislocation of the hip. The normal appearance of the peripheral os acetabuli may confuse interpretation and lead one to suspect that there has been a fracture of the

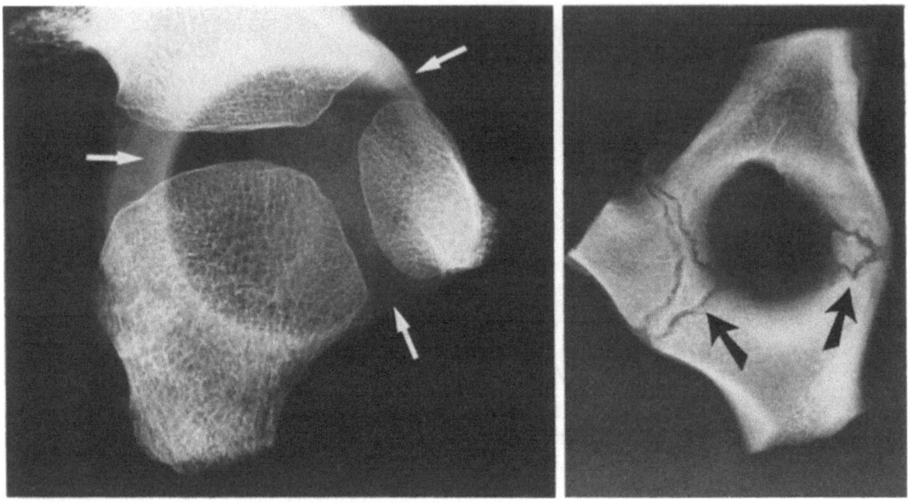

A B

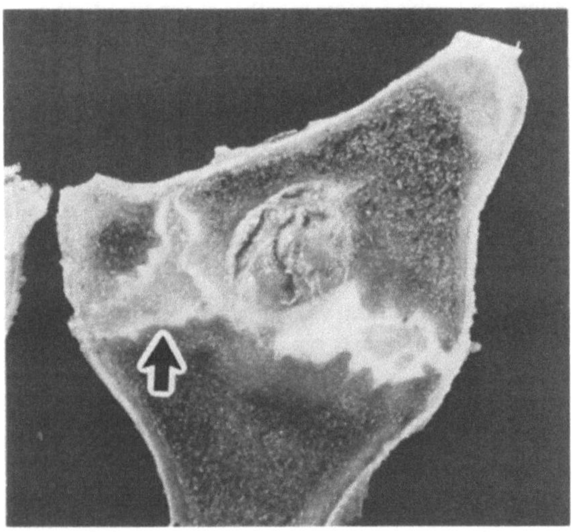

C

FIG. 7–3 Development of the triradiate cartilage. **A** Roentgenographic appearance at 3 years. The arrows depict the three arms of this cartilage sector. **B** Roentgenographic appearance of the development of secondary ossification centers (*arrows*) during adolescence. **C** Morphologic appearance of the specimen shown in **B.** The arrow indicates one of the secondary ossification centers within the triradiate cartilage.

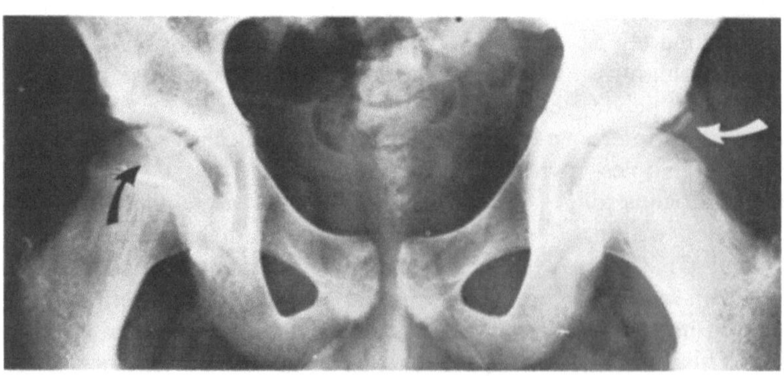

FIG. 7–4 Normal secondary ossification along the left posterosuperior rim (*white arrow*). Note the continuity of such secondary rim ossification with the triradiate secondary ossification (*black arrow*) in the right hip.

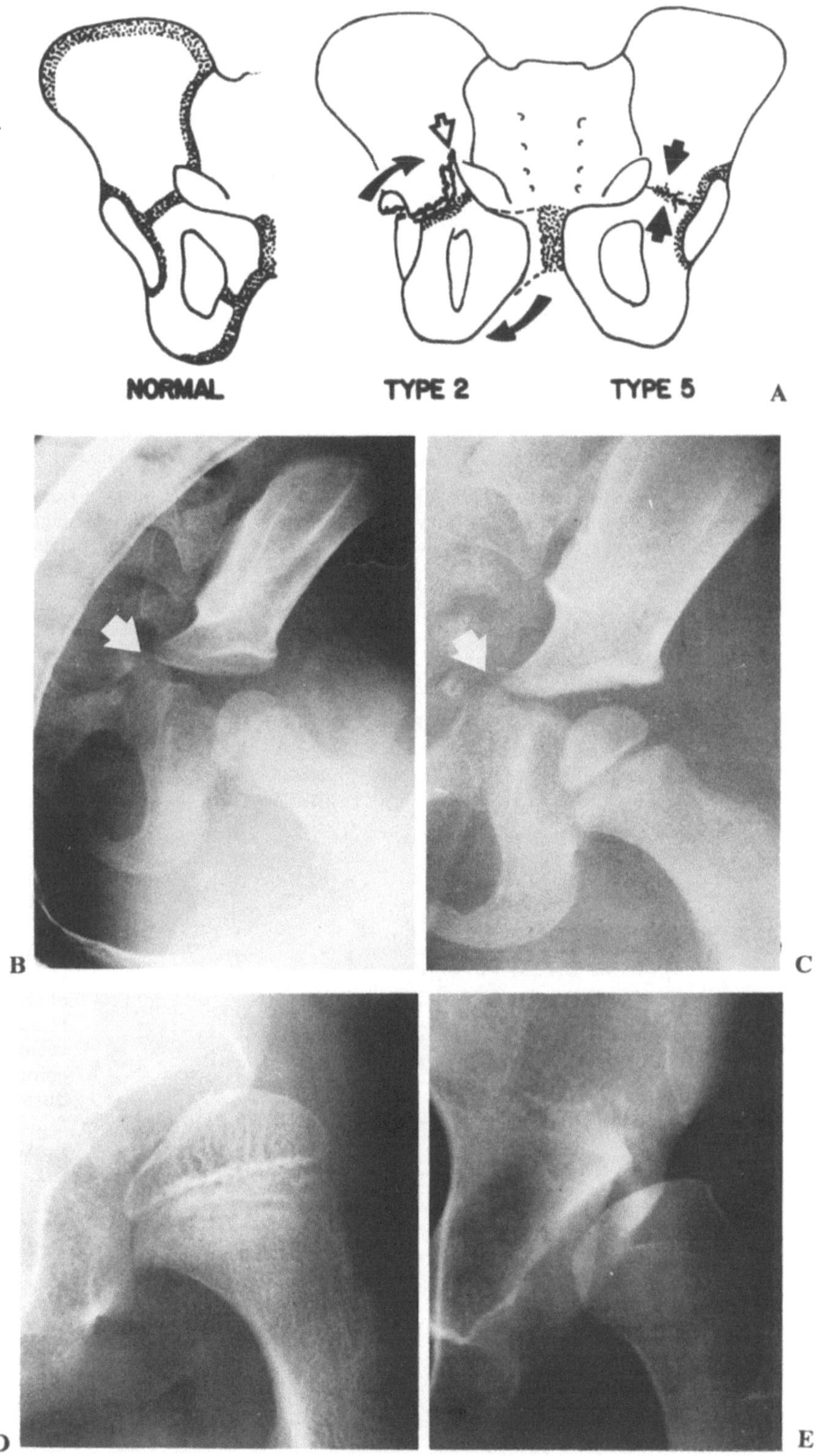

FIG. 7–5 **A** Schematic of types 2 and 5 triradiate fractures. Solid arrows indicate probable directions of deforming forces. Open arrow shows the metaphyseal fragment characteristic of the type 2 pattern. **B** Roentgenogram of the hip of a 2-year-old girl sustaining multiple trauma, including brain injury, femoral shaft fracture, sacroiliac disruption (but without obvious ramus fracture), and sciatic nerve damage. The possibility of triradiate injury (*arrow*) was considered as the lower area of disruption (in the absence of a ramus fracture), although roentgenographic confirmation was not possible during the initial evaluation. **C** However, within 6 months she was beginning to develop an osseous bridge (*arrow*). **D** Two years after injury the triradiate cartilage closed and the femoral head was subluxating. She will undoubtedly require reconstructive surgery as she gets older. E. Similar patient at skeletal maturity, 11 years after triradiate injury; note the shallow acetabulum and subluxated, deformed proximal femur.

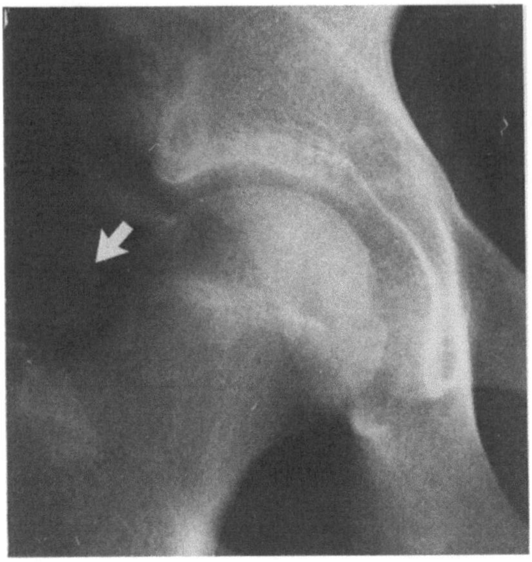

A

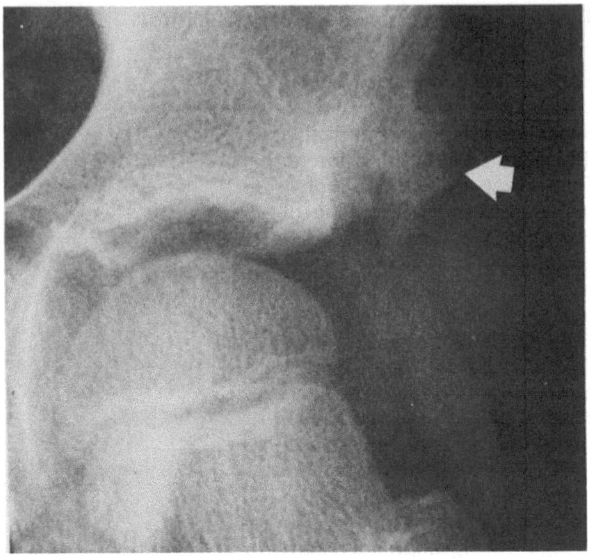

B

FIG. 7–6 **A** Avulsion fracture (*arrow*) of the anterior inferior iliac spine. **B** In a similar injury, without roentgenographic evidence of avulsion at the time of initial pelvic injury, an exostosis (*arrow*) formed several weeks later as the cartilaginous rim healed progressively to the underlying pelvis.

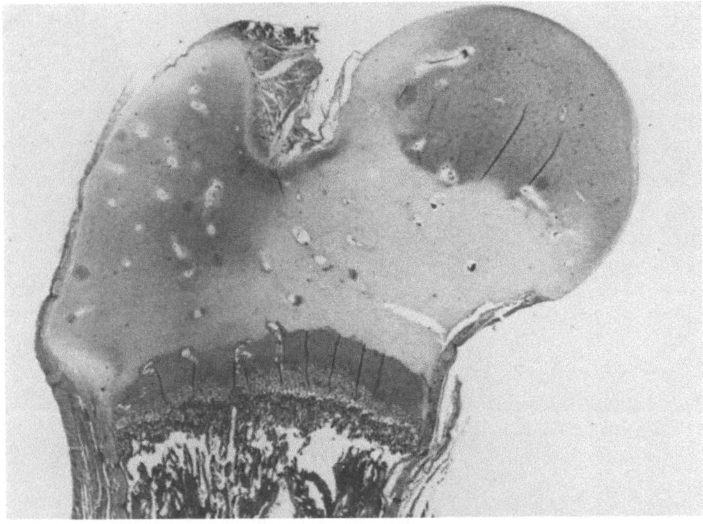

A

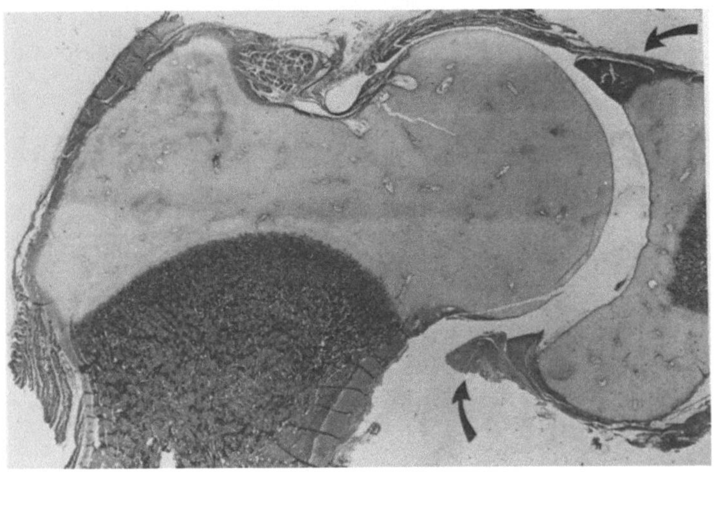

B

FIG. 7–7 **A** Section of the proximal femur of a 7-month-old fetus, showing the transverse orientation of the common physis. **B** In the newborn physeal contour changes are just beginning in the central and subcapital regions. Note the extensive vascularity (cartilage canals) throughout the common chondroepiphysis. Arrows indicate the fibrocartilaginous labrum. **C** Specimen roentgenogram showing the chondroepiphysis which is not usually evident during evaluation for trauma in infants. The arrows indicate the femoral neck at the attachments of the capsule (*c*).

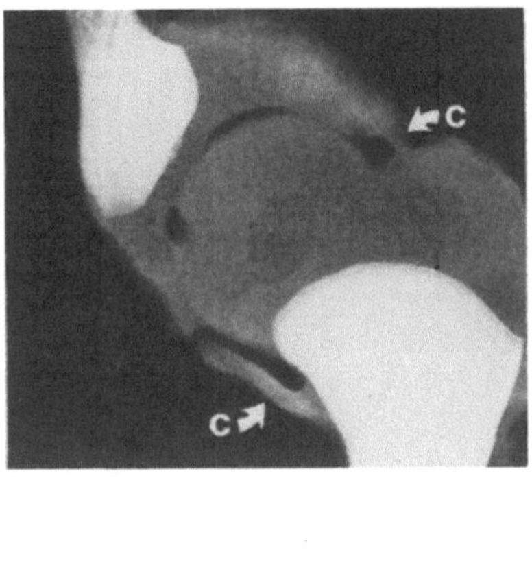

C

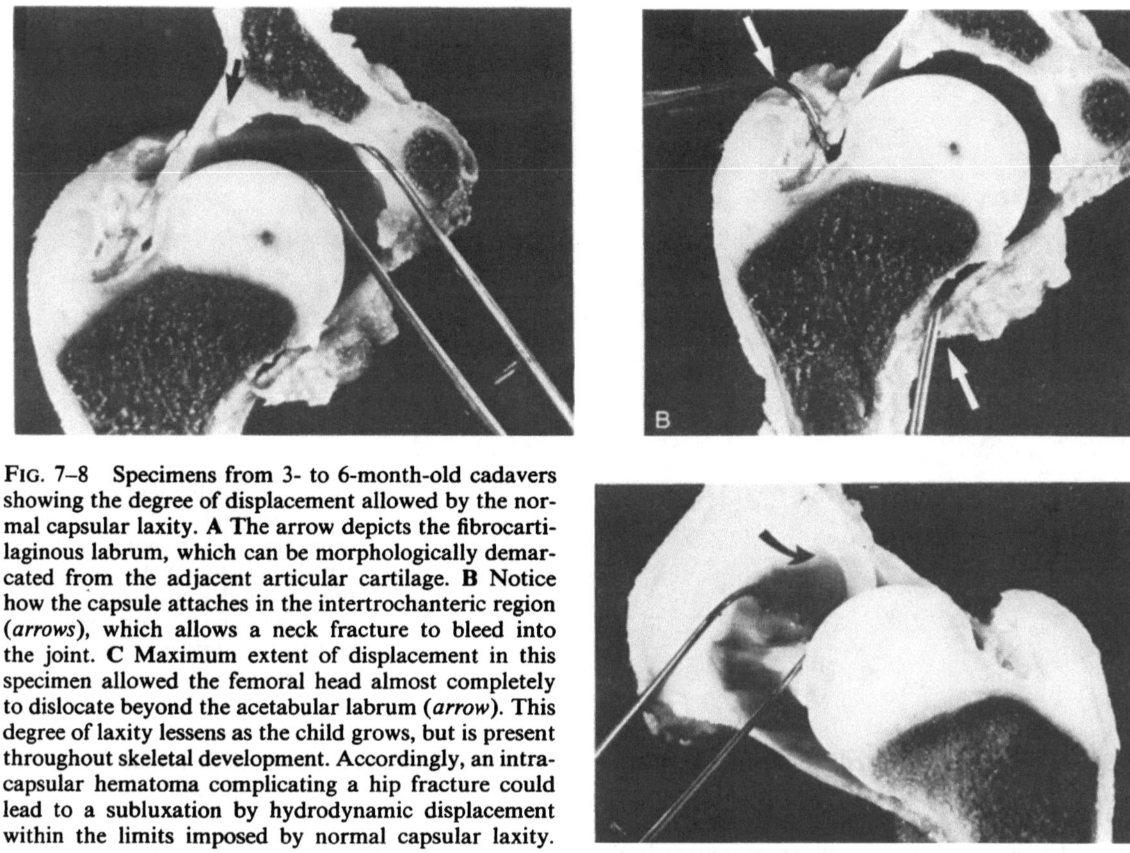

FIG. 7–8 Specimens from 3- to 6-month-old cadavers showing the degree of displacement allowed by the normal capsular laxity. **A** The arrow depicts the fibrocartilaginous labrum, which can be morphologically demarcated from the adjacent articular cartilage. **B** Notice how the capsule attaches in the intertrochanteric region (*arrows*), which allows a neck fracture to bleed into the joint. **C** Maximum extent of displacement in this specimen allowed the femoral head almost completely to dislocate beyond the acetabular labrum (*arrow*). This degree of laxity lessens as the child grows, but is present throughout skeletal development. Accordingly, an intracapsular hematoma complicating a hip fracture could lead to a subluxation by hydrodynamic displacement within the limits imposed by normal capsular laxity.

posterior rim, when in actuality this is only a normal biological development. The inferior iliac spine, which is a composite part of the superior acetabular rim, may be avulsed in the cartilaginous phase. In such a situation, it is impossible to diagnose the actual injury until callus formation subsequently makes the diagnosis certain several weeks later (Fig. 7–6B).[39] One must suspect this type of injury when there is considerable pain and guarding around the hip in a child who has sustained major pelvic trauma.

Proximal Femur

Morphology

Neonate At birth the proximal femur is a composite chondroepiphysis of the greater trochanter and capital femur (Fig. 7–7). Morphologically there is a spherical femoral head, variable anteversion, and virtually no femoral neck. Since the tip of the greater trochanter is level with the femoral articular surface, the normal morphology initially is characterized by a *neutral* articulotrochanteric distance (ATD). However, in each ensuing developmental period, the ATD becomes increasingly positive commensurate with elongation of the femoral neck. The hip capsule attaches along the intertrochanteric region superiorly, anteriorly, and posteriorly, and just above the lesser trochanter inferiorly. On the acetabular side, the capsule attaches just beyond the fibrocartilaginous labrum, making this rim and its transverse acetabular ligament continuation intracapsular. The capsule is loose during this period. If the hip joint is fluid-filled, as in a traumatic joint effusion, this capsular laxity may readily allow lateral displacement, which should not be mistaken for congenital hip dysplasia (Fig. 7–8).

Three to Six Months Secondary ossification begins in the capital femur by 4 to 6 months (Fig.

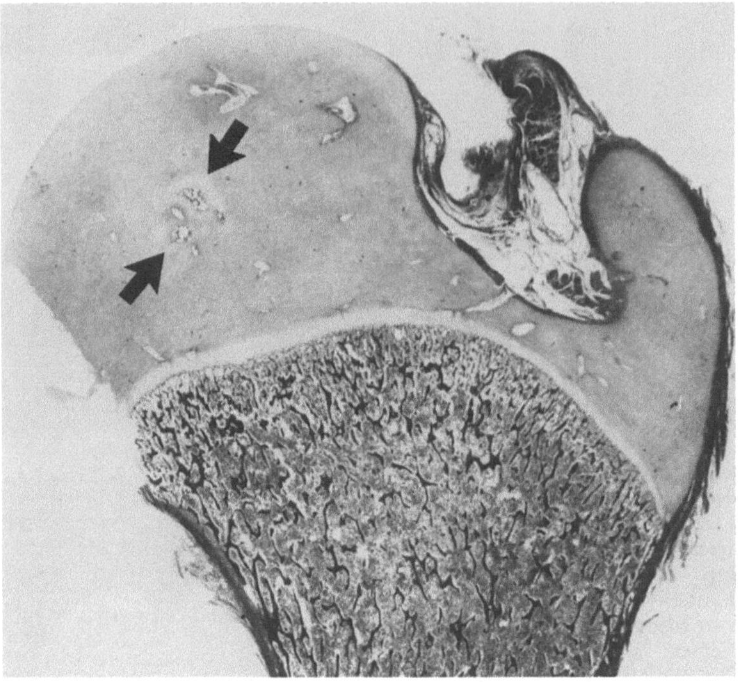

FIG. 7–9 Early development of capital femoral ossification center from two foci (*arrows*). These will rapidly coalesce. Note the separation of capital femoral and trochanteric regions by the intraepiphyseal cartilaginous bridge as the femoral neck develops.

7–9). This centrally located, spherical ossification center expands centrifugally (eventually conforming to the hemispheric shape of the articular and physeal contours). This ossification center is dependent upon an intact vascular supply for both its initial and continued development. Any temporary or permanent decrease in the normal pattern of blood flow, as in a femoral neck fracture, will have variable effects upon the ability of the capital femoral ossification center to continue its normal pattern of maturation.

Two major morphologic changes commence during this period—development of the femoral neck through a more rapid growth of the subcapital portions of the physis and metaphysis, and development of the capital femoral secondary ossification center. The hip continues to have a significant degree of capsular laxity. As the femoral neck develops, more of the medial metaphysis becomes intracapsular. Growth of the acetabular labrum makes it increasingly important in stabilizing the hip. There is a continued susceptibility to vascular damage as the femoral neck develops. Since this is the period of initial appearance of the secondary ossification center, which depends upon an adequate blood supply derived primarily through the posterosuperior vessels, occlusion of or traumatic damage to these vessels during a fracture or dislocation may seriously impair this stage of chondro-osseous transformation.

Six to Twelve Months The femoral neck continues elongation and establishes a discrete area which may be defined as the capital femoral physis (Fig. 7–10). With elongation of the femoral neck there is increasing separation of the capital femoral and greater trochanteric regions, although there remains a relatively large amount of cartilage in the intraepiphyseal region. As the neck develops, the superior articular surface of the capital femur gradually becomes more proximally situated than the greater trochanter, establishing a *positive* articulotrochanteric distance.

One to Two Years The femoral neck elongates, leading to narrowing and lengthening of the intraepiphyseal cartilage zone (Fig. 7–11). The physis of the intraepiphyseal region still contains a preponderance of columnar cells typical of compression-responsive physeal cytoarchitecture. The increased growth of the medial physis leads to a more specific definition of the capital femoral physis. The secondary ossification center expands, adapting to the hemisphericity of the surrounding articular surface. Where it is juxtaposed to the physis and metaphysis, the secondary center flat-

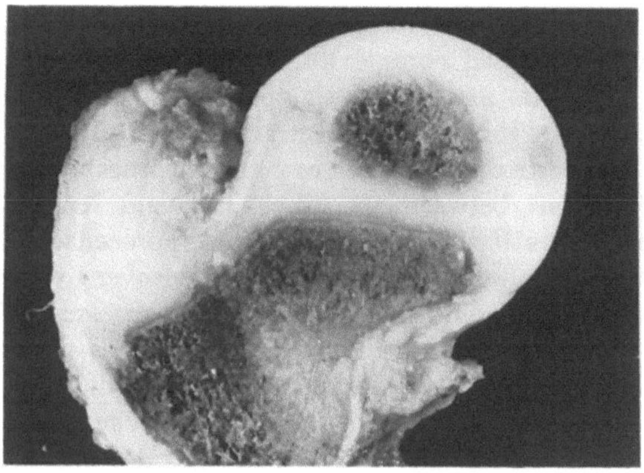

A

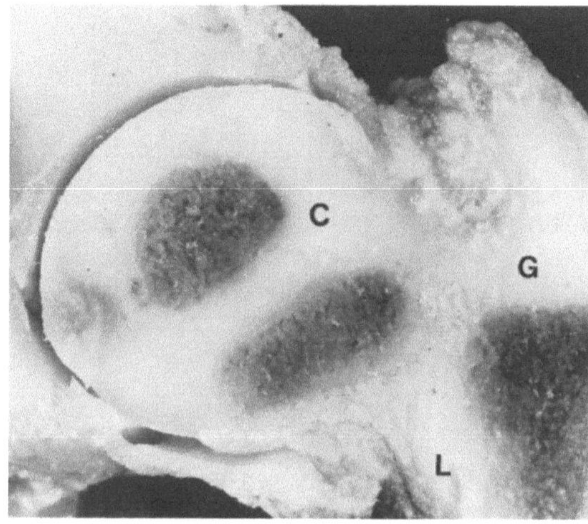

B

FIG. 7–10 **A** By 8 to 10 months a well-formed capital femoral ossification center is present. **B** Posterior slab section shows continuity of epiphyseal cartilage among the capital femoral (*C*), greater trochanteric (*G*), and lesser trochanteric (*L*) regions.

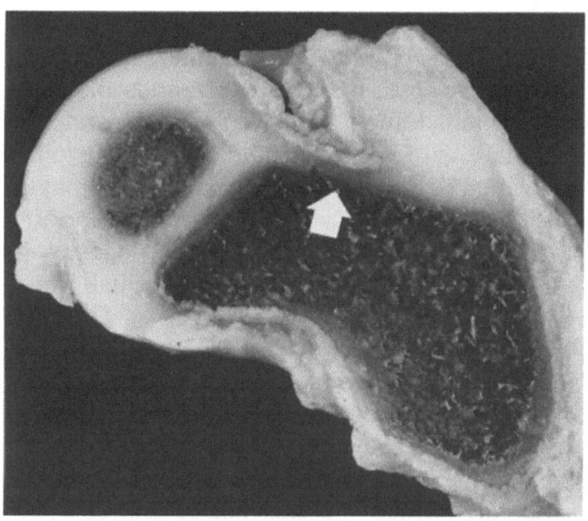

A

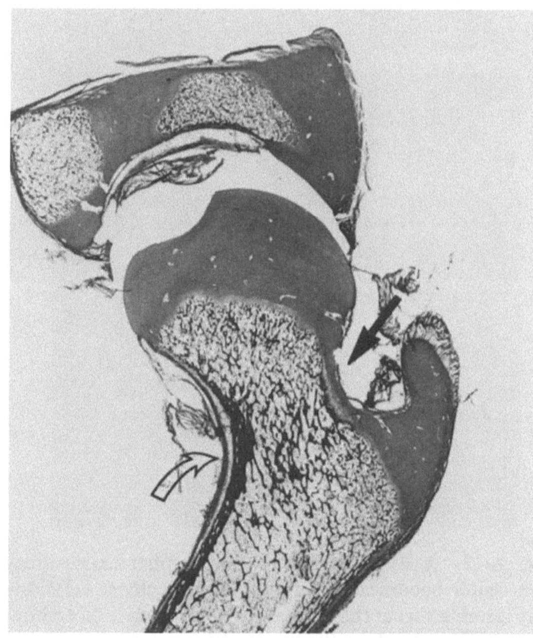

B

FIG. 7–11 **A** By 1 year the femoral neck is a well-developed structure with a posterosuperior cartilaginous continuity (*arrow*). **B** Histological section showing early development of the calcar (*open arrow*) along the inferior femoral neck. Note thickening of the trabecular bone within the intertrochanteric region. The solid arrow indicates the cartilaginous continuity along the developing neck.

tens and establishes a bipolar growth zone between the capital femoral ossification center and metaphysis. The medial physis, in response to normal hip joint mechanics (joint reaction forces), begins to angulate and develop mamillary processes, giving the physis an undulated appearance that increases resistance of the physis to shear stresses.[13,40] The ligamentum capitis femoris enters a deepening fovea capitis. The capsule exhibits decreasing laxity.

Three to Four Years The femoral neck continues longitudinal and interstitial growth (Fig. 7–12). The intraepiphyseal cartilage is thinner, although a discrete posterosuperior region remains as a definite mass of cartilage between trochanter and fem-

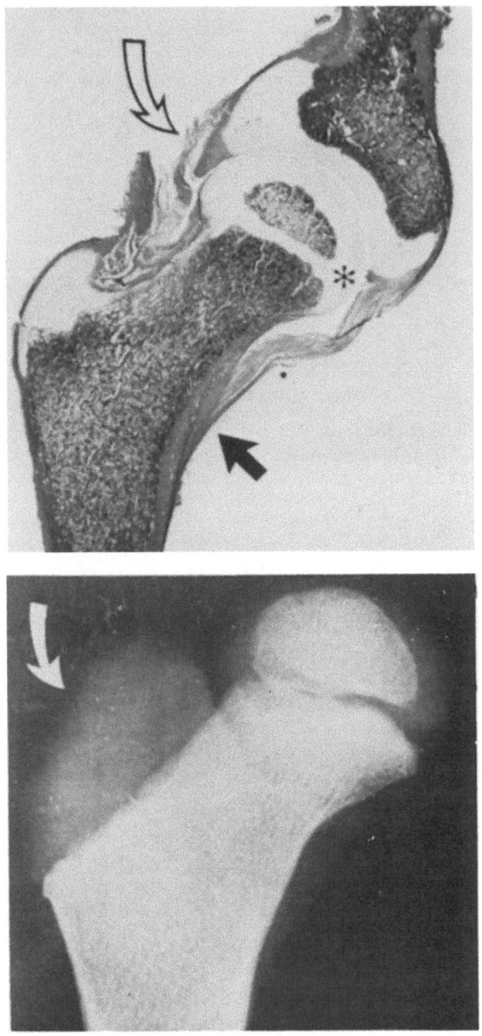

FIG. 7–12 **A** By 3 years the initially spherical ossification center becomes hemispherical as a closer relationship develops with the capital femoral physis. Note how the capsule extends to the base of the neck (*solid arrow*). The acetabular rim is completely within the joint (*open arrow*). Lappet formation is evident medially(*). **B** Roentgenogram of specimen from a 6-year-old. Note the completely cartilaginous greater trochanter (*arrow*).

oral head. The greater trochanter develops a secondary ossification center just above the lateral metaphysis. This may appear as a single center, or initially may form multiple, small ossific foci which rapidly coalesce. Ossification then extends into the remainder of the trochanteric epiphysis. The trochanteric physis is developing an undulated appearance, similar to the capital femoral physis. Again, this appears to be a response to shearing biological stresses imposed by the hip musculature. The increased complexity of the undulations of the capital femoral physis appears to be directly related to thinning of the intraepiphyseal cartilage. This particular zone serves certain biomechanical functions between the trochanter and femoral head. As it thins, some of these biomechanical functions must change, and be taken over by the developing undulations (mamillary processes) of the capital femoral physis. The metaphysis shows increasing development of medial trabecular patterns along the superior femoral neck. The articulotrochanteric distance increases, reflecting the faster growth rate of the capital femoral physis relative to the trochanteric physis. The capital femoral secondary ossification center enlarges in a hemispherical fashion. However, as it approaches the fovea capitis, an indentation develops. This is a normal developmental pattern and in no way indicates pathological change in the medial femoral head.

Five to Eight Years The secondary ossification center of the greater trochanter expands and often develops an additional ossification center near the proximal end of the trochanter, comparable to the ossification pattern in the proximal tibial epiphysis and tibial tuberosity. This accessory secondary center rapidly fuses with the main secondary center. The ossification center of the capital femur enlarges to fill most of the epiphysis. The area juxtaposed to the fovea capitis develops a distinct indentation in the ossification center (Fig. 7–13). Interdigitating mamillary processes develop as discrete regions of the capital femoral physis. By the end of this stage of development, the proximal femur has formed the final anatomical contours of a functionally separate femoral head and greater trochanter (although still anatomically connected), and neck–shaft angle. Most of the subsequent growth through adolescence will comprise remodeling of trabecular patterns and integrated enlargement of the capital femur and trochanters. By the end of this stage, the discrete trabecular arching patterns along the superior femoral neck are established.

Nine to Twelve Years There are no significant morphological changes during this period. Instead, growth comprises continued maturation of the ossification centers of the trochanter and capital femur and widening and maturation of the femoral

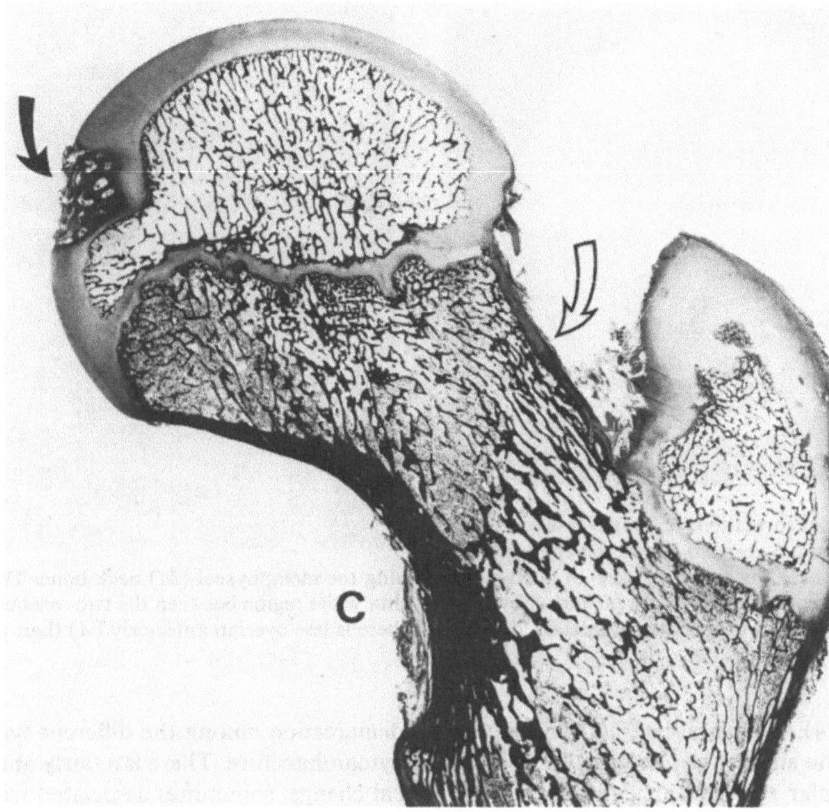

FIG. 7–13 By 10 years all structures are well developed. The capital femoral ossification center develops a normal indentation where the ligamentum capitis femoris attaches (*solid arrow*). The growth plate is undulated, with discrete mamillary processes. The superior neck region is thinning (*open arrow*). The calcar (*c*) is thick and oriented with the other internal trabecular patterns. Trabecular orientation is also more evident in the capital femoral ossification center (middle region).

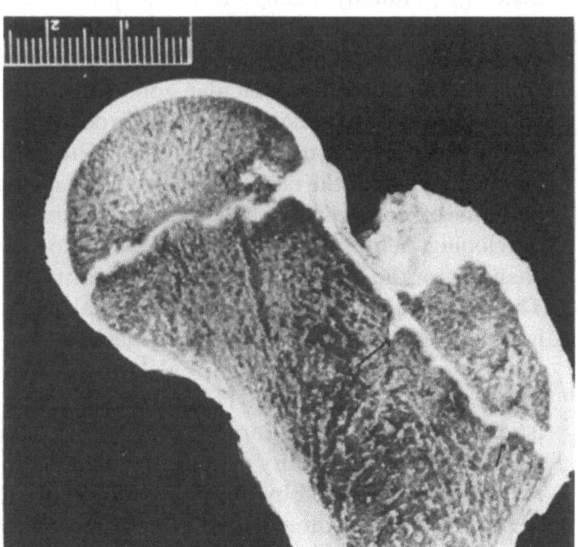

A

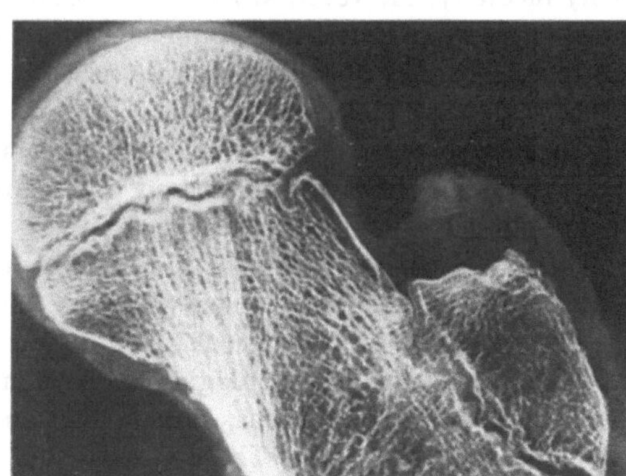

B

FIG. 7–14 By 12 years the internal trabecular systems are well oriented to both compression and tension stresses. A Slab section. B Roentgenogram. Note the upward continuity of the main compression-responsive trabeculae from the calcar toward and into the capital femur.

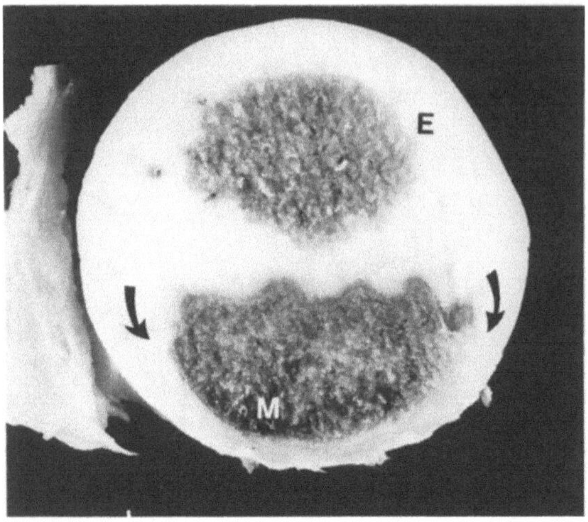

A

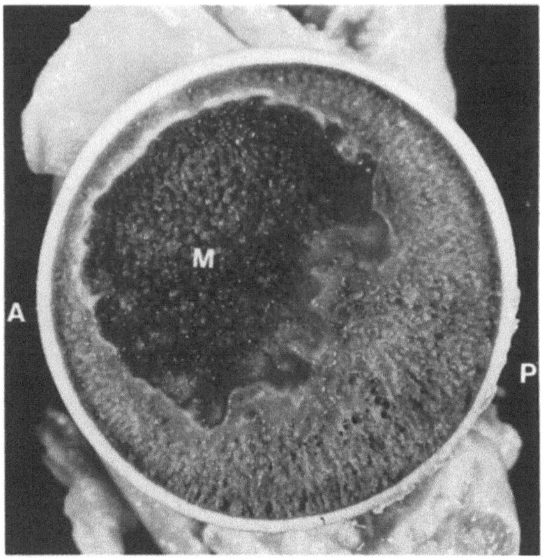

B

FIG. 7–15 Lappet formation. A Transverse section of femoral head from a 6-year-old shows the epiphysis (*E*) overlapping (*arrows*) the femoral neck of metaphysis (*M*). B Similar section from a 14-year-old shows the capital femoral ossification center completely overlapping the metaphyseal (*M*) neck bone. The physis is the thin white region between the two osseous regions. Note there is less overlap anteriorly (*A*) than posteriorly (*P*).

neck (Fig. 7–14). The triradiate cartilage is narrowing, as is the amount of cartilage between the ossified acetabular roof and articular surface. Interdigitation of the mamillary processes into the metaphysis becomes increasingly complex. The capital femoral epiphysis extends over and around the metaphysis anteriorly, medially, and posteriorly. This creates the impression, when viewing an intact femoral specimen, that the articular surface covers both epiphysis and metaphysis, especially medially. However, when a slab section is viewed, it is evident that both epiphysis and articular surface extend over the metaphysis (Fig. 7–15). This is termed *lappet formation.* Where this epiphyseal extension over the metaphysis occurs, the growth plate turns abruptly and may exhibit changes in cell column formation patterns.

The most striking change at the cellular level occurs in the intraepiphyseal growth plate along the posterosuperior femoral neck. This region develops a significant fibrocartilaginous component and changes to membranous, rather than endochondral, bone formation. There is extensive microvascularity in the superficial layers of the fibrous tissue along the posterosuperior femoral neck, and a distinct changing pattern of histology (Fig. 7–16). Along the femoral neck there are areas of fibrous tissue, fibrocartilage, and columnar cartilage, with all forming bone, and with no distinct demarcation among the different types of cellular cytoarchitecture. There is a fairly abrupt histological change, sometimes associated with an osseous extension analogous to the osseous ring of the zone of Ranvier, demarcating the lateral portion of the capital femoral physis from the intraepiphyseal physis. The cell columns are obliquely oriented away from the center of the intraepiphyseal region, and appear to follow tensile stress patterns. In the midportion of the intraepiphyseal region, the histology gradually changes from oblique cell columns to fibrocartilage making bone by membranous ossification. The tissue layers in this region comprise an outer fibrovascular zone (analogous to periosteum), a middle layer of fibrocartilage, and an inner layer of membranous bone. The cellular changes reflect the changes reflect the changing patterns of compression and tension within the developing femoral neck, comparable to the changes in the developing tibial tuberosity.[36,47] The major function of the intraepiphyseal region is to allow widening of the femoral neck.

Thirteen to Sixteen Years This period characteristically is one of initial rapid growth which may be related to susceptibility to slipped capital femoral epiphysis, followed by physiological closure of the physis. Of the three active growth regions of the proximal femur, the capital femoral physis is

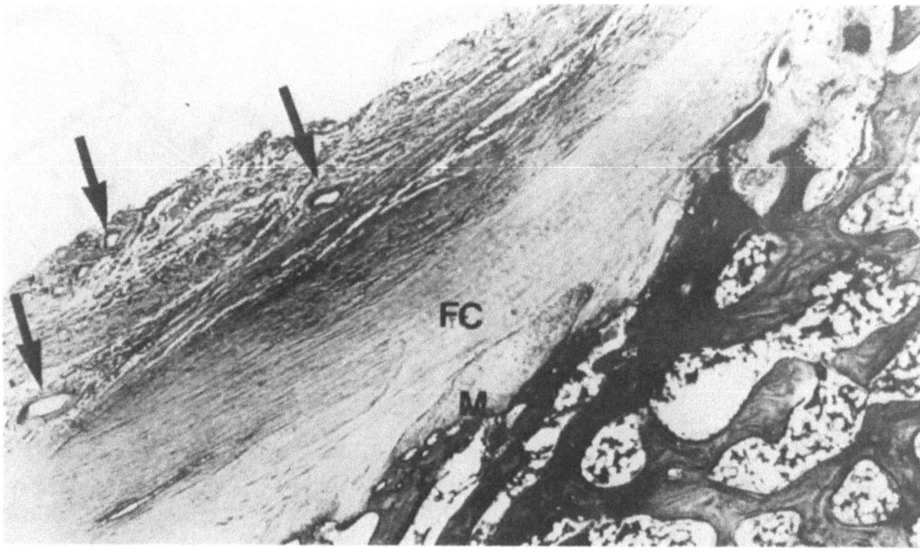

FIG. 7–16 Histology of the femoral neck in an adolescent. Multiple vessels are present (*arrows*). The cartilage modulates from columnar cartilage to fibrocartilage (*FC*), which is probably more mechanically adapted to the variable tensile stresses in this region as the cartilage thins.

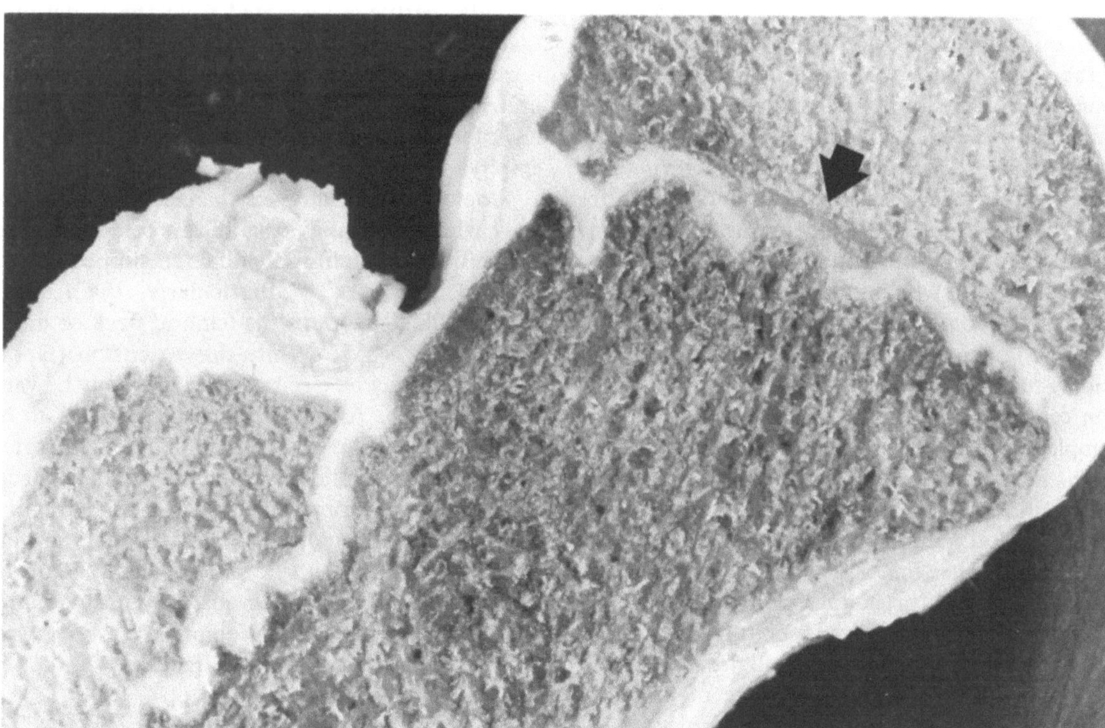

FIG. 7–17 Beginning central changes of osseous thickening above the physis (*arrow*) indicate the earliest stages of closure, which proceeds from central to peripheral in this region. Note the greater trochanteric physis has not commenced comparable changes.

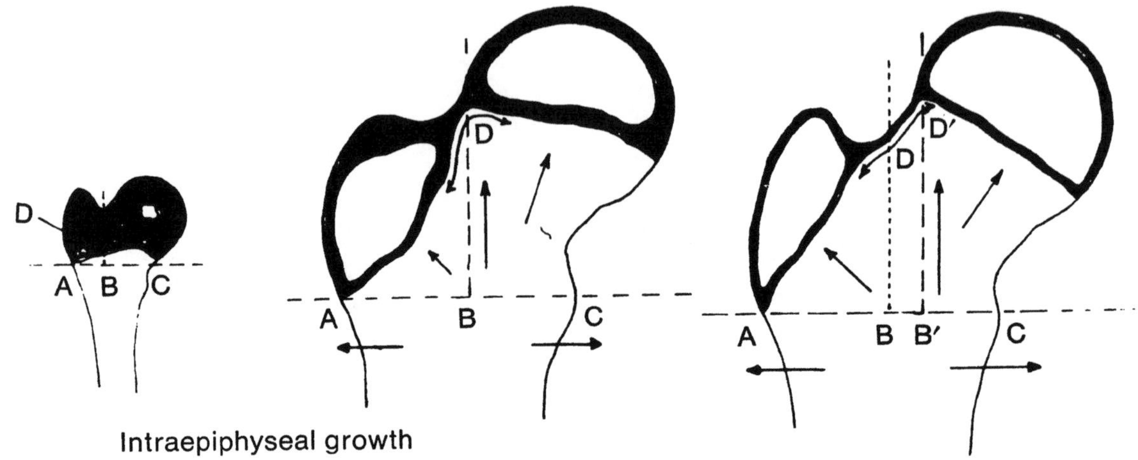

FIG. 7–18 Schematic of patterns of growth at birth (*left*), 7 years (*center*), and 14 years (*right*). Preferential growth in the *BC* segment initially establishes the capital femoral physis. As the neck develops further, the *D-D*[1] growth region contributes to width, as well as length of the neck.

the first to close, with the trochanters closing several months later. Histologically the process is most evident centrally with increasing thickness of the subchondral bone plate of the epiphyseal ossification center and similar thickening of the trabecular bone of the underlying metaphysis. The growth plate becomes less functional, forms cell clones, rather than cell columns, and the entire plate thins (Fig. 7–17). The dense osseous regions on either side of the attenuating physis are joined by small bridges which gradually increase in size. This fusion progresses in a centrifugal fashion, incorporating the entire capital femoral physis and leading to a fusion between the epiphyseal ossification center and metaphysis. As fusion is nearing completion in the capital femur, a similar process begins in the greater trochanteric physis. Growth may continue in the greater trochanter after cessation of capital femoral growth. In situations such as slipped capital femoral epiphysis, which often is associated with premature cessation of growth of the capital femoral physis, continued trochanteric growth may lead to loss of the articulotrochanteric distance, and in the case of moderate to severe slips, may contribute to an overgrowth of the trochanter leading to a neutral or negative ATD.

As the capital femoral ossification center expands, most of the epiphyseal cartilage will be completely replaced to leave only a thin layer of articular cartilage separated from the underlying maturing subchondral plate by the tidemark. This normal thinning of the cartilage may be misinterpreted radiographically as a pathological narrowing of the joint space in slipped capital femoral epiphysis.[48]

Anatomically, there are changes in the femoral neck which may play a significant role in the susceptibility of certain individuals to slipped capital femoral epiphysis.[13,40] Particularly, the femoral head cartilage overlaps the femoral neck or metaphysis (Fig. 7–15). While this extension (lappet formation) may be circumferential, it may be variably extended. Anterior extension appears to be the most variable, which may make this region less able to withstand posteriorly directed displacement (shearing) forces. The intertrochanteric and subtrochanteric regions have a rectangular appearance in cross section,[14] a factor which should be considered when planning corrective osteotomies for slipped capital femoral epiphysis or coxa vara complicating a femoral neck fracture.

Neck Development

Throughout development the capital femoral and trochanteric epiphyses have a cartilaginous conti-

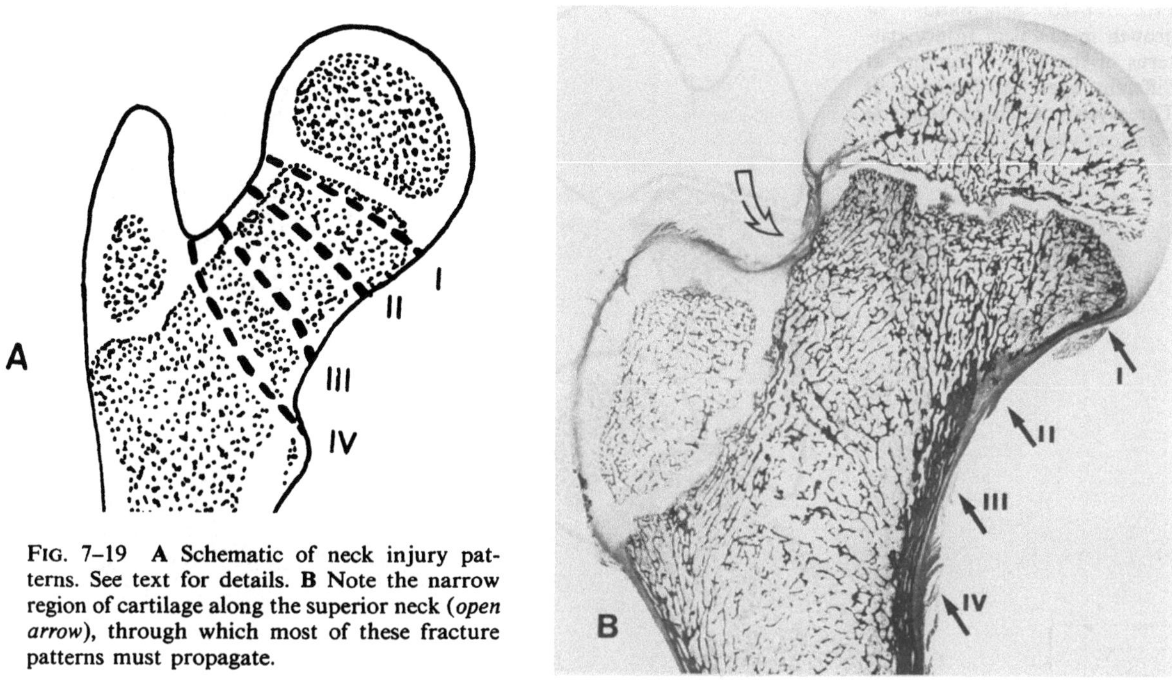

FIG. 7–19 **A** Schematic of neck injury patterns. See text for details. **B** Note the narrow region of cartilage along the superior neck (*open arrow*), through which most of these fracture patterns must propagate.

nuity along the posterosuperior femoral neck. Selective growth of both the capital femoral and intraepiphyseal physes leads to the establishment of a well-defined femoral neck (Fig. 7–18). While this intraepiphyseal region changes with time, thinning as the child grows, it is essential for normal latitudinal growth (i.e., width) of the femoral neck. Damage, as in a femoral neck fracture, may seriously impair the capacity of the neck to develop normally. Furthermore, the blood vessels course along the posterosuperior femoral neck, have a variable intracartilaginous course, and are more susceptible to injury if the fracture to the subcapital or neck region propagates into the intraepiphyseal (neck) cartilage.

The primary spongiosa initially formed during neck development is not completely oriented to biological forces across the hip joint. However, the more biomechanically responsive secondary spongiosa forms trabecular patterns oriented to compression and tension forces.[41,43,44,49] This process becomes increasingly evident during adolescence, when the characteristic patterns become well formed. Initially the dominant area of trabecular orientation goes from the calcar to the middle region of the capital femoral physis. Arching patterns develop along the superior neck, bridging between greater trochanter and capital femur. The last trabecular area to develop a specific orientation is the bone within the capital femoral ossification center.

The development of the femoral neck brings about changes in the contour of the capital femoral physis. Initially this is transversely directed, but during the first year begins to exhibit preferential growth in the medial and middle sections. As these regions develop, the capital femoral physis becomes more medially (varus) and posteriorly oriented. This pattern eventually may predispose to slipped capital femoral epiphysis. Undulations and mamillary processes develop in the physis. These probably serve as a biological anchor to minimize or prevent displacement due to shear stresses.[13,40,58,59]

The mild posterior tilt of the capital femoral physis is extremely important for the biological "correction" of anteversion. Normally rotational deformities, such as those present after a physeal fracture, do not spontaneously correct (i.e., derotate). However, the posterior and varus tilt of the physis allows the femoral neck to grow "backward" relative to the bicondylar axis of the distal femur, thus progressively decreasing the amount of anteversion from the characteristic 40° in the young child to 15° by the end of skeletal development.

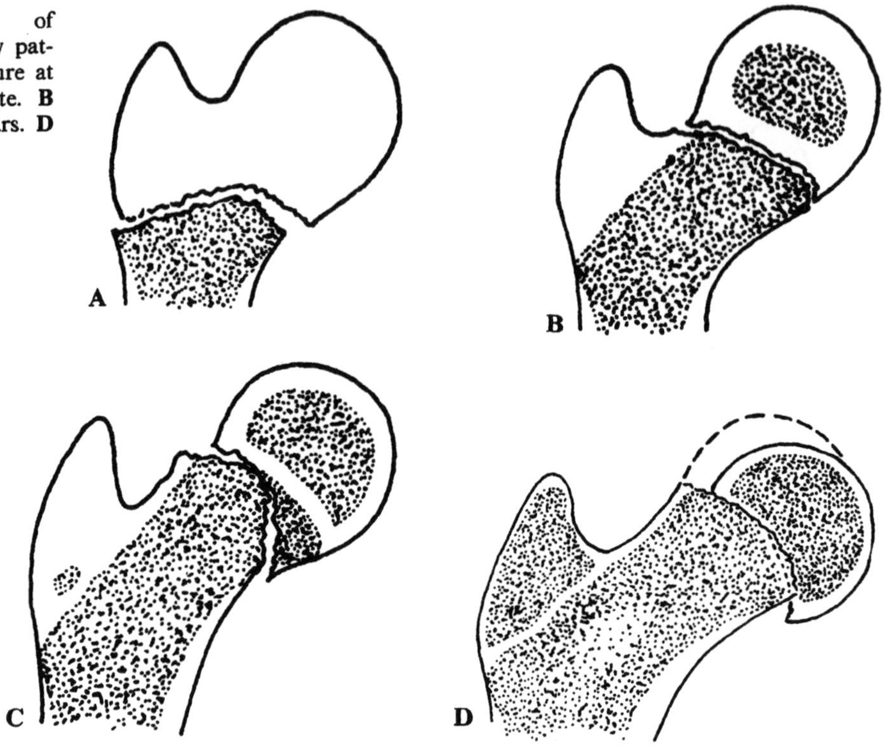

FIG. 7–20 Schematic of growth mechanism injury patterns of the type I fracture at different ages. **A** Neonate. **B** Three years. **C** Eight years. **D** Fourteen years.

Injury Patterns

Proximal femoral fractures are infrequent prior to skeletal maturity.[1,2,5,8–11,19–28,30,32,33,50–58,60,65,66] Proximal femoral fracture may occur at birth, and diagnostically must be separated from congenital hip dysplasia.[17,29,34,61,62,64] The injury may be seen in an abused infant. In young and old children considerable violence is required, and there often are accompanying injuries. In adolescence, an acute injury represents one end of the spectrum of slipped capital femoral epiphysis. Pathological fractures may occur in many diseased states, including renal osteodystrophy, hypothyroidism, juvenile rheumatoid arthritis, septic arthritis, and malignancies.

There are several important differences between proximal femoral fractures in adults and children. Since the combined, circumferential periosteal/perichondrial tube is much stronger, fractures are not always significantly displaced.[13,40,46] In particular, the presence of the cartilaginous intraepiphyseal bridge along the superior and posterior neck tends to prevent significant displacement of the physis, unless this epiphyseal cartilage is also disrupted, a factor that is impossible to discern with standard roentgenographic techniques. A potential complication, ischemic necrosis, may affect, specifically or in combination, the epiphysis, the metaphysis, and the physis. Ischemic damage will obviously have very different effects on the immature proximal femur than a similar complication in the mature bone of an adult.

Classification As in the adult fractures occur at different levels along the femoral neck (Fig. 7–19). However, because the femoral neck is actively elongating, certain types cannot occur at younger ages, and a given type may vary with age and extent of femoral neck development.

The type I injury may assume several different patterns contingent upon the age of the patient (Fig. 7–20). During the neonatal period and the first year of life the entire proximal femoral chondroepiphysis, including capital femur, intraepiphyseal region, and greater trochanter, will traumatically separate as a contiguous unit. The lesser trochanter also may be included, depending upon the mechanism of injury. Increased medial cell column disruption may cause localized type V injury, with the potential for temporary or permanent growth arrest and a progressive, traumatic coxa vara.

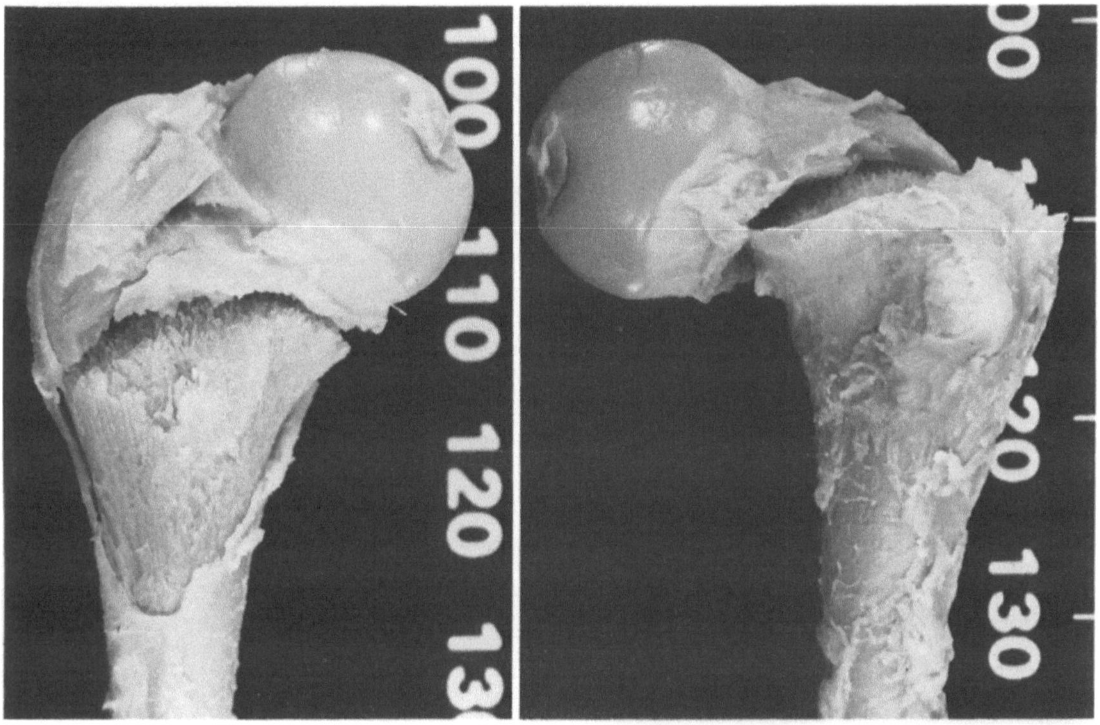

A B

As the femoral neck progressively develops, the fracture pattern changes and increasingly localizes to the capital femoral region. The fracture line may extend from the intertrochanteric notch superiorly across the intraepiphyseal cartilage, and along the capital femoral physis (type III), or partially along the capital femoral physis and finally into the metaphysis of the femoral neck (type IV). During adolescence fracture primarily involves the capital femoral physeal/metaphyseal interface, crossing the remnants of the intraepiphyseal region.

Type II (transcervical) is a fracture through the midportion of the femoral neck. Type III (cervicotrochanteric) occurs through the base of the femoral neck. Type IV (peritrochanteric) is between the base of the femoral neck and the lesser trochanter.

In the younger child limited development of the length of the neck is going to affect the pattern of fracture, at least from the standpoint of defining types II, III, and IV. However, treatment is not significantly different in any, and the risks of complications such as ischemic necrosis and coxa vara are reasonably high in all types. It is extremely important to remember that there is a variably thick cartilaginous continuity along the posterosuperior neck, and that the fracture may propagate into and through this, essentially making types

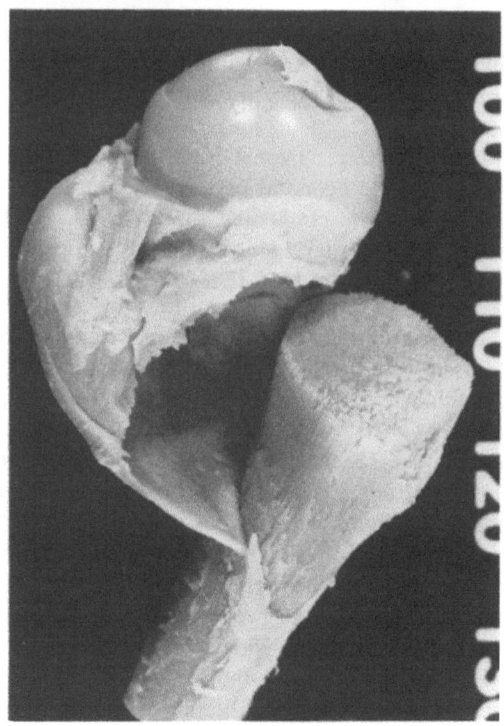

C

FIG. 7–21 Experimental neonatal fracture. **A** Notice fracture line extending completely across the physeal–metaphyseal interface, and the disruption of the anterior periosteum. **B** As the shaft laterally displaces, the chondroepiphysis tilts posteriorly and into varus. **C** Notice the intact periosteum posteriorly.

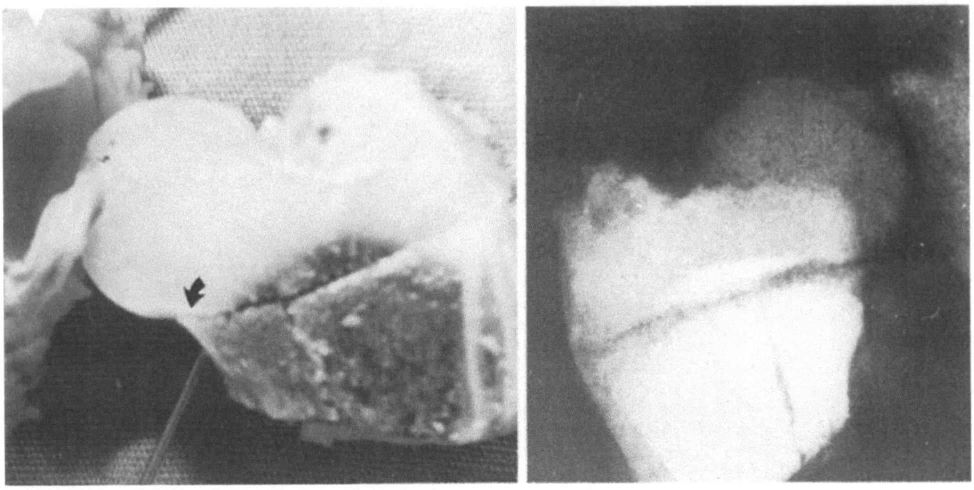

A B

FIG. 7–22 Experimental neonatal fracture. **A** Note medial crushing where fracture propagates into the physis (*arrow*). **B** Roentgenogram.

II, III, and IV each a growth mechanism injury that mandates accurate anatomical reduction to prevent potential growth deformity.

Neonatal Injury Type I fractures may occur at birth or in the neonatal period. They must be distinguished from congenital hip dysplasia (CHD), which has a similar roentgenographic appearance. However, unlike CHD, these injuries usually are associated with pain on examination of the hip.

Milgram obtained postmortem specimens from children dying from disease not affecting the skeleton.[31] Manipulative epiphyseal separation was produced by simultaneously rotating and bending the specimens. Microscopically the zone of separation was variably through the hypertrophic cell layer. Meier reported two cases of children with epiphysiolysis consequent to birth trauma.[30] One of these children died several weeks later, and autopsy showed marked callus formation around the shaft with a fracture through the region just below the common growth plate separating the entire proximal femoral epiphysis from the shaft.

Similar experiments in our Skeletal Development Laboratory have shown an epiphysiolysis, *not* a dislocation, will result (Fig. 7–21). The separation generally occurs through or below the zone of hypertrophic cartilage. Medial physeal cell column disruption and propagation into the epiphysis were noted experimentally (Fig. 7–22), and certainly offer an explanation for the localized type 5 growth mechanism injury which may infrequently occur and lead to a deformity such as coxa vara.

Slipped Capital Femoral Epiphysis This injury may be an acute traumatic separation of a previously normal epiphysis.[2,13–15,18,58] However, the distinction between acute and chronic conditions often may be quite difficult. Slipped capital femoral epiphysis (Fig. 7–23), whether acute or chronic, should be considered a fracture selectively involving the capital femoral physis. The epiphysis and physis are displaced posteriorly and then into varus. The discrete anatomy of the area mechanically predisposes to this pattern of failure.[14]

Anatomy and Treatment The prognosis for union is excellent in a child with an undisplaced fracture. However, this fracture area, similar to the lateral condyle of the distal humerus, carries a reasonable risk of delayed union, nonunion, and malunion. When a displaced or potentially unstable fracture is reduced and held only in a cast, coxa vara may still occur due to isometric muscular contractures in the cast.

The hardness of a child's bone and the small size of the femoral neck limit acceptable fixation devices. Large nails are to be condemned, as they

C
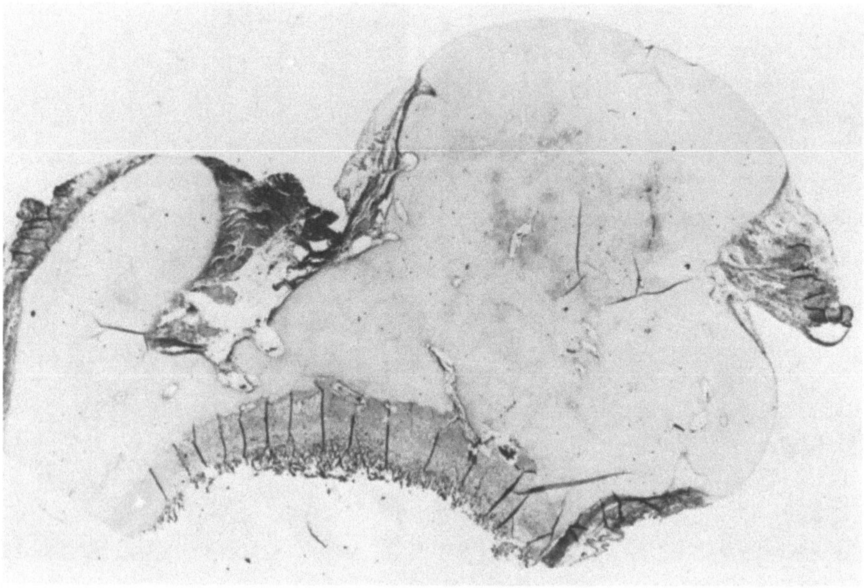

FIG. 7–22 C Histological section.

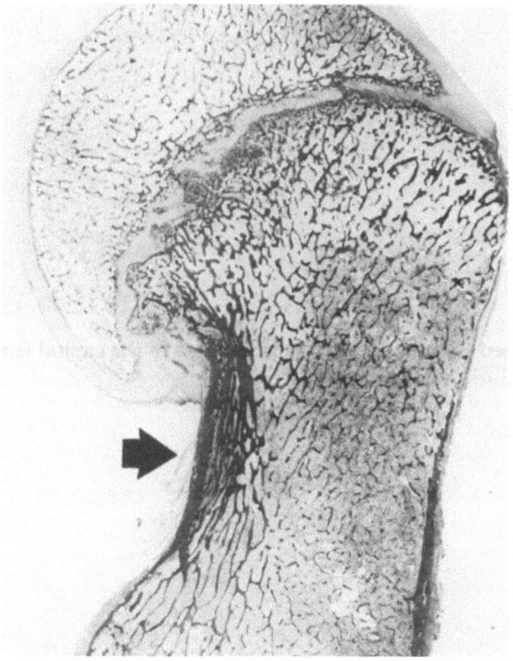

FIG. 7–23 Slipped capital femoral epiphysis. Note the posterior direction of the slip (*open arrow*) and augmentation of the calcar (*solid arrow*) in this chronic lesion.

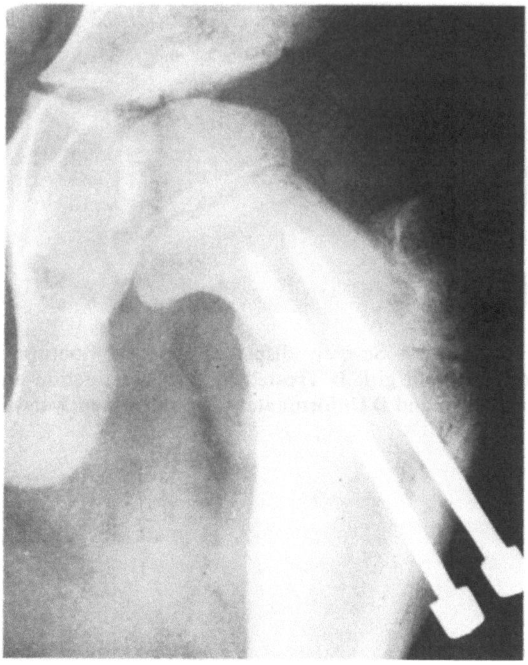

FIG. 7–24 Intertrochanteric (type IV) fracture in an 11-year-old with congenital insensitivity to pain. Notice that the pins cross the fracture but not the physis.

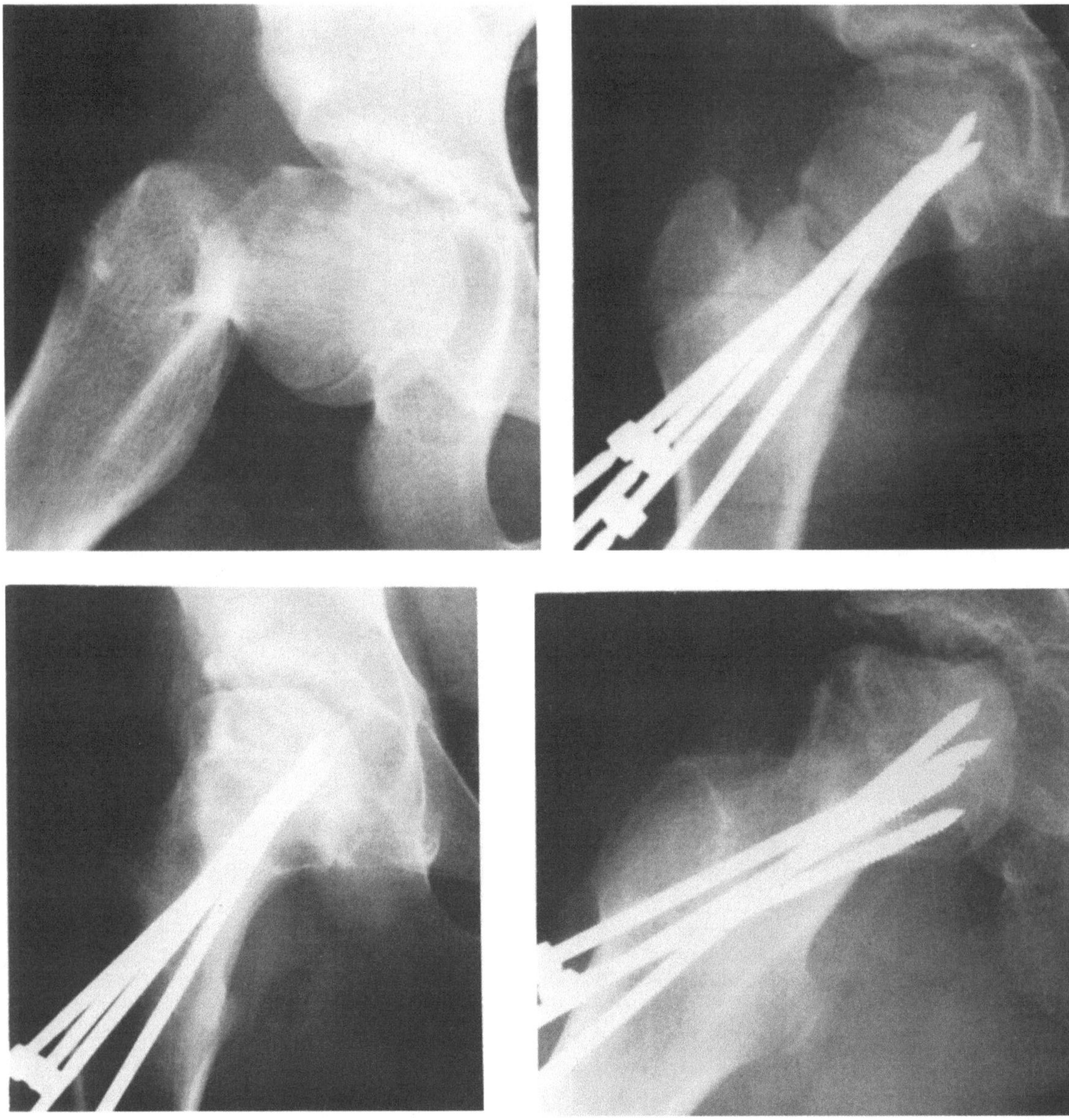

A B C D

FIG. 7–25 **A** Severely displaced type III fracture in a 13-year-old girl. **B** Treated by closed reduction and pinning. **C** and **D** Unfortunately, she subsequently developed ischemic necrosis and collapse of the capital femoral ossification center.

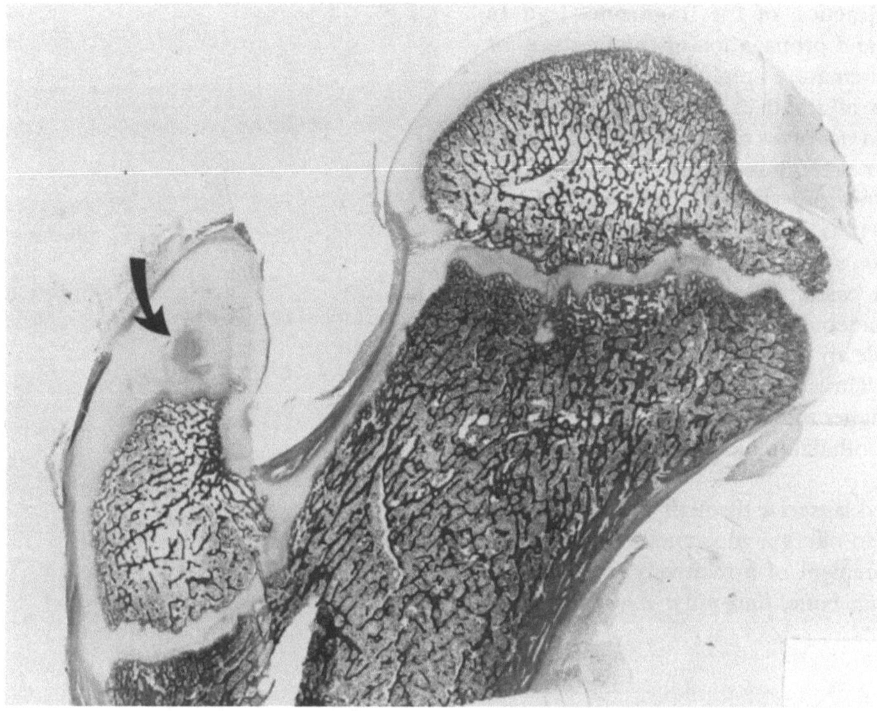

A

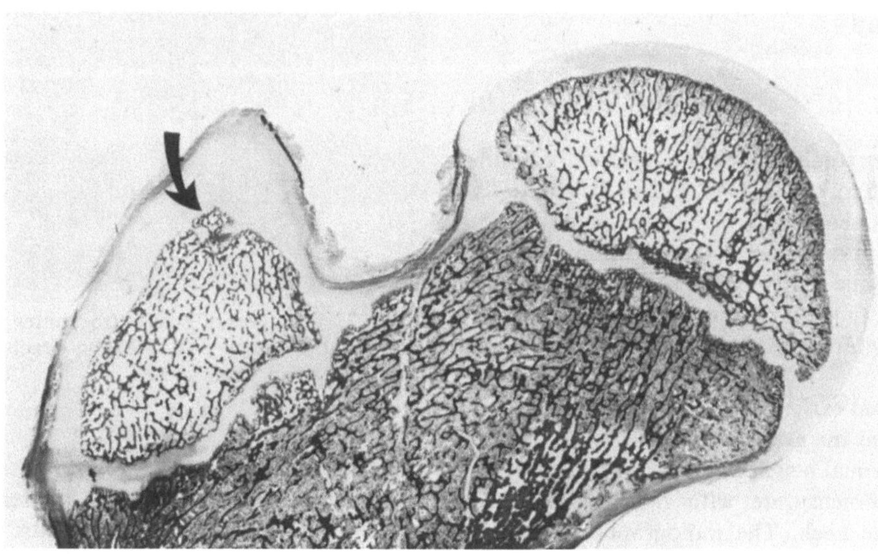

B

FIG. 7–26 Development of greater trochanter. **A** Accessory ossification may develop at the tip (*arrow*). **B** This fuses (*arrow*) to the main center. These variations should not be misinterpreted as fractures.

may cause distraction of the fragments, lead to fragmentation and propagation of the fracture, or predispose to premature epiphysiodesis. Threaded pins or screws of small caliber should be used, but these should *not* cross the physis (which would create a risk for premature epiphysiodesis), unless the patient is nearing skeletal maturity (Fig. 7–24 and 7–25). It is usually unnecessary to cross the growth plate, except in some high cervical fractures. In such cases, pins with a smooth shaft should be considered, and should be removed as soon as possible to avoid interfering with subsequent growth. Threaded pins crossing the growth plate cause a higher rate of premature epiphysiodesis than do smooth fixation pins of the same diameter.

A child-sized lagscrew through a predrilled and tapped hole also offers a good method. However, it requires placement of a relatively large device, displacing much bone, and must *never* cross the physis.

Trochanters

Morphology

The greater trochanter begins secondary ossification at age 5 to 7 years (Fig. 7–26). This initially is present just above the trochanteric physis. With further maturation secondary ossification proceeds cephalad into the remainder of the epiphyseal cartilage. Epiphysiodesis occurs from age 16 to 19 years, usually after the capital femoral region has closed.

As discussed earlier, the tip of the cartilaginous trochanter and the articular surface of the capital femur are of equal height at birth. A positive ATD develops commensurate with development and growth of the neck. The radiographic measurement of the ATD is really a measurement of the difference of the secondary ossification centers, not the true ATD of the still unossified portions of the cartilage. The greater trochanter, being surrounded by well-vascularized perichondrium, grows latitudinally and longitudinally from this tissue, but the major longitudinal growth is from the physis.

The lesser trochanter does not secondarily ossify until adolescence, and fuses from age 16 to 19 years.

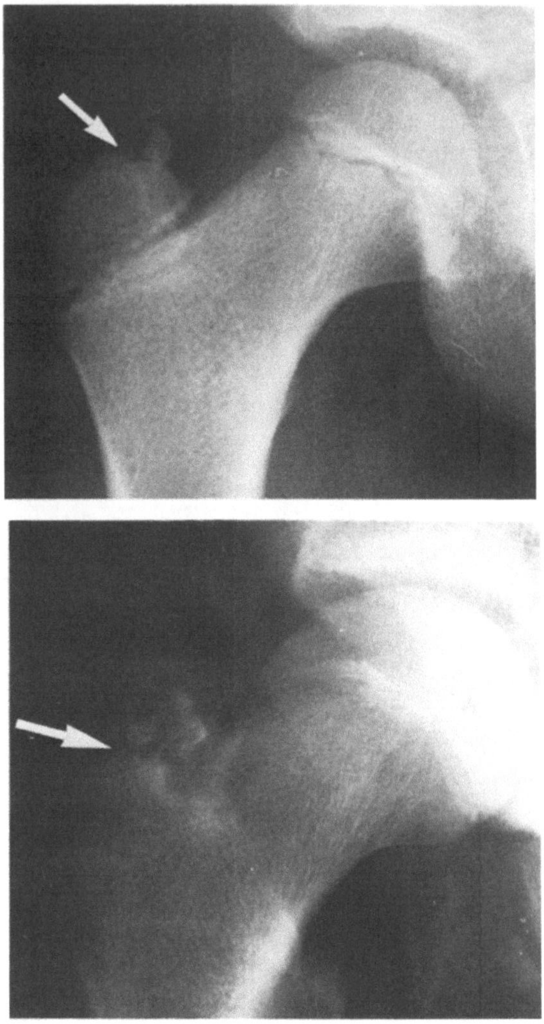

A

B

FIG. 7–27 Fractures of greater trochanter. **A** Avulsion injury to tip (*arrow*). **B** Healing fracture (*arrow*) through center of ossification.

Injury Patterns

Fractures involving the trochanters are unusual, but they do occur and one must be familiar with the developmental anatomy in order to make the diagnosis and render appropriate treatment. The cartilaginous proximal portion may be injured without any corroborating roentgenographic evidence.

Fractures may occur through the upper end or midportion of the developing ossification center (Fig. 7–27). These generally result from a direct blow or avulsion, and often are undisplaced. An injury must be carefully distinguished from normal variations in which an accessory ossification

FIG. 7–28 **A** Avulsion fracture of entire trochanter (*arrow*) accompanying anterior hip dislocation. **B** Schematic of injury. **C** Similar injury to the right hip in another child at 7 years led to premature growth arrest and overgrowth of the femoral neck several years later.

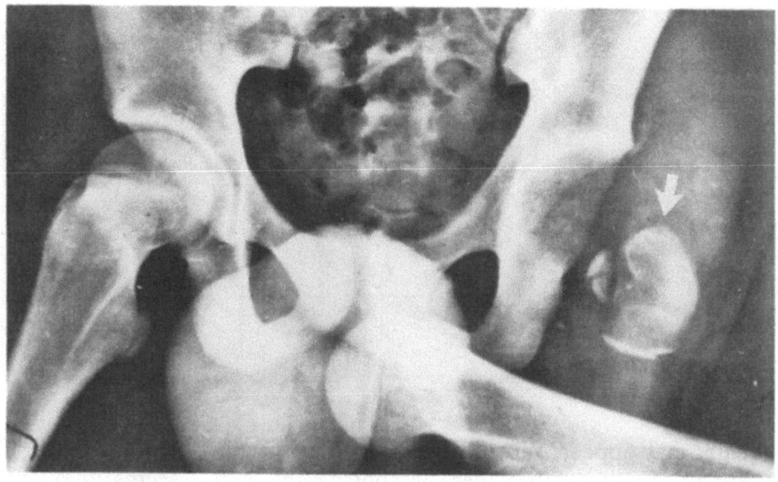

A

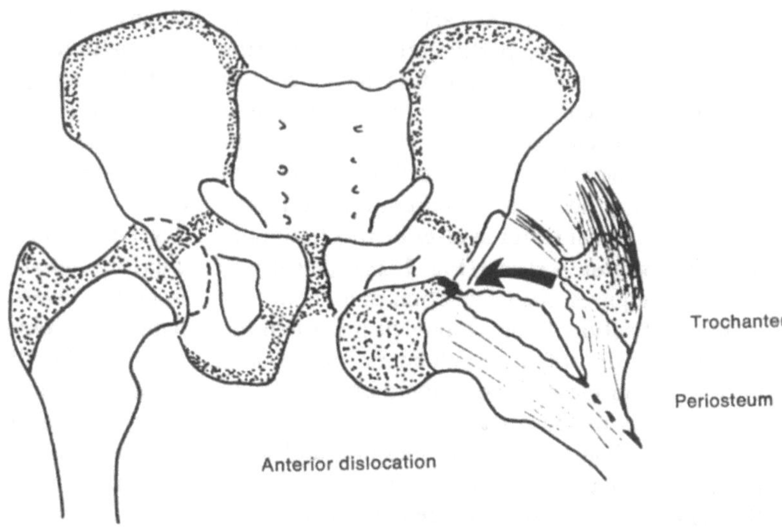

B

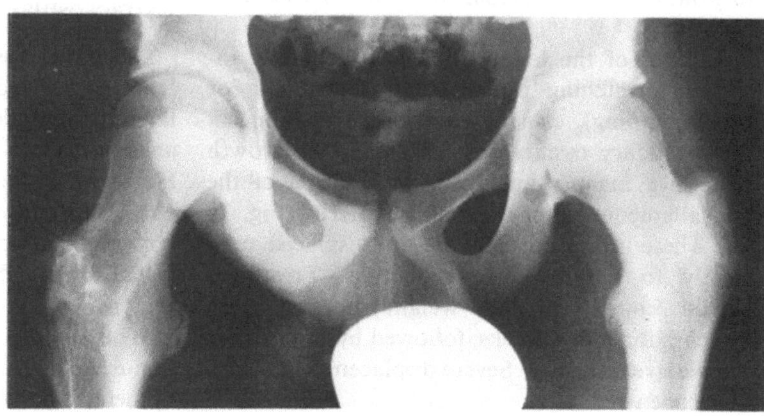

C

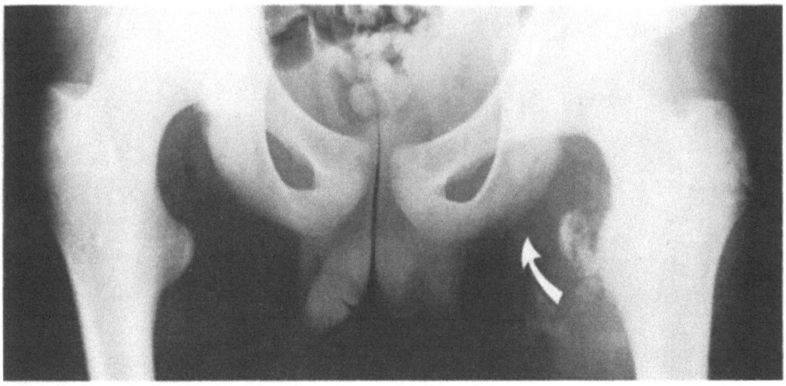

FIG. 7–29 Fracture of the lesser trochanter (*arrow*) in an adolescent.

center may appear. When there is significant separation, it is likely that there is considerable soft tissue disruption as well as cartilaginous damage.

On rare occasions, particularly with anterior hip dislocations, the entire greater trochanter may be avulsed from the remainder of the proximal femur.[37] This occurs because all the musculotendinous and periosteal attachments of the greater trochanter remain intact as a composite lateral unit, while the proximal femur avulses forward, slipping out of the periosteal sleeve (Fig. 7–28). This injury generally requires open reduction and some type of internal fixation. Efforts should be made to minimize penetration of the trochanteric physis with pins. Any fixation methods should appreciate the fact that this region must continue to grow in a longitudinal fashion. When it does not, and when there is premature growth arrest of the region, the remainder of the proximal femur may continue to grow, leading to an elongated femoral neck (Fig. 7–28).

Injuries of the lesser trochanter generally involve a stretching injury (such as running or broad-jumping), causing avulsion of portions of the secondary ossification center and/or growth plate in a manner analogous to avulsion of the medial epicondyle of the distal humerus (Fig. 7–29). These injuries usually are not displaced sufficiently to require open reduction. Treatment should consist of non-weight bearing with crutches for 3 to 4 weeks, followed by progressive muscle strengthening. Severe displacement may require open reduction.

Vascularity

As in most biological morphology, vascular distribution to the proximal femur shows considerable individual variation within a reasonably general pattern.[12,34,35,42,44,63] The proximal femur seems uniquely susceptible to vascular disorders at any and all stages of postnatal development and maturation. An understanding of the complex and changing patterns of macroscopic and microscopic circulation of the proximal femur during postnatal skeletal maturation is essential to an adequate appreciation of the role of this vasculature in both normal morphological and physiological developmental patterns, as well as abnormal, vascular-mediated growth patterns encountered in ischemic (avascular) necrosis of slipped capital femoral epiphysis, femoral neck fracture, and traumatic hip dislocation. This predisposition may be ascribed primarily to the gradual development of an intracapsular course for those discrete, increasingly limited blood vessels supplying the capital femoral epiphysis and physis.

Extracapsular Circulation

The extracapsular blood supply to the proximal femur is derived principally from the medial and lateral circumflex arteries. There are numerous anastomoses to vessels external to the hip joint. However, while anatomical connections are present, compromise of one or more major extracapsular vessels at specific areas may jeopardize functional blood flow from adjacent anastomotic regions.

The predominant blood supply of the proximal femur, no matter what the stage of postnatal development, is derived from the deep (profunda) femoral artery, which gives origin to two major branches—the lateral and medial circumflex arteries. The lateral circumflex artery invariably arises from the profunda femoris artery. The medial circumflex artery usually originates from the profunda femoris artery, but may arise as an indepen-

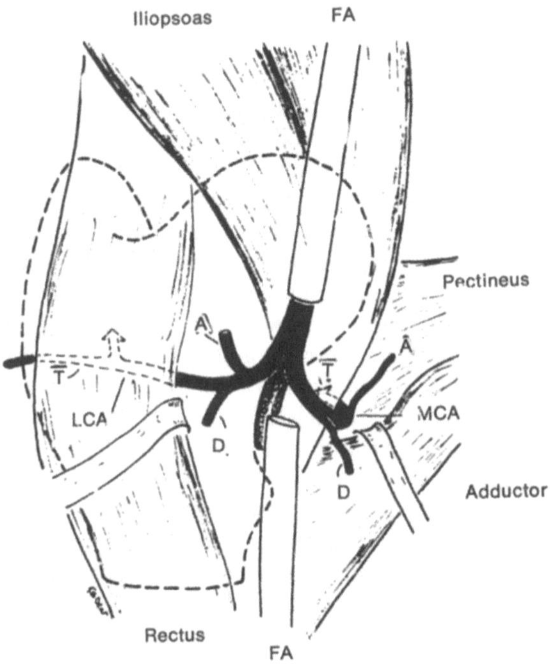

FIG. 7–30 Schematic of origin of main blood vessels to the proximal femur. *FA*, femoral artery; *MCA*, medial circumflex artery; *LCA*, lateral circumflex artery; *A*, ascending branches; *D*, descending branches; *T*, transverse branches.

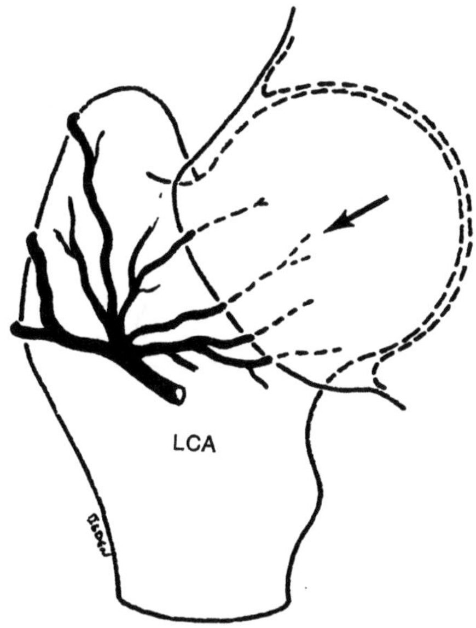

FIG. 7–31 Schematic of lateral circumflex artery (*LCA*), which primarily supplies the greater trochanter, but does send some anterior branches (*arrow*).

dent vessel directly from the main femoral trunk. The origin and initial course of these femoral circumflex vessels are depicted in Fig. 7–30.

The lateral circumflex artery crosses to the long head of the rectus femoris. Beneath this muscle the transverse branch gives rise to an artery that courses to the underlying anterolateral proximal femur near the insertion of the hip capsule. Upon reaching the proximal femur, this transverse branch of the lateral circumflex artery gives off several branches that penetrate the anterior and lateral portions of the greater trochanter and much of the anterior portion of the capital femur along the capsular insertion (Fig. 7–31). During the first year of life the lateral circumflex branches supply a considerable portion of the anterior chondroepiphysis. However, with growth (particularly the development of the femoral neck) the lateral circumflex artery increasingly supplies the greater trochanter, anterior femoral neck, and metaphysis, and decreasingly contributes to the intracapsular capital femoral circulation.

The medial circumflex artery crosses the medial portion of the iliopsoas muscle. This initial course

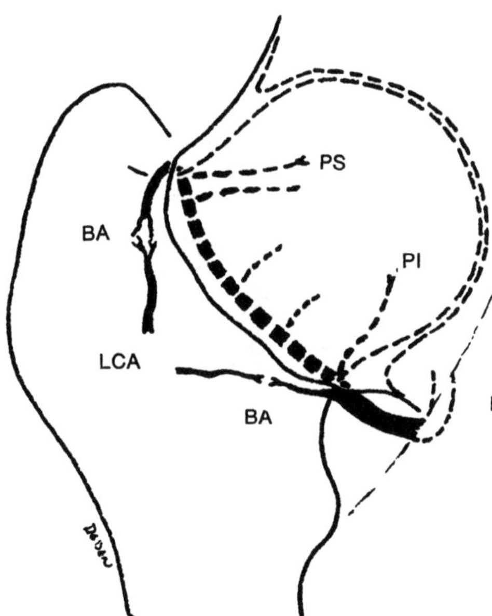

FIG. 7–32 Schematic of basal anastomosis (*BA*), which is derived from both medial (*MCA*) and lateral (*LCA*) circumflex arteries. *PS*, posterosuperior vessels; *PI*, posteroinferior vessels.

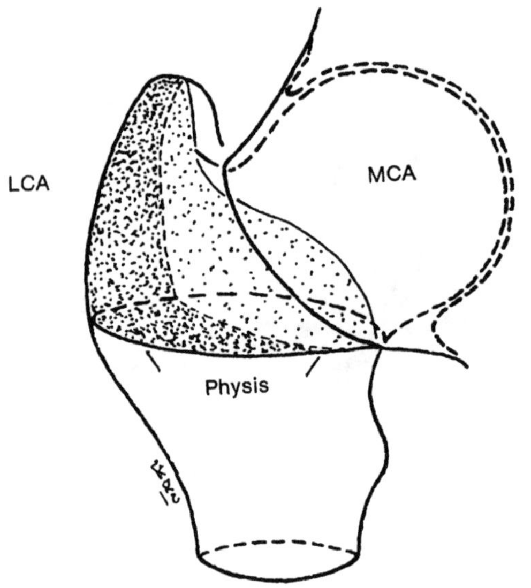

FIG. 7–33 Schematic of relative contributions of medial (*MCA*) and lateral (*LCA*) circumflex arteries to epiphyseal and physeal regions. The LCA area is stippled.

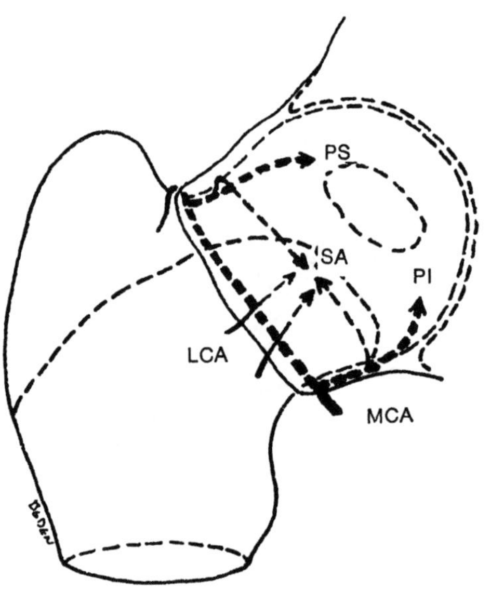

FIG. 7–34 Schematic of subsynovial (intracapsular) anastomosis (*SA*), which is derived from the posterosuperior (*PS*) and posteroinferior (*PI*) branches of the medial circumflex artery (*MCA*). The lateral circumflex artery (*LCA*) contributes very little anteriorly to this anastomosis.

is highly variable. The main branch of the medial circumflex artery goes between the iliopsoas and pectineus/adductor group, wrapping completely around the iliopsoas tendon to reach the posteromedial side of the proximal femur, between the inferomedial capsular insertion and the lesser trochanter. A small branch courses anteriorly along the capsular insertion, while the major portion of the medial circumflex artery traverses the posterior intertrochanteric notch as the intraepiphyseal artery, crosses to the anterosuperior portion of the intertrochanteric groove, and anastomoses with the terminal ramifications of the lateral circumflex artery, creating the first of three important proximal femoral anastomoses (Fig. 7–32). This pericapsular, variably complete, vascular ring is the basal or trochanteric anastomosis. In contrast to the intracapsular and intraepiphyseal circulations, which change continually during postnatal development, the extracapsular circulation along the intertrochanteric regions changes anatomical relationships very little with subsequent proximal femoral development, remaining just outside the capsule throughout development.

Intracapsular Circulation

At birth there is a bipartite circulation to the entire proximal femoral chondroepiphysis, with minimal contribution from the artery of the ligamentum capitis femoris. The two circumflex vessels supply approximately equal portions of the greater trochanteric and capital femoral epiphyseal cartilage and physis, with the medial circumflex artery supplying the posterior half and the lateral circumflex artery supplying the anterior half (Fig. 7–33).

With growth the most significant factor relative to the contributions of the medial and lateral circumflex arteries to the proximal femoral circulation is the postnatal development of the femoral neck. This causes a relative medial displacement of the capital femoral epiphysis and necessitates major modifications of the circulatory patterns.

The lateral circumflex branches increasingly dominate as the blood supply to the developing intracapsular metaphysis. As the articular surface and underlying epiphysis gradually overlap the anterior and inferior metaphysis, there are fewer areas where the anterior vessels can penetrate. This probably is a major factor in the regression of anterior epiphyseal blood supply. The anterior

FIG. 7–35 Posterosuperior vessels. **A** Epiphyseal (*solid arrow*) and physeal (*open arrow*) vessels in a 7-year-old. **B** Single vessel (*arrow*) in a 12-year-old.

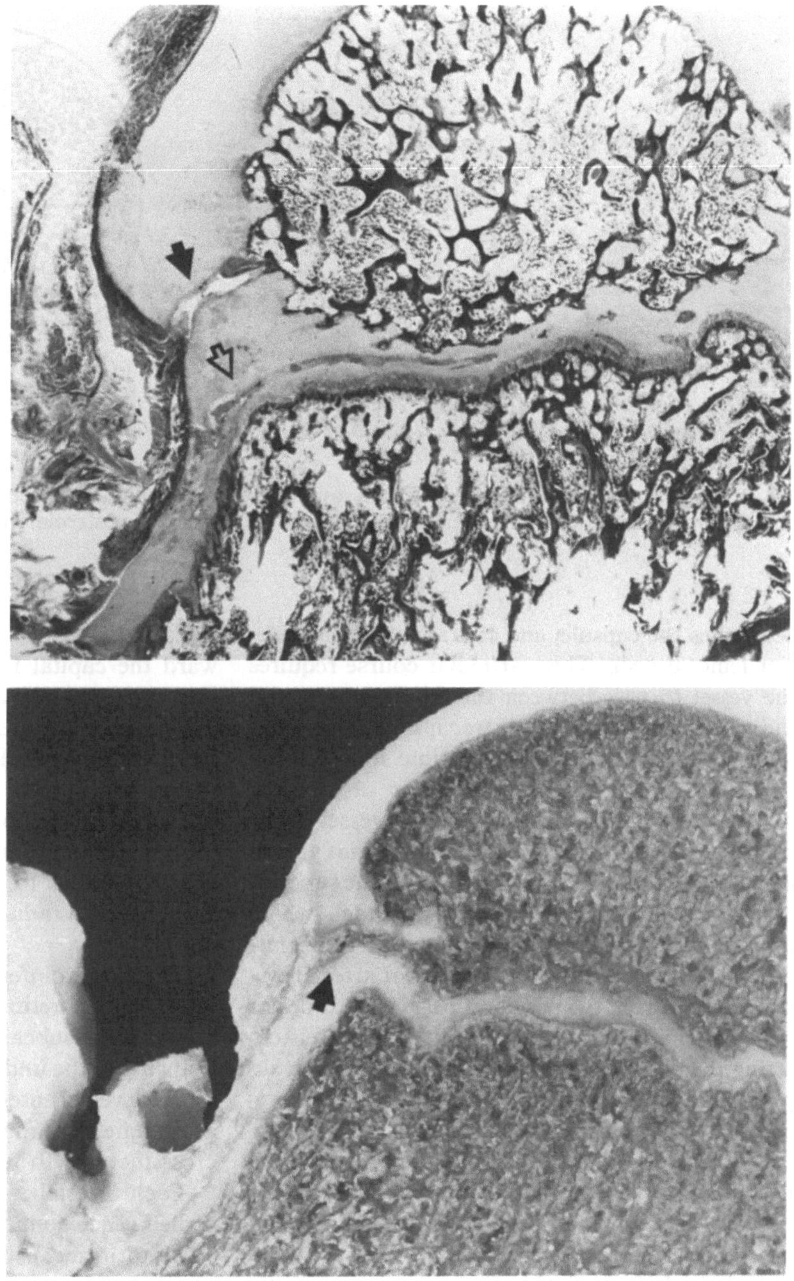

A

B

metaphyseal arteries also contribute to the subsynovial anastomosis, which is found along the subcapital region adjacent to the articular surface (Fig. 7–34). By 3 to 5 years of age, the anterior branches primarily supply the metaphysis, and the anterior portion of the subsynovial anastomosis becomes less prominent. The gradual regression of the anterior epiphyseal supply characterizes normal postnatal vascular development of the proximal femur.

The medial circumflex branches provide the majority of the circulation of the capital femur throughout development. Two primary circulatory systems develop, with both systems being posterior. The first vessel arises from the medial circumflex artery near the level of the lesser trochanter,

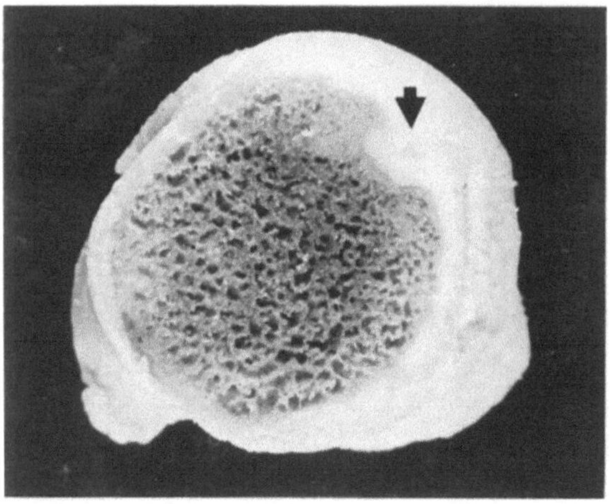

A

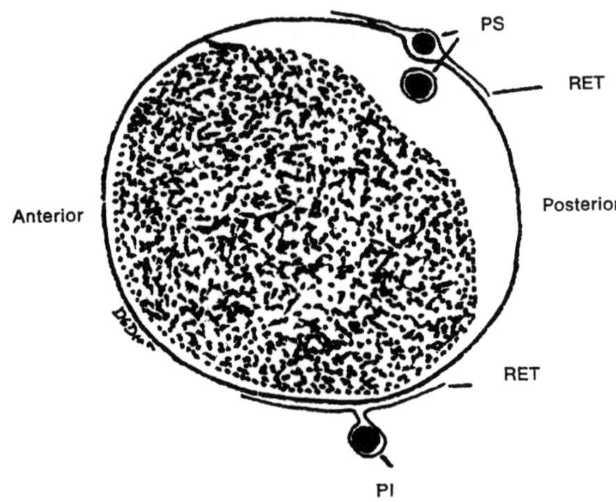

B

FIG. 7–36 Intracartilaginous course of posterosuperior vessel (*arrow*) along femoral neck. **A** Slab section. **B** Schematic. *RET,* retinaculum; *PS,* posterosuperior vessels; *PI,* posteroinferior vessels.

penetrates the capsule, and courses along the inferior femoral neck. This particular course requires the vessel to pass between the femoral neck and the closely juxtaposed, extracapsular, iliopsoas tendon, which makes it susceptible to occlusion in certain positions (e.g., traumatic dislocation, whether anterior or posterior). This vessel is the posteroinferior artery. The more important vessels penetrate the capsule and course along the superior region of the femoral neck. This system, which is usually comprised of at least two or more arteries, is defined as the posterosuperior arterial system. Even during the perinatal period the superior region is characterized by several large vessels entering the chondroepiphysis (Fig. 7–35). Both superior and inferior systems contribute to the aforementioned subsynovial anastomosis.

With progressive development of the femoral neck each of these medial circumflex–derived vascular systems must gradually elongate to accommodate the increasing distance between the joint capsule and sites of penetration into the capital femoral cartilage. The sites of entry are always directly into the epiphyseal cartilage without penetrating physeal or articular cartilage.

The posterosuperior vessels may be contained within a retinacular reflection, may be between retinaculum and cartilage, or may even be intracartilaginous (Fig. 7–36), a factor which must be considered when femoral neck fractures involve this posterosuperior cartilage. These multiple vessels tend to be quite fixed in their anatomical location, particularly if the majority of the course toward the capital femoral epiphysis is within the intraepiphyseal cartilaginous connection. Accordingly, they are more susceptible to injury, whether from a femoral neck fracture or a cuneiform osteotomy for slipped capital femoral epiphysis. At the superior subcapital sulcus the vessels continue into the femoral head in a smooth, curvilinear course parallel to the physis. Intracartilaginous branches then radiate from these primary penetrating vessels.

The posteroinferior artery courses in a much more mobile retinacular reflection and goes directly to the subcapital sulcus, giving off minimal branches to the underlying epiphysis and metaphysis. This vessel enters the epiphysis directly. Again, at no time does the posteroinferior artery directly cross the growth plate.

Each arterial system is accompanied by thin-walled venae comitantes, which may be more sensitive to intracapsular pressure changes than the arteries.

The developing femoral neck derives blood supply from two primary sources. The metaphysis is supplied principally by the anterior retinacular branches derived from the lateral circumflex artery. The intraepiphyseal cartilaginous bridge between the capital femur and greater trochanter is supplied by branches from the posterosuperior arteries (Fig. 7–37). Such a pattern thus maintains the characteristic, relative independence of epiphyseal and metaphyseal circulations. However, the cartilaginous bridge along the posterior femoral neck progressively thins.

Sinusoidal anastomoses between epiphyseal (medial circumflex) and metaphyseal (lateral circumflex) circulations are more common than in other regions of the proximal femur. These anastomoses seem to be venous, and undoubtedly play a role in patterns of vascular drainage from the capital femoral region.

Another important feature is the relationship of the blood vessels to the joint capsule. Along the intertrochanteric notch the blood vessels are external to the joint capsule. Vessels penetrate the capsule at its level of insertion into the epiphyseal cartilage along the posterosuperior intertrochanteric notch. A few small branches course within the capsule itself, but these vessels are not directly involved in the blood supply of the proximal femur. Therefore, capsulotomy or traumatic damage to the capsule, as in a hip dislocation, should not affect the blood supply of the proximal femur as long as the underlying, and anatomically separate, posterosuperior and posteroinferior vessels are not specifically damaged.

Intraepiphyseal Circulation

The developing chondroepiphysis is quite vascular, being supplied through structures termed cartilage canals.[34,35,37,38] An understanding of the microanatomy and physiology of these canals is fundamental to understanding the nature of the epiphyseal and physeal cartilage, dynamic tissues with considerable cellular activity. The initial phases of development of the secondary ossification center of the chondroepiphysis take place immediately adjacent to cartilage canals, similar to the process of vascular irruption that led to the development of the primary ossification center embryologically.

These canals have several important characteristics. First, and most important, they supply discrete regions within the epiphysis, with virtually no anastomosis between canalicular systems of adjacent regions. Second, while the canals enter the epiphysis at fairly regular intervals along the growth plate periphery of most epiphyses, they have progressively limited entry into the capital femoral epiphysis. Third, the canals may serve as an additional source of chondroblasts for interstitial enlargement of the epiphysis. Fourth, the canals are surrounded by a dense area of cartilage and intercellular matrix that probably renders an internal microsupport system to the chondroepiphysis and protects the canals from collapse during load-bearing stress. And fifth, the canals play an integral role in the development of the secondary ossification center. Each of the aforementioned factors plays a causal role in the development of the highly variable presentations of avascular (ischemic) necrosis and delayed healing following trauma, such as a fracture through the neck of the femur or hip dislocation.

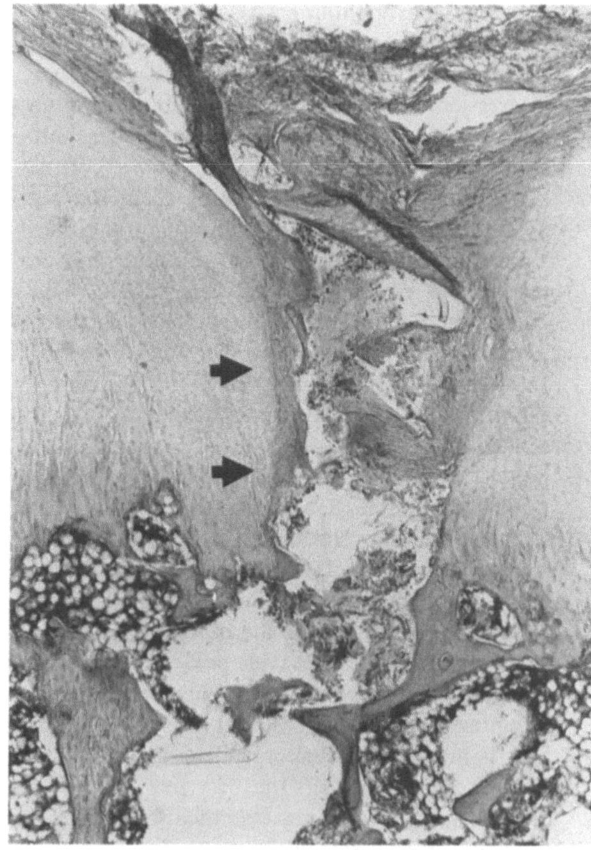

FIG. 7–37 Vessels crossing the posterosuperior intraepiphyseal cartilage of femoral neck (*arrows*) to directly enter the metaphysis.

During the perinatal period the growth plate is a relatively planar, transversely oriented structure under the entire proximal femoral chondroepiphysis. Blood vessels from the basal anastomosis enter the epiphyseal cartilage directly along the capsular insertions, anteriorly and posteriorly, without any significant intracapsular course. Small vessels also directly penetrate the epiphysis external to the capsule to supply the neck and greater trochanter. Throughout postnatal development the greater trochanter will maintain this multiple vessel system, whereas the capital femur undergoes a regression from multiple, small penetrating vessels until only a few major vessels supply the entire capital femur.

The small branches originating from the pericapsular plexuses of the medial and lateral circumflex vessels enter the proximal femoral chondroepiphysis in penetrating cartilage canals. These penetrating canals occur at intervals along the periphery of the physis, along the line of junction of the joint capsule with the perichondrium in the intraepiphyseal (intertrochanteric) groove, and through the perichondrium over the greater trochanter.

With postnatal development of the femoral neck, the extracapsular patterns of penetration are essentially unchanged, while the intracapsular patterns change significantly. Penetrating vessels become fewer in number as the multiple, minimally branched vessels progressively coalesce at the original sites of penetration to create arborized systems stemming from a few dominant vessels. Although there is increasing interconnection at the sites of penetration, and within the first few millimeters of cartilage, the terminal ramifications continue to be end-arterial systems.

The canal systems are dispersed throughout the chondroepiphysis, except for a narrow area under the differentiating articular cartilage, which derives most metabolic exchange directly from the joint fluid. The canals are most numerous in the central region, where the secondary ossification center will eventually form, and along the physis (in the germinal zone).

The cartilage canals vary extensively in their morphology, although all have one artery, one or more veins, and surrounding connective tissue and capillaries. The major variability is the degree of capillarity within the canal and the degree of cartilage maturation (i.e., ground substance, calcification, cellular hypertrophy) in the canal wall. The capillaries are either peripheral networks along the course of the artery or glomerular tufts at the termination of the artery and canal.

The canals vary in length. Those along the growth plate periphery tend to be short, rarely branch, and generally end in a modified capillary loop. Longer canals extend more deeply into the chondroepiphysis, frequently branch, and are surrounded by a capillary network. The capillaries form glomerular structures of varying complexity, both along the course of the canal as well as terminally. The canals are characterized by the arterioles dividing into diffuse periarterial capillary loops that rejoin to form venules. At the terminations of the long canals the arterioles divide into highly branched structures. These more complex, glomerular like structures are most frequent in the area of those germinal and dividing chondrocytes forming the preossification centers of the capital femur and greater trochanter.

With increasing age many of the cartilage canals show increased amounts of glycosaminoglycan deposition along the canal periphery, with this being most evident in canals adjacent to the preossification center. The changes are undoubtedly necessary for calcification and ossification, which may occur along canal systems as an isolated phenomenon or as an extension of the normal process of enlargement of the ossification center. The canals undergoing these chemical changes in the matrix also exhibit hypertrophy of the cartilage cells, in contrast to the undifferentiated cell pattern initially present at the canal margins.

The initial pattern of distribution of each cartilage canal is end-arterial, with no anastomosis between canal networks shortly after penetration of the major stem vessels into the epiphysis. This relative independence of the major arborizations is an important concept for understanding the highly variable appearance of ischemic complications. However, once the secondary ossification center of the capital femur is established, many cartilage canal systems enter it and form a variable intraepiphyseal anastomosis. However, this particular anastomosis may be the least functional, and certainly may not be sufficiently functional to allow one vascular system (e.g., the posteroinferior vessels) to acutely distribute to the area of bone and cartilage supplied by another system (e.g., the posterosuperior vessels). Interchange of blood flow at this anastomotic level may not be rapid enough, or quantitatively sufficient, to prevent the relatively rapid cellular death of bone (ossification center) and physeal cartilage, both of which are more dependent upon a functioning vascular supply than the undifferentiated cartilage. There may, however, be sufficient flow to maintain growth of the undifferentiated cartilage, which characteristically enlarges despite significant changes in the ossification center, physis, and even metaphysis.

Perhaps the most important role of the intracar-

FIG. 7–38 Development of capital femoral ossification center. **A** Early cartilage hypertrophy prior to ossification. Note the large number of surrounding cartilage canal systems. **B** Early ossification around a central arterial supply.

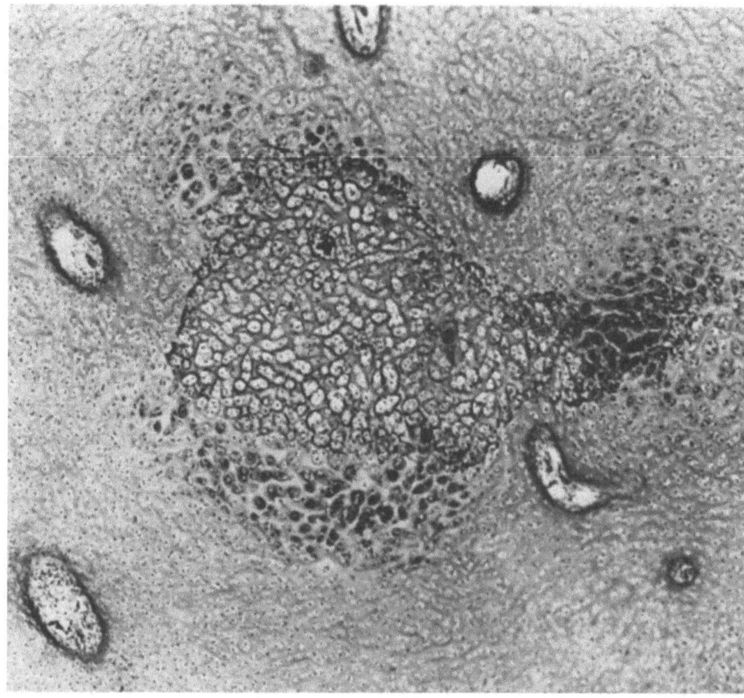

A

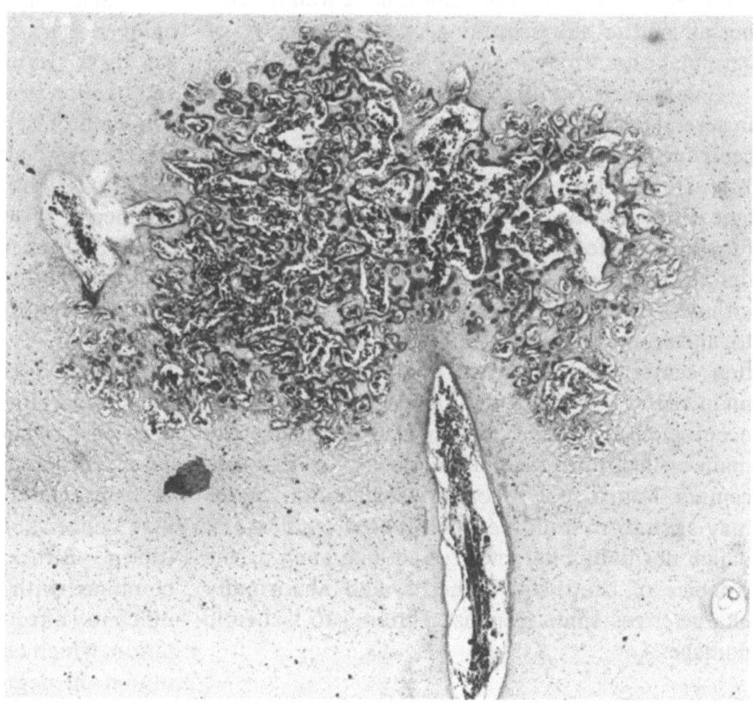

B

tilaginous microvascular system is the establishment and progressive enlargement of the secondary ossification center. The earliest stage of formation of the ossification center is cellular hypertrophy (Fig. 7–38), which is analogous to the same step in the formation of the primary ossification center. However, in contrast to the prenatal primary process, postnatal secondary epiphyseal ossification occurs around a central capillary unit, or glomerulus. This area of cellular hypertrophy is usually surrounded by several cartilage canals, only one of which contributes to the penetrating glomerulus (although any one of them may be capable of this initial vascularization). The hypertrophic cells, in the presence of proper biomechanical stimulation and vascularization, undergo progressive changes of calcification and ossification, concomitant with centrifugal enlargement of the spherical ossific nucleus. The most central area, surrounding the blood vessels, is the ossified region. Peripheral to and immediately surrounding this zone of ossification is a spherical zone of hypertrophied chondrocytes. Further out cells are arranged radially in short columns. Circumscribing all of the aforementioned cells is a layer of germinal chondrocytes.

Enlargement of the ossification center occurs in several ways. First, there is a constant spherical, centrifugal expansion of the initial center that involves the transformation of undifferentiated cartilage into cells capable of further modulation and functional differentiation. Second, the previously described process of formation of an ossific nucleus around a capillary complex may occur peripheral to, and separate from, the main secondary ossification center, with eventual coalescence into the main center as it expands. Third, ossification may occur along cartilage canal walls, extending the main ossification center or connecting ossification centers. Fourth, the secondary ossification center may arise from multiple small foci of ossification, which normally characterizes an area such as the trochlea of the distal humerus, and abnormally characterizes some response patterns to ischemic damage.

Circulation and Femoral Neck Injury

The primary factor predisposing the proximal femur to vascular insult, whether during treatment for congenital deformities or following trauma, appears to be the transition from multiple vessels to limited vessels. Most of the anterior epiphyseal and physeal contributions from the lateral circumflex artery are redirected to supply the anterior metaphysis. Concomitantly, branches of the medial circumflex artery enlarge and elongate, coeval with the elongation of the femoral neck. These vessels initially course external to cartilage and bone, covered by retinacular folds. With further development the posteroinferior vessels are encased in retinacular folds, while the posterosuperior vessels remain between cartilage and retinaculum, and may even course within the intraepiphyseal cartilage. Both the posterosuperior and posteroinferior vessels have significant vascular roles in capital femoral development, with the posterosuperior arteries being essential to proper postnatal ossification and growth of the capital femur and intraepiphyseal neck. Thus, traumatic vascular damage of these specific vessels may have significant effects on proximal femoral growth and development.

Avascular (ischemic) necrosis of the capital femoral epiphyseal ossification center has been recognized as a serious complication encountered following the initial stages of treatment of congenital subluxation or dislocation of the hip.[7,34,35] Similar problems of ischemic necrosis may occur following fractures or dislocations of the developing hip (Fig. 7–25). Certainly the criteria for the presence or absence of this complication have emphasized radiographic changes in the secondary ossification center of the capital femur.[3,4,39] However, other areas such as the physis and metaphysis also must be assessed.

The use of the term avascular necrosis to refer to vascular insult in these traumatic conditions may be a misnomer. The compromise in blood supply may selectively involve only certain areas of the proximal femur, may be of variable duration, may conceivably originate from venous occlusion (due to intracapsular tamponade) rather than or combined with arterial occlusion, and may be significantly affected by the degree of collateral circulation, which certainly varies considerably depending on the degree of chondro-osseous maturation. Ischemic necrosis would seem a preferable term. The basic patterns of ischemic necrosis encountered in congenital hip disease are described by Bucholz and Ogden,[7] and similar patterns may exist in the traumatic situation,[16,52,54] although there is more variability and a greater involvement

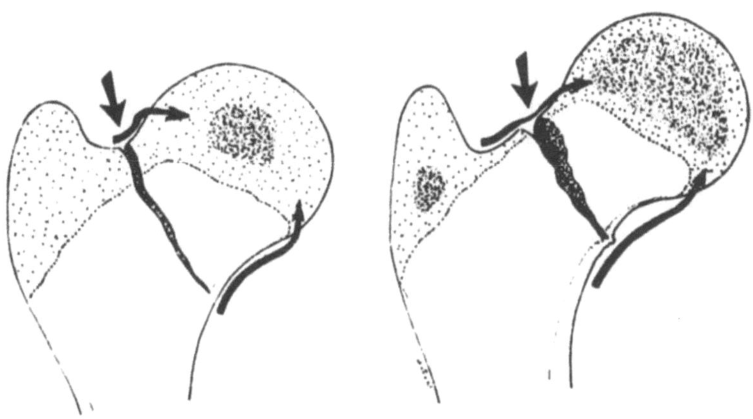

FIG. 7–39 Schematic of patterns of fracture propagation into the radiolucent cartilage (*stippled*) along the femoral neck at 2 and 11 years. Note how the posterosuperior vessels may be damaged (*arrows*).

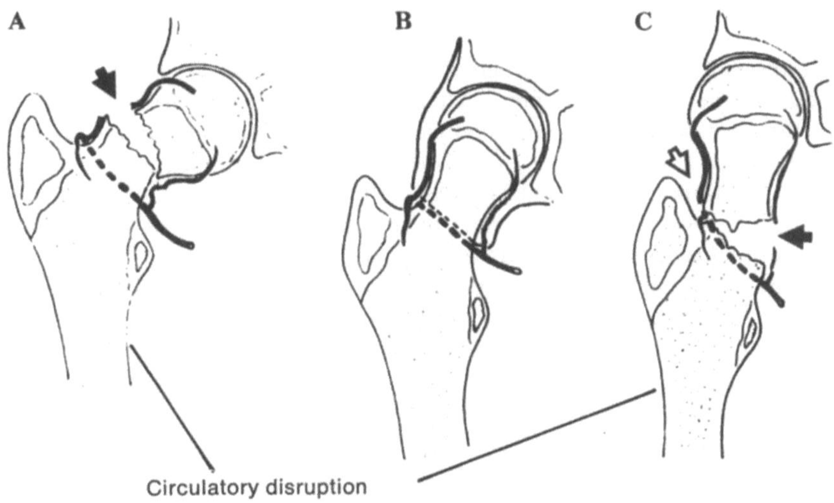

FIG. 7–40 Schematic of effect of angular deformity on the normal blood supply. **A** Varus. **B** Normal. **C** Valgus. Varus deformity will more likely damage the posterosuperior vessels (*solid arrow*), whereas valgus deformity will more likely damage the posteroinferior vessels (*solid arrow*), with the posterosuperior vessel (*open arrow*) less likely to be damaged.

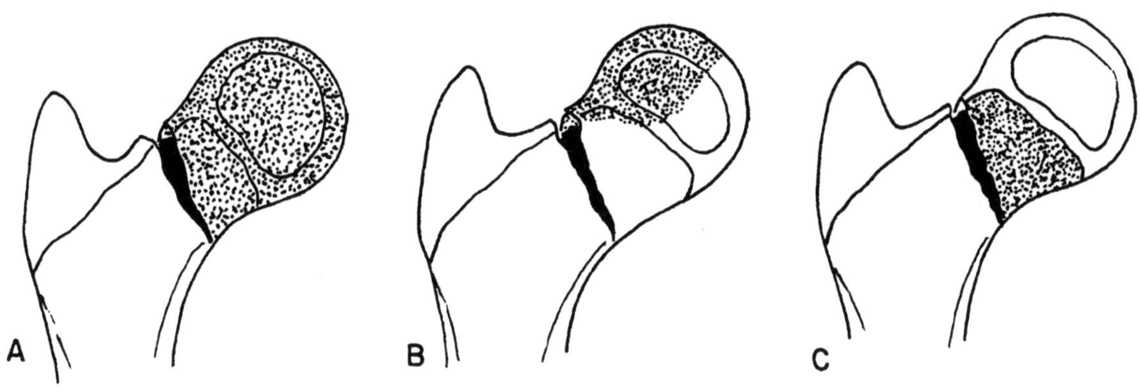

FIG. 7–41 Schematic of patterns of ischemic necrosis (*stippled areas*). **A** Damage of all vessels disrupts supply to metaphysis, physis, and epiphysis. **B** Selective posterosuperior damage may affect only the lateral portion of the capital femur (epiphysis and physis). **C** Selective damage to the nutrient metaphyseal vessels, with no damage to the posterosuperior and posteroinferior systems, may lead to selective ischemic change only in the metaphysis.

of the bone of the femoral neck, particularly in the older child with a femoral neck injury.

The extent of continuation of the fracture line into the posterosuperior bridging cartilage cannot be visualized (Fig. 7–39). The posterosuperior vessels course within, or affixed to, this cartilage. Leaving a fracture in varus not only increases risk of nonunion, but also may attenuate this key vascular system and lead to chronic ischemia (Fig. 7–40). The posteroinferior vessels within the more mobile, pedunculated inferior retinaculum are much less susceptible to damage, unless there is severe deformity or displacement of the proximal fragment. Excessive valgus may attenuate the posteroinferior vessels.

The presumed cause of necrosis is damage to or occlusion (partial, temporary) of the anterior, posterosuperior, and posteroinferior vessels passing along the neck of the femur. It is not clear whether ischemia results from complete division of all vessels, kinking of those vessels that remain intact, or tamponade by hemarthrosis within the hip capsule. Such tamponade may have a more significant effect on venous drainage than arterial, and may affect capillary exchange in a retrograde manner. Such tamponade also raises the question of efficacy of decompression, either by needle aspiration or capsulotomy.

There appear to be three roentgenographic patterns of ischemic necrosis (Fig. 7–41). One is a total involvement of the epiphysis, physis, and metaphysis extending from the level of fracture. The second is anterolateral involvement of the capital femur. The third represents involvement of the anterior vessels from the lateral circumflex artery, with involvement of only the metaphysis, with an uninvolved epiphysis.

Premature fusion of the capital femoral physis is sometimes an early sign of ischemic necrosis. Premature epiphyseal fusion may result in shortening of the leg and relative coxa vara, a short neck, and a weak lever arm for the hip abductor muscles.

In contrast, increase in circulation consequent to the trauma may produce a coxa magna, which is poorly covered if the acetabulum does not similarly expand. This is a good prognostic sign, as it implies more than adequate circulation, rather than ischemia.

Vascular complications may occur following undisplaced as well as displaced fractures of the femoral neck in children. It is possible that extension of the fracture line through the cartilaginous bridge of the intraepiphyseal region results in damage to a major blood vessel (Fig. 7–39). Transcervical fractures appear more likely to undergo necrosis than cervicotrochanteric fractures. Displaced transepiphyseal fractures have the poorest prognosis, with development of ischemic necrosis as high as 80%. The incidence of ischemic necrosis in those 10 years of age or younger is 21%, whereas in those over 10 years of age it is 47%.[39]

Hip-injured children probably should have a bone scan several months after healing of the injury, and have this repeated approximately a year after the injury to assess any possible vascular damage or compromise. A bone scan at the time of injury or within the first month may be difficult to interpret because of new bone formation from the healing fracture, as well as the changes consequent to injury and immobilization in the femoral head. The first roentgenographic signs of ischemic necrosis are a mild sclerotic appearance and the head does not grow compared to the opposite side. The cartilage space widens. These signs are present long before gross fragmentation and deformity of the head.

If there is any suggestion of ischemic change, and if there seems to be a gradually appearing roentgenographic accompaniment, due consideration should be given to premature epiphysiodesis of the greater trochanter to minimize overgrowth and loss of the normal articulotrochanteric difference.

Bibliography

1. Allende, G., and Lesama, L. G.: Fractures of the neck of the femur in children. J. Bone Joint Surg., 33A:387, 1951.
2. Barash, H. L., Galante, J. O., and Ray, R. D.: Acute slipped capital femoral epiphysis. Clin. Orthop., 79:96, 1971.
3. Barquet, A.: Avascular necrosis following traumatic hip dislocation in childhood. Factors of influence. Acta Orthop. Scand., 53:809, 1982.
4. Barquet, A.: Natural history of avascular necrosis following traumatic hip dislocation in childhood. A review of 145 cases. Acta Orthop. Scand., 53:815, 1982.
5. Bonvallet, J. M.: Sur un cas exceptionnel de luxation traumatique de la hanche de l'enfant, associée à un décollement épiphysaire complet et à une fracture du noyan ciphalique. Rev. Chir. Orthop., 51:723, 1965.
6. Bucholz, R. W., Ezaki, M., and Ogden, J. A.: In-

jury to the acetabular triradiate cartilage. J. Bone Joint Surg., 64A:600, 1982.
7. Bucholz, R. W., and Ogden, J. A.: Patterns of ischemic necrosis of the proximal femur in nonoperatively treated congenital hip disease. In: The Hip. Proceedings of the Hip Society, Vol. 6. St. Louis, Mosby, 1978.
8. Butler, J. E., and Cary, J. M.: Fracture of the femoral neck in a child. J.A.M.A., 218:398, 1971.
9. Canale, S. T., and Bourland, W. L.: Fracture of the neck and intertrochanteric region of the femur in children. J. Bone Joint Surg., 59A:431, 1977.
10. Chigot, P. L., and Vialas, M.: Fractures du col du femur chez l'enfant. Ann. Chir. Infant., 4:209, 1963.
11. Chong, K. C., Chacha, P. B., and Lee, B. T.: Fractures of the neck of the femur in childhood and adolescence. Injury, 7:111, 1975.
12. Chung, S. M.: The arterial supply of the developing proximal end of the human femur. J. Bone Joint Surg., 58A:961, 1976.
13. Chung, S. M., Batterman, S. C., and Brighton, C. T.: Shear strength of the human femoral capital epiphyseal plate. J. Bone Joint Surg., 58A:94, 1976.
14. Clark, C. R., Southwick, W. O., and Ogden, J. A.: Slipped capital femoral epiphysis and correction by biplane osteotomy. AAOS Instructional Course Lectures. St. Louis, Mosby, 1979.
15. Duncan, J. W., and Lovell, W. W.: Anterior slip of the capital femoral epiphysis. Clin. Orthop., 110:171, 1975.
16. Durbin, F. C.: Avascular necrosis complicating undisplaced fractures of the neck of the femur in children. J. Bone Joint Surg., 41B:758, 1959.
17. Elizalde, E. A.: Obstetrical dislocation of the hip associated with fracture of the femur. J. Bone Joint Surg., 28:838, 1946.
18. Fahey, J. J., and O'Brien, E. T.: Acute slipped capital femoral epiphysis. J. Bone Joint Surg., 47A:1105, 1965.
19. Feigenberg, Z., Parker, M., Levy, M., Seelenfreund, M., and Fried, A.: Fractures of the femoral neck in childhood. J. Trauma, 17:942, 1977.
20. Grassi, G., and Nigrisoli, P.: Traumatic separation of the upper femoral epiphysis in a child aged two. Ital. J. Orthop. Traum., 2:135, 1976.
21. Hoeksema, H. D., Olsen, C., and Rudy, R.: Fracture of femoral neck and shaft and repeat neck fracture in a child. J. Bone Joint Surg., 57A:271, 1975.
22. Imhauser, G.: Zur pathogenese und therapie der jugendlichen huftkopflosung. Z. Orthop., 88:3, 1957.
23. Jacob, R., and Niemann, K.: Fractures of the hip in childhood. South. Med. J., 69:629, 1976.
24. Kampner, S. L., and Wissinger, H. A.: Anterior slipping of the capital femoral epiphysis. J. Bone Joint Surg., 54A:1531, 1972.
25. Cay, S. P., and Hall, J. E.: Fracture of the femoral neck in children and its complications. Clin. Orthop., 80:53, 1971.
26. Kohli, S. B.: Fracture of the neck of the femur in children. J. Bone Joint Surg., 56B:776, 1974.
27. Lam, S. F.: Fractures of the neck of the femur in children. J. Bone Joint Surg., 53A:1165, 1976.
28. Lindseth, R. E., and Rosene, H. A.: Traumatic separation of the upper femoral epiphysis in a newborn infant. J. Bone Joint Surg., 53A:1641, 1971.
29. McDougall, A.: Fracture of the neck of the femur in childhood. J. Bone Joint Surg., 43B:16, 1961.
30. Meier, A.: Geburtstraumatische epiphysenlosung am proximalen femurende. Arch. Kinder., 116: 267, 1939.
31. Milgram, J. W., and Lyne, E. D.: Epiphysiolysis of the proximal femur in very young children. Clin. Orthop., 110:146, 1975.
32. Miller, W.E.: Fracture of the hip in children from birth to adolescence. Clin. Orthop., 92:155, 1973.
33. Mortens, J., and Christensen, P.: Traumatic separation of the upper femoral epiphysis as an obstetrical lesion. Acta Orthop. Scand., 34:239, 1964.
34. Ogden, J. A.: Anatomic and histologic study of factors affecting development and evolution of avascular necrosis in congenital dislocation of the hip. In: The Hip. Proceedings of the Hip Society, Vol. 2. St. Louis, Mosby, 1974.
35. Ogden, J. A.: Changing patterns of proximal femoral vascularity. J. Bone Joint Surg., 56A:941, 1974.
36. Ogden, J. A.: Osgood-Schlatter's disease and development of the tibial tuberosity. Clin. Orthop., 116:183, 1976.
37. Ogden, J. A.: Development and growth of the musculoskeletal system. In Albright, J. A., and Brand, R. (eds.): The Scientific Basis of Orthopaedics. New York, Appleton, 1979.
38. Ogden, J. A.: Chondro-osseous development and growth. In Urist, M. (ed.): Fundamental and Clinical Bone Physiology. Philadelphia, Lippincott, 1980.
39. Ogden, J. A.: Skeletal Injury in the Child. Philadelphia, Lea & Febiger, 1982.
40. Ogden, J. A.: Injury to growth mechanisms of the immature skeleton. Skel. Radiol., 6:237, 1981.
41. Ogden, J. A.: Dynamic pathobiology of congenital hip dysplasia. In Tachdjian, M.O. (ed.): Congenital Hip Disease. Edinburgh, Churchill Livingstone, 1982.
42. Ogden, J. A.: Normal and abnormal circulation. In Tachdjian, M. O. (ed.): Congenital Hip Disease. Edinburgh, Churchill Livingstone, 1982.
43. Ogden, J. A.: Congenital dysplasia of the hip. In Resnick, D., and Niyamura, G. (eds.): Diagnosis

of Bone and Joint Disorders. Philadelphia, Saunders, 1981.
44. Ogden, J. A.: Hip development and vascularity. Relationship to chondro-osseous trauma in the growing child. In: The Hip. Proceedings of the Hip Society, Vol. 9. St. Louis, Mosby, 1981.
45. Ogden, J. A.: Prenatal and postnatal development of the hip. In Katz, J. F., and Siffert, R. S. (eds.): Management of Hip Disorders in Children. Philadelphia, Lippincott, 1983.
46. Ogden, J. A.: Skeletal growth mechanism injury patterns. J. Ped. Orthop., 2:371, 1982.
47. Ogden, J. A., Hempton, R. F., and Southwick, W. O.: Development of the tibial tuberosity. J. Bone Joint Surg., 56A:1539, 1974.
48. Ogden, J. A., Simon, T., and Southwick, W. O.: Cartilage space width and slipped capital femoral epiphysis. Yale J. Biol. Med., 50:17, 1977.
49. Osborne, D., Effman, E., Broda, K., and Harrelson, J.: The development of the upper end of the femur, with special reference to its internal architecture. Radiology, 137:71, 1980.
50. Peltokallio, P., and Kurkipaa, M.: Fractures of the femoral neck in children. Ann. Chir. Gynaec. Fenn., 48:151, 1959.
51. Pforringer, W., and Rosemeyer, B.: Fractures of the hip in children and adolescents. Acta Orthop. Scand., 51:91, 1980.
52. Ratliff, A. H. C.: Fractures of the neck of the femur in children. J. Bone Joint Surg., 44B:528, 1962.
53. Ratliff, A. H. C.: Traumatic separation of the upper femoral epiphysis in young children. J. Bone Joint Surg., 50B:757, 1968.
54. Ratliff, A. H. C.: Fractures of the neck of the femur in children. Orthop. Clin. North Am., 5:903, 1974.
55. Rigault, P., Iselin, F., Moureau, J., and Judet, J.: Fractures du col du femur chez l'enfant. Rev. Chir. Orthop., 52:325, 1966.
56. Rouiller, R., Griffe, J., and Crespy, G.: Epiphyseolyse femorale superieure apres fracture basicervicale. Resultat apres trois ans. Rev. Chir. Orthop., 57:65, 1971.
57. Sonheim, K.: Fracture of the femoral neck in children. Acta Orthop. Scand., 43:523, 1972.
58. Speer, D. P.: Experimental epiphysiolysis: an etiologic model of slipped capital femoral epiphysis. Trans. Orthop. Res. Soc., 3:47, 1978.
59. Speer, D. P.: Experimental epiphysiolysis: Etiologic models of slipped capital femoral epiphysis. In: The Hip. Proceedings of the Hip Society, Vol. 10. St. Louis, Mosby, 1982.
60. Stougard, J.: Post-traumatic avascular necrosis of the femoral head in children. J. Bone Joint Surg., 51B:354, 1969.
61. Touzet, P., Rigault, P., Padovani, J. P., Pouliquen, J. C., Mallet, J. F., and Guyonvarch, G.: Les fractures du col du femur chez l'enfant. Rev. Chir. Orthop., 65:341, 1979.
62. Towbin, R., and Crawford, A. H.: Neonatal traumatic proximal femoral epiphysiolysis. Pediatrics, 63:456, 1979.
63. Trueta, J.: The normal vascular anatomy of the human femoral head during growth. J. Bone Joint Surg., 39B:358, 1957.
64. Weigel, K., and Conforty, B.: Die traumatische Epiphysenablosung am oberen Femurende beim Neugeborenen. Z. Orthop., 112:1286, 1974.
65. Weiner, D., and O'Dell, H.: Fractures of the hip in children. J. Trauma, 9:62, 1969.
66. Wilson, J. C.: Fractures of the neck of the femur in children. J. Bone Joint Surg., 22:531, 1940.

CHAPTER 8

Anteversion of the Femur

PETER D. PIZZUTILLO, G. DEAN MACEWEN, AND ALFRED R. SHANDS

The term "anteversion of the femur" has been used interchangeably with "medial femoral torsion" and "antetorsion" in the orthopedic literature. At various times, they may have identical meaning or may refer to different degrees of torsional relationships. In this chapter, the term "anteversion of the femur" will be used exclusively to describe in degrees the anterior position of the head–neck axis with respect to the bicondylar axis of the distal femur (Fig. 8–1). When the head–neck axis is parallel or posterior to the bicondylar axis of the femur, "retroversion" is described.

Most individuals demonstrate anteversion of the femur as a normal anatomical finding. Increased levels of anteversion are normally noted at birth and slowly regress to a definable range in the adult. It is usually either the persistence of high infantile degrees of anteversion or the existence of degrees of anteversion that exceed expected values for a given age and sex that is the source of clinical problems.

The evolution of a slowly increasing degree of anteversion in the femur of the embryo has been well documented,[19] but the actual forces involved are not known. It has been suggested that the medial rotation of the lower limb buds causes fetal anteversion of the femur; however, no definite cause has been identified.

At the Alfred I. duPont Institute, a 20-year follow-up study involving 1990 examinations was done, using the Dunlap–Shands method of measuring anteversion.[4,25] Evaluation of 864 anteversion studies of normal children revealed an average angle of anteversion of 32° at birth that gradually regressed to an average angle of 15° by 16 years of age. A graphic demonstration of this study (Fig. 8–2) has commonly been used as the standard for normal development. It is worth noting that there is little change in the angle of anteversion during the first year of life. This absence of change, which has also been observed in older, nonambulatory children, is thought to be indirect evidence that muscular forces generated while walking are necessary for the regression of anteversion.[17] Morscher studied 120 hips of normal children and noted that the plane of the proximal femoral physis was not perpendicular to the axis of the femoral neck, but rather deviated from this axis to face posteriorly (Fig. 8–3). On the basis of his observations, Morscher suggested that muscular and gravitational forces applied to the proximal femur will cause the neck to grow posteriorly toward a relative position of retroversion and will thus diminish the existing degree of anteversion.[17]

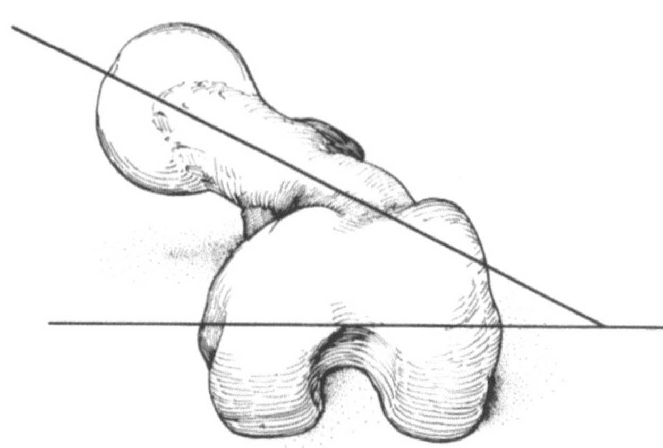

FIG. 8–1 The head-neck axis of the femur is directed anteriorly from the bicondylar axis.

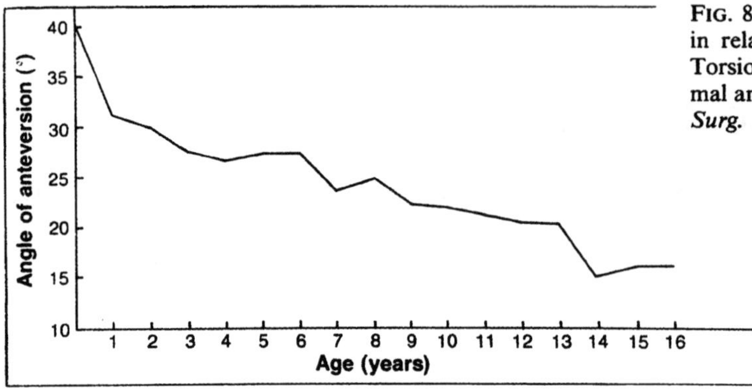

FIG. 8–2 The change in anteversion is plotted in relation to increasing age (Fabry G, et al: Torsion of the femur: a follow-up study in normal and abnormal conditions. *J. Bone and Joint Surg.* 55A:1726–1738, 1973).

Method of Measurement

Clinical examination of patients with unrestricted hip motion will provide an approximate measure of the degree of anteversion by comparing internal and external rotation of the extended hip. Children with increased femoral anteversion demonstrate significantly greater internal rotation of the hip than external rotation (Fig. 8–4). An anteroposterior (AP) radiograph of the hips in neutral rotation typically reveals an apparent coxa valga (Fig. 8–5), which decreases when the hips are internally rotated to yield a more accurate assessment of the neck–shaft angle (Fig. 8–6).[22] Fluoroscopic examination has been used by Rogers [21] and by Stewart and Karshner [27] to document anteversion but has been abandoned because of increased exposure to radiation and difficulty in reproducing results.

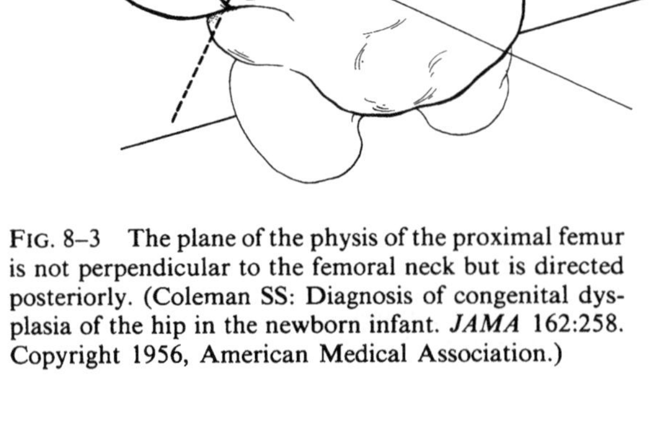

FIG. 8–3 The plane of the physis of the proximal femur is not perpendicular to the femoral neck but is directed posteriorly. (Coleman SS: Diagnosis of congenital dysplasia of the hip in the newborn infant. *JAMA* 162:258. Copyright 1956, American Medical Association.)

Many problems have been encountered in the development of techniques to precisely measure anteversion in patients and in dried bone specimens. Most of these relate to technicalities in defining the femoral neck axis and the ideal femoral shaft axis, since the femur is curved in more than one plane.[1,15,28]

In 1953, Dunlap and Shands [2] described a simple technique for radiographically documenting the angle of anteversion with minimum exposure to radiation. An inexpensive positioning apparatus (Fig. 8–7) is used for consistent reproducibility. A posteroanterior radiograph of the hips and pelvis is obtained with the patient lying prone, with hips fully extended and knees flexed to 90° (Fig. 8–8). The neck–shaft angle, or the apparent angle of inclination, is measured directly from this radiograph.

The patient is then turned to the supine position and the lower extremity is placed in the positioning device (Fig. 8–9). Adjustable leg supports allow both hip and knee flexion to 90° and the thigh is abducted 20°. A reference bar is extended from the positioning apparatus and placed just lateral to the greater trochanter. A lateral radiograph of the hip is obtained and the apparent angle of torsion is determined by measuring the angle formed by the central axis of the femoral neck and the reference bar representing the transcondylar axis of the femur (Fig. 8–10). The true angle of anteversion is derived by plotting the apparent angle of torsion and the angle of measured inclination on a graph devised by Webber [2] (Fig. 8–11).

In addition to the Dunlap–Shands [2] technique and other biplanar techniques,[3,9,13,18,24] axial transverse tomography has been used to determine anteversion. This method is reliable but involves special equipment, increased radiation exposure, a co-

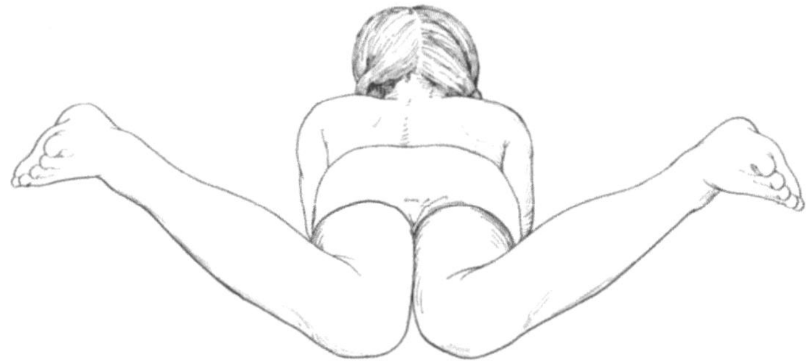

FIG. 8–4 With the hips in extension, internal rotation of the hips will significantly exceed external rotation.

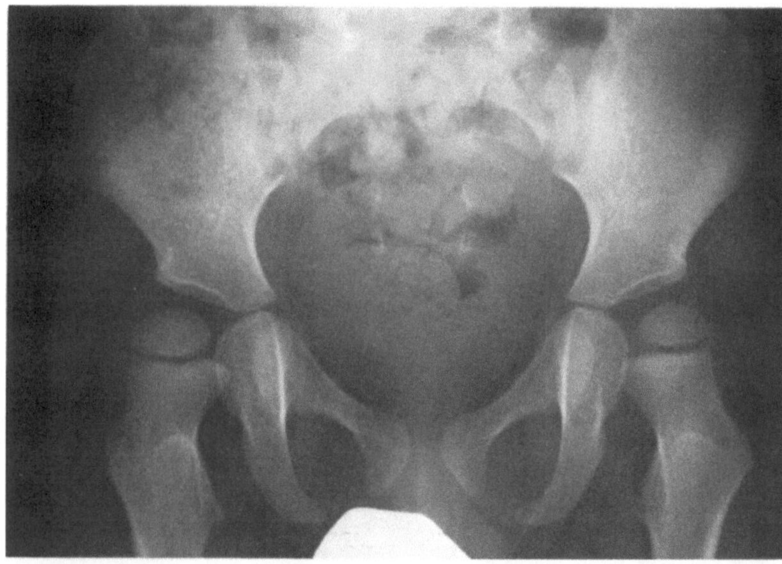

FIG. 8–5 An AP radiograph of the hips and pelvis demonstrates apparent valgus of the proximal femur.

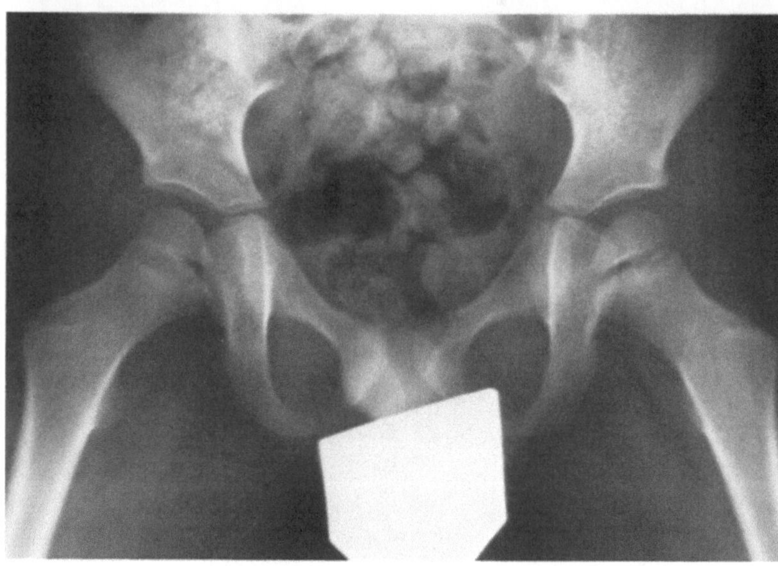

FIG. 8–6 An AP radiograph of the hips and pelvis with the hips in internal rotation reveals a more accurate assessment of the femoral neck-shaft angle.

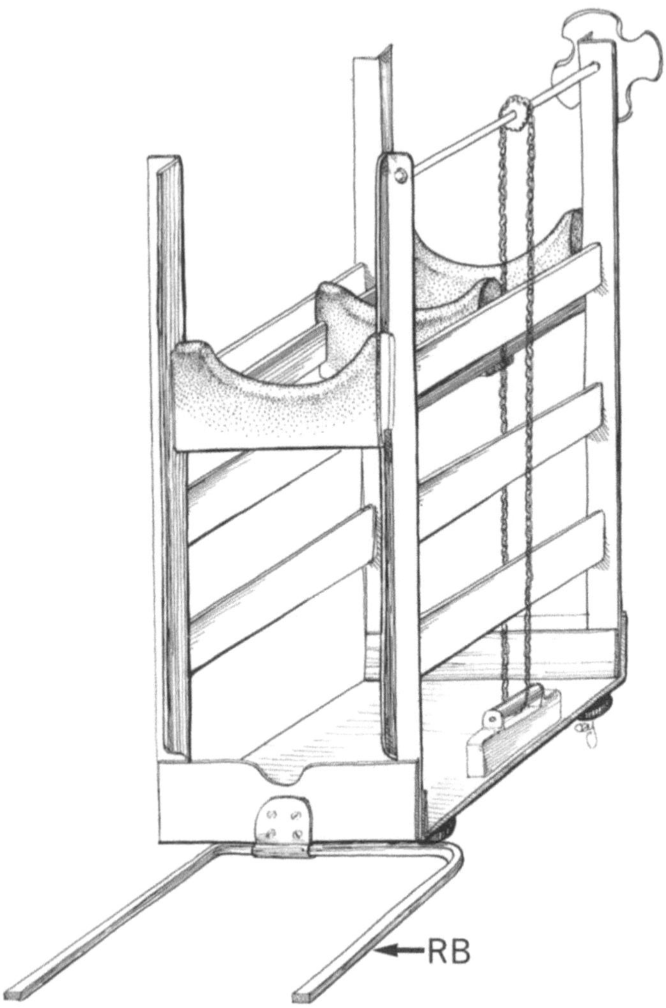

FIG. 8–7 The positioning apparatus used for the Shands-Dunlap technique of determining anteversion.

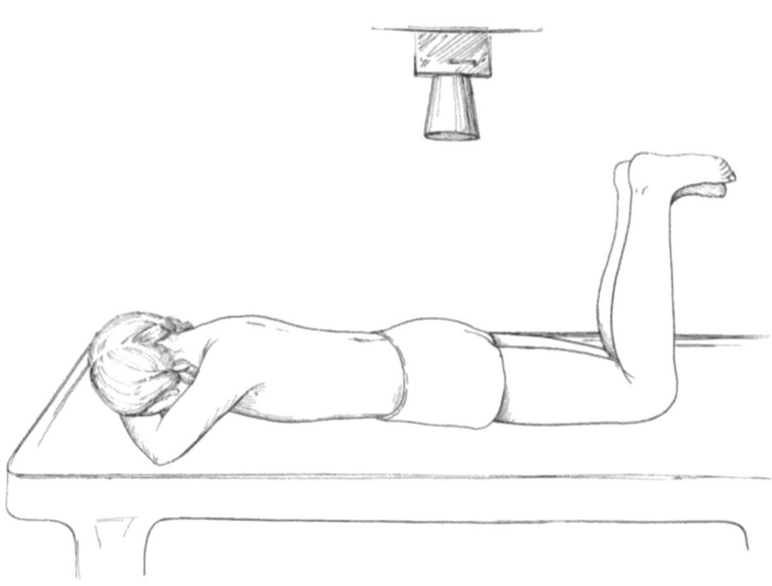

FIG. 8–8 A PA radiograph of hips and pelvis is obtained with the patient lying in the prone position to determine the measured angle of inclination.

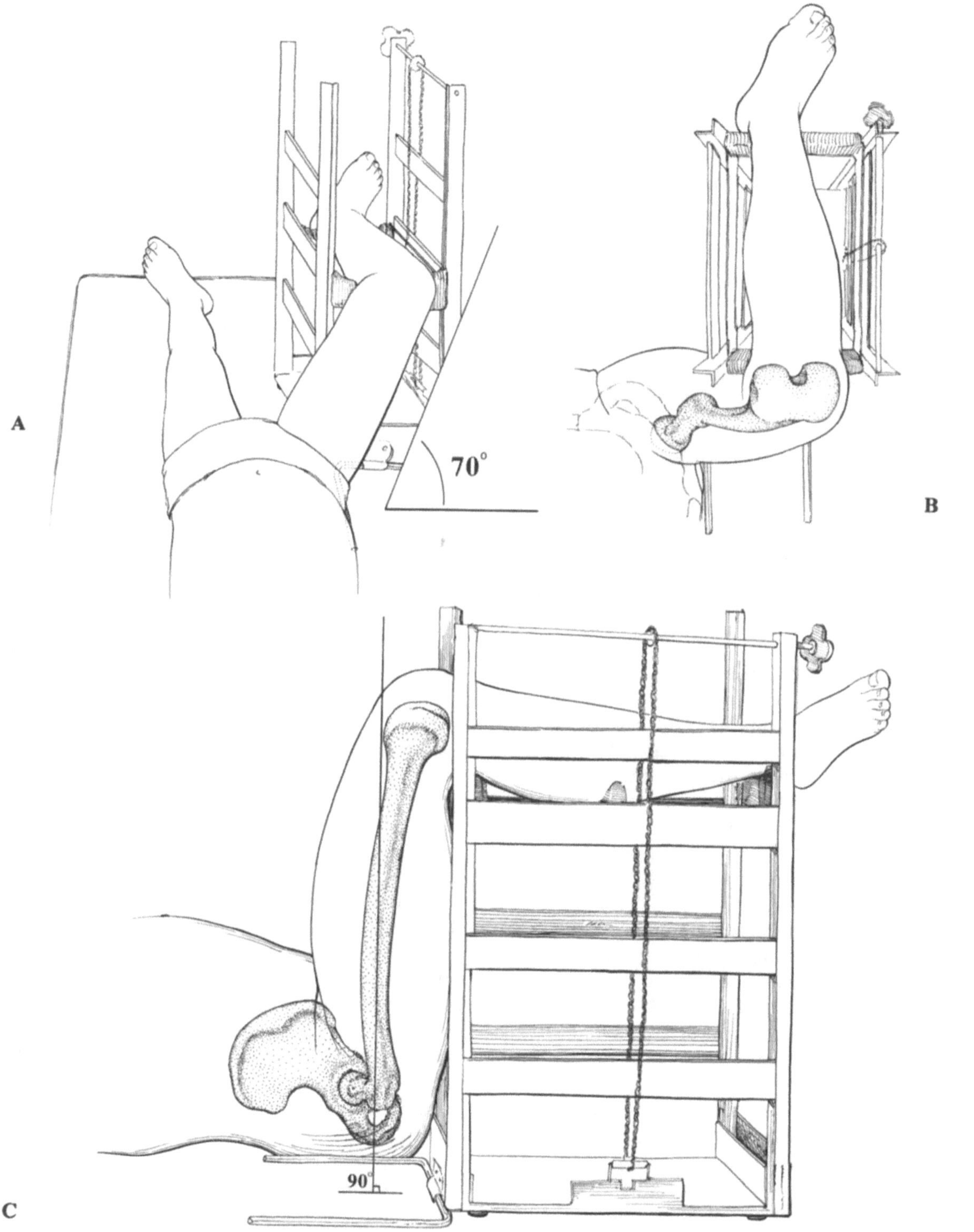

FIG. 8–9 The position of the patient in the apparatus demonstrates 90 degrees of hip and knee flexion and 20 degrees of abduction of the hip.

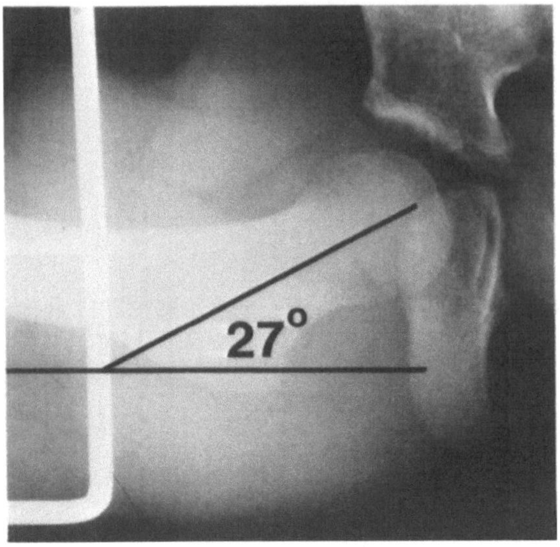

FIG. 8–10 The measured angle of anteversion is determined from the axis of the neck to the reference bar of the apparatus.

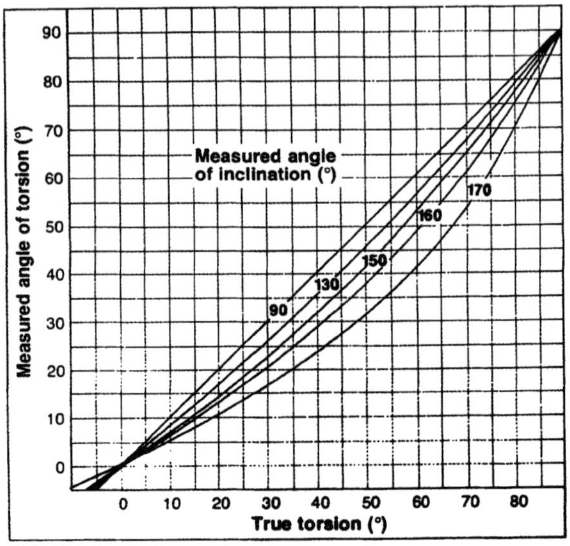

FIG. 8–11 Webber graph (Dunlap K, et al: A new method for determination of torsion of the femur. *J. Bone and Joint Surg.* 35A:289–311, April, 1953).

operative patient, and limitations imposed by leg size and girth.[5,8] Biplanar and axial techniques are comparable in accuracy, with a range of error of 5–10°.[14,23]

Computerized analysis of the angle of femoral anteversion has been reported by Henriksson.[6] His technique circumvents many intrinsic problems by employing three radiographs: an AP view of the hip, a lateral view of the hip, and a lateral view of the knee. Each radiograph is subjected to template analysis with computerized integration of data to determine ideal axes and angles. Henriksson has reported an accuracy of ±3° for the angle of anteversion.

Computerized axial tomography (CAT) is capable of defining the angle of anteversion by comparison of the femoral neck axis with the bicondylar axis of the femur (Fig. 8–12).[20,30] This requires cooperation of the patient or a positioning device to maintain the same alignment of the leg during the entire study.[7] Although this method of analysis is not usually indicated in the evaluation of the child with idiopathic femoral anteversion, it can be extremely helpful in determining the degree of anteversion in the child with restricted hip motion or with complex torsional deformities of the lower extremity. Limited motion of the hip will not only impede a good clinical estimation of anteversion, but will also prevent accurate evaluation by radiological methods that require precise positioning of the lower extremities. Coexisting torsional changes involving the hip, distal femur, and ankle of the same limb are often quite difficult to analyze by clinical examination and are better described by CAT analysis.

Developmental Variations

Infants commonly present an external rotation attitude of the lower extremities that parents may interpret as turning-out of the foot. This position is usually due to external rotatory contracture of the hip that spontaneously resolves once independent ambulation is mastered. As the contracture resolves, the child frequently develops increasing internal rotation of the hip and existing femoral anteversion may be clinically expressed by an intoeing gait.[31] During ambulation, the patella will orient inwardly and will emphasize the proximal source of internal rotation (Fig. 8–13). Toeing-in is exaggerated during running activities and during walking when the child is fatigued. There is a tendency to sit in the reverse tailor's position as a consequence of the rotation of the hip joint (Fig. 8–14). The duPont Institute study involving 432 normal children revealed a progressive decrease in anteversion from 32° at birth to 23° at 7 years of age and 15° at 16 years of age.[4,25]

In addition to those children who undergo ex-

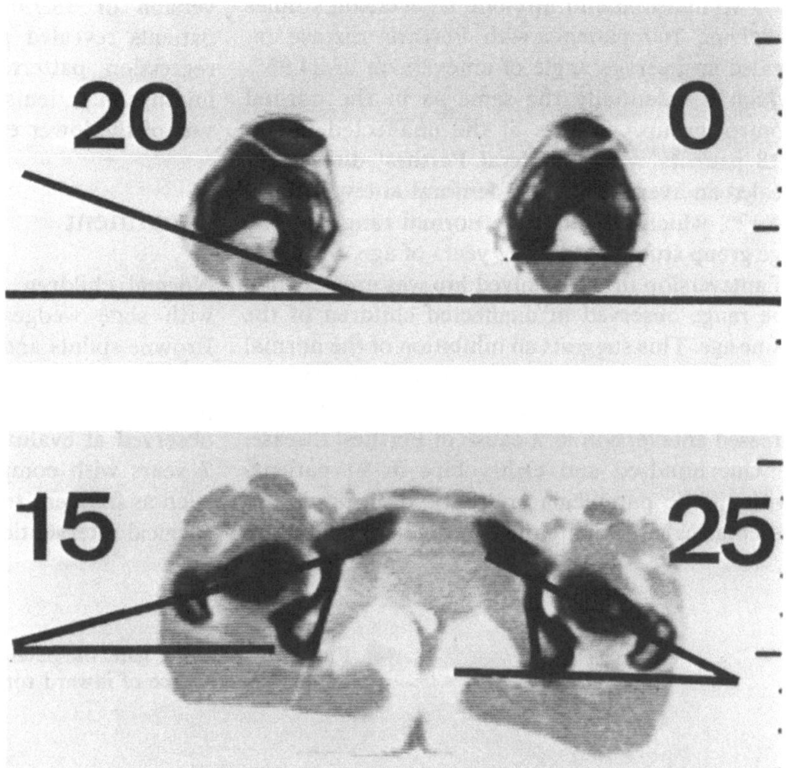

FIG. 8–12 CT scan reveals increased anteversion of the left hip of 35 degrees by adding the angle of the femoral neck (15 degrees) to the angle formed by the bicondylar axis (20 degrees).

pected remodeling of the femur, there is another group of normal children with degrees of anteversion that exceed the expected range for their age and sex. These children demonstrate a persistent in-toeing gait and have a reported incidence of 13.6% in the general population.[16] Fabry et al.[4] studied 175 patients with persistent in-toeing and found an average angle of anteversion of 42.68° (using the Dunlap–Shands technique) at initial evaluation. When reevaluated 5.5 years later, the average angle of anteversion in this group was 39.48°. It was interesting to observe that while no significant change in anteversion occurred during the study period, half of the group exhibited a normal walking pattern when reexamined. The authors postulated that compensatory external rotation of the lower leg was responsible for the observed improvement in gait. Kobyliansky's study [12] of corresponding femurs and tibias of 50 cadavers documented that increased femoral anteversion is frequently associated with compensatory external tibial torsion. Thus, many children with in-toeing gait and persistent high levels of femoral anteversion will spontaneously remodel their lower legs and improve their gait pattern.

The angle of femoral anteversion is increased in certain orthopedic pathological states, such as congenital dislocation of the hip, Perthes' disease, cerebral palsy, and talipes equinovarus; and is usually decreased in coxa vara and congenital short femur.[4,10,11,25,29] The clinical significance of femoral anteversion was emphasized when it was recognized as an important factor in the treatment of congenitally dislocated hips. The duPont study [4] revealed that the average angle of anteversion in 209 congenitally dislocated hips was 43°, which is 15.8° greater than expected. Follow-up evaluation revealed an insignificant decrease to 38°. In patients with unilateral hip dislocation, the unaffected hip was also measured and initially demonstrated an average angle of anteversion of 44.62°. Six years later the angle of anteversion had only decreased to an average of 41.59°. These findings suggest that derotation osteotomy of the femur may be required to maintain stability once it has been achieved in certain patients with congenital dislocation of the hip. Furthermore, spontaneous regression to a more normal range of anteversion does not usually occur in patients with congenital dislocation of the hip.

Two hundred and fifty-one anteversion studies involving 160 patients with Perthes' disease revealed an average angle of anteversion of 24.96°, which is essentially the same as in the normal control group.[4] Studies of the unaffected hip in 118 patients with unilateral Perthes' disease revealed an average angle of femoral anteversion of 25.12°, which is within the normal range for the age group studied. After 12 years of age, the angle of anteversion in the involved hip was greater than the range observed in unaffected children of the same age. This suggests an inhibition of the normal torsional remodeling of the femur secondary to the Perthes' process and does not implicate increased anteversion as a cause of Perthes' disease.

One hundred and eighty hips in 91 patients with spastic paraplegia or spastic diplegia due to cerebral palsy exhibited an average angle of anteversion of 38.79°.[4] Follow-up study of these patients revealed persistent anteversion with no regression pattern. Morscher observed similar findings in patients with flaccid and spastic paralysis of the lower extremities.[17]

Treatment

Normal children with anteversion were treated with shoe wedges, twister cables, and Denis–Browne splints and were compared with a similar but untreated control group. No significant improvement in the angle of femoral anteversion was observed at evaluation. Children over the age of 7 years with complaints of functional disability, such as frequent tripping and falling, may require surgical intervention. They almost always demon-

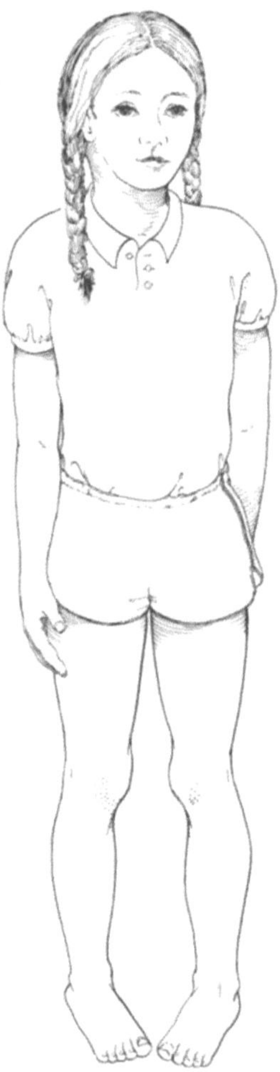

◀ FIG. 8–13 During gait, the patella will orient inwardly and indicate the proximal source of inward rotation.

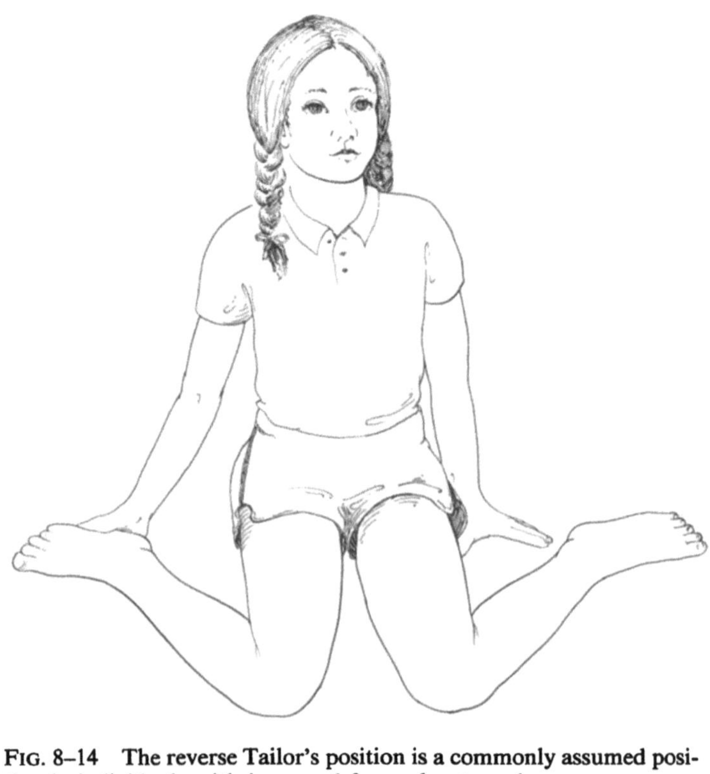

FIG. 8–14 The reverse Tailor's position is a commonly assumed position in individuals with increased femoral anteversion.

strate less than 15° of external rotation of the extended hip and little or no attempt at compensatory external tibial torsion.

The concern that persistent increased femoral anteversion is a cause of osteoarthritis of the hip and knee [16] has never been substantiated, and thus there is no good evidence in support of prophylactic correction of anteversion.[10,32]

Derotation osteotomy of the femur has been described at the intertrochanteric and subtrochanteric levels of the proximal femur and at the supracondylar level of the distal femur.[24] In the child under 10 years of age, supracondylar osteotomy can be performed with a minimum of surgical trauma and cosmetically superior incisional scars. Supracondylar osteotomy of the femur in the older child may be complicated by knee joint stiffness or loss of stability due to a thin periosteal sleeve. Therefore, a proximal approach to the femur is favored in the older child.

Staheli [26] reported a 15% rate of significant complications with various techniques of derotation osteotomy. This high rate should serve as a warning against surgery for casual considerations and demands accurate preoperative assessment and precise surgical technique to avoid pitfalls.

Summary

Anteversion of the femur exists as a phase of natural development of the lower limb, and in most children regresses to values with no clinically expressed problems. In those children with persistent high angles of anteversion, the early problem of in-toeing gait is corrected by compensating external tibial torsion. Brace treatment has not been effective in reducing the angle of anteversion, and fortunately only a small percentage of children with persistent anteversion will require surgical derotation of the femur to improve their functional status.

Increased angles of anteversion are seen in children with congenital dislocation of the hip, Perthes' disease, cerebral palsy, and talipes equinovarus; decreased angles are found in patients with coxa vara and congenital short femur. This observation has been helpful in planning successful treatment programs for many of these patients.

A variety of techniques has been suggested for the measurement of the angle of anteversion. When motion of the hip is restricted or when complex torsional deformities are present, CAT scan analysis is very helpful in determining true angles. When motion of the hip is not restricted, the Dunlap–Shands technique provides a safe, inexpensive, and reproducible method of assessing femoral anteversion.

Bibliography

1. Bentley, H. B.: Radiographic morphometry of the femoral shaft. Radiography, 44:233, 1978.
2. Dunlap, K., Shands, A. R., Jr., Hollister, L. C., Gaul, J. S., Jr., Streit, H. A.: A new method for determination of torsion of the femur. J. Bone Joint Surg., 35A:289, 1953.
3. Dunn, D. M.: Anteversion of the neck of the femur. J. Bone Joint Surg., 34B:181, 1952.
4. Fabry, G., MacEwen, G. D., Shands, A. R., Jr.: Torsion of the femur: a follow-up study in normal and abnormal conditions. J. Bone Joint Surg., 55A:1726, 1973.
5. Fisher, R. L., Duncan, A. S., and Bronzino, J. D.: The application of axial transverse tomography to the measurement of femoral anteversion. Clin. Orthop., 86:6, 1972.
6. Henriksson, L.: Measurement of femoral neck anteversion and inclination. Acta Orthop. Scand., Suppl. 186:1, 1980.
7. Hernandez, R. J., Tachdjian, M. O., Poznanski, A. K., Dias, L. S.: CT determination of femoral torsion. Am. J. Radiol., 137:97, 1981.
8. Hubbard, D. D., Staheli, L. T.: The direct radiographic measurement of femoral torsion using axial tomography. Clin. Orthop., 86:16, 1972.
9. Iwamoto, M., Basmajian, J. V., Strom, C. H.: A method for determining femoral neck–shaft and anteversion angles. Arch. Phys. Med. Rehabil., 53:253, 1972.
10. Jani, L.: Idiopathic anteversion of the femoral neck. Int. Orthop., 2:283, 1979.
11. Katz, J. F.: Femoral torsion in Legg-Calve-Perthes disease. J. Bone Joint Surg., 50A:473, 1968.
12. Kobyliansky, E., Weissman, S. L., Nathan, H.: Femoral and tibial torsion. Int. Orthop. 3:145, 1979.
13. Konig, G.: A practical method for the determination of the angle of antetorsion and neck–shaft angle of the femur. Z. Orthop., 110:76, 1972.
14. LaGasse, D. J., Staheli, L. T.: The measurement of femoral anteversion. Clin. Orthop., 86:13, 1972.
15. Magilligan, D. J.: Calculation of the angle of anteversion by means of horizontal lateral roentgenography. J. Bone Joint Surg., 38A:1231, 1956.
16. McSweeny, A.: A study of femoral torsion in children. J. Bone Joint Surg., 53B:90, 1971.

17. Morscher, E.: Development and clinical significance of the anteversion of the femoral neck. Reconstr. Surg. Traumat., 9:107, 1967.
18. Ogata, K., Goldsand, E. M.: A simple biplanar method of measuring femoral anteversion and neck–shaft angle. J. Bone Joint Surg., 61A:846, 1979.
19. Ohji, T.: A study of the torsion of lower extremity in human embryo. Mippon Seikeigeka Gakkai Zasshi 53(3):321, 1979.
20. Peterson, H. A., Klassen, R. A., McLeod, R. A., Hoffman, A. D.: Use of computed tomography in dislocation of the hip and femoral neck anteversion in children. J. Bone Joint Surg., 63B:198, 1981.
21. Rogers, S. P.: A method for determining the angle of torsion of the neck of the femur. J. Bone Joint Surg., 13:821, 1931.
22. Rogers, S. P.: Observations on torsion of the femur. J. Bone Joint Surg., 16:284, 1934.
23. Ruby, L., Mital, M. H., O'Connor, J., Patel, U.: Anteversion of the femoral neck. J. Bone Joint Surg., 61A:46, 1979.
24. Ryder, C. T., Crane, L.: Measuring femoral anteversion: the problem and the method. J. Bone Joint Surg., 35A:321, 1953.
25. Shands, A. R., Jr., Steele, M. K.: Torsion of the femur. J. Bone Joint Surg., 40A:803, 1958.
26. Staheli, L. T., Clawson, D. K., Hubbard, D. D.: Medial femoral torsion: experience with operative treatment. Clin. Orthop., 146:222, 1980.
27. Stewart, S. F., Karshner, R. G.: Congenital dislocation of the hip. A method of determining the degree of antetorsion of the femoral neck. Am. J. Roentgenol., 15:258, 1926.
28. Tan, C. K.: A photographic method of measuring the obliquity, neck angle, and angle of torsion of the human femur. Singapore Med. J., 13(5):235, 1972.
29. Telesczynski, M.: Torsion of the femur and congenital hip dislocation, Chir. Narz. Ruchu Ortop. Pol., 34:337, 1969.
30. Weiner, D. S., Cook, A. J., Hoyt, W. A., Jr., Oravec, C. E.: Computed tomography in the measurement of femoral anteversion. Orthopaedics, 1:299, 1978.
31. Weiner, D. S., Weiner, S. D.: The management of developmental femoral anteversion: sham or science? Orthopaedics, 2:492, 1979.
32. Zinn, W. M.: Reflections on degenerative hip disease. Ann. Phys. Med., 10:209, 1970.

CHAPTER 9

Fractures in Children

RAYMOND G. TRONZO

Fractures of the hip in childhood and early adolescence are rare injuries. Few orthopedic surgeons individually have much experience with these fractures. Therefore, we must depend on a collective source of knowledge for an understanding of these fractures. They are categorically devastating injuries. Since the adult presentation is entirely different from that in children, it would be wrong to transfer our knowledge of fractures of the hip in adults to fractures of the hip in children. Similarly, experience with fractures in children generally should not be transposed to the management of specific fractures of the hip in children. For example, fractures of the distal radius in children may heal without medical assistance through growth remodeling, leaving the child with no functional disability. Such is not the case when dealing with childhood hip fractures: varus deformity in about one-third of cases and premature closure of the femoral neck epiphyses in over 10%.

General Characteristics of Hip Fractures in Children

Hip fractures are formidable injuries frequently ending in disastrous results. Blount [1] stated, "True fractures of the proximal end of the femur are so rare no one has great experience with them. They are usually indifferently treated with bad results." Even today with aggressive, prompt treatment, avascular necrosis can occur as well as growth distortions, resulting in life-long effects to the patient; all of which is beyond the control of the treating surgeon.

Collective series are small when one scans the literature, averaging about 20 patients. Sources usually referred to are those of Morrissey,[3] Pforringer and Rosemeyer,[4] Boitzy,[2] and Ratliff.[5] The latter author has the largest individual experience totaling 30 patients. Ratliff also collected 168 cases with 170 fractures from interested members of the British Orthopaedic Society. His analysis of this study was presented at the Ninth Meeting of the Hip Society in 1981.[5]

Incidence

In a 12-year period from 1947 to 1959, seven patients under 17 years of age were admitted to the Manchester Royal Infirmary. In the same period, 900 adults were admitted with fractures of the hip producing a ratio of 1:130.

Age

The age range was from 2 to 16 years, with the majority between ages 11 and 16; there was a slight preponderance of boys over girls. Only Boitzy [2] and Pforringer and Rosemeyer [4] distinguished between childhood and adolescence. They defined children as from age 1 to 11 and adolescents as from age 12 to 18. The latter investigators found that the results in adolescents were poorer.

Mechanism of Injury

The majority of these children sustained severe injuries. The most common accidents involved being knocked over in a traffic accident, falling from a height, and falling from a bicycle. A small number had sustained relatively minor injuries through slipping while walking or being pushed over by another child. Interestingly, few children sustained hip injury while engaged in sports. Of particular importance is the possibility of delayed diagnosis. One infant had a birth injury which was not recognized until a week later. Another child slipped while walking, experienced pain, and was examined a week later when the diagnosis was made. Thus, these injuries are not only treacherous but sinister.

In Ratliff's series,[5] 31% sustained various other significant injuries, most important of which were head injuries. Of note is the association of fractures of the pelvis. Other serious complicating injuries were rupture of the spleen, bladder, and kidney.

One may observe fracture of the superior pubic ramus on the same side as a fractured femoral neck. Ratliff determined that in 25 children severe bruising of the lateral hip was noted, which must be a consideration in planning surgery. Such would indicate that the mechanism of injury was not rotational as in adults, but a result of direct trauma to the lateral aspect of the hip joint.

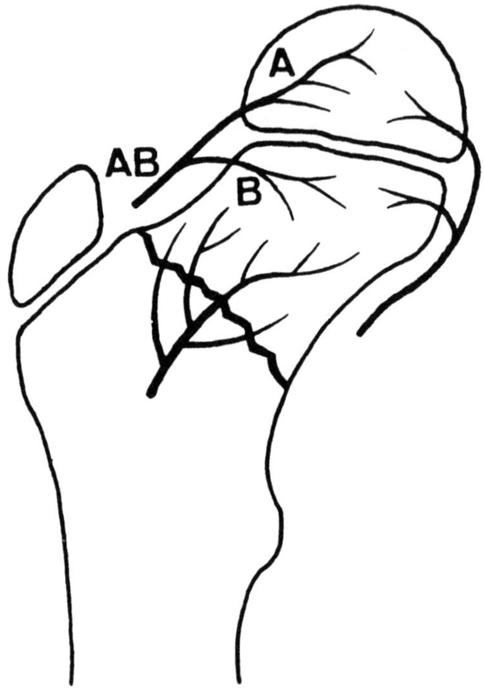

FIG. 9–1 The lateral epiphyseal vessels are important arteries to the femoral head and neck (*AB*). Of lesser importance are the superior metaphyseal arteries.

Unique Characteristics of the Upper Femur in a Child

The vascular supply to the child's hip is different from that in adults (Fig. 9–1). There is no blood supply directly connecting the femoral head with the femoral neck. Owing to their interarticular position, the head and neck do not receive blood from the surrounding tissue but must be supplied by vessels traversing the neck of the femur under the thick periosteum. An injury at this site may disrupt these sensitive vessels, causing damage to the capital epiphysis and/or the distal portion of the femoral neck, and resulting in avascular necrosis and/or early closure of the epiphysis. The vessels of ligamentum teres femoris are an insufficient supply for the epiphysis. However, upper femoral necrosis can still occur even after an undisplaced intertrochanteric fracture in a region where blood supply supposedly is less precarious and more luxurious.

The femoral neck in children is thick and tough. Consequently, it does not comminute when fractured. The periosteum is likewise thick and tough. When a fracture is displaced, from violent trauma, the periosteum is twisted and may cause vascular damage by compression of the vessels. Reduction of the fragments is thus made difficult, and aggressive action via early, prompt open reduction should be considered.

The dense bone in the femoral neck also makes penetration with internal fixation difficult. The smaller diameter of the neck also limits the fixation device in that it must be smaller than that used in adults.

The epiphyseal plate when damaged frequently closes; this may result in varus deformity of the femoral neck. Closure of the upper epiphysis may also produce early closure at the distal femoral epiphysis and even at the femoral epiphysis, resulting in a significantly shorter limb.

Classification by Anatomical Site

Colonna first publicized a classification,[5] based on one conceived by Delbet, which is still commonly used (Table 9–1). Ratliff[5] suggested that transcervical and cervicotrochanteric or basilar fractures should be grouped together since their characteris-

TABLE 9.1 Types of Hip Fractures

Type I: Transepiphyseal fractures are rare and must be distinguished from acute slips which occur in abnormal capital epiphyses; therefore, acute juvenile epiphysiolysis is to be excluded here (Fig. 9–2).
Type II: Transcervical or cervical fractures are by far the most common type (Fig. 9–3).
Type III: Cervicotrochanteric or basicervical fractures are located at the base of the neck and do not involve the trochanteric epiphysis. In children the transition from the trochanteric region to the neck is more abrupt than in adults. Completely disconnecting fractures are therefore more frequent (Fig. 9–4).
Type IV: Trochanteric fractures carry the same general good prognosis as in adults but unfortunately are seen far less frequently (Fig. 9–7).

tics are similar, both in complications and in mode of treatment. Ratliff claimed that before reduction it is nearly impossible to distinguish a transcervical fracture from a basilar neck fracture. He emphasized the need for a true lateral view in order to properly assess the status of the reduction. This was emphasized earlier in Chapter 4. The lateral radiograph is as important as the AP view and is an essential part of the diagnosis and treatment of this condition.

It is necessary to distinguish these fractures by displacement as this is an important consideration in their treatment. Seventy percent will be displaced. Displacement of the capital femoral epiphysis must be distinguished from a slipped epiphysis. The former is an acute, traumatic separation in an otherwise normal upper femur which is not the case in slipped capital femoral epiphysis. A displaced epiphysis also carries the poorest prognosis because of the high rate of complications. Fortunately it is very rare and occurs in children usually under the age of 9. It results from severe violence.

Complications

Ratliff found that one or more complications occur in 69% of cases.[5] They even occur in 33% of initially undisplaced fractures. Prognosis depends on the amount of vascular damage. It may well be that the fate of the upper femur is determined at the time of impact.

Complications are as follows:

1. Avascular necrosis.
2. Coxa vara.
3. Growth disturbances of the upper femoral neck and knee from early epiphyseal closure.
4. Delayed union.
5. Nonunion.
6. Shortening of the injured leg.
7. Sciatic nerve palsy.

Treatment

Treatment should reflect a prompt, aggressive attitude on the part of the surgeon. Such a bold approach is recommended by Pforringer and Rosemeyer: "Irrespective of the type of fracture it was found that immediate operative treatment leads to the best results."[4] In children as well as in adolescents, the risk of avascular necrosis, premature closure of the epiphysis, nonunion, and coxa vara deformity is less following immediate operative treatment.

A valuable tool, image intensification of the fluoroscopic x-ray, has been improved for greater efficiency in the last 2 years. Image intensifiers aid in anatomical reduction and near perfect pin placement, both of paramount importance in this injury. This modality should help improve previous poor results.

An additional mode of treatment has been proposed by Boitzy, Müller, and Weber.[2] These workers achieved a low incidence of avascular necrosis in their cases by opening the capsule and draining the hematoma. They felt that the hematoma produced a tamponade effect causing avascular necrosis. Boitzy, Muller, and Weber, therefore, *open all fractures,* displaced and undisplaced, to perform this procedure and to supplement the reduction with internal fixation so that insidious displacement will not occur. Their method is bold and may not be accepted by more conservative surgeons.

The assumption underlying this bold treatment could not be confirmed by a recent study. Drake and Meyers[6] studied the intracapsular pressure in 13 acute femoral neck fractures. A Bell and Howell transducer was coupled with a standard voltmeter so that voltage measured correlated in a direct ratio with pressure in mm Hg, i.e., 10 volts equalled 100 mm Hg. The total volume aspirated from the hip joint preoperatively never exceeded 5 ml of blood, the pressures varying from 0–68 mm Hg. These findings suggested that preop-

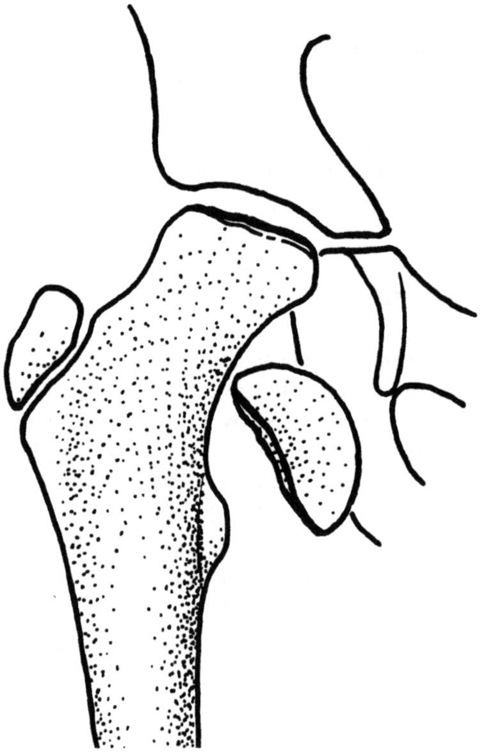

FIG. 9–2 Transepiphyseal fracture, type I. (Courtesy of Dr. Boitzy.)

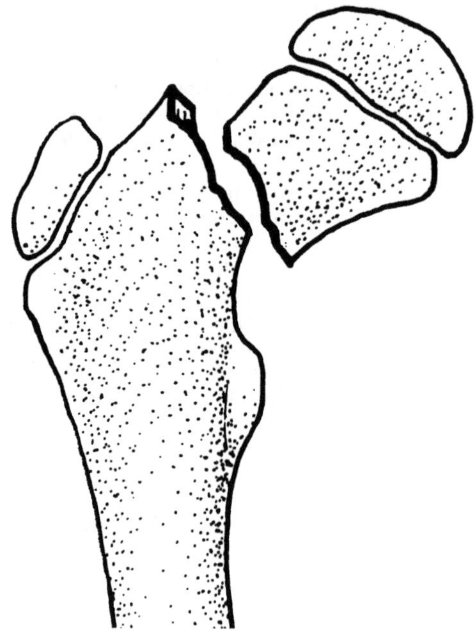

FIG. 9–3 Transcervical fracture, type II. These are slightly more common than the basal fractures. (Courtesy of Dr. Boitzy.)

erative aspiration of the joint is unlikely to influence the vascularity of the femoral head since the volume of the hemarthosis was so small and the measured intraarticular pressure fell well below the diastolic pressure level.

The method of internal fixation proposed here is a contribution of the Swiss surgeons (ASIF). The use of heavy screws should prevent delayed and nonunion not only by holding the fragments firmly but by compressing them together. The Coventry screw as modified at the Campbell Clinic has gained wide attention in this country (Fig. 9–5). It was originally designed for fixation of pediatric intertrochanteric osteotomies. However, it lends itself well to fixation of children's hip fractures.

The treating surgeon should be able to prevent delayed union and nonunion, which in turn are the major factors in producing coxa vara. He should be able to prevent late displacement of certain fractures but he probably will not be able to prevent avascular necrosis. However, he may be able to guide this process to a better eventual outcome by early recognition through bone scanning and possible early aggressive treatment.

Transepiphyseal Separations

Most all transepiphyseal separations are displaced (Fig. 9–2). They can be difficult to manipulate. Prompt reduction and internal fixation should be done; the reduction should be as anatomical as possible if the lesion cannot be opened. If it cannot be reduced anatomically, an anterior Calahan incision should be used and the fragments *eased* into position. Smooth Steinmann pins should be used to transfix the fragments: three should be sufficient. They should be removed after being in place 1 month with the child protected in a body cast for another month. These lesions heal rapidly.

The epiphysis is reduced closed and pinned from the lateral side. At the time of surgery, a catheter should be placed in the capsule by skidding the catheter and its internal trocar along the anterior neck into the capsule.

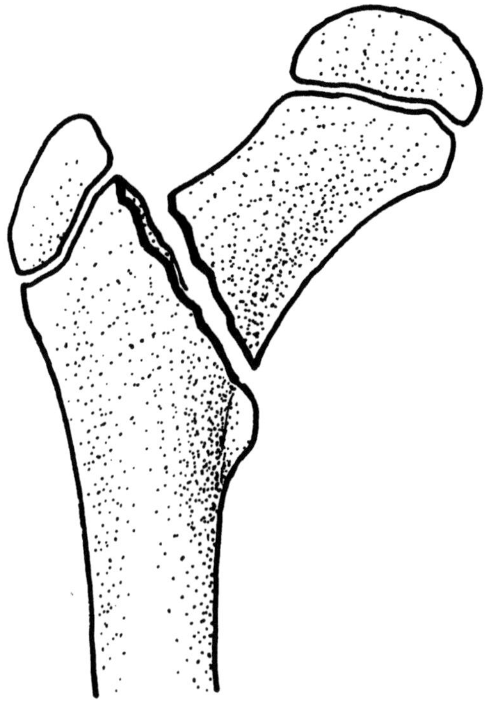

FIG. 9–4 Basal or cervicotrochanteric fracture, type III. (Courtesy of Dr. Boitzy.)

Transcervical and Cervicotrochanteric (Basicervical) Fractures

Undisplaced Fractures These fractures should be fixed by closed pinning using the ASIF screws. A catheter can be passed along the anterior neck through the incision used for the pins so that the trocar will lead the catheter into the capsule for drainage of the hematoma.

Displaced Fractures (*Figs. 9–3 and 9–4*) The fracture is reduced closed and, if a near anatomical reduction is achieved, fixed with 2 or 3 ASIF screws. The Coventry screw used in intertrochanteric osteotomies was designed at the Children's Institute in Coventry, England. It has been modified at the Campbell Clinic and can also be used as a single screw for these fractures. Because the femoral neck is so hard, predrilling and pretapping instruments complement the Campbell Clinic System (Fig. 9–5).

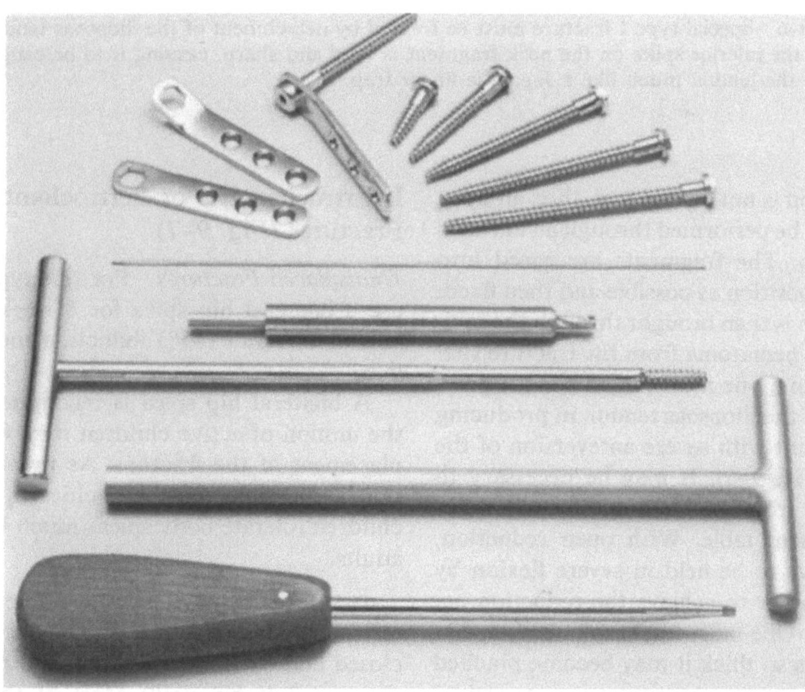

FIG. 9–5 The Campbell pediatric compression screw system comes in variously angled side plates with three or four holes, plus screws of various length and a drill and tap, all of which is an improved version of the Coventry, England, system.

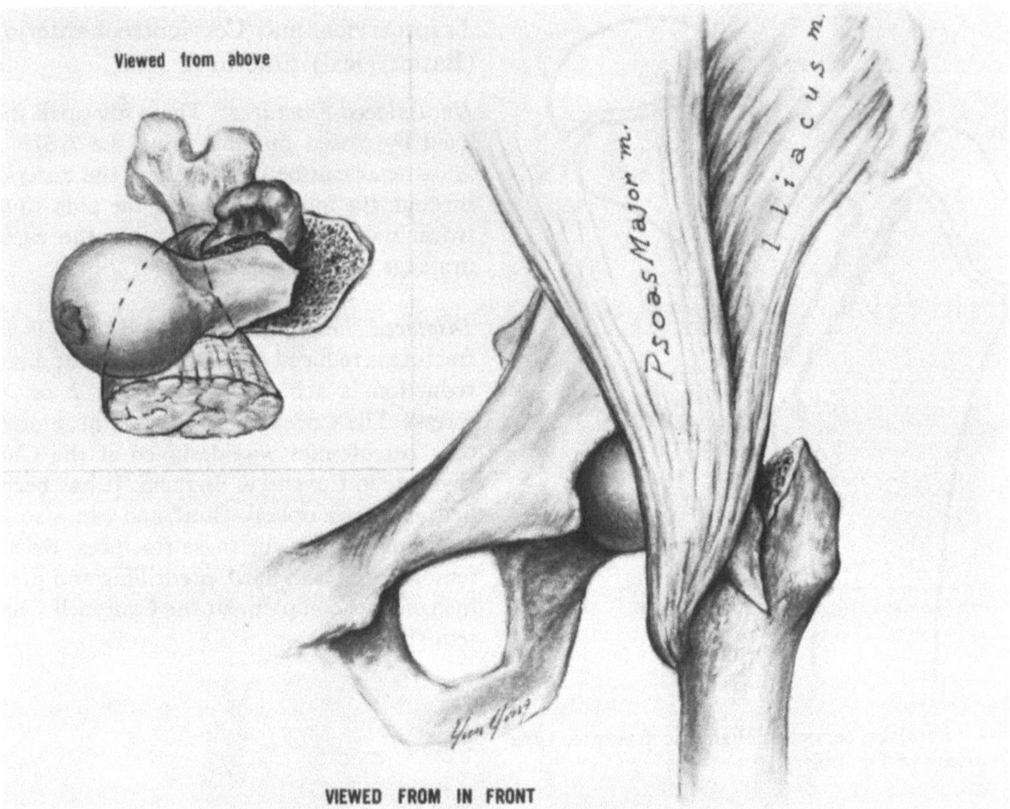

FIG. 9–6 Special type I fracture must be treated by detachment of the iliopsoas tendon when the inferior spike on the neck fragment is long and sharp, causing it to be caught under the tendon much like a Japanese finger-trap.

If the reduction is not anatomical, then an open reduction should be performed through an anterior Calahan incision: The fragments are eased into as anatomical a position as possible and then fixed. A hemovac drain is then brought through the incision to drain the hematoma from the fracture site.

In the reduction, one must remember the powerful influence of the iliopsoas tendon in producing varus displacement with severe anteversion of the femoral neck (Fig. 9–6). It may be necessary to move the patient from the fracture table to a regular operating room table. With open reduction, the hip may have to be held in severe flexion by an assistant in order to achieve the reduction before it is pinned. One must further remember that the periosteum is so thick it may become pinched between the fragments, preventing proper reduction. This, too, may be an appropriate reason for an open reduction in an attempt to avoid nonunion.

Intertrochanteric or Pertrochanteric Fractures (Fig. 9–7)

Undisplaced Fractures For this type of fracture, use a bilateral hip spica for 8 weeks. The hip is held in moderate (45°) abduction and neutral rotation.

A bilateral hip spica is recommended because the motion of active children may well cause displacement of the fracture. As much immobilization as possible must be achieved, especially as children tolerate body spicas much better than do adults.

DISPLACED FRACTURES The displaced intertrochanteric fracture should be manipulated closed and fixed with a screw and plate. (Do not use an adult hip nail!) Most of the current orthopedic manufacturers produce the Coventry screw or its equivalent (Fig. 9–5).

Although theoretically the intertrochanteric

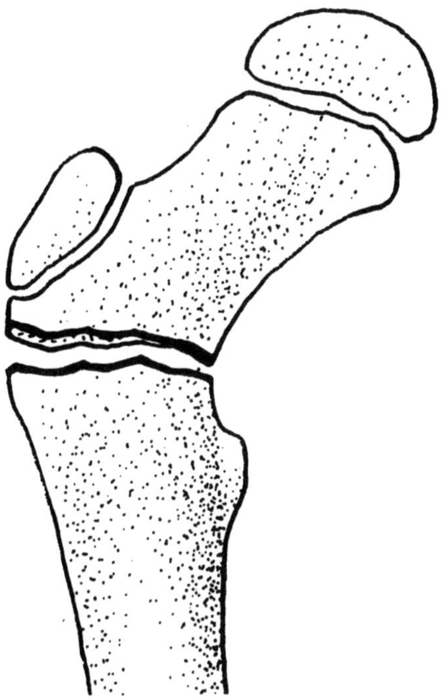

FIG. 9–7 Trochanteric fractures (pertrochanteric or intertrochanteric), type IV, carry the best prognosis.

fracture should lie outside the confines of the capsule, a catheter should still be inserted into the hip joint to drain any possible hematoma which may become trapped and produce the tamponade effect described by Weber and his colleagues.

The implants should be removed as soon as the fracture shows evidence of healing, usually after 10 to 12 months.

Further Surgical Considerations

These injuries should be treated as emergencies in order to evacuate the hematoma and prevent contractures of the joint capsule which may impede the reduction. The Swiss group treats the hip fracture as an emergency. They also recommend that any reduction on the fracture table should be gentle with very little stretching in order to avoid any or further damage to the delicate femoral vessels.

These workers advocate a Watson-Jones approach which can lead to difficulty in visualizing the femoral neck. The author prefers an anterolateral incision of Calahan where the anterior joint capsule can be opened and the hip visualized. If one does not wish to extend the incision to the lateral cortex a separate incision can be made in order to insert the pins from the lateral intertrochanteric area into the neck. This is especially true when trying to gently reduce a separated femoral epiphysis—the Watson-Jones approach will not provide the proper exposure. One may also initially use air instruments to drill a small Steinmann pin across the fracture site. This will lock the fracture together until the heavy ASIF screws can be inserted into the neck; the pin is then removed. Interoperative antibiotics should be used to prevent any infection which may occur from surgery.

The length of the screws should reach the epiphyseal plate but not beyond in order to prevent premature closure (Fig. 9–8).

Treatment of Complications

Avascular Necrosis

Ratliff[5] was the first to categorize the pattern of avascular necrosis of the upper end of the femur (Figs. 9–9 to 9–11).

Avascular necrosis is the most common complication. It occurs promptly and can be detected as early as 3 months postinjury.

In some patients, severe, diffuse collapse can occur with subluxation of the hip. Occasionally a segmental necrosis may occur in the dome. In others, revascularization may occur without any significant collapse, but the head is left with a curious coarse trabecular appearance. Unfortunately the particular response to avascular necrosis is unpredictable. The child with a fractured femoral neck, displaced or undisplaced, should have a bone scan done at 3 months, at 6 months, and then at 12 months for its earliest possible detection.

Ratliff found no good results after type I necrosis. He found no evidence to suggest that this type was related to the direction of the fracture line, any one type of injury mechanism, or any particular method of treatment. It was associated with half of the cases of nonunion. Type II necrosis was uncommon and there is little information to help determine the course of treatment. Type III necrosis is likewise seldom seen and may be the most benign of the various types. It also is associated with premature fusion and resulting varus deformity; thus its treatment may be geared to the correction of the varus deformity should it

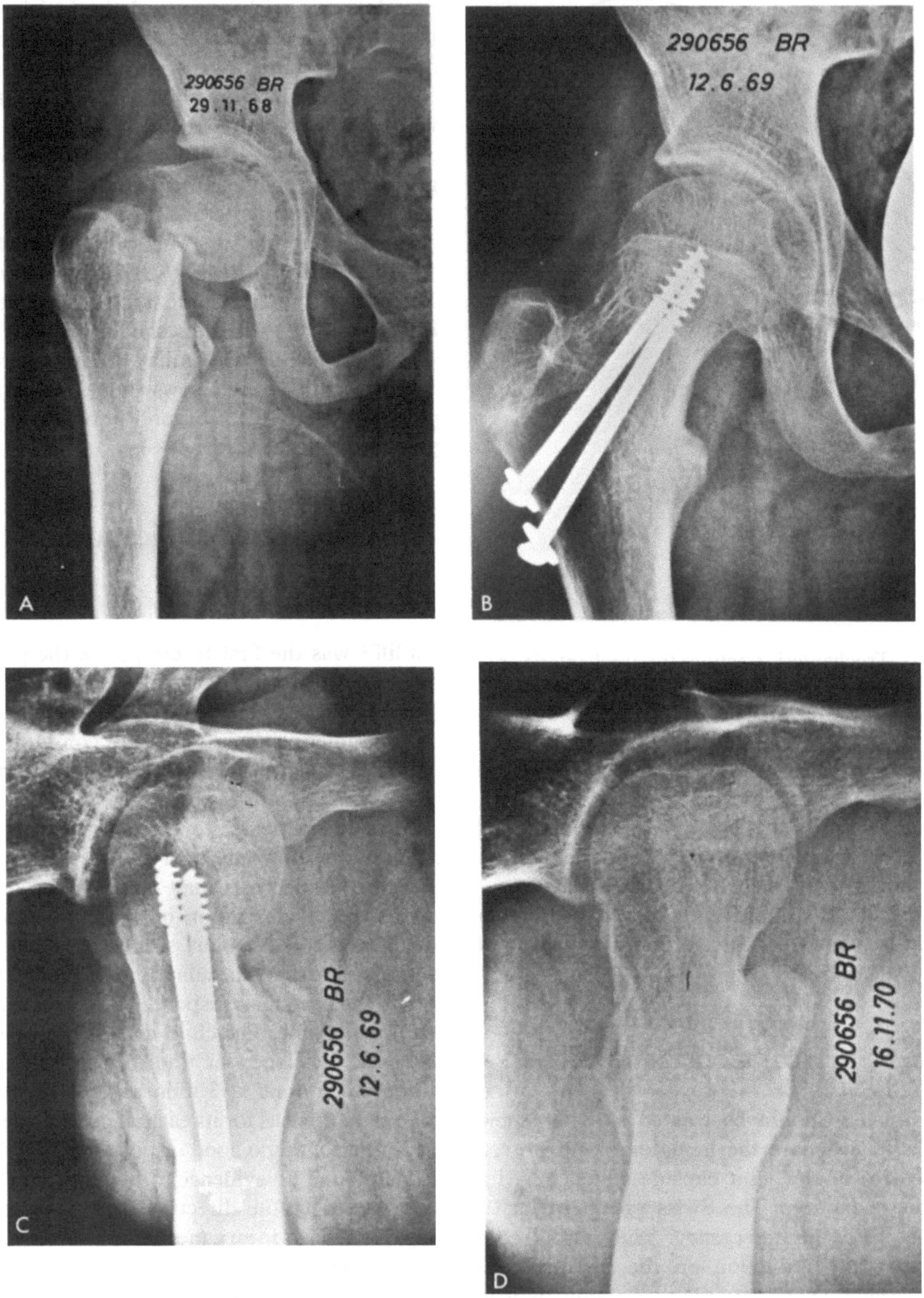

FIG. 9–8 **A** Transcervical fracture. **B** and **C** Open reduction is performed and an anterior arthrotomy done to relieve the hemarthrosis. Note that the pins do not cross the epiphyseal line. **D** and **E** Excellent healing without the troublesome varus deformity.

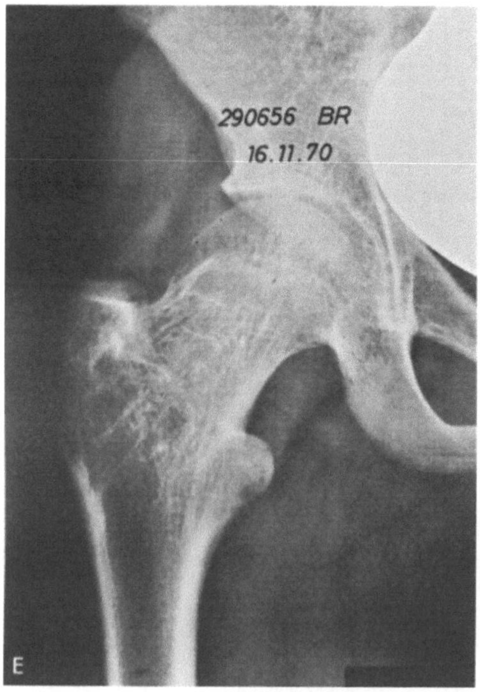

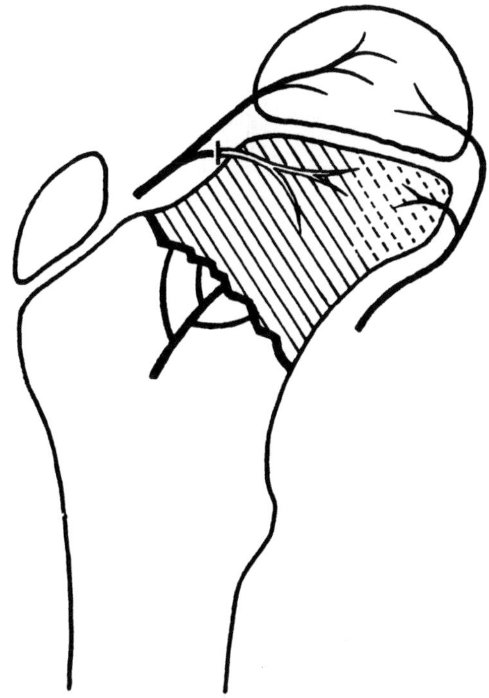

FIG. 9–10 Necrosis limited by the plate proximally and by the fracture itself distally.

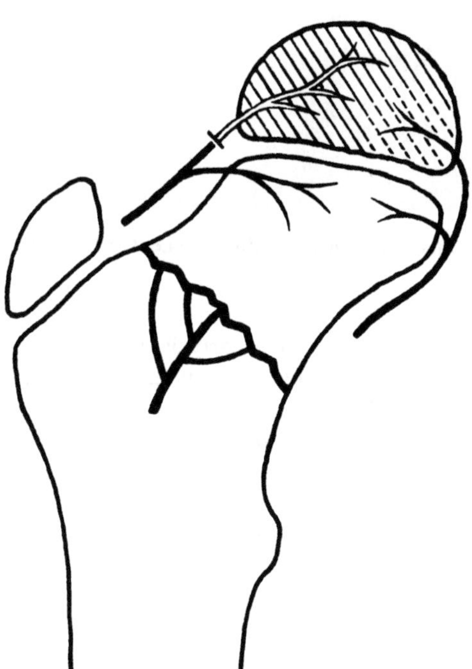

FIG. 9–9 Necrosis limited by the epiphyseal plate.

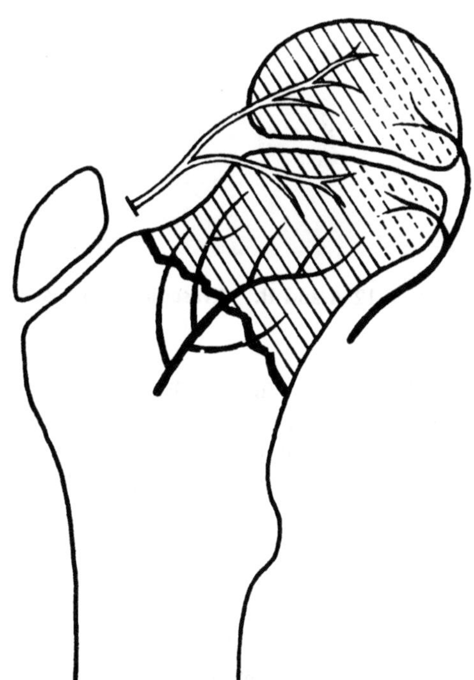

FIG. 9–11 Combination of the two, leaving the entire head and neck necrotic.

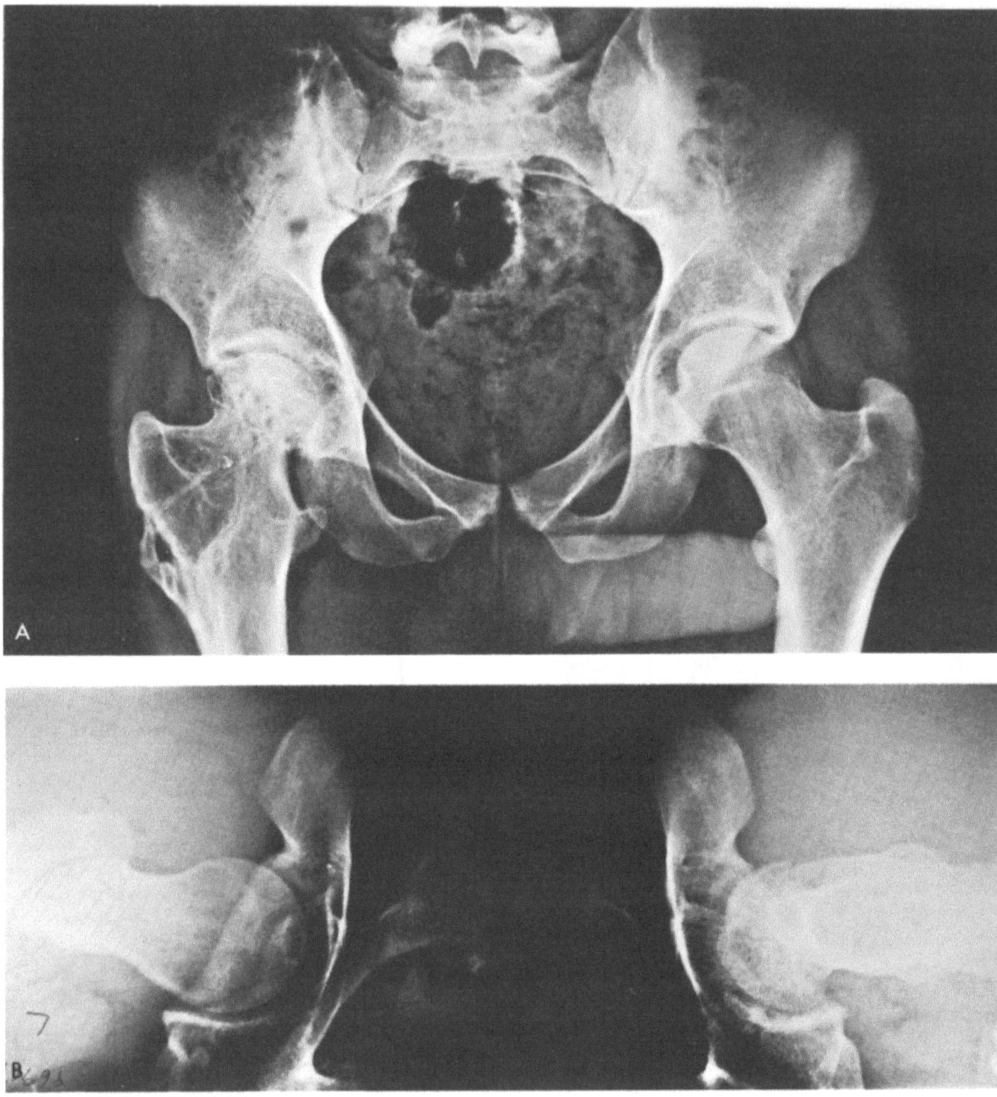

FIG. 9–12 **A** and **B.** Avascular necrosis successfully treated with an *early* displacement osteotomy.

occur with premature fusion. The earliest radiological sign of avascular necrosis is an increased density of the area in question, which appears shortly after the fracture. As the process progresses there are varying degrees of collapse. These are late and may be prevented by information gained from bone scanning. One method of treatment is an early displacement osteotomy (Fig. 9–12). The case illustrated was done by Dr. Boitzy. None of the published studies discussed the alternate possibility of a pelvic osteotomy. This is a viable alternative which will cover the head and shift the relationship of the weight-bearing surfaces.

An osteotomy done early is a bold approach; however, procrastination may be disastrous. If the bone scan shows early necrosis, coverage of the femoral head should be extended with an osteotomy of the Salter type. The extra coverage will take weight off the hip, hopefully preventing late collapse and early arthritis. Circulation to the head may also improve.

Coxa Vara

If coxa vara is associated with nonunion, it should be promptly corrected by subtrochanteric osteotomy with displacement of the proximal fragment over the center of the shaft (Fig. 9–12). If the fixation device was weak and tenuous, causing the nonunion, it should be replaced by the sturdier, mechanically more efficient ASIF screws or a Coventry type of screw and plate. A bone graft across the site may be considered. Ratliff recommended using the fibula for such a procedure.[5]

Ratliff also made an important point that coxa valga should not be allowed to be left too severe because it will not correct itself with growth, as is the case with coxa vara, usually.

Coxa vara unassociated with delayed union or nonunion should be treated with observation; if the epiphyses are still open this will most likely correct itself spontaneously. If it progresses, an early subtrochanteric osteotomy should be done.

Delayed Union

In delayed union the hip has not healed within 6 months. Appropriateness of the fixation device should be evaluated and some compressive apparatus considered. If delayed union is seen in a case treated without internal fixation but with cast immobilization, the author suggests open repair of the fracture with compression and possibly a bone graft. There is as yet no information available about electrostimulation of delayed union in children.

Arthritic Changes

There is no hard information available about possible disabling arthritis in these patients. One would expect this to occur as patients become older, in the late 20s or early 30s. Total hip replacement is still controversial in this setting. The author would consider a displacement osteotomy or a Salter osteotomy before contemplating artificial replacement of any kind.

Premature Closure

Morrissey[3] has stated the following:

"The incidence of epiphyseal closure varies with different authors, ranging from 15% in Ratliff's series to 62% in the series of Canale and Bourland. Several interrelated factors are associated with the occurrence of premature closure of the epiphyseal plate and it is difficult to separate them. However, the main ones include the type of fixation and occurrence of avascular necrosis.

Canale and Bourland have clearly shown that in the case of Knowles' pins, if these penetrate or cross the epiphyseal plate, premature fusion is more likely than if they do not. There is no evidence, however, to indicate that the same would be true if smooth pins were used. Another form of treatment, the spica cast, is also associated with a significant number of cases of premature closure of the plate, in the treatment of both displaced and nondisplaced fractures."

Of particular interest are the three patients in Ratliff's series who sustained closure of the distal femoral epiphyseal plate after prolonged cast immobilization.[5]

Just as it is difficult to pinpoint one aspect of treatment in the incidence of premature epiphyseal closure, it is also difficult to directly implicate avascular necrosis. Although there is a much higher incidence of epiphyseal closure in those patients with avascular necrosis, there is also a greater incidence of displaced fractures, thus indicating that more severe trauma may be involved.

The leg discrepancy with which the patient is left after premature closure of the plate will depend on the age of the patient and the occurrence of avascular necrosis. Avascular necrosis may contribute to shortening in an absolute manner by collapse in height and in a relative manner by flexion–adduction deformity. Since the proximal femoral epiphysis accounts for only approximately 15% of the growth of the entire leg, significant discrepancy due to plate closure alone is to be expected only in younger children.

Subtrochanteric Osteotomy

Ratliff[5] states the following:

Recently this operation has been advocated in the primary treatment of intracapsular fractures in adults. It has been used for cases in which the risk of nonunion is increased, such as when the fracture line is steep, there is marked comminution, or the displacement cannot be reduced by manipulation.

Primary subtrochanteric osteotomy was performed in six patients in this series because of the inability to obtain a good position with manipulative reduction. Four of these six children had good or fair results; the two poor results were caused in one patient by severe avascular necrosis and in the other by nonunion of the fracture despite the osteotomy.

Several conclusions can be drawn from this small series:

1. Remarkable remodeling of the upper end of the femur with growth may occur after an osteotomy. This was noteworthy when the osteotomy was low

and when a gap was left between the inferior part of the neck of the femur and the upper part of the distal fragment. Remodeling cannot occur if the distal fragment is placed close under the neck of the femur; in these cases shortening may result.
2. A late varus deformity may develop at the site of the osteotomy, even after union. The tendency for a varus position to develop should be anticipated when performing this operation, and the distal fragment should deliberately be placed in marked abduction.
3. A primary osteotomy is a useful procedure that may have to be performed when manipulative reduction has not been successful. . . .

Gupta, Chaturvedi, and Pruthi stressed the use of a primary osteotomy in a large series of cases and stated that 71% of these patients had good results with a transcervical fracture. They also emphasized that considerable remodeling can occur at the upper end of the femur after this operation. I could find no other reference in the literature to this method of treatment for these fractures.

Bibliography

1. Blount, W. P.: Fractures in Children. Baltimore, Williams & Wilkins, 1955.
2. Boitzy, A.: Fractures of the hip in children. In Tronzo, R. G. (ed.): Surgery of the Hip, 1st ed., Philadelphia, Lea & Febiger, 1973, p. 551.
3. Morrissey, R.: Hip fractures in children. Clin. Orthop., 152:202, 1980.
4. Pforringer, W., Rosemeyer, B.: Fractures of the hip in children and adolescents. Acta Orthop. Scand., 51:91, 1980.
5. Ratliff, A. H. C.: Fractures of the neck of the femur in children. In: Proceedings of the Ninth Meeting of the Hip Society. St. Louis, Mosby, 1981, p. 188.
6. Drake, J. K., Meyer, M. H.: Intracapsular pressure and hemarthrosis following femoral neck fractures. Clin. Orthop., 182:172–176, 1984.

CHAPTER 10

Congenital Coxa Vara

WALTER A. HOYT, JR., BARRY J. GREENBERG, AND ARNE MELBY III

Fiorani,[30] in 1881, published the first clinical description of a lesion of the hip due to bending of the neck of the femur, after observing 15 patients, mostly children, with slight limps which had commenced soon after ambulation. Similar observations of this particular adduction bowing of the femur were reported by Muller [65] in 1889. Hofmeister,[42] in 1894, with a classical description of the adduction deformity, suggested the name *coxa vara* for this condition. Kredel,[53] in 1896, was the first investigator to describe obvious *congenital coxa vara,* which he observed in two children also exhibiting other malformations, such as congenital pes equinovarus. As originally intended, the term *coxa vara* denotes a particular adduction deformity of the shaft of the femur in relation to the head and neck. Most contemporary definitions of this deformity include a decrease of the angle between the neck and shaft of the femur, designated as the angle of inclination.

The lack of a standard system of classification, publication of various theories of the etiology of coxa vara, varying age of onset of this deformity, and individual investigator bias have resulted in marked confusion of terms used to describe and discuss coxa vara deformities in children. Various authors have referred to this same condition as infantile, developmental, cervical, idiopathic, and congenital coxa vara. We, as have many investigators,[2,5,23,26,31,38,39,40,41,43,55,80,95] prefer to denote this condition, congenital, since it is our opinion that in congenital coxa vara, the delay in the manifestation of the deformity is essentially temporal, with the primary etiological factor being present in utero, or at birth.

Amstutz and Wilson [3] proposed a system of classification based on etiological concepts, which in many instances is arbitrary, but nevertheless provides an understanding of the various characteristics of this deformity. Two broad categories were selected by Amstutz and Wilson for differentiating the types of coxa vara deformities: (1) the congenital type and (2) the acquired type. Congenital types are further classified as to types that occur as localized congenital disturbances associated with or without bowing or shortening of the femur, and types that occur with generalized growth disturbances such as osteochondrodystrophy, cleidocranial dysostosis, dysplasia epiphysealis multiplex, and achondroplasia. The acquired types are classified as to etiological factors such as vascular compromise and insult, infection, trauma, metabolic disorders, and tumor. The type of congenital coxa vara described in this chapter has been referred to by others as developmental, infantile, and cervical, and is presented as an isolated localized growth disturbance, usually diagnosed when the child begins to ambulate, in which a decrease of the angle of inclination of the proximal femur is observed, without shortening or bowing of the femur.

It is the purpose of the following discussion to present sufficient fundamental information so that the reader will thoroughly understand the pathogenesis of this deformity, be able to recognize it, treat it, and differentiate it from other abnormalities of the proximal end of the femur. Lack of such fundamental knowledge on the part of the clinician can result in severely disabling deformities, as shown in Figs. 10–1 to 10–3, which depict, in sequence, progressive deformity and joint deterioration of unrecognized or untreated coxa vara.

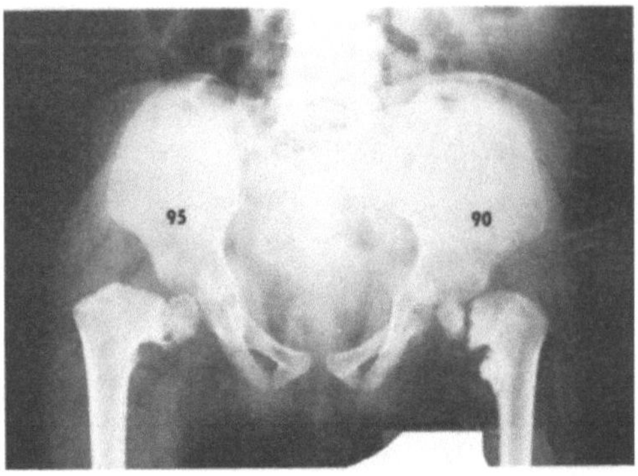

FIG. 10–1 A 4-year-old patient with bilateral coxa vara. Angles of inclination 95° and 90°, respectively.

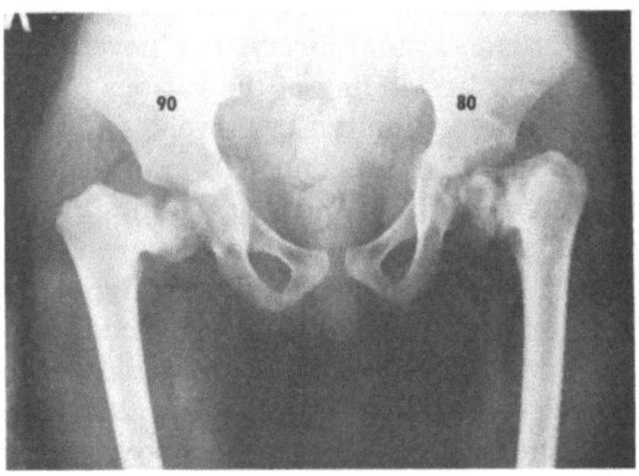

FIG. 10–2 Same patient as in Fig. 10–1, now aged 6 years. Angles of inclination 90° and 80°, respectively.

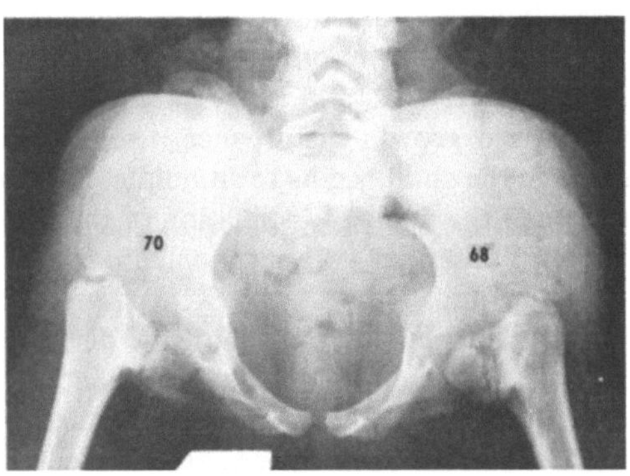

FIG. 10–3 Same patient as in preceding figures, now aged 8 years. Angles of inclination 70° and 68°, respectively.

Incidence

Congenital coxa vara is relatively rare, estimated by Johanning at one case per 25,000 live births.[47] The frequency of coxa vara is low, compared with the frequency of other orthopedic lesions, being reported by several hospitals to represent less than 1% of their total orthopedic admissions. Unilateral involvement is more common than bilateral, with reported ratios as follows: Pylkkanen,[76] 1.9 to 1; Magnusson,[62] 2.2 to 1; and Zimmermann,[96] 3.0 to 1. The incidence of coxa vara is not influenced by sex or race. In cases of unilateral involvement, either the left or right femur may be involved with equal frequency.

Prior to 1974, it was not universally accepted that congenital coxa vara was a familial condition. However, the fact that the occurrence of this deformity was reported in identical twins,[23,24,80] siblings,[1,8,59,75] parents,[2] and near relatives [59] suggested familial tendencies. In 1974, Say et al.[84] published their observations on 94 patients with congenital coxa vara and 25 unaffected relatives living in the Turkish village of Gonyeli, in Cyprus. Clinical and radiological studies were made, and a pedigree covering 13 generations was made from information given by the local populace. The pedigree, comprising over 300 subjects, showed classical autosomal dominant inheritance. In addition to the congenital coxa vara of varying severity, almost all of the affected individuals exhibited short stature with bowing of the lower extremities, and some of the individuals had relative iliac hypoplasia and protrusio acetabuli.

Etiology

As described by Morgan and Somerville,[64] in the newborn infant, the femur basically consists of a calcified shaft, containing actively proliferating nutrient vessels, which is closed at both ends by cartilaginous epiphyses. Although each epiphysis has one or more vascular islands which become the ossific nuclei, the epiphyseal plate, per se, is not yet fully formed. The proximal femoral metaphyseal plate has the appearance of a transverse crescentic line, composed histologically of cartilage columns interposed between the bony end plates of the epiphysis and the metaphysis. It consists of two parts: a medial cephalic segment and a lateral trochanteric segment. Shortly after birth, the medial cervical portion matures, and ossification of the femoral head is seen to occur during the first year of postnatal life, with resulting elongation of the femoral neck. Since this initial spurt of growth of the femoral neck is not opposed, the femoral neck angle is more vertical, a normal condition known as infantile coxa valga. As the infant starts to ambulate, particularly with use of the hip abductors, the lateral portion of the plate matures, with the appearance of the greater trochanteric epiphysis as a separate growth center. Thus, there are two separate areas where rapid growth occurs proximally, which interact, according to Compere et al.[19] to determine the femoral neck angle and the length of the proximal diaphysis. Furthermore, there are normal physiological forces which tend to promote a varus or valgus attitude of the femoral neck. With weight bearing, body weight produces varus deformation, and the hip rotators and hip adductors produce valgus deformation.

Amstutz and Wilson [3] reviewed the study by Von Lanz and Mayet, which showed that differential epiphyseal growth and interrelated physiological forces usually combine to result in a gradual decrease in the angle of inclination during growth and development. Von Lanz and Mayet determined the mean angle of inclination to be 148° at 1 year of age, which gradually, with growth and development, decreased to a mean of 120° in the aged. By definition, coxa vara is a decrease of the normal angle of inclination. Pylkkanen [76] reported an angle less than 110° to be pathological; however, individual variation as well as variation with age does occur.

Despite what is now thoroughly known regarding the normal sequence of events in the growth and development of the femur and hip joint, the precise etiology of coxa vara remains unknown. Numerous investigators, based upon clinical, roentgenological, histopathological, and experimental studies, have proposed varying theories of the etiology of coxa vara, implicating inborn genetic errors, congenital anomalies, vascular insults, developmental errors, traumatic events, or biomechanical insufficiencies. It is our opinion that there are several etiological factors to account for coxa vara deformities, in that to date no one etiological factor has been proven to cause all types of coxa vara observed, particularly as classified by Amstutz and Wilson.[3]

As shown in Fig. 10–4, one type of coxa vara

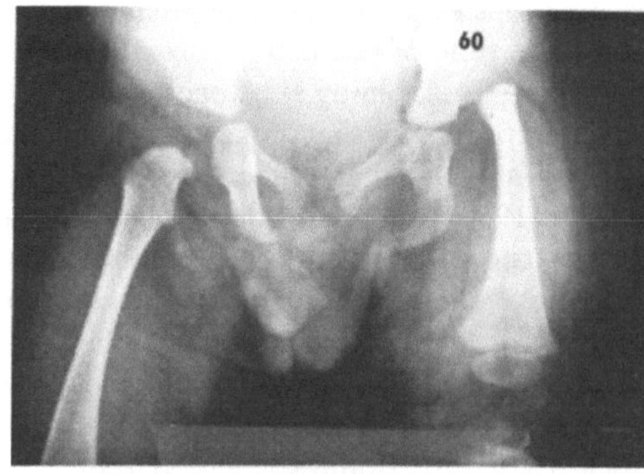

FIG. 10–4 Association of congenital coxa vara with proximal focal femoral deficiency.

may be diagnosed at birth or shortly thereafter, due to the concomitant shortening of the femur.[31,32,79] In addition, other associated congenital abnormalities, such as pes equinovarus, may be present.[53,71] Having had the opportunity to examine femoral heads removed for the treatment of coxa vara, Hoffa,[41] in 1905, and Helbing,[39] in 1906, observed histological defects of endochondral ossification, and concluded that coxa vara was congenital in origin. Hoffa [41] concluded that the bone lacked bioplastic energy as a result of a bone disease during intrauterine development which destroyed the growth capacity of the epiphyseal plate. Helbing [39] concluded that coxa vara was due to a complete absence of, or delay in, ossification. Schwarz,[86] also observing the defect of endochondral ossification, believed that the bending of the femoral neck was due to lack of space in the uterus or to pressure exerted by the uterine wall. Nilsonne [68] concluded that coxa vara is congenital in origin, and develops as a result of a disturbance of the embryonic circulation in the area of the femoral neck. A recent study by Chung and Riser [17] added substance to these earlier theories of congenital vascular insufficiency; they were able to demonstrate that the endochondral ossification defect noted in the growth plate of the proximal femur was associated with a reduction in the number and caliber of intraosseous arteries supplying the metaphyseal side of the epiphysis, and extraosseous medial ascending cervical arteries on the surface of the femoral neck. Kreuz [54] and Zimmermann [96] concluded that congenital disturbance of endochondral ossification of the epiphysis was the probable cause of coxa vara, which was more recently confirmed by Pylkkanen,[76] in his study of 25 biopsies of the vertical fissure defect removed at the time of corrective osteotomy.

Drehmann,[21,22] Golding,[31] Joachimstahal,[46] and Reiner [78] proposed that coxa vara was the first stage of a congenital defect of the femur. Erlacher,[26] in 1950, proposed that dysplasia of the hip was the true cause, resulting in a congenital malformation of the entire hip point, in addition to a varus deformity of the femur. Further evidence in favor of a true congenital etiology of coxa vara is the occasional familial occurrence observed in identical twins,[24,80] siblings,[1,8,59,75] parents,[2] or near relatives.[59] Furthermore, Say and associates [84] have demonstrated a classical autosomal dominant inheritance pattern for coxa vara, in their study of over 300 residents of a Turkish village.

In contrast to the theories of congenital origin, many theories have been proposed that are concerned with the statics and dynamics of the hip joint, particularly those present and produced when the child begins to ambulate.[3,33,76] In favor of these theories is the fact that most cases are first diagnosed when the child begins to ambulate, with the observation of a painless limp in cases of unilateral involvement, or the characteristic waddling gait seen with bilateral involvement. For practical purposes, these theories may be classified as developmental. Fairbank,[27,28] in 1928, was the first investigator to clearly separate these patients from the congenital group, and coined the term, "infantile" or "cervical" coxa vara. Observing the triangular fragment, in many cases bilateral, he postulated that a developmental error was the cause, with formation of the fragment from a separate ossification center. While Armstrong [4] later confirmed the findings of Fairbank, Walter [90-92] concluded that coxa vara may result from a physiological reaction of the bone to an unphysiological, shearing stress of weight bearing in the presence of a femoral neck defect. Walter further substantiated his opinion by the fact that after corrective osteotomy, the abnormal bony lesion would quickly heal. Babb et al.[5] concluded that the responsible developmental triangular fragment was an osteochondritic lesion, which probably was vascular and of congenital origin. Simons,[87] Pauwels,[73] Strauss,[88] and Magnusson [62] believed that the vertical fissure developed as an insufficiency fracture, which in the absence of trauma would progress to formation of a true pseudarthrosis without treatment.

Pauwels,[74] has stated that coxa vara is purely developmental, and is "congenital" only in the sense that there is some mechanical and biological insufficiency in the neck of the femur. This insufficiency reduces the load-bearing capacity of the femoral neck, and results in progressive deformation of the femoral neck into a varus attitude. This enhances the detrimental effects of bending stress with continued load, in addition to increasing slide stress as the epiphysis assumes a more oblique position. The net result is further varus deformation and shortening of the neck of the femur, with concomitant displacement of the femoral head medially. Histologically, Pauwels observed reabsorption of the calcified columns of the epiphyseal cartilage as a result of the deformation of the femoral neck, and indicated this as the cause for the neck shortness. He noted that further reabsorption leads to narrowing of the femoral neck and formation of the vertical fissure defect. Pauwels observed that this gap is not a *Y*- or *V*-shaped split of the epiphyseal plate, but is of mechanical origin due to reabsorption (fatigue fracture type). Although Pauwels clearly defined the biomechanics and pathogenesis of coxa vara, he did not elucidate the primary etiology, and his study did not determine when the alteration occurred, or in which area of the epiphyseal plate the deformation occurred. Patella and Bancale [72] studied the angular relationship between the cephalic and trochanteric growth plates, defining this as the angle of the femoral growth cartilage, which is about 125°, and is exactly equal to the femoral–neck angle. They proposed that whereas the cephalic segment is normally subjected to compression forces, and the trochanteric segment is normally subjected to tension forces, slowing or cessation of growth in one section, while it continues normally in the other, will result in angular and morphological changes. Patella and Bancale [72] determined that these changes occurred in the epiphyseal plate zones of proliferating and hypertrophied cells, so that not only is varus observed, but in addition, longitudinal growth of the femur is retarded.

Elmslie,[25] in 1907, was the first investigator to suggest trauma as the cause of coxa vara, occurring at the time of birth or shortly thereafter. Morgan and Somerville [64] described congenital coxa vara in an infant born to a mother who had incurred abdominal injury in a fall during her pregnancy. They concluded that coxa vara was a result of intrauterine injury, which resulted in the formation of a lesion which caused interruption of ossification of the femoral neck. Furthermore, they concluded that if this lesion, which they presumed was vascular, was distal to the trochanter, congenital coxa vara would develop with shortening of the femur, whereas if the lesion was proximal to the trochanter, varus deformity without shortening would occur. McDougall,[63] in 1961, published his study of fracture of the neck of the femur in children, and described the occurrence of progressive coxa vara in 13 out of 24 treated fractures. McDougall also showed, in the untreated cases, that union of the proximal fragment to the base of the neck of the femur, or to the medial side of the shaft, does occur, despite continuous shearing stress across the fracture with weight bearing. Blockey [10] described three cases of coxa vara in which trauma appeared to be the cause of the deformities; from his experience, as well as his knowledge of McDougall's study,[63] he concluded that the vertical fissure line is a fracture which eventually heals, with or without treatment. A similar opinion has been expressed by Rang,[77] who theoretically reconstructed the events that occur in the manifestation of infantile coxa vara.

Evidence has been found, experimentally, which appears to confirm the traumatic etiology of coxa vara. Based on animal experiments in which they induced a limited subchondral fracture of the head or neck of the femur in a manner which produced various forms of aseptic necrosis, Nagura [66] and Kosuge [67] concluded that coxa vara should be regarded as aseptic osseous necrosis, and that the entity was traumatic in origin. Compere et al.[19] demonstrated in animal experiments that when the epiphyseal plate of the femoral head is traumatized its growth is arrested, and a coxa vara deformity results. In addition, they showed that a coxa valga deformity is produced when the greater trochanteric epiphysis is traumatized. This observation was further substantiated by Laurent,[58] who demonstrated experimentally that the greater trochanteric epiphysis adds nothing to the length of the femur, but only interacts with the capital femoral epiphysis to determine the femoral-neck angle.

To determine the potential of the three proximal femoral epiphyses, and their contribution toward the architectural configuration of the proximal femur, this author [44] conducted an extensive, multiphasic laboratory study with dogs. The greater and lesser trochanteric epiphyses were subjected to two separate procedures: (1) excision and denervation of the attached muscles, and (2) total excision of the individual epiphyses. The capital femoral epiphysis was subjected to removal of varying amounts of plate. The most pertinent findings of this study were as follows:

1. The capital epiphysis is the only proximal femoral epiphysis responsible for longitudinal growth.
2. Following total excision of the greater trochanteric epiphysis, a typical coxa valga deformity of the proximal femur developed.
3. Partial excision of the subcapital epiphyseal plate produced a characteristic coxa vara deformity, the extent of the varus being directly related to the area and amount of excision.
4. The lesser trochanteric epiphysis is a traction epiphysis of minor importance and does not contribute significantly to the proximal femoral architecture.

Figure 10–5 shows the typical coxa vara deformity of the proximal femur which developed in a dog after partial excision of the inferior portion of the capital epiphysis. In this series of experiments, a marked difference in the angles of inclination was observed. In addition, there was a variable effect observed on the angle of declination (anteversion, retroversion), a difference in overall length of the femur, and in many cases, marked overgrowth of the greater trochanter. The variation in the degree of coxa vara produced is believed due to the extent of involvement of the epiphyseal plate by the experimental trauma, although supportive data for this postulate were not available.

However, in an analysis of 75 clinical cases of coxa vara, we observed a relationship between the degree of varus deformity and the extent of involvement of the subcapital epiphyseal plate. Figure 10–6 is a composite drawing of the presurgical roentgenograms in these cases. This analysis revealed that as the size of the triangular fragment increases, the area of involvement of the epiphyseal plate by the disease process (vertical fissure defect) decreases, as does the degree of varus deformity. Conversely, the smaller the triangular fragment, the greater is the area of involvement of the epiphyseal plate and the degree of varus deformity. In this study, evidence was not apparent to substantiate or refute previously proposed theories that weight bearing creates mechanical shearing forces which then act through a defect to result in varus deformation of the femoral neck. In their

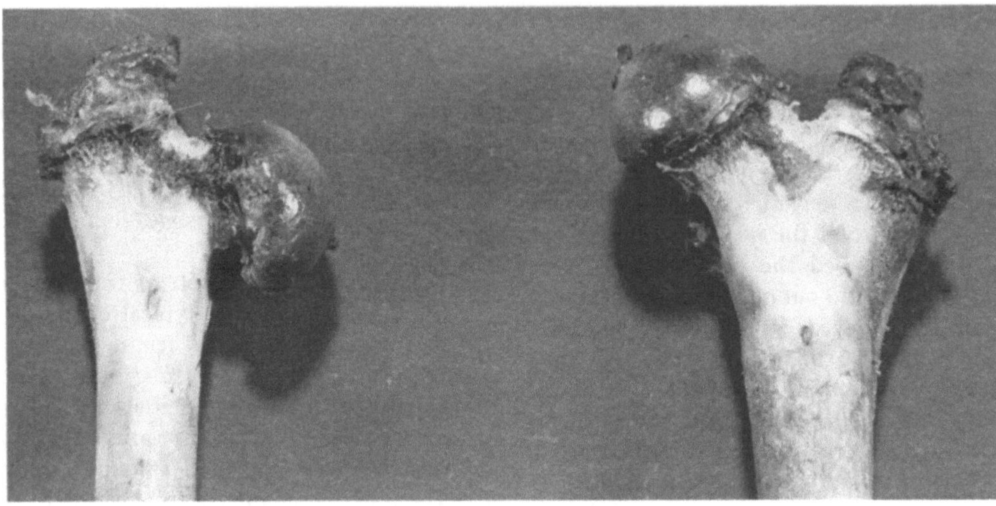

FIG. 10–5 Proximal femora of a 7-month-old dog 6 months after partial excision of the inferior portion of the capital epiphysis. Inclination angle on left 107° and right (control) 130°.

review of 17 cases of isolated congenital coxa vara, Amstutz and Wilson [3] observed that the wider and more vertical the fissure defect, the more severe the varus, and the more marked the shortening of the femoral neck.

More recent evidence indicates that the greater trochanteric epiphysis may be responsible, in part, for longitudinal growth of the femur. Based upon their clinical observations, Morgan and Somerville [64] state that increase in length of the femur is a result of interaction of both the capital and greater trochanteric epiphyses, in addition to their determination of the angle of inclination. In 1967, Weissman [94] reported his result in treating a 3.5-year-old female, who had incurred destruction of her femoral head by a septic process at the age of 2 months. In addition to absence of the femoral head, she had a significant length discrepancy measuring 3 cm. Weissman transplanted the trochanteric epiphysis into the acetabulum via an incomplete transverse osteotomy. On follow-up examination performed 6.5 years later, the trochanteric epiphysis was observed to have the appearance of a round ball which filled the acetabulum, and the functioning trochanteric epiphysis resembled the opposite normal capital epiphysis. The angulation caused by the original osteotomy was not apparent due to active remodeling that had occurred. Of major significance was that the previously observed length discrepancy had resolved, and the femurs were equal in length. Salvati [82] has also successfully utilized the greater trochanter and its epiphysis to replace femoral heads destroyed by sepsis in six children.

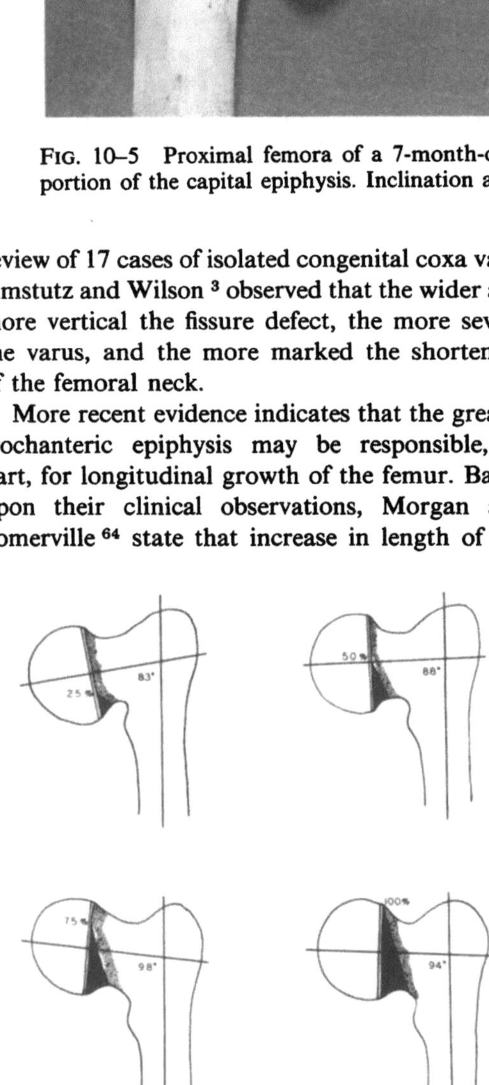

FIG. 10–6 Composite drawing showing the variation of the extent of coxa vara with the size of the triangular fragment.

Working with three groups of rats, Savastano and Bliss,[83] in 1975, provided evidence to support the active influence of the greater trochanteric epiphysis on the length of the femur, as suspected by Morgan and Somerville.[64] In their control group I, unilateral partial subtrochanteric osteotomies of the femur were performed. Group II rats underwent unilateral ablation of the epiphysis of the greater trochanter, and Group III rats underwent unilateral ablation of the capital femoral epiphysis. The animals were sacrificed 10 weeks after surgery, and the operated femurs were compared to their unoperated counterparts. Group I rats did not demonstrate any observable difference in the length or angle of inclination. Group II rats did not demonstrate any observable difference in length; however, the operated specimens did show a valgus tendency of the neck–shaft angle. Group III rats did not demonstrate any observable difference in length; however, the operated specimens did show a varus tendency of the neck–shaft angle. From their study, Savastano and Bliss concluded that the greater trochanteric epiphysis does have a growth potential, and that this growth potential can be utilized when the capital femoral epiphysis is damaged.

Pathological Findings

It is certainly not the lack of interest, but rather the low incidence and difficulty in obtaining appropriate biopsy material that account for the limited number of published histological investigations and descriptions of coxa vara. The first studies were published by Hoffa,[41] in 1905, and by Helbing,[39] in 1906, who described their observations of the intact femoral heads that were removed to facilitate placement of the femoral shaft into the acetabulum. Similar observations were published by Schwarz,[86] Camitz,[14] and Delitala.[20] All of these investigators agreed that coxa vara occurs as a result of a defect in endochondral ossification, based upon observations of a large amount of fibrous tissue, rather than cancellous bone, within the femoral metaphysis, causing inherent weakness of the femoral neck and inability to support loads. Of interest, in light of what is known today, is that even though he had no supportive pathological evidence, Schwarz [86] proposed that the triangular fragment formed as a result of vascular insufficiency of the femoral neck, causing the coxa vara deformity to develop.

In 1960, Pylkkanen [76] provided a significant study of the pathological findings in 25 patients with coxa vara. His study was of 25 surgical biopsies of the vertical fissure defect taken at the time of intertrochanteric osteotomy. He did not, however, have the opportunity to study the growth plates, secondary centers of ossification, or articular cartilage specimens. In most of his specimens, he noted the presence of a uniform cartilaginous plate which corresponded to the transverse zone of rarefaction visible on the roentgenograms. Although the cartilage resembled that of the epiphyseal plate, he observed a markedly disturbed cellular arrangement and a weakened, severely disturbed process of endochondral ossification. He observed atrophic metaphyseal bone, which sometimes contained islets of cartilage, lying immediately adjacent to the cartilage. Furthermore, throughout the areas of both cartilaginous and osseous tissue, he observed invasion by significant amounts of connective tissue. In a comprehensive review, the histopathological changes he observed were classified according to the degree of severity judged clinically and roentgenologically. He observed that in individuals with severe clinical disability and extensive radiographic deterioration, the histological changes were usually marked, whereas in cases where the lesion was clinically and roentgenologically mild, the histological changes were also mild.

As the disease progressed with increasing age, he observed that the histological changes were, in general, more marked in older patients than in younger ones. Based upon his observations, Pylkkanen concluded, as did other investigators before him,[7,13,34,95] that the cause of congenital coxa vara is a disturbance in ossification and growth which originates in the medial part of the proximal femoral epiphyseal plate. The deposition of groups of cartilage cells within the metaphyseal bone of the femoral neck results in a weakness in the neck and a disturbance and delay in ossification. Furthermore, he proposed that when ambulation is begun, the forces which the femoral neck must withstand are increased, and because of the weakness of the neck, the varus deformity gradually develops and progresses. However, Pylkkanen was not able to determine the precise etiology of the coxa vara; namely, the event or factor resulting in defective endochondral ossification.

In 1978, Chung and Riser [17] published their study of the pelvis and proximal femora of a child with coxa vara who died of unrelated causes. At the time of autopsy, they injected the femoral artery of the affected side with barium sulfate, and the femoral artery of the normal side with latex. Appropriate sections of the specimens were prepared and studied. They observed, in the affected right femur, that while there was a normal vascular pattern within the central portion of the ossification center, blood vessels to the metaphyseal side of the growth plate were decreased in number and caliber. Furthermore, in comparison to normal lateral ascending cervical arteries, a decrease in the number and size of the medial ascending cervical arteries and intraosseous blood vessels in the subchondral region was observed.

In their histological preparations, Chung and Riser observed a similar striking defect of endochondral ossification of the affected femur, as observed by previous investigators,[20,39,41,76] but in addition, they observed an endochondral defect of ossification of the "normal" side, although less striking in appearance. Furthermore, they observed abnormal endochondral cartilage formation in the secondary centers of ossification, the growth plates, and the trochanters, as well as in the growth plates of the iliac crests and ischial tuberosities. Their histological studies revealed that the epiphysis had the appearance of a partial split, with separation and formation of the vertical defect, identifiable radiographically as the fissure defect, and isolation of the triangular fragment, having the appearance of a Salter type II fracture fragment. They concluded that coxa vara develops locally in an individual with a generalized growth plate disorder and may be precipitated by, or results in, a deficiency in the vascular supply to the affected part, which may also be precipitated by trauma, as suggested by the fracture appearance of the triangular fragment.

Pathogenesis

In reviewing the various theories that have been proposed pertaining to the etiology of congenital coxa vara, the pathological findings, and the experimental studies, it is apparent that there are several potential causes for the common idiopathic form of coxa vara. There is no doubt that in many cases there is a clear, recognizable cause, such as trauma, infection, generalized growth disturbance, rickets, and so on. However, for the most part the etiology remains obscure. Nevertheless, regardless of the etiology, there may be a common mechanism to account for progression of the deformity.

Rang [77] compares the mechanism of infantile coxa vara to that of slipped upper femoral epiphysis that occurs in adolescents. He concludes that trauma results in rupture of an inherently fragile growth plate, with resultant displacement of the femoral head. New bone is then formed by the epiphysis in its displaced position of varus, forming the triangular fragment which is observable roentgenographically, with concomitant shortening and widening of the femoral neck. Furthermore, since pseudarthrosis formation is a common sequela of adult intracapsular fractures of the femoral neck, Rang concludes that the presence of a persistent pseudarthrosis in infantile coxa vara is an anticipated event.

Although our experimental study showed that coxa vara can result from surgical trauma to the capital femoral epiphysis, with the severity of the varus deformity correlating to the area of epiphyseal trauma, it did not clearly identify the etiology as observed in the young child. It is our opinion, as has been also expressed by other investigators,[37,48,70,76,77] that in cases of isolated coxa vara, either unilateral or bilateral, there is faulty maturation of the cartilage of the femoral neck with irregular ossification. As a consequence of weight bearing through this area of insufficiency, as postulated by Pauwels,[73] the vertical defect forms, isolating the triangular fragment. Continuing weight-bearing forces cause shear forces through the vertical defect, increasing as the defect grows more perpendicular in direction, with resulting progression of the varus deformity. Our review of 75 clinical cases correlated the size of the triangular fragment with the severity of the deformity, revealing that the fragment appears to protect the epiphyseal plate as well as to affect the orientation and direction of the vertical fissure defect. Pseudarthrosis ensues with further progression, with displacement of the femoral head below the level of the greater trochanter, and eventually below the level of the lesser trochanter. Furthermore, this appearance of a flame-shaped trochanter is caused, in part, by unrestricted overgrowth of the greater trochanteric epiphysis. Diaphyseal and acetabular dysplasia occurs in late cases of severe varus deformity, and rapid deterioration of the hip joint occurs.

History and Physical Examination

As stated, coxa vara deformity does not develop until after birth, and usually not until the age of walking. Most patients with coxa vara are first

Age	0–1	2	3	4	5	6	7	8	9	10	11	12	13	14	15	16	17	OVER 20
No. of Patients		3	10	9	5	1	9	5	6	9	5	6	4	10	2	2	2	10

FIG. 10–7 Ages when first seen by orthopedist, excluding cases with congenital shortening.

brought to the attention of an orthopedist when they are noted to have a peculiar, painless, lurching limp when the involvement is unilateral, or a peculiar, painless waddling gait when bilateral deformities are present.[9] This characteristic waddling gait is similar to that seen in an individual with bilateral dislocation of the hips. On initial evaluation, a careful history should be recorded, to determine if the case in point is one of congenital coxa vara, or if the etiology is traumatic, infectious, or metabolic in origin. One should also inquire as to the presence of the disease process in parents, siblings, and near relatives.

For the purpose of this discussion, the author had the opportunity to review 98 case histories of individuals evaluated and treated for congenital coxa vara by orthopedists of the Piedmont Orthopedic Society. Figure 10–7 shows the ages at which these 98 patients were first seen by an orthopedist for complaints of an abnormal limp or gait. The lack of concentration of cases in any one age group does not allow valid conclusions to be made as to time of onset of the disease process. It is disconcerting, however, to realize how late in life and in the disease process these patients were first examined for definitive care. Figure 10–8 depicts the age when these same patients were first observed to have an abnormal gait, this information being obtained by direct questioning of the patient or family members. As the majority of these patients were first noted to have an abnormal gait at the time of initial weight bearing, it can be concluded that the disease process is active at the time of initial weight bearing.

On physical evaluation of these individuals, in addition to careful and complete examination of the lower extremities, the examiner should evaluate the entire patient for the presence of other congenital malformations and systemic disorders. Depending upon the age of the patient, the severity of the disease process, and the extent of involvement by the deformity, one, several, or all of the following physical findings may be observed and recorded:

1. A gluteus medius type of painless limp with unilateral involvement.
2. A peculiar, painless, waddling gait with bilateral involvement.
3. Shortness of stature.
4. Positive Trendelenburg's test.
5. Lumbar lordosis, most marked with bilateral involvement.
6. Leg length discrepancy which is more apparent with unilateral involvement.
7. A widened perineum most marked with bilateral involvement.
8. Prominence of the greater trochanter with narrowing of the distance between the origin and insertion of the hip abductors.
9. Contracture of the hip.
10. Limitation of abduction of the hip joint.
11. Limitation of internal rotation of the hip joint.
12. Limitation of extension of the hip joint.
13. Limitation of external rotation of the hip joint.
14. Limitation of flexion of the hip joint.
15. Limitation of adduction of the hip joint.

Age	Unknown	At weight bearing	3	4	5	6	7	8	9	10	11	12
No. of Patients	11	42	9	10	6	4	1	3	1	6	2	3

FIG. 10–8 Ages when abnormality first noticed, according to histories.

Radiological Examination

In the initial evaluation of individuals presenting with congenital coxa vara, anteroposterior (AP) roentgenograms of both hips should be made with the patient supine. Any apparent leg length discrepancy should be confirmed by scanogram technique. Laminograms of the involved hip(s) may be helpful to further elucidate the deformity. In individuals with a significant leg length discrepancy, the spine should be evaluated for lordosis, as well as scoliosis, with appropriate roentgenograms being made when indicated.

Examination of a roentgenogram of an individual with advanced congenital coxa vara (Fig. 10–12) reveals that in addition to a decrease in the angle of inclination, a triangular piece of bone is present in the femoral neck, inferior and in juxtaposition to the femoral head. This piece of bone is bounded by two radiolucent bands, traversing the neck and forming an inverted *Y*. As shown in Fig. 10–6, larger fragments will have the appearance of an inverted *V*. The inner band is the capital femoral epiphyseal plate, while the lateral line is an abnormal area of increased radiolucency, which is the site of faulty maturation of cartilage within the femoral neck, as well as irregular calcification.

The normal angle of inclination, previously defined as the angle between the neck and the shaft of the femur, is 135°. As shown in Figs. 10–1 to 10–3, unrecognized or untreated coxa vara is a progressive, disabling deformity. Figure 10–9 is a graph illustrating the fact that the varus deformity progresses during growth, as a result of weight-bearing forces being exerted on the weakened area of the femoral neck. This graph was drawn after measuring the angle of inclination on the initial roentgenograms of the 98 patients previously cited, and is a plot of that information vs. the age of the patients at the time of initial evaluation by an orthopedist. The gradual progression of coxa vara as age advances is clearly demonstrated. On the other hand, some of the patients in this study did not conform to this progressive pattern, the discrepancy possibly being explained by individual variation of the disease process.

As the varus deformity progresses with growth, as a result of weight-bearing forces, sequential roentgenograms will demonstrate the progression and deterioration of the hip joint. The significant radiographic findings observed, in the approximate order of their appearance, are as follows:

1. Varus deformity of the neck.
2. Progression of the epiphyseal plate toward a vertical position.
3. Appearance of the transverse zone of rarefaction, or fissure of the neck.

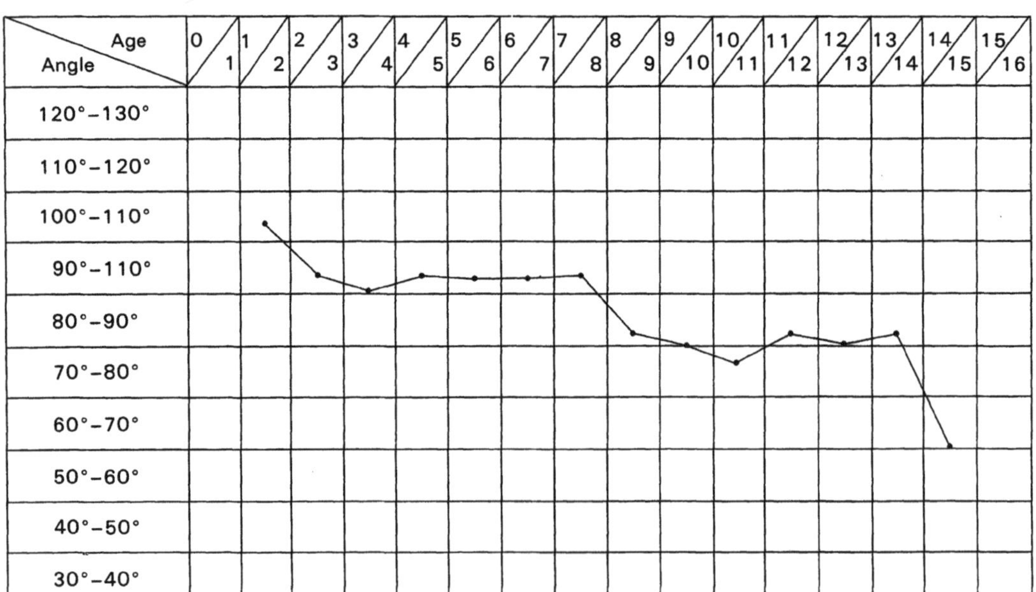

FIG. 10–9 Mean angle measurements of all hips at time first seen, to show progression of varus deformity with age.

4. Formation of a triangular fragment within the femoral neck, the so-called *Y* or *V* fragment.
5. Progression of the varus deformity.
6. Enlargement of the greater trochanter.
7. Narrowing of the femoral shaft.
8. Shortening of the femoral shaft.
9. Deformity of the femoral shaft.
10. Deformity of the acetabulum.
11. Spontaneous healing of the femoral neck fissure and triangular fragment (occasionally).
12. Complete deterioration of the proximal end of the femur (occasionally).

These findings will be separately discussed and illustrated in order to demonstrate the natural progression of congenital coxa vara without surgical intervention. The severity of the disease process, as estimated radiographically, may vary in the same patient in cases of bilateral involvement, and may or may not correlate to the age of the patient, clearly demonstrating the individuality of this problem.

Figure 10–10, a roentgenogram of the pelvis and hips of a 3-year-old child, clearly demonstrates the initial radiographic finding of varus deformity of the head and neck as the earliest manifestation of the disease process. In addition, progression of the epiphyseal plate from its normal horizontal position to a more vertical position is observed. Although varus deformity of the neck is the initial radiographic finding, there may well be a stage of this disease, designated as the prevarus state, that occurs prior to the development of the varus deformity. Because of the cartilaginous nature of the neck, roentgenographic evidence is lacking to support this supposition.

The next state commonly observed radiographically in the natural progression of congenital coxa vara is the appearance of the transverse zone of rarefaction or fissure defect in the neck of the femur, juxtaposed to the femoral capital epiphysis (Fig. 10–11). The size, location, and direction of this defect will vary with the severity of the disease process. In many cases the defect may be seen to be very narrow, whereas in other cases it will appear to be broad with calcified flecks scattered throughout. The position of the defect in the neck, and its obliquity as it traverses the neck, generally do not conform to any regular, predictable pattern. In some cases, the defect may lie immediately adjacent to the capital femoral epiphysis for its entire length, while in other cases it is seen to traverse the neck obliquely, lying adjacent to the epiphysis in the upper or lateral portion of the neck and then cutting obliquely across the neck away from, or distal to, the epiphyseal plate. However, it is significant that in every case, a portion of the defect lies immediately adjacent to the epiphysis. Therefore, by induction or biomechanical interference, the defect significantly alters epiphyseal growth potential, resulting in progression of the varus deformity and further deterioration of the proximal femur.

With the appearance of the fissure defect in the neck of the femur, the triangular fragment, referred to as the inverted *Y* or *V* fragment, is seen to appear as the neck calcifies. As illustrated in Fig. 10–12, the inner side of this fragment is the epiphyseal plate, while the outer border is the

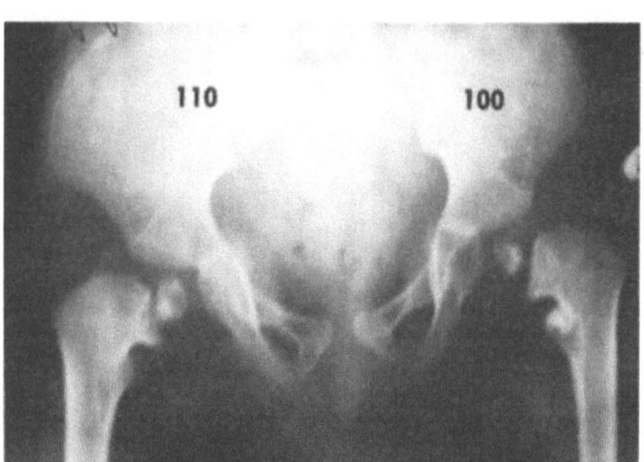

FIG. 10–10 Varus deformity (bilateral) in a child aged 3 years, with progression of the epiphyseal plate toward a vertical position.

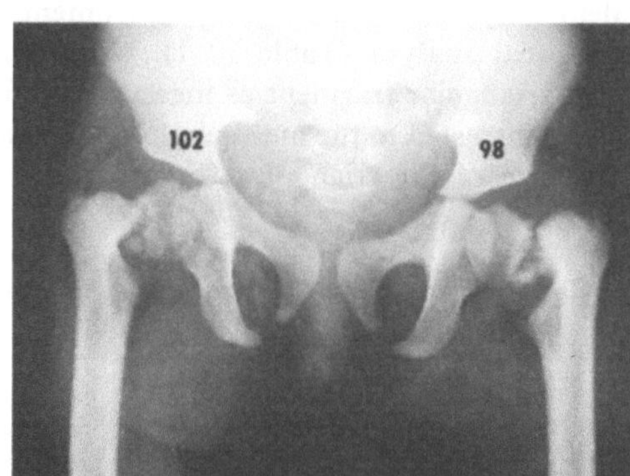

FIG. 10–11 Transverse zone of rarefaction or fissure of the neck appearing after varus deformity and progression of the epiphyseal plate toward a vertical position.

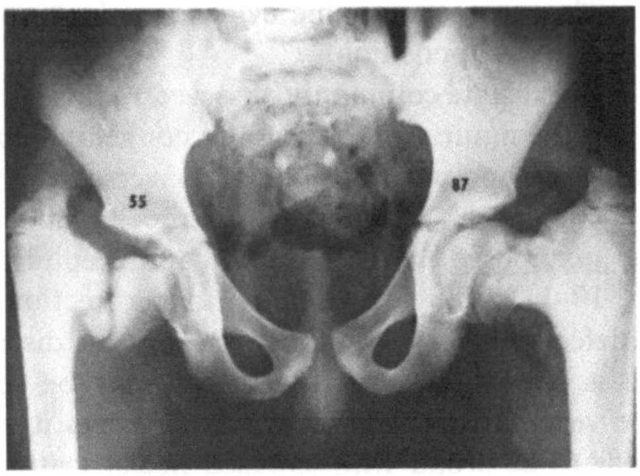

FIG. 10–12 Formation of a triangular or *Y* fragment.

fissure or rarefied zone. The size of the triangular fragment varies considerably from case to case, as well as in the same individual with bilateral involvement. Figure 10–12 shows a small triangular fragment on the right side with the major portion of the defect lying immediately adjacent to the epiphyseal plate, while on the left side there is a large triangular fragment with the major portion of the defect lying remote from the epiphyseal plate. It is important to note that, even with the large fragment, the defect has some direct contact with the superior portion of the growth plate. Figure 10–6 shows the inverse relationship between the size of the triangular fragment and the angle of inclination of affected femurs in 75 individuals. The triangular fragment appears then to provide a protective barrier, by virtue of its position between the epiphysis and the fissure defect. Therefore, in those femurs with small triangular fragments, the major portion of the fissure defect lies adjacent to the epiphysis, resulting in a greater varus deformity. This fact is further documented by a statistical analysis (Table 10–1), where the size of the triangular fragment as measured in 68 patients is contrasted to the mean angle of inclination. The size of the triangular fragment is expressed as a percentage representing the ratio of the measured length of the border of the triangular fragment juxtaposed to the epiphyseal plate, and the total diameter of the plate measured as the length of the superior-inferior axis on an AP roentgenogram.

TABLE 10–1 Comparison of size of triangular fragment with mean angle measurement (68 hips)

Size of Triangular Fragment	Number of Hips	Average Angle
0–25%	32	83°
25–50%	13	88°
50–75%	14	98°
75–100%	9	94°

Magnusson,[62] Pauwels,[73] and other investigators [87,88,91] have proposed that the fissure defect of the femoral neck and the triangular fragment represent an insufficiency fracture of the neck due to abnormal shearing forces resulting from weight bearing in the varus position. Furthermore, they implicated these shearing forces as the primary etiological factor causing progression of the deformity. Although mechanical shearing force created by weight bearing and acting through the defect may account for the coxa vara deformity, our observations of the size and position of the triangular fragment suggest that retardation of the normal growth pattern and potential of the capital femoral epiphysis may be due to the proximity or apposition of the fissure defect to the epiphysis. The more intimately the defect lies to the epiphyseal plate, the more it appears to interfere with the orderly growth one would normally anticipate. A large triangular fragment appears to protect the epiphysis, thus allowing it to exert its growth potential more normally. Therefore, while the "shearing" theories have merit, and undoubtedly may account for some of the varus progression observed, it is likewise apparent that a more significant cause of the varus deformity is the failure of normal growth activity of the capital epiphysis.

As observed in Fig. 10–13, with progression of the coxa vara deformity, enlargement of the greater trochanter will occur. Studies have indi-

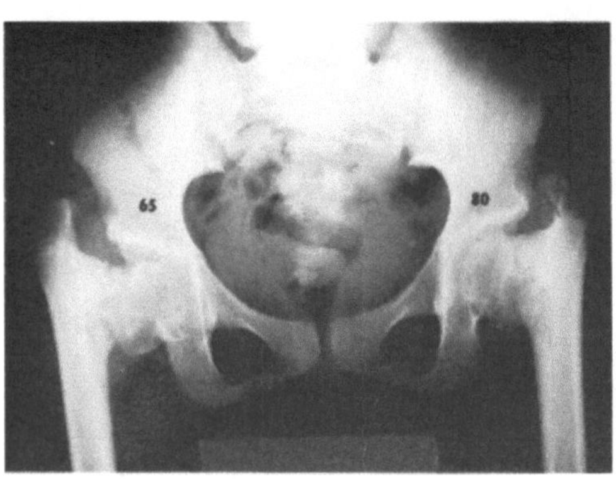

FIG. 10–13 Disproportionately larger size of greater trochanter as related to the rest of the proximal femur.

TABLE 10–2 Comparison of size of greater trochanter with size of triangular fragment (68 hips)

	Size of Triangular Fragment			
	0–25%	25–50%	50–75%	75–100%
Enlarged greater trochanter	25	3	6	2
Normal greater trochanter	11	8	12	1

cated that initially this is a relative enlargement, due primarily to the varus position of the head and neck. As the condition continues to progress, the relative enlargement becomes more apparent as a fixed deformity. Comparing the size of the triangular fragment to the greater trochanter, Table 10–2 reveals that the smaller the triangular fragment (more extensive involvement of the capital epiphysis by the fissure defect), the greater the tendency for overgrowth and enlargement of the greater trochanter. There appears to be an intriguing balance between these two growth centers under normal circumstances. This balance is disturbed in coxa vara, and the restraining influence on the greater trochanteric epiphysis as exercised by the capital femoral epiphysis is partially lost. When this balance is upset, the proximal femoral configuration is altered and overgrowth of the greater trochanter occurs.

With enlargement of the greater trochanter and continuing progression of the deformity, narrowing of the femoral shaft, shortening of the neck, deformity of the femoral head, and deformity of the acetabulum will be observed (Fig. 10–14). The extent of shortening of the femoral neck will vary with the extent of the fissure defect and the length of time it is present. In other words, the larger and wider the defect, and the longer it remains before closure, the more the femoral neck will shorten. At the same time, the head of the femur, being depressed into the inferior reaches of the acetabulum by the varus position, will show initially some degree of osteoporosis, and ultimately the femoral head becomes deformed. The acetabulum, lacking the growth stimulation of a normally placed and normally formed femoral head, will then become secondarily deformed.

The final phase or stage of congenital coxa vara without surgical intervention may be radiographi-

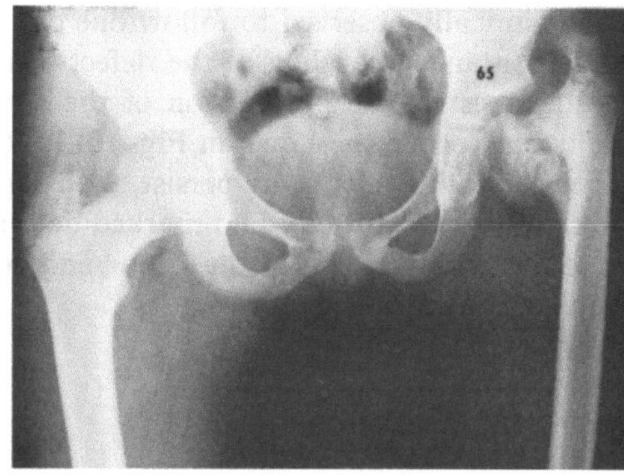

FIG. 10–14 Narrowing of the shaft, shortening of the neck of the femur, deformity of the head, and deformity of the acetabulum.

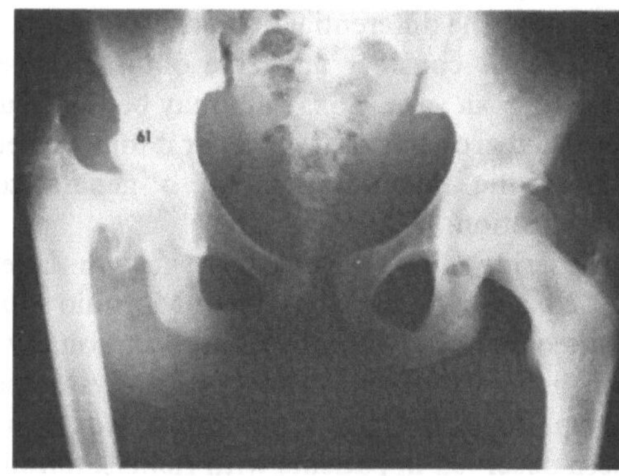

FIG. 10–15 Spontaneous healing of the defect with arrest of the varus progression.

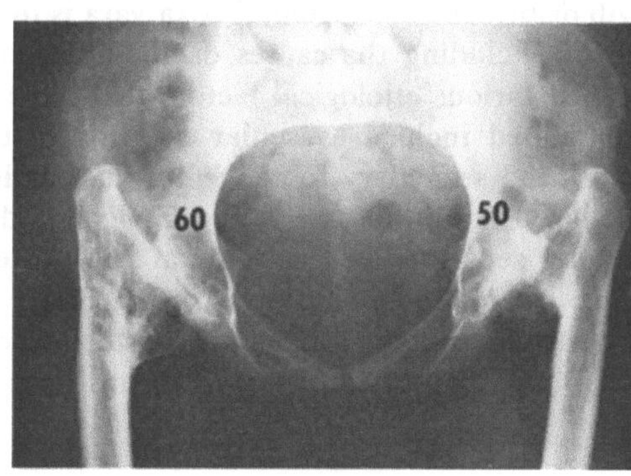

FIG. 10–16 Persistence of the defect, progression of the deformity, and deterioration of the proximal end of the femur.

cally and clinically observed to follow one of two courses. Spontaneous healing of the defect in the neck with arrest of the progression of the varus deformity may occur, as shown in Fig. 10–15. On the other hand, the defect may persist, with rapid progression of the deformity and marked deterioration of the proximal end of the femur and acetabulum, as shown in Fig. 10–16.

Differential Diagnosis

Congenital coxa vara as discussed in this chapter is a distinct clinical entity, initially appearing as a varus deformity of the proximal femur at the time of early weight bearing. At the time of initial evaluation, in the differential diagnosis of the problem, one must consider and rule out the causes of acquired coxa vara. Coxa vara may be the result of a localized growth disturbance, or it may present as one of the manifestations of a generalized growth affection.

Considering first generalized growth affections,[85] coxa vara is usually seen in Morquio's disease (osteochondrodystrophy), and occasionally is seen in achondroplasia, cleidocranial dysostosis, and dysplasia epiphysealis multiplex. Coxa vara has been observed in patients with rickets, familial osteopetrosis,[50] primary hypoparathyroidism,[36] and hypothyroidism.

Unilateral coxa vara in an individual in which all other joints are normal represents a localized growth disturbance. Congenital coxa vara is diagnosed by excluding the causes of acquired coxa vara. The various etiological factors that have to be considered include avascular necrosis of the femoral head secondary to congenital dislocation of the hip, Perthes' disease,[16] and Gaucher's disease; joint sepsis as well as femoral neck osteomyelitis; traumatic epiphysiolysis, particularly in the battered child; osteoporosis–osteomalacia (rickets); and fibrocystic disease (fibrous dysplasia).

Treatment

As previously shown, untreated congenital coxa vara will follow one of two courses. Either there will be spontaneous healing of the defect with arrest of the progression of the varus deformity,[45,76] or the defect will persist, the deformity will progress, and there will be rapid, disabling deterioration of the hip joint. However, one should not be lulled into a state of complacency in regard to this problem, as the reported cases of spontaneous resolution are rare, and a watch-and-wait attitude will usually end in a disastrous result.

Historically, futile attempts have been made to treat congenital coxa vara nonsurgically. Fiorani,[30] thinking that the coxa vara resulted from systemic rickets, recommended antirachitic therapy, in addition to relief from weight bearing with crutches or a supporting bandage. Throughout the early part of the twentieth century, nonoperative treatment was recommended by many, based on their theories of femoral neck insufficiency. Elmslie [25] recommended immobilization in a position of abduction and internal rotation, followed by the use of a Thomas splint for at least 6 weeks. Nilsonne [69] and Le Mesurier,[59] recommended the use of traction for this condition. However, as reported by Bade [6] and Zadek,[95] these methods of nonoperative treatment were, for the most part, completely valueless in the treatment of coxa vara.

There are two fundamental postulates which must be fulfilled in order to achieve successful treatment of coxa vara: (1) adequate correction of the varus deformity, and (2) closure of the defect in the neck of the femur. Correction of the varus deformity changes the stress on the vertical fissure defect in the femoral neck from shear to compression, minimizes shortening of the femur length which has occurred, and tends to reestablish the proper tension–length relationship of the abductor muscles. Closure of the defect in the neck of the femur will prevent recurrence of the deformity.

Oliver Wendell Holmes once stated that "the life of the law has not been logic, it has been experience." Experience has shown that there are no effective nonoperative methods which will correct the varus deformity and promote closure of the defect. The only effective method, to date, which corrects the varus deformity and promotes closure of the defect, is surgery, by means of a subtrochanteric or intertrochanteric osteotomy of the femur. In 1888, Keetley [49] was the first person to attempt operative correction of a coxa vara deformity, utilizing a subtrochanteric cuneiform osteotomy to achieve considerable improvement in his patient. In 1896, Kraske [52] was the first person to perform a cuneiform osteotomy of the neck of the femur for correction of this deformity; however, the results were not satisfactory, and this method was soon abandoned. Femoral neck osteotomies, by and large, are technically difficult to perform, require internal fixation to maintain position of correction of the fragments, and are associated with a high failure rate because of nonunion and avascular necrosis of the femoral head. Zimmermann,[96] Langenskiold,[56] Magnussen,[62] Pylkkanen,[76] and other investigators have reported the difficulty in obtaining, and maintaining, an acceptable valgus correction by high femoral osteotomy.

During the twentieth century, it has become apparent and widely accepted that corrective subtrochanteric or intertrochanteric osteotomy, with or without the use of temporary or permanent internal fixation, is the treatment of choice for congenital coxa vara.* In addition, many investigators [38,43,51,59,95] advocate the use of drilling or bone graft to promote premature closure of the epiphyseal plate. In reviewing the many types of intertrochanteric and subtrochanteric osteotomies that have been described for correction of coxa vara, and the various internal fixation implants that have been designed or modified for this purpose, it becomes apparent that no one method has been totally satisfactory in every case.

The dilemma that confronts the orthopedic surgeon in the treatment of congenital coxa vara is not necessarily what to do, but rather how and when to do it. Factors that must be considered in making a treatment decision include the age of the patient, the severity of the deformity, degree of disability and impairment of function, and whether the varus deformity is progressive or static. Moreover, the relationship of these factors to each other is extremely important. Based upon these factors, and regular, interval evaluations of the patient, general guidelines for the treatment of coxa vara have been recommended [2,89] for patients with mild deformities, based upon the angle of inclination, the width and direction of the vertical fissure, and the absence of documented progression. These investigators [2,89] recommend a conservative, nonoperative approach for mild deformities in which the angle of inclination is greater than 90 to 100°, the vertical fissure defect is narrow and forms an angle of 60° or less with the horizon, and no progression of varus is noted. They advocate the use of a shoe lift to correct significant leg length discrepancy, passive exercises to correct any hip contractures, and frequent evaluations to watch for any progression of the deformity. Although Zimmermann [96] reported that the progression of the varus deformity can be controlled by conservative means, this has certainly not been our experience, nor the experience of others.[2,3,89] As described by Tachdjian,[89] the use of a quadrilateral ischial socket orthosis may be helpful, not to prevent progression of the deformity, but rather to protect the femoral neck from weight-bearing forces when corrective osteotomy has to be delayed for one reason or another. Barr [7] and Noble and Hauser [70] have recommended that surgery be postponed until puberty because of the tendency of the deformity to recur after osteotomy. However, in delaying treatment, the deformity may become so severe that correction will be impossible to achieve, and secondary dysplastic changes in the hip or pseudarthrosis of the neck will develop, for which there is no effective treatment.

As previously stated, successful treatment of congenital coxa vara demands adequate correction of the deformity and closure of the defect in the femoral neck. As opposed to a watch-and-wait attitude in mild deformities as determined by the angle of inclination, the width and orientation of the vertical fissure defect, and the age of the patient, as has been expressed by other investigators, it is our opinion that in all cases of congenital coxa vara in which there is radiographic evidence of a vertical fissure defect in the femoral neck, regardless of width or orientation, an abduction subtrochanteric osteotomy should be performed as early as possible, in order to achieve a good functional result and to prevent progression of the deformity. It is the presence of this defect, and not the angle of inclination, that is the indication for surgery, for it has been our experience that if there is a defect, one can anticipate progression. If for some reason surgical osteotomy must be delayed, then we agree with Tachdjian [89] in providing relief to the femoral neck from weight-bearing forces by the use of a quadrilateral ischial socket orthosis.

It has been our experience, and it is therefore our opinion, that satisfactory correction of a congenital coxa vara deformity with closure of the vertical fissure defect can be accomplished by a subtrochanteric abduction osteotomy of the affected femur, with stabilization of the fragments by the use of Steinmann pins incorporated in the postoperative hip spica cast. The following operative technique is advocated.

* See Refs. 1–3,5,11,12,15,18,24,29,31,35,38,43,55,57,60–62, 73,75,76,80,81,89,93

Depending on the size of the patient, the patient should be in a supine position on a regular operative table, or a fracture table may be used for larger patients. The trochanteric region and the proximal shaft of the femur are surgically accessible through a routine midlateral longitudinal incision. Although the vastus lateralis can be detached from the linea aspera and reflected anteriorly, a midline division is easier, and if limited to the proximal portion does not result in significant neurovascular muscular necrosis. Using roentgenographic control, the level of the osteotomy is accurately determined, and should be perpendicular to the longitudinal axis of the femur just below the lesser trochanter. The osteotomy may be completed by using power instruments, or manually by osteotome and mallet, care being exercised in minimizing the amount of periosteal stripping and in protection of the more medial structures. Using appropriate roentgenographic control, heavy Steinmann pins are inserted into the proximal and distal fragments after the osteotomy is completed. The Steinmann pin in the proximal fragment should be advanced up to, but not into or through, the capital femoral epiphysis, to avoid damage to and premature closure of the plate. The Steinmann pin in the distal fragment should secure both the lateral and medial cortices of the femur. By careful and slow manipulation of the Steinmann pins, and by abducting the leg if a fracture table is used, a valgus position should be obtained at the osteotomy site. Overcorrection of the deformity is recommended, to allow for some recurrence of the deformity postoperatively that occurs with remodeling and healing. The amount of overcorrection may vary from case to case, depending on the severity of the deformity and the age of the patient, but the general recommendation is 15–20°. If femoral abduction causes the distal fragment to displace medially with rotation of the proximal fragment into varus, or if overriding of the fragments occurs, an adductor tenotomy should be done by open or subcutaneous technique.

In a review of 28 corrective osteotomies performed for coxa vara, Weighill [93] observed that inadequate correction occurred only in those children in whom an adductor tenotomy had been omitted, and demonstrated in his review how tightness of the adductor muscles causes mechanical malposition of the fragments following intertrochanteric and subtrochanteric osteotomy. The incision(s) may be closed in a routine fashion after hemostasis is obtained, with appropriate suction drainage to prevent hematoma formation subcutaneously. Using roentgenographic control, the desired position of correction is verified, manually abducting the leg and manipulating the protruding ends of the Steinmann pins if necessary. While this position is maintained, a hip spica cast is applied from the nipple line to the toes on the affected side and to just above the knee on the contralateral side, with secure incorporation of the Steinmann pins. If within the first 7 to 10 days postoperatively, loss of the position of correction occurs, or if a more valgus position is desired, the cast may be wedged accordingly.

The patient should be immobilized in the cast until there is roentgenographic evidence that the osteotomy has firmly united, at which time the cast should be removed. The Steinmann pins may be removed at the same time; however, drainage or pain may necessitate prior removal. As a rule, prophylactic antibiotics are not recommended to prevent pin tract infection, for if infection develops, more than likely it will be a very resistant strain. On the other hand, if a pin tract infection does develop, then one must culture the organism, prescribe appropriate antibiotics, and if drainage persists, remove the offending pin.

Generally, bony union of the osteotomy is obtained within 8 to 12 weeks. After the cast and pins are removed, mobilization of the hip joint is gradually achieved by a program of graduated exercises. When adequate mobility of the hip joint has been achieved, the patient may begin to ambulate with crutches; partial weight bearing of the affected side is allowed until there is roentgenographic evidence of complete healing of the fissure defect of the femoral neck, at which time full unrestricted activity may be resumed.

The operative technique for the correction of congenital coxa vara which we advocate is illustrated in Figs. 10–17 to 10–19. Figure 10–17 shows the pelvis and hips of a young child with bilateral involvement, the angles of inclination being 85°. Figure 10–18 is a roentgenogram made several days after bilateral subtrochanteric osteotomies were performed, and shows that the angles of correction achieved were 150° and 170°. Figure 10–19 is a roentgenogram of the same individual made several years later, demonstrating some loss of correction with remodeling; however, the final result of 140° and 135° was quite acceptable, and the

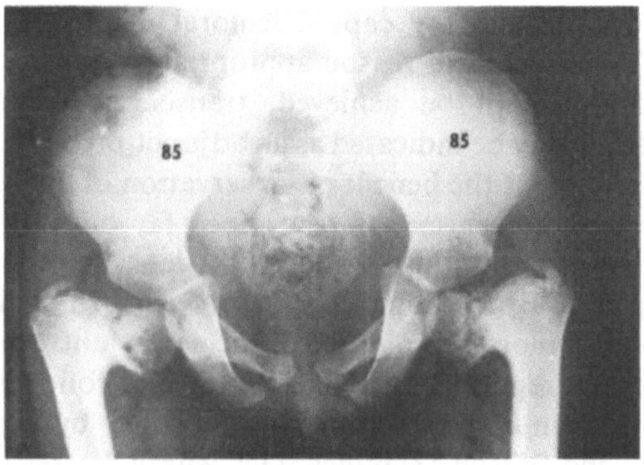

FIG. 10–17 Subtrochanteric osteotomy, preoperative evaluation.

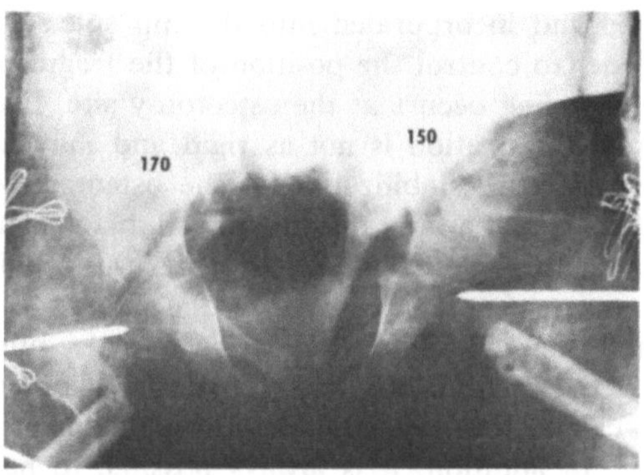

FIG. 10–18 Subtrochanteric osteotomy, postoperative correction.

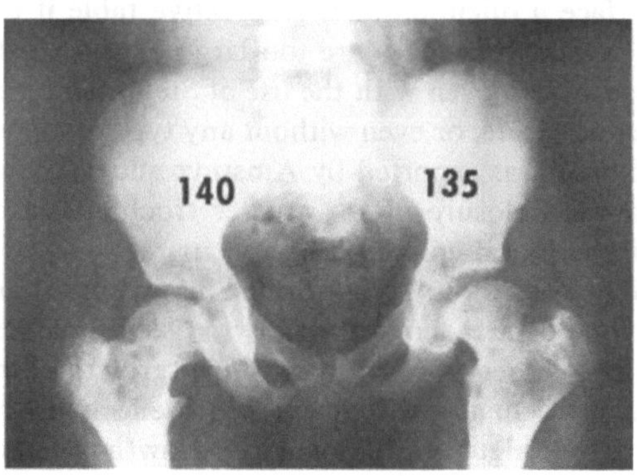

FIG. 10–19 Subtrochanteric osteotomy, follow-up evaluation.

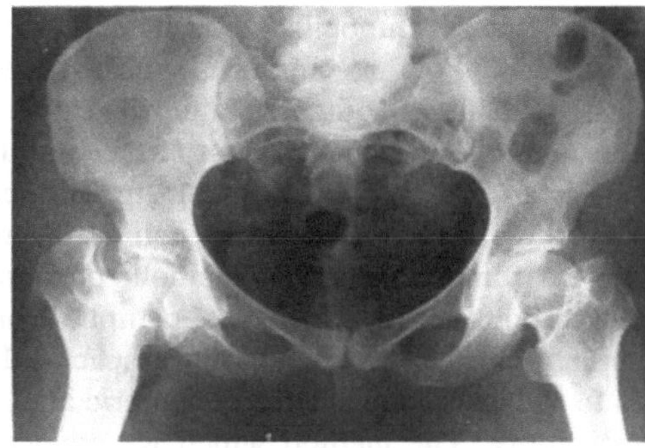

FIG. 10–20 39-year follow-up of a case of bilateral congenital coxa vara after bilateral abduction osteotomies at age 9 years.

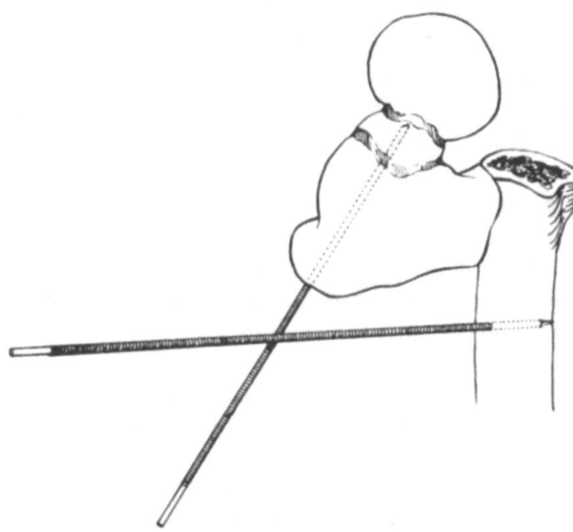

FIG. 10–21 Technique of subtrochanteric osteotomy, valgus position of proximal fragment, and proper placement of Steinmann pins to avoid injury to the capital femoral epiphysis.

individual had a normal, painless gait with unrestricted full range of motion of both hip joints. Figure 10–20 is a 39-year follow-up for an individual who had bilateral congenital coxa vara deformities corrected at the age of 9 by bilateral subtrochanteric abduction osteotomies. There is a satisfactory correction bilaterally, and surprisingly, little arthritis of the hip joints is observed. Figure 10–21 is an artistic rendering showing proper pin placement to avoid injury to the capital femoral epiphysis.

As discussed by Amstutz and Wilson,[3] in their clinical review and in their review of the many surgical techniques proposed for the correction of coxa vara, of the many exacting principles of surgery, four are of paramount importance. These are (1) control of the proximal fragment; (2) adduction of the proximal fragment or abduction of the distal fragment, or both; (3) provision for stability of the fragments in the corrected position;

and (4) adequate immobilization. The surgical technique which we recommend satisfies these requisites, and these requisites should be satisfied if the reader chooses to use another technique.

Aside from the complications of any surgical procedure involving the hip joint such as wound infections, thrombophlebitis and embolic phenomena, muscle contractures, and so on, complications have been reported which are more specifically related to the technique of subtrochanteric abduction osteotomy. The method which we advocate is no exception. During the initial postoperative period, persistent or recurrent varus may be observed, as a result of failure to obtain satisfactory correction at the time of surgery, settling of the fragments, or active muscle displacement. With incorporation of the Steinmann pins in the hip spica cast as advocated, wedging of the cast may correct this problem. Of greater concern is the fact that following removal of the cast, mobilization of the hip joint, and initiation of weight bearing, recurrence of the deformity is observed. This complication will occur if full weight bearing is allowed prior to the anticipated closure of the fissure defect, and when the defect fails to close at all, allowing then for continuation of the disease process.

It is obvious that the younger patient at the time of surgery requires a more radical degree of correction, than does the older patient. Le Mesurier [59] proved that bone grafting per se, as the surgical treatment, does not affect the degree of the deformity or arrest progression. However, as an adjunct to osteotomy, in selected cases, to prevent recurrence of the deformity, bone grafting may be indicated. It has been our experience that at the time of surgery, adduction of the proximal fragment with abduction of the distal fragment rotates the linear vertical fissure defect of the femoral neck into a horizontal position, thereby decreasing the shearing stress through this area of insufficiency. With protected weight bearing as advocated, the defect is seen to spontaneously close within 1 year. At the time of surgery, determination of the epiphyseal angle should be made to confirm the adequacy of correction, as it has been shown by Haraldsson [37] and others that if the epiphyseal angle is greater than 30°, coxa vara tends to recur, and the tendency increases as the epiphyseal angle increases. This measurement is made of the angle of intersection of two lines, one drawn horizontally through the *Y*-cartilage, and one drawn through the capital femoral epiphysis. If for some technical reason appropriate valgus correction cannot be achieved, transcervical bone grafting may be indicated as an adjunct procedure, realizing that the benefit of preservation of correction and prevention of recurrence far outweighs the risk for the development of a leg length discrepancy. Even though premature closure of the capital femoral epiphysis can occur in untreated cases, as reported by Pylkkanen,[76] and following subtrochanteric osteotomy, as reported by Amstutz and Wilson,[3] significant leg length discrepancies were not observed.

In the operative technique which we advocate, percutaneous Steinmann pins are judiciously placed and incorporated into the hip spica cast in order to control the position of the fragments while healing occurs at the osteotomy site. Even though the fixation is not as rigid and may not provide secure stabilization of the osteotomized fragments that an intramedullary rod, blade plate, or spline provides, this technique has the definite advantage of not requiring a second operation to remove the internal fixation device, and also minimizes the risk of injury to the greater trochanteric and capital femoral epiphyses through operative error. In addition, it is always possible to have available Steinmann pins of necessary length and diameter, whereas the assortment of sizes of internal fixation devices is limited, and the surgeon may face a dilemma at the operative table if the only available devices are too large or too small. Nevertheless, even with the use of Steinmann pins as we advocate, or even without any type of metallic fixation, as reported by Amstutz and Wilson,[3] premature closure of the greater trochanteric or capital femoral epiphysis can occur.

When osteotomy is performed in a young child, or if the capital femoral epiphysis is traumatized and closes prematurely, marked overgrowth of the greater trochanter will occur, which effectively reduces the valgus angle. Some overgrowth is beneficial, if the vertical defect and epiphysis have ossified, as this overgrowth tends to restore abductor muscle leverage. Excessive overgrowth, on the other hand, is detrimental, affecting the mobility and stability of the hip joint. Therefore, if the overgrowth becomes excessive, an epiphysiodesis should be performed without further procrastination.

A more frequently seen complication of the transtrochanteric osteotomy procedure is the development of a coxa valga deformity postoperatively. This complication occurs when the greater trochanteric epiphysis is traumatized and closes prematurely. The gradual change to valgus is due to continued growth potential of the capital femoral epiphysis after healing of the cervical defect, without the normal restraining influence of the greater trochanteric epiphysis. The development of a coxa valga deformity after traumatization of the greater trochanteric epiphysis might erroneously lead one to believe that isolated greater trochanter epiphysiodesis without osteotomy will cause valgus correction to occur. Langenskiold and Salenius [56] reported the results of greater trochanter epiphysiodesis in 30 children, and concluded that the results were unreliable because of unpredictable growth potential of the femoral capital epiphysis, as well as varying age of the individual and degree of varus deformity. In other words, the value of this type of isolated procedure is dependent upon an active capital femoral epiphysis, capable of exerting its growth potential through an intact femoral neck. Growth potential of the capital femoral epiphysis is restricted as long as the vertical defect remains open, and therefore there is no logical reason to believe that greater trochanter epiphysiodesis, without abduction osteotomy and closure of the vertical fissure defect, will be effective.

Observing the natural course of the disease process following surgery, a properly performed osteotomy as advocated brings about two major changes: (1) correction of the varus deformity to a valgus position, and (2) healing of the vertical fissure in the femoral neck with preservation of the angular correction achieved. A number of cases may show some loss of correction in the months and years after surgery due to remodeling that occurs with healing, or due to continuation of the disease process until the vertical fissure defect heals. The interval required for the defect to heal cannot be accurately predicted, but it may heal in as little as 4 months. Almost all of the defects should be healed by 1 year after surgery.

In the clinical evaluation of the patient after satisfactory subtrochanteric osteotomy, one generally sees an improvement in active and passive range of motion of the affected hip, and a conversion from a positive to a negative Trendelenburg's test. The previously noted discrepancy in leg length may become less apparent, especially with unilateral involvement. On the other hand, if the deformity recurs due to persistence of the fissure defect, a repeat osteotomy is recommended. In the rare individual in whom the fissure defect persists and for all practical purposes develops into a true pseudarthrosis, bone-grafting procedures, with or without the use of internal compression–fixation devices, may be tried. However, to date, these salvage methods have for the most part been unsuccessful. It must be emphasized again that improvement in the clinical picture requires a properly performed subtrochanteric abduction osteotomy, and the fissure defect of the neck must be closed before unrestricted activity is allowed.

It is not within the scope of this chapter to discuss the development of disabling hip joint problems that may be the eventual sequelae of congenital coxa vara in the adult. As described, hip dysplasia occurs with severe coxa vara. Other chapters in this text will provide additional information pertaining to these problems, specifically in regard to diagnosis and treatment.

Bibliography

1. Almond, H. G.: Familial infantile coxa vara. J. Bone Joint Surg., 38B:539, 1956.
2. Amstutz, H. C., and Freiberger, R. H.: Coxa vara in children. Clin. Orthop., 22:73, 1962.
3. Amstutz, H. C., and Wilson, P. D., Jr.: Dysgenesis of the proximal femur (coxa vara) and its surgical management. J. Bone Joint Surg., 44A:1, 1962.
4. Armstrong, J. R.: Case of infantile coxa vara, with notes on etiology. Lancet, 1:1498, 1935.
5. Babb, F. S., Ghormley, R. K., and Chatterton, C. C.: Congenital coxa vara. J. Bone Joint Surg., 31A:115, 1949.
6. Bade, A.: Zur abgrenzung der verschiedenen formen von coxa vara. Z. Orthop. Chir., 59:53, 1933.
7. Barr, J. S.: Congenital coxa vara. Arch Surg., 18:1909, 1929.
8. Barrington-Ward, L. E.: Double coxa vara with other deformities occurring in brother and sister. Lancet, 1:157, 1912.
9. Becton, J. L., and Diamond, L. S.: Persistent limp in congenital coxa vara. South. Med. J., 60:921, 1967.
10. Blockey, N. J.: Observations on infantile coxa vara. J. Bone Joint Surg., 51B:106, 1969.
11. Blount, W. P.: Blade-plate internal fixation for high femoral osteotomies. J. Bone Joint Surg., 25:319, 1943.
12. Borden, J., Spencer, G., Jr., and Herndon, C. H.: Treatment of coxa vara in children by means of

a modified osteotomy. J. Bone Joint Surg., 48A:1106, 1966.
13. Burckhardt, E.: Zur histologic der coxa vara infantum. Helv. Chir. Acta, 13:123, 1946.
14. Camitz, H.: Etude comparee sur la coxa vara dite congenitale et osteochondrite coxale juvenile (coxa plana). Acta Chir. Scand., 73:521, 1934.
15. Carter, H. R., and Vitale, C. C.: Developmental coxa vara. Canad. J. Surg., 3:324, 1960.
16. Chen, S. C.: Infantile coxa vara with superimposed Perthes-like change. Proc. R. Soc. Med., 61:667, 1968.
17. Chung, S., and Riser, W.: The histological characteristics of congenital coxa vara. Clin. Orthop., 132:71, 1978.
18. Cleveland, M., Bosworth, D. M., and Pietra, A. D.: Subtrochanteric osteotomy and spine fixation for certain disabilities of the hip joint. J. Bone Joint Surg., 33A:351, 1951.
19. Compere, E. L., Garrison, M., and Fahey, J. J.: Deformities of the femur resulting from arrestment of growth of the capital and greater trochanteric epiphyses. J. Bone Joint Surg., 22:909, 1940.
20. Delitala, F.: Sulla coxa vara congenita. Contributo anatomo-patologico. Arch. Orthop., 30:382, 1913.
21. Drehmann, G.: Die coxa vara. Ergebn. Chir. Orthop., 2:452, 1911.
22. Drehmann, G.: Zur frage der angeborenen coxa vara. Klin. Wschr., 47:1752, 1910.
23. Duncan, G. A.: Congenital and developmental coxa vara. Surgery, 3:741, 1938.
24. Duncan, G. A.: Congenital coxa vara occurring in identical twins. Amer. J. Surg., 37:112, 1937.
25. Elmslie, R. C.: Injury and deformity of the epiphysis of the head of the femur: coxa vara. Lancet, 1:410, 1907.
26. Erlacher, P.: Die dysplasie als krankheitsursache. Z. Orthop., 79:269, 1950.
27. Fairbank, H. A. T.: Coxa vara due to congenital defect of the neck of the femur. J. Anat., 62:232, 1928.
28. Fairbank, H. A. T.: Infantile or cervical coxa vara. In: The Robert Jones Birthday Volume, A Collection of Surgical Essays. London, Oxford University Press, 1928.
29. Ferguson, A. B., Jr.: Orthopaedic Surgery in Infancy and Childhood, 3rd ed. Baltimore, Williams & Wilkins, 1968.
30. Fiorani, G.: Sopra una forma speciale di zoppicamento. Gazz. Osp., 2:717, 1881.
31. Golding, F. C.: Congenital coxa vara. J. Bone Joint Surg., 30B:161, 1948.
32. Golding, F. C.: Congenital coxa vara and the short femur. Proc. R. Soc. Med., 32:641, 1938.
33. Gullemin, A.: Quelques observations de la coxa vara essentielle et d'osteochondrite. Rev. Orthop., 11:51, 1924.
34. Gutig, C., and Herzog, A.: Der berginn der sogenannten coxa vara congenita aseptische schenkelhalsnekrose. Beitr. Klin. Chir., 156:551, 1932.
35. Haas, S. L.: Lengthening of the femur with simultaneous correction of coxa vara. J. Bone Joint Surg., 15:219, 1933.
36. Hafezi, F.: Recurrent congenital coxa vara associated with primary hypoparathyroidism. Clin. Orthop., 79:127, 1971.
37. Haraldsson, S.: The epiphyseal angle in coxa vara infantum and its relation to results. Acta Orthop. Scand., 39:76, 1968.
38. Hark, F. W.: Congenital coxa vara. Amer. J. Surg., 80:305, 1950.
39. Helbing, C.: Die coxa vara. Z. Orthop. Chir., 15:502, 1906.
40. Hilgenreiner, H.: Zur Genese der coxa vara. Med. Klin., 5:159, 1931.
41. Hoffa, A.: Die angeborenen coxa vara. Dtsch. Med. Wschr., 31:1257, 1905.
42. Hofmeister, F.: Coxa vara, a typical form of. Beitr. Klin. Chir., 12:245, 1894.
43. Horwitz, T: The treatment of congenital (or developmental) coxa vara. Surg. Gynecol. Obstet., 87:71, 1948.
44. Hoyt, W. A., Jr., Troyer, M. L., Reef, T., and Shiek, S.: The proximal femoral epiphyses: experimental and correlated clinical observation of their potential. J. Bone Joint Surg., 48A:1026, 1966.
45. Jerre, T.: Spontaneous recovery in coxa vara infantum. Acta Orthop. Scand., 25:149, 1955.
46. Joachimstahal, G.: Ein fall von congenitalein herzfehler combiniert mit angeborenen oberschenkeldefect. Klin. Wschr., 37:172, 1900.
47. Johanning, K.: Coxa vara infantum. I. Clinical appearance and aetiological problem. Acta Orthop. Scand., 21:273, 1951.
48. Johanning, K.: Coxa vara infantum. II. Treatment and results of treatment. Acta Orthop. Scand., 22:100, 1952.
49. Keetley, C. B.: Coxa vara. Lancet, 1:115, 1900.
50. King, R. E., and Lovejoy, J. F.: Familial osteopetrosis with coxa vara. J. Bone Joint Surg., 55A:381, 1973.
51. Kleinberg, S.: The treatment of early epiphyseolisthesis at the hip by drilling and delayed weight-bearing. Bull. Hosp. Joint Dis., 13:94, 1952.
52. Kraske, P.: Uber die operative behandlung der statischen schenkelhalsverbiegung. Zbl. Chir., 6:121, 1896.
53. Kredel, L.: Coxa vara congenita. Contralb. Chir., 23:969, 1896.
54. Kreuz, L.: Kritische betrachtungen zur morphologic der angeborenen coxa vara. Arch. Orthop. Chir., 28:106, 1930.
55. Langenskiold, F: On pseudarthrosis of the femoral neck in congenital coxa vara. Acta Chir. Scand., 98:568, 1949.

56. Langenskiold, F., and Salenius, P.: Epiphysiodesis of the greater trochanter. Acta Orthop. Scand., 38:199, 1967.
57. Lasserre, C.: Subtrochanteric oblique osteotomy in coxa vara with temporary external fixation of fragments. J. Bone Joint Surg., 13:296, 1931.
58. Laurent, L. B.: Growth disturbances of the proximal end of the femur in the light of animal experiments. Acta Orthop. Scand., 28:256, 1959.
59. Le Mesurier, A. B.: Developmental coxa vara. J. Bone Joint Surg., 30B:595, 1948.
60. LoCoco, S., Pusateri, W., and Newman, W. H.: Intramedullary fixation after subtrochanteric osteotomy for coxa vara and coxa valga deformities in children. South. Med. J., 66:1379, 1973.
61. MacEwen, G. D., and Shands, A. R., Jr.: Oblique trochanteric osteotomy. J. Bone Joint Surg., 49A:345, 1967.
62. Magnusson, R.: Coxa vara infantum. Acta Orthop. Scand., 23:284, 1954.
63. McDougall, A.: Fracture of the neck of the femur in childhood. J. Bone Joint Surg., 43B:16, 1961.
64. Morgan, I. E., and Somerville, E. W.: Normal and abnormal growth of the upper end of the femur. J. Bone Joint Surg., 42B:264, 1960.
65. Muller, E.: Torsion of the femoral neck during the growth period. A new disease picture. Beitr. Chir., 4:137, 1889.
66. Nagura, S.: Zur atiologie der coxa vara, zugleich beitrag zur kenntnis der transformation der knochen. Arch. Klin. Chir., 199:533, 1940.
67. Nagura, S., and Kosuge, S.: Die pathogenese und das wesen der pertsschen krankheit. Arch. Klin. Chir., 191:345, 1938.
68. Nilsonne, H.: Contributions as to the knowledge of congenital coxa vara. Acta Radiol., 3:383, 1924.
69. Nilsonne, H.: On congenital coxa vara. Acta Chir. Scand., 64:217, 1929.
70. Noble, T., and Hauser, E.: Coxa vara. Arch. Surg., 12:501, 1926.
71. Oger, J.: Abnormalities of the femur with bilateral coxa vara. J. Belg. Med. Phys. Rhum., 14:115, 1959.
72. Patella, V., and Bancale, R.: Anatomical, pathological, and clinical aspects of epiphyseal detachment, congenital coxa vara, and epiphysiolysis (slipped epiphysis) in relation to the development of the proximal femoral growth cartilage. Ital. J. Orthop. Traumatol., 3:239, 1977.
73. Pauwels, F.: Zur therapie der klinischen coxa vara. Z. Orthop., 64, 1936.
74. Pauwels, F.: In: Biomechanics of the Normal and the Diseased Hip. New York, Springer-Verlag, 1976.
75. Peabody, C. W.: Subtrochanteric osteotomy in coxa vara. Arch. Surg., 46:743, 1943.
76. Pylkkanen, P. V.: Coxa vara infantum. Acta Orthop. Scand., 48(Suppl.):1, 1960.
77. Rang, M.: In: The Growth Plate and Its Disorders. Edinburgh, Livingston, 1969.
78. Reiner, M.: Ueberden congenitalen femurdefect. Z. Orthop. Chir., 9:544, 1901.
79. Ring, P. A.: Congenital short femur (simple femoral hypoplasia). J. Bone Joint Surg., 41B:73, 1959.
80. Roberts, W. M.: End result study of congenital coxa vara treated by Haas trochanteric osteotomy. South. Med. J., 43:389, 1950.
81. Sage, F. P.: Congenital anomalies. In: Campbell's Operative Orthopaedics, 6th ed. St. Louis, Mosby, 1980.
82. Salvati, E. A.: Septic arthritis of the hip in infancy: treatment of the sequelae and long-term results. In: Proceedings of the Seventh Open Scientific Meeting of The Hip Society. St. Louis, Mosby, 1979.
83. Savastano, A., and Bliss, T.: Contribution of the epiphysis of the greater trochanter to the growth of the femur. Int. Surg., 60:280, 1975.
84. Say, B., Taysi, K., Pirnar, T., Tokgozoglu, N., and Inan, E.: Dominant congenital coxa vara. J. Bone Joint Surg., 56B:78, 1974.
85. Schmidt, A.: Zur atiologie der coxa vara und der perthesschen krankheit. Z. Orthop. Chir., 1:55, 1892.
86. Schwarz, E.: Uber die coxa vara congenita. Beitr. Klin. Chir., 87:685, 1913.
87. Simons, B.: Die sogenannte coxa vara congenita. Beitr. Klin. Chir., 161:205, 1935.
88. Strauss, A.: Die atiologie der huftgelenkdeformitaten. Z. Orthop., 68, 1938.
89. Tachdjian, M.: In: Pediatric Orthopaedics. Philadelphia, Saunders, 1972.
90. Walter, H.: Die patholgie und klinik der coxa vara. Verh. Dtsch. Orthop. Ges., 24:8, 1929.
91. Walter, H.: Sogenannte angeborene coxa vara durch umlagerung der pseudarthrosenzone geheilt. Zbl. Chir., 40:2359, 1933.
92. Walter, H.: Zur genese der coxa vara. Med. Klin., 29:1071, 1931.
93. Weighill, F.: The treatment of developmental coxa vara by abduction subtrochanteric and intertrochanteric femoral osteotomy with special reference to the role of adductor tenotomy. Clin. Orthop., 116:116, 1976.
94. Weissman, S.: Transplantation of the trochanteric epiphysis into the acetabulum after septic arthritis of the hip. J. Bone Joint Surg., 49A:1647, 1967.
95. Zadek, I.: Congenital coxa vara. Arch. Surg., 30:62, 1935.
96. Zimmermann, M.: Untersuchungen uber krankheitsbild und aetiologie der sogenannten coxa vara congenita oder coxa vara infantum. Z. Orthop., 68:389, 1938.

CHAPTER 11

Legg-Calvé-Perthes Disease

WALTER B. GREENE

In 1910 Arthur Legg [45] of Boston, Jacques Calvé [8] of Paris, and George Perthes [55] of Germany independently published papers describing a hip disorder occurring in children that healed with flattening of the femoral head. Idiopathic osteonecrosis of the femoral head occurring in children has subsequently been known as Legg-Calvé-Perthes disease, or, as it is commonly termed, Legg-Perthes disease. Of all hip disorders, Legg-Perthes' disease is without a doubt the least understood and most vigorously debated.

The purpose of this chapter will be to describe a management plan for the patient with Legg Perthes' disease. In order to do this, an understanding of the natural history of the disorder and some discussion of its etiology will also be necessary. Two facts should be remembered throughout our discussion: First, the syndrome is self-limited, in that the femoral head heals with or without treatment. Second, as orthopedic surgeons we cannot influence the rate of healing, but rather our treatment plan must provide optimal conditions for minimizing hip joint deformity while the osteonecrosis is resolving. As in all pediatric hip disorders, this must be done with consideration of the total child as well as consideration of future problems.

Epidemiology, Etiology, and Pathology

The usual age of onset is 4 to 8 years, but may be anywhere from 2 to 12 years of age. Males are four to five times more likely to have the disease and blacks are rarely affected. Unilateral involvement is the rule and occurs in approximately 90% of cases. Bilateral involvement and a higher percentage of females are found in the younger age groups.[22]

The incidence of the disorder in England varies from 5.5 to 11.1 per 100,000 children under 15 years,[2] the variation depending on the region of the country. In 1964 the reported incidence in Massachusetts was 5.7 per 100,000 children.[50] Regional variation in the United States would probably be greater than that of England because areas having a greater percentage of black children in the population would show a lower overall incidence.

In most cases, genetic factors and hormonal problems have not been found.[22,78] A delay in skeletal maturation is a frequent finding,[22,28,31,34,78] and in fact the relatively advanced skeletal maturation of blacks and females may explain the lower incidence of the disease in this population. Short stature may also be seen, although not to the same degree as the delay in skeletal maturation.[22,28,31] Using detailed anthropometric measurements, Burwell et al.[7] found impairment of most linear measurements and hypothesized that Legg-Perthes' disease could be a primary abnormality of femoral head growth associated with a functional overload of the femoral capital epiphysis causing a secondary vascular compromise.

The traditional theory of etiology is that interruption of the blood supply to the femoral capital epiphysis is the primary factor in Legg Perthes' disease. Trueta [76] and Chung [12] have studied the arterial supply to the proximal femur of the growing child. The epiphyseal vessels come from the medial and lateral circumflex arteries. The medial femoral circumflex artery supplies the medial, posterior, and lateral ascending cervical arteries while the lateral circumflex artery supplies the anterior ascending cervical arteries. Other names for the ascending cervical arteries are the retinacular or metaphyseal vessels. The ascending cervical arteries traverse the articular capsule and then branch to form epiphyseal and metaphyseal vessels. Both Trueta and Chung have shown that most of the epiphyseal blood supply comes from branches of the lateral ascending cervical artery. The interval between the greater trochanter and capsule is extremely narrow in children less than 8 years old and is a possible area of constriction to the lateral ascending cervical artery.

Variation in the vascular supply may explain some of the age, race, and sex characteristics in Legg Perthes' disease. Chung [12] found the number of ascending cervical vessels to be significantly decreased in children aged 3 to 10 years compared to the 0- to 2-year-old group, and in older black children there were more anterior and medial ascending cervical branches. The intraarticular arterial ring that may be formed by the ascending cervical arteries was more often incomplete in males, although with respect to age and race there was no difference in the completeness or incompleteness of the arterial ring. However, the difficulty in correlating anatomical variation in epiphyseal blood supply to the occurrence of Legg Perthes' disease is twofold: (1) insufficient number of detailed anatomical dissections at different ages to allow statistical comparison, and (2) our present inability to outline the epiphyseal circulation in patients with Legg Perthes' disease.

More than one episode of infarction may be necessary to produce the typical changes seen in Legg-Perthes' disease. This concept is supported by experimental studies,[68] and in three of four autopsy cases, the femoral head pathology was also consistent with more than one episode of vascular interruption.[19,37,49] Inoue et al.[36] found histological evidence of double infarction in 51% of femoral head biopsy specimens from patients with Legg-Perthes' disease. In this study, the pathological findings suggested that the first episode of infarction was an extrinsic event which involved the whole femoral head, whereas the subsequent episodes of infarction were patchily distributed without total head involvement. Extrinsic compression of the capital epiphyseal blood supply may occur; however, obvious sources for extrinsic pressure such as recognizable trauma or transient synovitis have not been typically observed in this disorder.[22]

Whatever the primary event, death of bone cells initiates the changes of osteonecrosis, revascularization, and reossification. The pathology of the femoral head deformity in Legg Perthes' disease is based on the changes which occur during the process of revascularization and reossification. Experimental studies have been helpful in the understanding of this pathology.[29,30,63] After osteonecrosis, revascularization begins and is subsequently followed by reossification. Reossification in the area of cancellous bone starts by the deposition of woven bone on the dead trabeculae. The woven bone may then be replaced by lamellar bone or the repair process may proceed with resorption of the dead trabeculae followed by replacement with new bone. This repair process would cause thickening of the trabeculae, a finding confirmed in autopsy studies.[19,37,49] In the subchondral region, compact bone makes the process of reossification more difficult since bone resorption must proceed any bone formation. When bone resorption progresses faster than bone repair, "walls" of fibrous tissue develop and these areas of fibrous tissue may impede deposition of woven bone. The subchondral bone that has undergone initial repair is at risk for collapse since the woven bone is biologically plastic to mechanical stresses. Shear stresses on the femoral head coupled with bone resorption may result in a subchondral fracture that is seen on roentgenograms as the crescent sign (Figs. 11–1 and 11–3A). If this biologically plastic bone can be maintained within the acetabulum, then the femoral head will heal without significant loss of its sphericity, even though it may have some residual coxa magna and coxa plana.

Residual femoral head deformities that may occur after healing of the avascular necrosis include coxa plana, coxa breva, and coxa magna. Coxa plana results from weight-bearing stresses causing collapse of the more biologically plastic bone that is formed during the initial phase of reossification. Coxa breva is related to ischemia of the epiphysis. Since the epiphyseal vessels supply the germinal cells of the physis, damage or occlusion of these vessels may affect the longitudinal growth contributed by the proximal femoral growth plate.[62] In ten patients having total head involvement Gage and Cary [25] found the average growth loss to be 7.0 mm, but some patients had greater than 20 mm of shortening. The blood supply to the greater

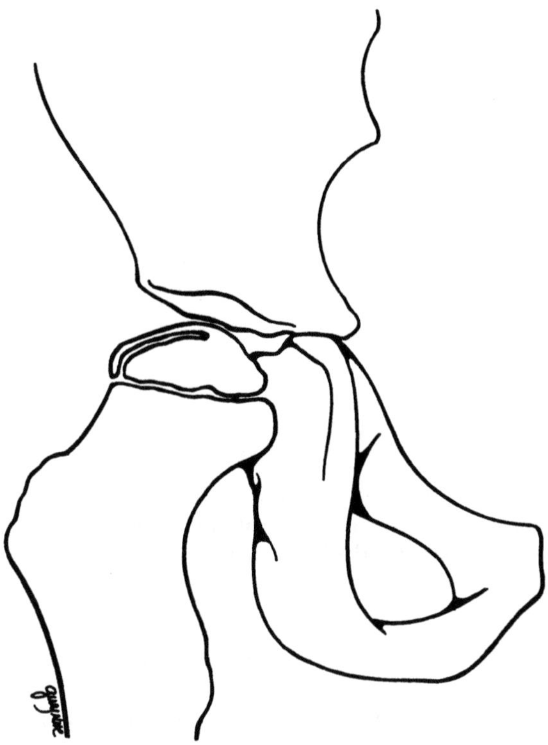

FIG. 11-1 Diagramatic representation of crescent sign. See also Fig. 11-3A.

trochanteric physis is not affected in Legg Perthes' disease, and relative overgrowth of the greater trochanter may cause a decreased articulotrochanteric distance and a slight decrease in the neck–shaft angle. Rarely is the greater trochanter so affected that abductor musculature insufficiency develops.[25] Widening of the femoral neck occurs because appositional growth in the metaphysis continues as its blood supply is unaffected.[62]

Coxa magna is probably related to cartilage hyperplasia. In the early radiodense or fragmentation stage, the femoral head appears small on plain radiographs, but arthrograms actually show overall enlargement of the femoral head, thereby demonstrating hyperplasia of the articular cartilage.[27] The ischemic bony femoral epiphysis cannot grow, but its articular cartilage can be nourished by the synovial fluid, and indeed a mild synovitis may actually stimulate articular cartilage growth. The synovitis associated with Legg Perthes' disease is described as mild because joint aspiration at arthrography has not revealed excessive synovial fluid under pressure. Arthrography has also shown increased thickness of the medial acetabular cartilage without loss of contact or subluxation of the femoral head.[27] The acetabular cartilage hyperplasia presumably also results from the mild synovitis. Cartilage hyperplasia causes both extrusion and enlargement of the femoral head. As the osteonecrosis resolves, the hyperplastic cartilage is replaced with bone and the ultimate result is a femoral head which heals with coxa magna.

Presentation

On presentation to the physician, the patient's usual chief complaint is a limp. This limp is initially painless or is associated only with aching in the proximal thigh at the end of the day. The limp has frequently been present for several months, and its insidious progression makes it difficult to pinpoint the onset of the disorder. The limp and complaints of pain have usually become more noticeable by the time of presentation.

Physical examination shows limitation of hip abduction, internal rotation, and extension. Thigh circumference measurements and palpation of the buttocks will confirm atrophy of the thigh and gluteal muscles. Unless the disease is in an advanced stage, the limitation of hip movement usually reflects the degree of synovitis and muscle spasm rather than bony abnormalities. Rarely does the past history indicate any episodes of trauma or transient synovitis. Laboratory studies including sedimentation rate are usually normal. Clinical suspicion of the disease can be confirmed by roentgenographic evaluation which begins with good anteroposterior (AP) and frog-leg lateral pelvis films.

With bilateral involvement, other disorders which simulate the roentgenographic appearance of Legg Perthes' disease must be considered. Gaucher's disease, sickle cell anemia, and hypothyroidism may produce x-ray changes which can be confused with Legg Perthes' disease, but in these disorders the roentgenographic findings and clinical picture are usually different enough that errors in diagnosis are not made. Some of the epiphyseal dysplasias may be more difficult to differentiate, and in particular a less severe form of multiple epiphyseal dysplasia or Stickler's syndrome (hereditary arthro-ophthalmopathy) has been misdiagnosed as Legg Perthes' disease (Fig. 11-2).[70] In patients with bilateral involvement,

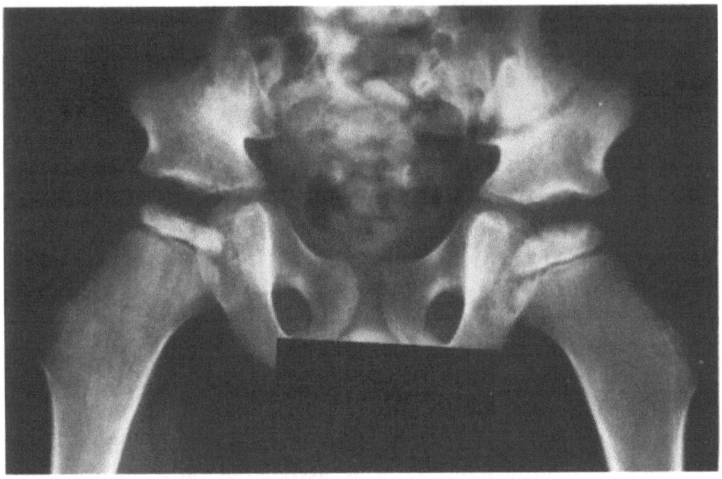

A

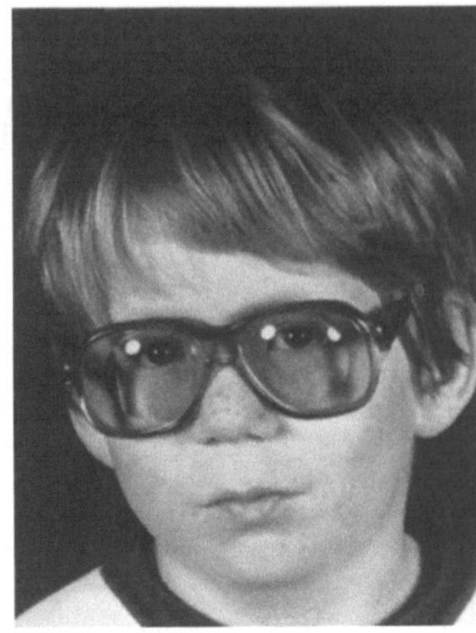

B

FIG. 11–2 **A** AP pelvis—3-year-old child. Disorder initially diagnosed as Perthes' disease and patient treated for several months in abduction brace without apparent healing. Subsequent correct diagnosis was Strickler's syndrome. Suggestive clinical features were bilateral femoral epiphysis involvement and requirement for thick-lens glasses. **B** Clinical photograph, age 5.

special attention should be directed to family history, the physical exam, and growth chart analysis. Routine x-rays to be considered in patients with bilateral involvement include views of the hands, spine, and knees. When indicated, further laboratory studies and roentgenographic evaluation may be necessary to exclude disorders simulating Legg Perthes' disease.

The overall radiographic appearance of the femoral epiphysis progresses through phases of increased density, fragmentation, reossification, and residual deformities (Fig. 11–3). Obviously these roentgenographic phases overlap and frequently the patient presents after extensive fragmentation has already occurred. In experimental studies, the first roentgenographic finding is decreased size of the osseous portion of the epiphysis;[63] however, in the clinical situation, this stage is rarely seen without some increased density. The increased density of the femoral head is both relative and absolute.[29,30] The associated osteopenia of the femoral metaphysis makes the femoral epiphysis appear relatively dense. The absolute increase in epiphyseal density results from new woven bone being laid down on dead but not resorbed trabeculae. In addition, the compaction or collapse in the area of osteonecrosis may produce increased density. Fragmentation results from resorption of the osteonecrotic bony trabeculae; the fibrous tissue and woven bone that replace the dead trabeculae are not dense enough to appear on x-ray. As further ossification and maturation of the healing bone occur, previous areas of fragmentation will be replaced by roentgenographically identifiable new bone. In the residual phase, the femoral head has been completely reossified and is left with a shape and contour ranging from a spherical head which is associated with long-term normal activity to a very irregular head which may cause a disabling arthritis at an early age.

Evaluation of the Patient with Perthes' Disease

Prior to undertaking treatment, the patient must be evaluated for the extent of osteonecrosis, the degree of skeletal maturity, the presence of subluxation or extrusion, and the degree of femoral head deformity already present. These factors are all prognostic indicators and need to be assessed before proper management can be instituted. It is also helpful to fully understand both the social and psychological aspects of the child and parents before deciding whether brace or surgical treatment is indicated.

The correlation between the extent of epiphyseal osteonecrosis and subsequent deformity in Legg Perthes' disease has been confirmed by many authors. Catterall[11] first popularized the concept of classifying the amount of femoral head necrosis, and his system remains the most accepted method of rating (Table 11–1).

In comparing patients who received no treatment with patients who were treated by a weight-relieving apparatus, Catterall [11] found that type I involvement did well whether treated or untreated. The good prognosis with type I femoral head necrosis has been confirmed by other studies; [3,38] however, if no treatment is elected for this group, careful follow-up must be maintained since the amount of femoral head deformity may change and necessitate more vigorous treatment. If the patient was under 4 years of age and had type II involvement, Catterall found that no treatment was acceptable, but some studies have indicated better results with treatment for Catterall type II involvement even in the younger child.[69] For types III and IV femoral head involvement, Catterall found better results with treatment regardless of age. Generally, other authors have agreed that Catterall types III and IV femoral head deformities have a poorer prognosis and need treatment regardless of age.[13,18,38,69] In fact, effectiveness of treatment should be analyzed only in patients having either Catterall type III or IV femoral head deformity, as type I and type II problems may do well without treatment.

The difficulty with the Catterall classification is that it can only be accurately determined after fragmentation has occurred. For the patient presenting late in the course of the disease this is no problem, but for the patient presenting early, the full extent of fragmentation in the Catterall classification may not be clear for 6 to 9 months (Fig. 11–4).[38,40,77] The extent of the crescent sign (Figs. 11–1 and 11–3a), a radiolucent defect probably representing a fracture in the subchondral bone, has been shown to correlate with the extent of femoral head osteonecrosis; [67] however, subchondral fissure may not always be present and may be difficult to quantify.

When patients present before radiographic classification is possible, 99m-technetium polyphosphate bone imaging can be helpful in both establishing the diagnosis and in determining the extent of osteonecrosis.[17,23,43,74] Obtaining AP and lateral images with pin-hole collimators provides better resolution in semiquantifying the area of osteonecrosis. LaMont et al.[43] have further quantified the extent of osteonecrosis by measuring radionuclide uptake of the femoral head and comparing these counts to normal bone. With advanced fragmentation, early revascularization obscures the scan, and bone imaging is not helpful in quantifying the osteonecrosis; however, at this time plain radiographs are sufficient to determine the Catterall classification.

The presence of subluxation or extrusion should be defined prior to instituting treatment and needs to be reassessed as treatment progresses. If extrusion is identified, then by definition the femoral epiphysis is not contained within the acetabulum. Klisic [42] defines extrusion or subluxation by measuring the acetabulum–head index. The index is the width of the covered epiphysis divided by the total width of the epiphysis, multiplied by 100 (Fig. 11–5). According to Klisic any ratio greater than or equal to 90 is contained, while a rating less than 90 is subluxated or extruded. The acetabulum–head index has the advantage of being a reproducible and objective measurement. The difficulty with this measurement as well as those described by other authors [18,32] is that the lateral epiphyseal segment may not be visible on plain radiographs at the time of diagnosis. In this situation, the amount of extrusion may be underestimated unless arthrography is used.

Several reports have documented that femoral heads without extrusion do much better than those with extrusion regardless of the age of presentation, type of Catterall classification, or type of treatment.[11,18,32,71] In the study by Green et al.[32] the Catterall type II femoral head deformity had 80% good results when the femoral head extrusion was 20% or less, but only 40% good results with extrusion greater than 20%. In more severe femoral head involvement (Catterall type III or IV), good results were obtained in 45% of cases without femoral head extrusion, but in only 8% of those cases with extrusion. Other signs of the head at

TABLE 11–1 Catterall Classification

I.	Only anterior portion of epiphysis involved. No collapse or sequestra formation.
II.	Only anterior portion involved, but to a greater extent. Collapse occurs in involved segment. Lateral wall intact.
III.	Only small portion medial aspect epiphysis not involved.
IV.	Total head involvement.

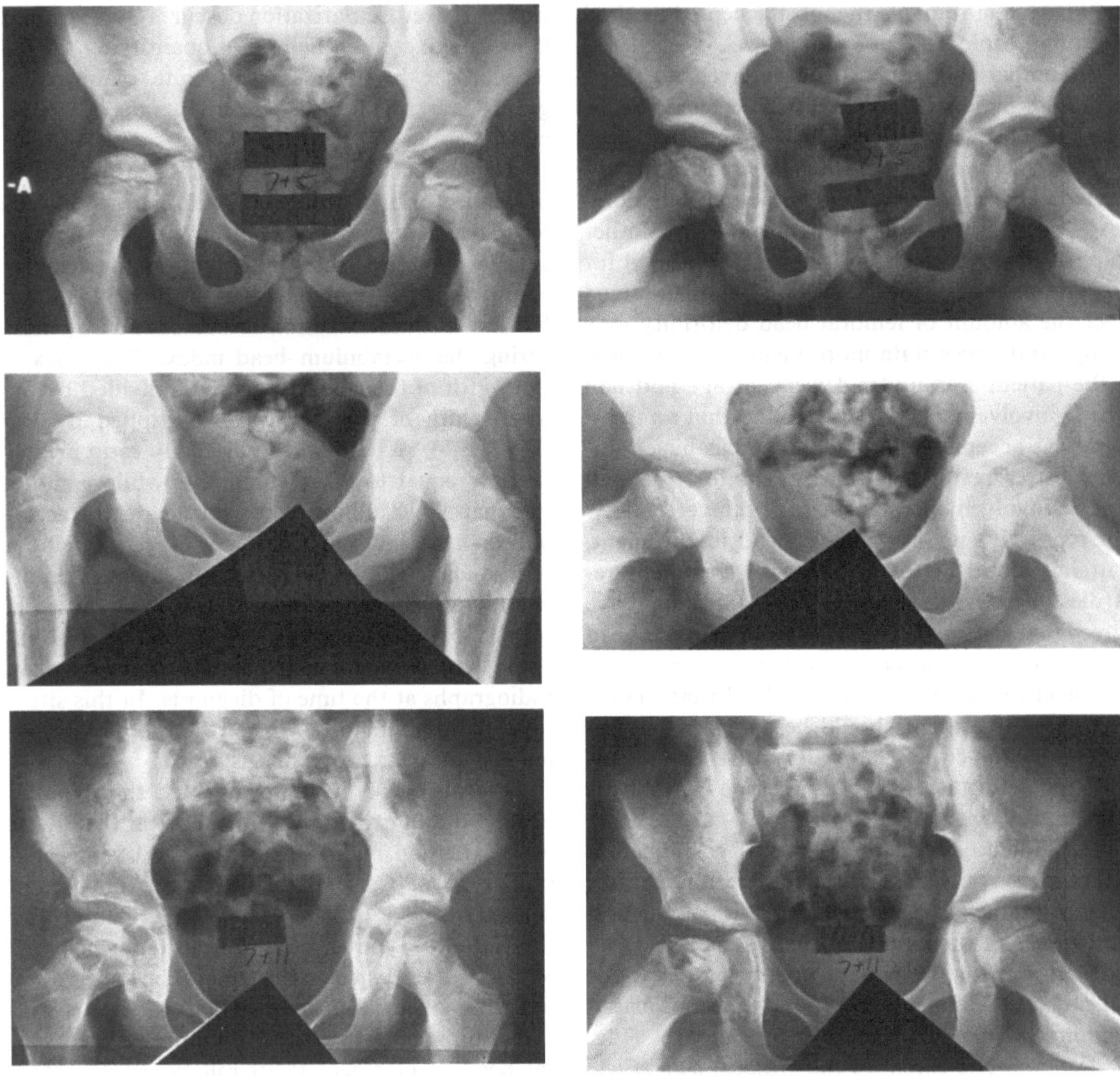

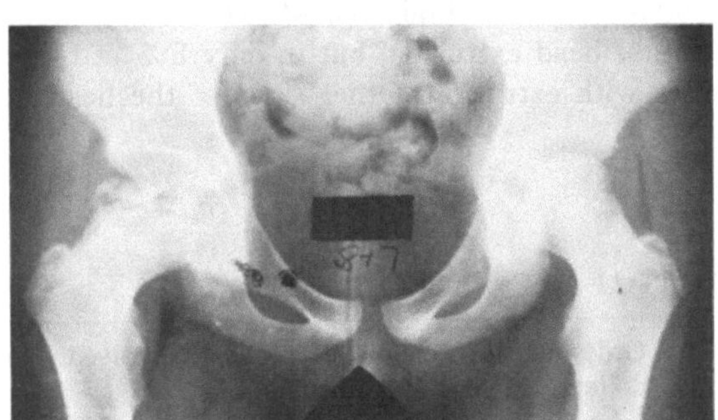

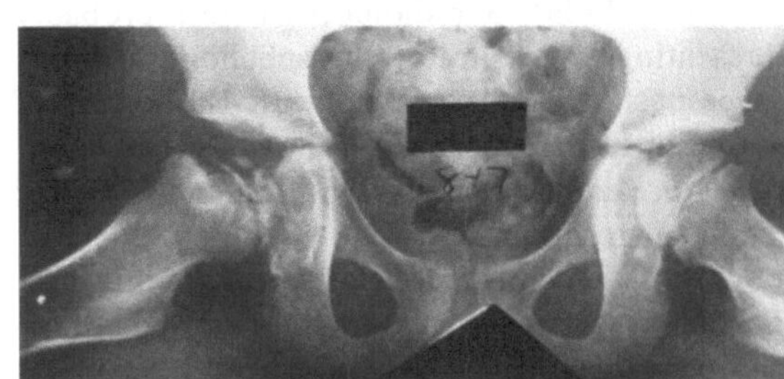

FIG. 11–3 **A** AP and lateral (frog-leg) pelvis. Male, aged 7 years and 5 months, presenting with Perthes' disease of the right hip. Roentgenograms show crescent sign, increased radiodensity, and mild epiphyseal extrusion with acetabulum–head index of 82. **B** AP and lateral (frog-leg) pelvis. Patient now 7 years and 8 months. Note increased sclerosis involving all of femoral head except medialmost corner. This would probably indicate Catterall type III deformity at this time, although classifying the type of femoral head deformity is still difficult. **C** AP and lateral (frog-leg) pelvis. Patient now 7 years and 11 months. Early fragmentation of the femoral epiphysis. Large metaphyseal cyst. **D** AP and lateral (frog-leg) pelvis. Patient now 8 years and 7 months. Early reossification of the lateral margin of the epiphysis. Author would not discontinue brace therapy until central sclerosis had been replaced.

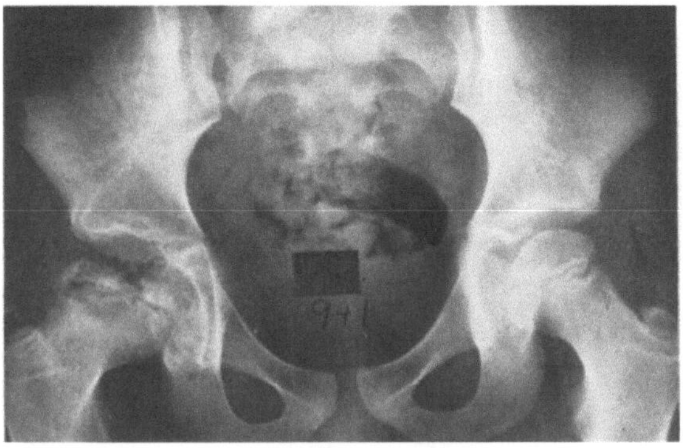
E

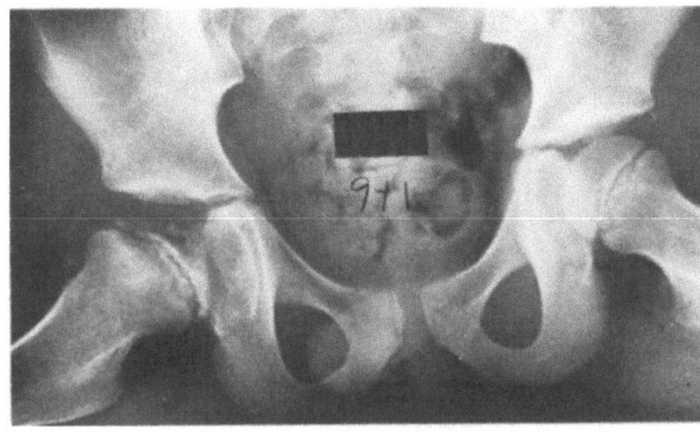
E′

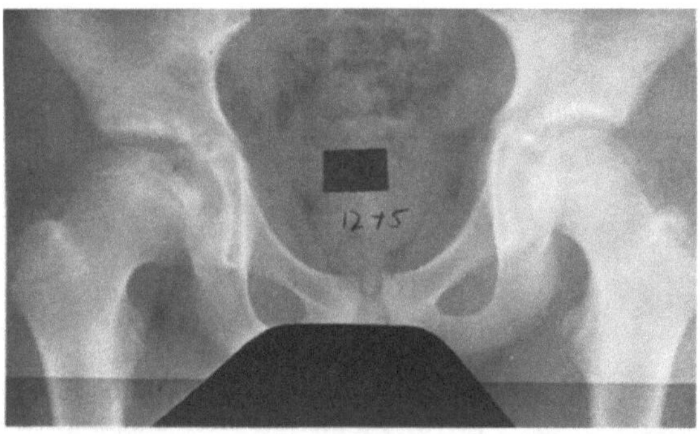
F

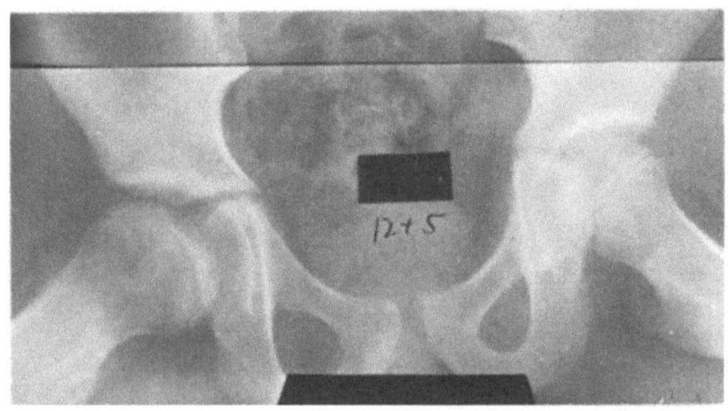
F′

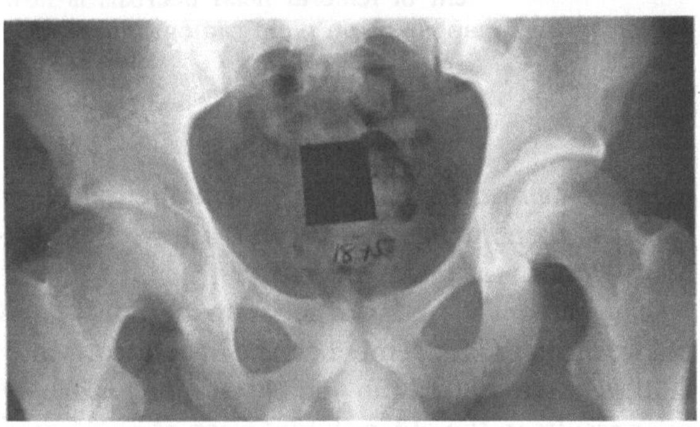
G

FIG. 11–3 Cont. **E** AP and lateral (frog-leg) pelvis. Patient now 9 years and 1 month. Reossification on anterior and lateral margins. Brace wearing could be discontinued. **F** AP and lateral (frog-leg) pelvis. Patient now 12 years and 5 months. Reossification still incomplete in central epiphyseal area. **G** AP pelvis. Patient now 18 years and 5 months. Residual deformity with 2 mm loss of sphericity on Mose circle. Although only a fair result by roentgenographic standards, clinical studies would indicate that this patient would have a good long-term functional status.[51,67]

risk, such as Gage's sign [24] (convex shape on the lateral border of the femoral neck), metaphyseal cysts, calcification lateral to the epiphysis, or a horizontal physis, are either inconsequential or another manifestation of subluxation.[42,65]

Arthrography can be helpful in determining subluxation and whether any femoral head flattening has occurred secondary to either collapse of the bony epiphysis or asymmetrical hyperplasia of the femoral head cartilage [26] (Fig. 11–6). Arthrography done with the aid of fluoroscopy also will identify the femoral head which is not containable either because a relatively mild asymmetry causes hinging of the femoral head on abduction or a more severe "saddle" type femoral head depression causes a complete block on attempted abduction.[61]

Determination of femoral head sphericity is mandatory when assessing long-term results of Legg Perthes' disease and is also helpful in the initial evaluation. Measurement of femoral head sphericity was first suggested by Goff [31] and later developed by Mose.[51] The Mose concentric circle templates (Fig. 11–7) allow reproducible assess-

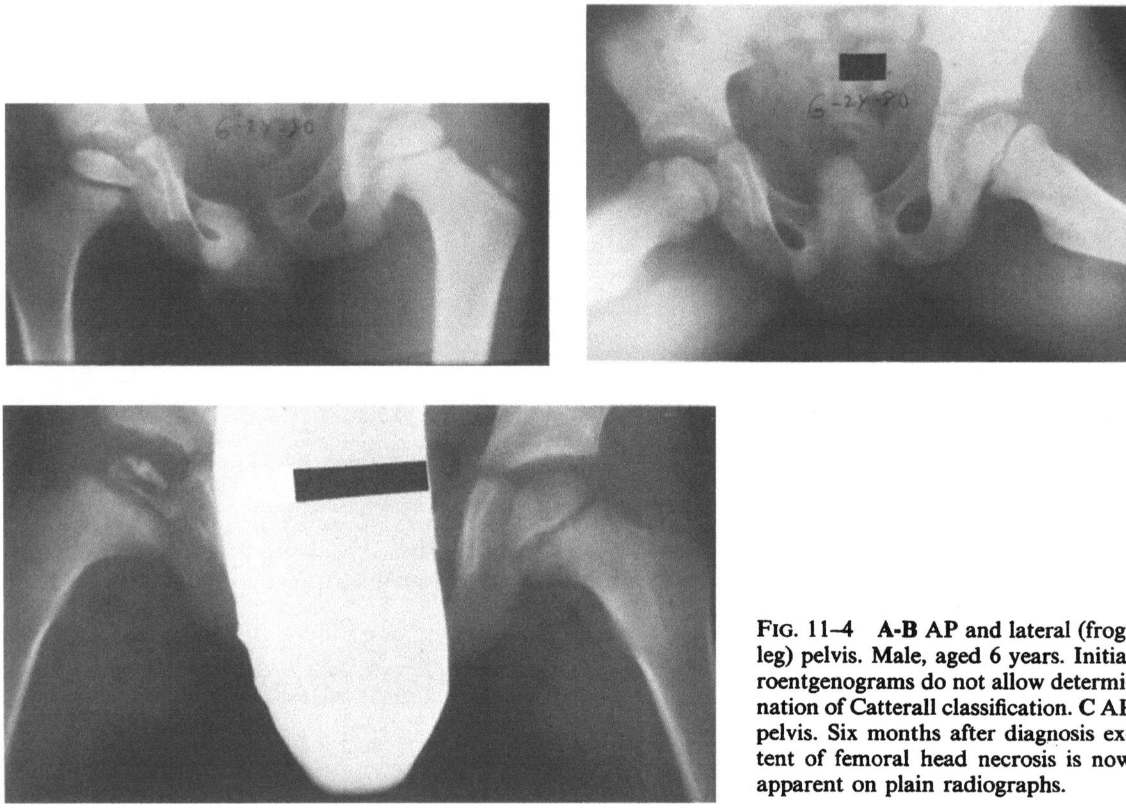

A B C

FIG. 11-4 **A-B** AP and lateral (frog-leg) pelvis. Male, aged 6 years. Initial roentgenograms do not allow determination of Catterall classification. **C** AP pelvis. Six months after diagnosis extent of femoral head necrosis is now apparent on plain radiographs.

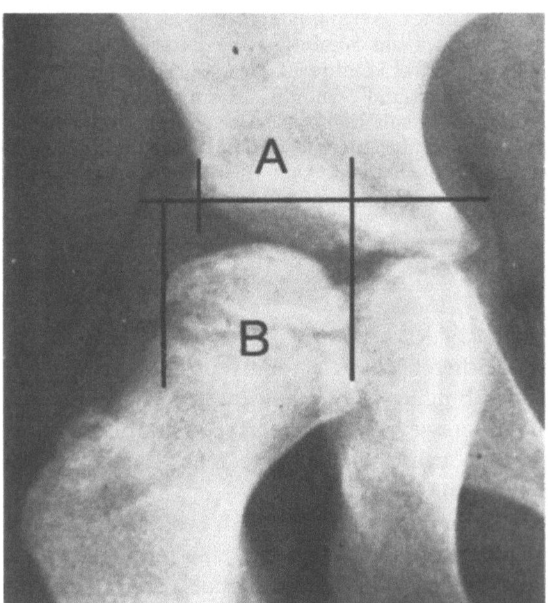

FIG. 11-5 Acetabulum–head index is measured as ($A - B$) × 100. In this radiograph the acetabulum–head index is 82.

ment of femoral sphericity. If fragmentation is present, then arthrography will allow measurement of femoral head sphericity.

The patient's age also needs to be considered before proper management can be instituted. Many studies have noted the increased percentage of poor results in the older child. Green et al.[32] found no good results in the child aged 8 or older who had epiphyseal extrusion of more than 20%. In a long-term study Stulberg and Salter [72] found that if the age of onset had been less than 6 years, patients had not developed symptomatic degenerative arthritis by middle age even if residual deformity was present; however, if the child was older than 10 years of age, symptomatic degenerative arthritis developed consistently if any residual deformity was present. The explanation that seems plausible is that in the younger age group, enough growth potential remains to allow remodeling of the acetabulum to conform with the nonspherical femoral head, whereas in the older child the remodeling potential of the acetabulum is limited. Whether children with skeletal immaturity do bet-

FIG. 11–6 **A-B** AP and frog-leg views of the left hip of a 6-year-old male with questionable femoral head collapse. **C-E** Arthrogram shows maintenance of femoral head sphericity, and with abduction, satisfactory containment is possible.

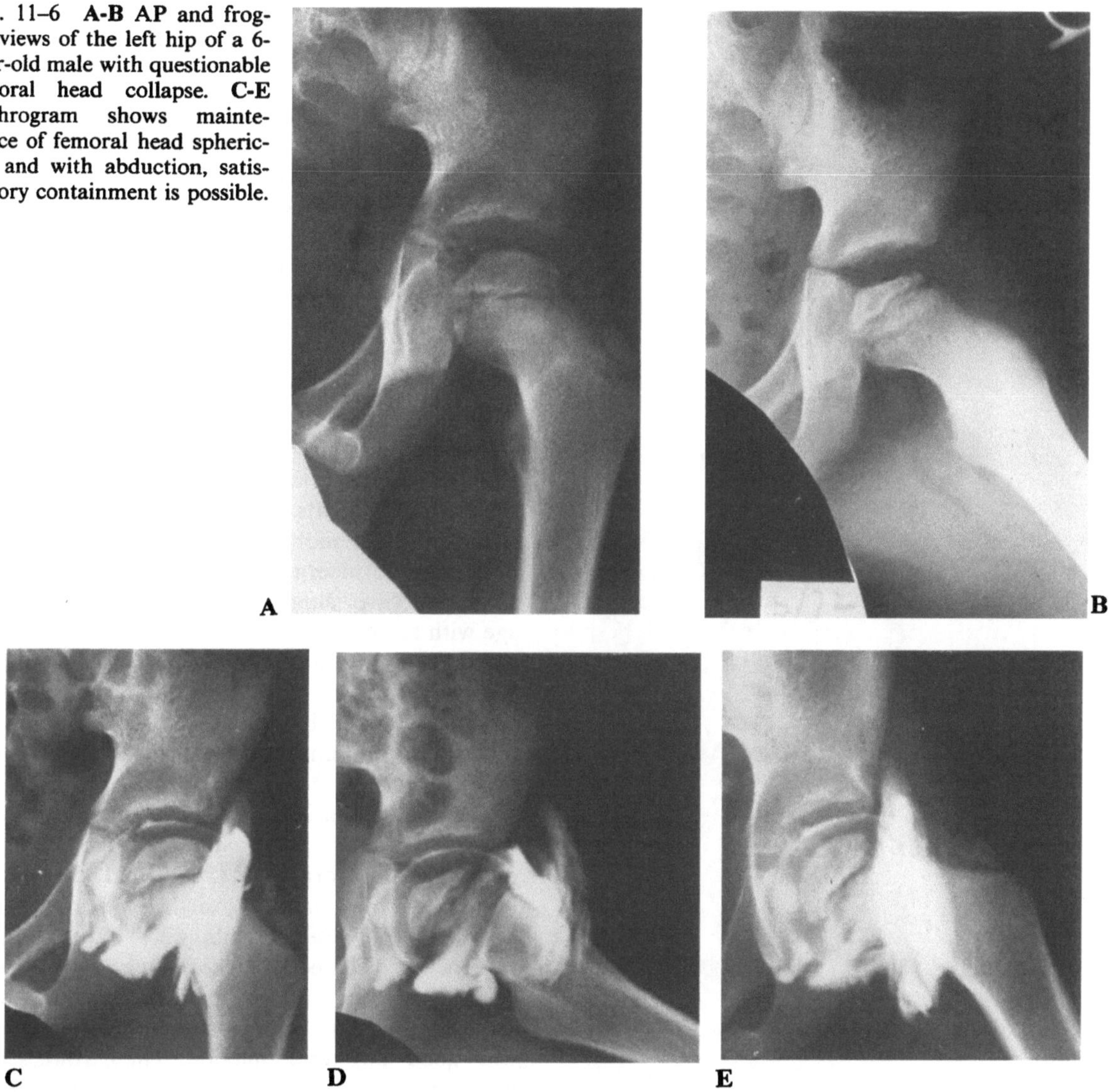

ter than patients whose skeletal age is equal to the chronological age is a question which has not been answered.

Treatment

Treatment for Legg Perthes' disease includes deciding who needs treatment, selecting the most appropriate therapy for the patient, and deciding when treatment can be stopped. The initial starting point for any patient is traction to regain lost hip abduction and internal rotation. The necessity for preliminary traction has been emphasized in many reports, and in the author's opinion cannot be underrated. With persistent synovitis and limitation of motion, ambulation either in an orthosis or after surgery is associated with persistent pain and joint stiffness. Although some of the surgical treatments for Legg Perthes' disease would apparently enable one to dismiss traction, this has not been shown to be the case, and all reports advocating surgical treatment still recognize the necessity for preliminary traction. Five to six pounds of skin traction are applied to each leg. As the synovitis subsides, the legs are gradually abducted until 45° of hip abduction and almost full internal rotation are obtainable. With severe femoral head involvement, traction frequently requires 2 to 3 weeks to obtain this motion. Although traction may be possible

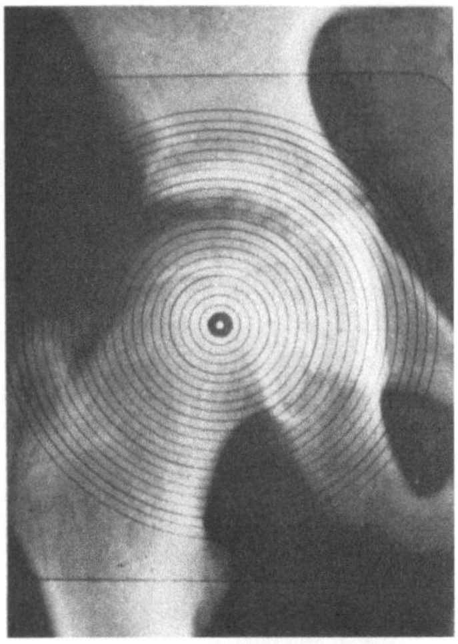

A

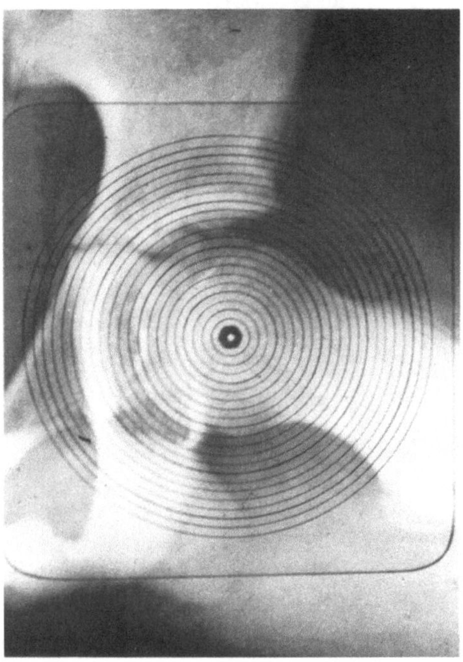

B

FIG. 11–7 A Method of Mose measurement, frontal view. B Method of Mose measurement, lateral view.

at home, in-hospital treatment is frequently necessary to obtain effective results.

After satisfactory motion has been regained, an isotopic bone image and arthrogram with fluoroscopy can be obtained. The bone scan is not done if the Catterall classification can be determined, but as noted before, this is impossible to do on plain radiographs in the early stages of the disease. Information sought on the arthrogram and fluoroscopy study includes (1) assessment of femoral head extrusion, (2) documentation that the area of osteonecrosis can be contained with a selected treatment program, and (3) whether any hinging of the femoral head against the acetabulum occurs with abduction (Fig. 11–6). With mild degrees of hinging, further traction or osteotomy may be required, but with a definite abduction block, containment treatment is not possible.[61]

The initial goal of treatment is to minimize development of femoral head deformity with an ultimate goal of preventing disabling osteoarthritis. Even after the osteonecrosis has healed, remodeling of the femoral head may continue until growth has been completed, the exception being the older child or a markedly irregular femoral head.[52] As anticipated, studies with long-term follow-up have shown that patients had no difficulty when the shape of the femoral head was spherical after healing.[53,71] Stulberg and Salter [72] found that patients did surprisingly well even to late middle age with an ovoid or flat femoral head which had corresponding abnormalities in the acetabulum. These patients had a "congruous incongruity," a term popularized by Curtis [15] to indicate abnormalities in the femoral head and acetabulum but overall matching congruity of the joint surfaces, a situation compatible with good long-term function. By contrast, patients with a flat femoral head but a normal femoral neck and normal acetabulum developed symptomatic coxarthritis during early adulthood.[72] These patients were by and large those who presented late, the average age at onset being 10.4 years. In this group the hip joint was aspherically incongruent, a situation incompatible with good long-term function. These studies are helpful in letting us know that a spherical femoral head should be the goal of treatment, but that some loss of sphericity may be compatible with good long-term function and minimal osteoarthritis even into late adulthood. This is important when one selects a treatment program because there are possible complications of any therapy, particularly surgical, and these should not outweigh the advantages of the selected treatment.

Observation

Some patients with Legg Perthes' disease will need no further treatment other than observation once a full range of motion has been regained. Most authors would agree that a Catterall type I femoral head involvement does as well without treatment as with treatment. In a child under 5 years of age with Catterall type II involvement, the question to treat or not to treat becomes more controversial. The author continues observation on those patients who have no evidence of extrusion or subluxation as defined by Klisic,[42] but will use containment methods of treatment for those demonstrating evidence of extrusion.

In patients where it is difficult to determine the Catterall classification, the isotopic bone image study can be used as a means to begin treatment by observation alone. With less than a 50% defect in the femoral head on the bone scan, and no evidence of extrusion, observation may be elected as a treatment alternative. Observation means that careful follow-up examinations including roentgenographic studies are obtained at frequent intervals. This is necessary because some patients may show progression of their femoral head deformity to either more extensive osteonecrosis or lateral extrusion, both of which would necessitate more vigorous treatment.

Treatment by Containment—Abduction Orthosis

Treatment by containment has been shown to produce the best results in patients with Legg Perthes' disease.[5,11,13,32,38,39] One theory explaining containment treatment is that with abduction and internal rotation of the proximal femur, the acetabulum will surround the femoral head epiphysis and maintain the spherical mold of the femoral head while the relatively plastic bone is replaced by lamellar bone.[66] Another theory is based on the concept that hyperplasia of the femoral articular cartilage occurs more extensively in the peripheral areas. The peripheral hyperplasia is associated with lateral extrusion and subsequent flattening of the femoral head. By abduction of the proximal femur the weight-bearing load is concentrated on the area of lateral overgrowth. Subsequent growth in the lateral area is inhibited by the increased compression from the margins of the acetabulum, as based on the Hueter-Volkmann law where bone growth is inhibited by compression, but stimulated by decreased pressure. In the abducted position, the central area of the femoral head has decreased pressure and therefore is stimulated to grow, resulting in retention, and in some cases, restoration of sphericity.[61]

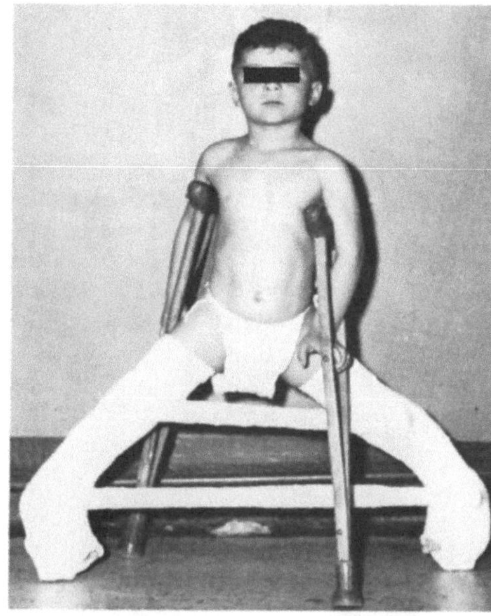

FIG. 11–8 Petrie abduction plaster casts.

Early programs of containment therapy frequently combined recumbency with abduction bracing.[5,16,31] Recumbency was used to diminish weight-bearing stresses on the femoral head. Prolonged recumbency in abduction resulted in satisfactory treatment for the femoral head deformity,[5] but necessitated long separation of the patients from their parents, family, and friends. With today's cost of hospitalization, prolonged recumbency may be standard for comparison but is not a viable treatment alternative.

Petrie and Bitenc [56] demonstrated that weight bearing in a fixed abduction plaster cast would allow effective treatment for Legg Perthes' disease without the need for 1 to 2 years of recumbency in a hospital. The Petrie cast was a significant advancement in the treatment of this disorder. The bilateral long-leg casts are attached with a spreader bar to keep the hips in 45° abduction and slight internal rotation (Fig. 11–8). The disadvantages of the Petrie cast are the need for continued replacement, resultant knee and ankle stiffness, and difficulty in personal hygiene with prolonged cast use.

Fixed abduction braces such as the Newington brace [16] and other similar orthoses [4,20] were another advancement in treatment. These braces simulate the concept of the Petrie cast with centraliza-

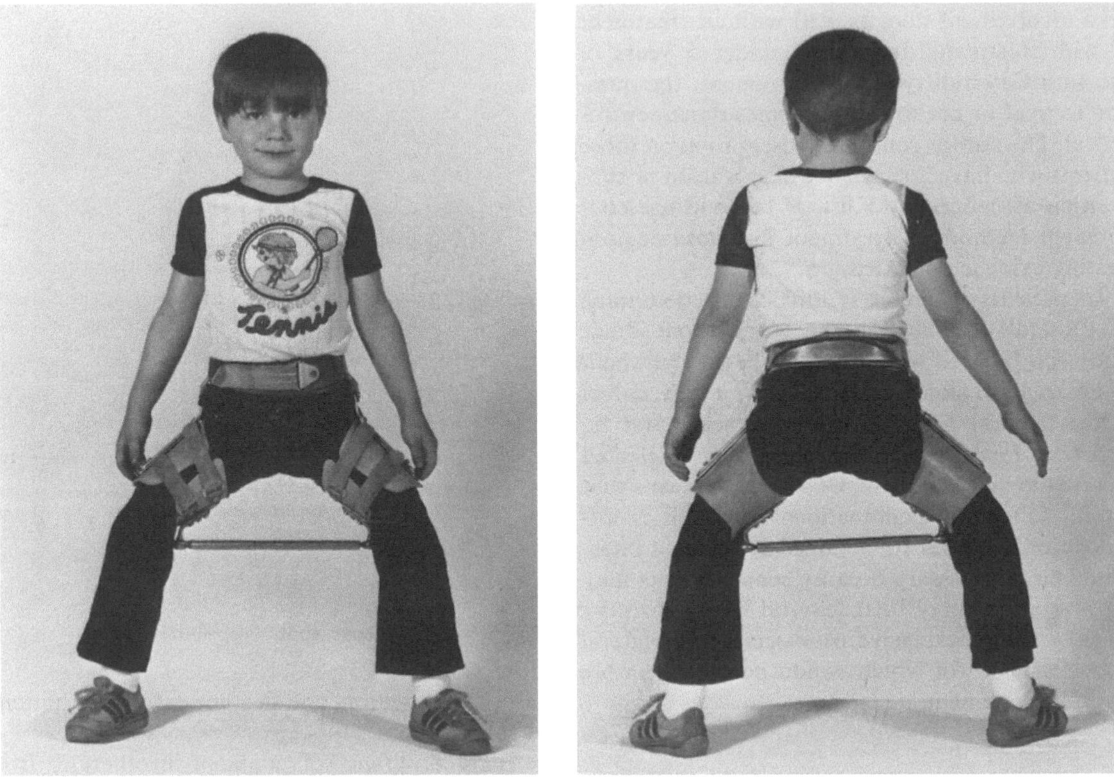

FIG. 11–9. **A** and **B** Five-year-old male in Scottish Rite abduction orthosis. Orthosis allows independent ambulation and participation in most play activities.

tion of the femoral head in the acetabulum by 45° of abduction and slight internal rotation, and like the Petrie cast, ambulation can be accomplished with crutches. The advantage of the brace is that bathing can be accomplished and knee and ankle motion maintained. The disadvantage of the fixed abduction brace is the size and weight of the orthosis. By incorporating the knee and ankle, the brace by necessity is relatively heavy and bulky. Like the Petrie cast, the Newington abduction brace does not allow ambulation in children under 5.5 years, since the younger children have inadequate upper extremity and trunk strength to control the orthosis.

The Scottish Rite abduction orthosis keeps the hips in abduction without incorporation of the knee or ankle.[57] The orthosis consists of a pelvic band, a single-axis hip joint, thigh cuffs, and a telescoping rod which joins the thigh cuff (Fig. 11–9). The telescoping rod limits adduction but will allow some abduction. The telescoping rod is also connected to the thigh cuffs with a universal joint which permits hip flexion and extension as well as some abduction and rotation. This brace is considerably lighter than the other, more extensive abduction braces and also has the advantage of unrestricted knee and ankle motion. The decreased weight and increased joint mobility enable the child not only to walk without crutches, but also extends activities to allow greater freedom for climbing and bike-riding activities. The light weight also makes the brace ideal for younger children, as they can ambulate quite effectively in this orthosis but were unable to do so with earlier braces. Since this brace is relatively new, comparison to other treatment modalities is still incomplete; however, early results are promising and indicate that the Scottish Rite orthosis has comparable results in maintaining femoral head sphericity.[57]

The fixed abduction orthosis has the theoretical disadvantage of limiting hip joint motion to only the flexion–extension plane while blocking the spin mobility seen with normal three-dimensional hip movement.[41] A fixed abduction orthosis may also concentrate abnormal stresses on certain areas of the femoral articular surface, thus leading to recurrent episodes of synovitis, adductor muscle spasm, and possible loss of containment. The Scottish Rite orthosis does not control internal rotation but this seemingly has not been a disadvantage, and in fact may be an advantage in that three-plane movement may promote femoral head sphericity.

The author uses the Scottish Rite orthosis as the preferred method of treatment for most patients with Legg Perthes' disease. The only exceptions to this treatment modality are the patients who are treated by observation as noted above, those who show lack of compliance in wearing the brace, or as discussed below, those patients who are not containable by abduction treatment. The ease of wearing the Scottish Rite orthosis and the greater activity levels possible in this brace have markedly decreased patient compliance difficulties, and in the author's experience, the social problems associated with compliance of brace wear are now restricted to noncompliant parents.

Ambulatory abduction brace treatment is begun after traction has been completed. Occasionally a short period in a Petrie cast may be beneficial in improving subsequent brace compliance. A standing pelvic roentgenogram in the brace is obtained to ensure that 40–45° of hip abduction and satisfactory containment have been achieved. Specific activities are not restricted except for jumping from heights. The brace is worn continuously except for bathing, dressing, and swimming. Swimming is allowed only in water which reaches at least to the nipple line.

Follow-up visits are usually every 3 to 4 months. Motion is assessed to determine if synovitis has recurred, a situation which is usually remedied by a short period of home traction. Some patients will develop an abduction contracture, and for this problem the author uses skin traction at night while maintaining abduction bracing during the day. During the follow-up clinic visits, roentgenograms are also assessed to determine whether containment is being maintained and to ascertain healing of the osteonecrosis.

Another development which has made brace treatment easier on the patient, his parents, and the orthopedic surgeon is the recognition that containment treatment can be discontinued before full reconstitution of the femoral head has occurred. Although discussed in 1934,[21] it was only in 1977 that the report by Thompson and Westin [75] clearly demonstrated the efficacy of discontinuing treatment once a buttress of reconstituted bone formed on the anterolateral portion of the femoral head. Another report advocated stopping treatment once the sclerotic bone is eradicated.[47] The author uses both concepts in determining the time to stop therapy. Once the dense bone has been completely resorbed, brace use is discontinued at night, and with formation of a buttress of new bone on the anterolateral portion of the epiphysis full weight-bearing activities are started (Fig. 11–3D and E). By using these indicators brace treatment has been considerably shortened and now ranges from 9 to 18 months, a factor which significantly enhances acceptance of brace treatment.

Braces such as the ischial weight-bearing models have not been proven to be effective.[54] Weight-relieving devices such as crutches or a Snyder sling are not as effective as a containment abduction orthosis. Although these devices do not provoke the nonphysiological stresses seen with ischial weight-bearing braces, they do not provide adequate containment and a child cannot be expected to consistently utilize them in the non–weight-bearing attitude. Kelly et al.[40] did find the Snyder sling to be acceptable for the child under 6 years of age; however, even in this age group the Scottish Rite orthosis is probably a better alternative as it not only provides effective containment of the femoral head, but also allows greater activity level and more effective ambulation than the Snyder sling.

Treatment by Containment—Surgery

The role of surgery in containment therapy for Legg Perthes' disease remains controversial. Both pelvic and femoral osteotomies have been advocated as the primary treatment modality; however, the superiority of either approach remains debatable. The theoretical studies by Rab et al.[58,59] raised questions about both pelvic and femoral osteotomies as adequate therapy. Rab et al.[58,59] used a computerized model to study containment and joint reaction forces in the theoretical young child's hip altered by an innominate osteotomy and a 15° varus plus 15° derotation osteotomy. Neither procedure altered the mechanical stress on the epiphysis, and with extensive necrosis both failed to significantly shield the necrotic area from stress. During gait, the varus derotation osteotomy increased lateral and anterior femoral head cover-

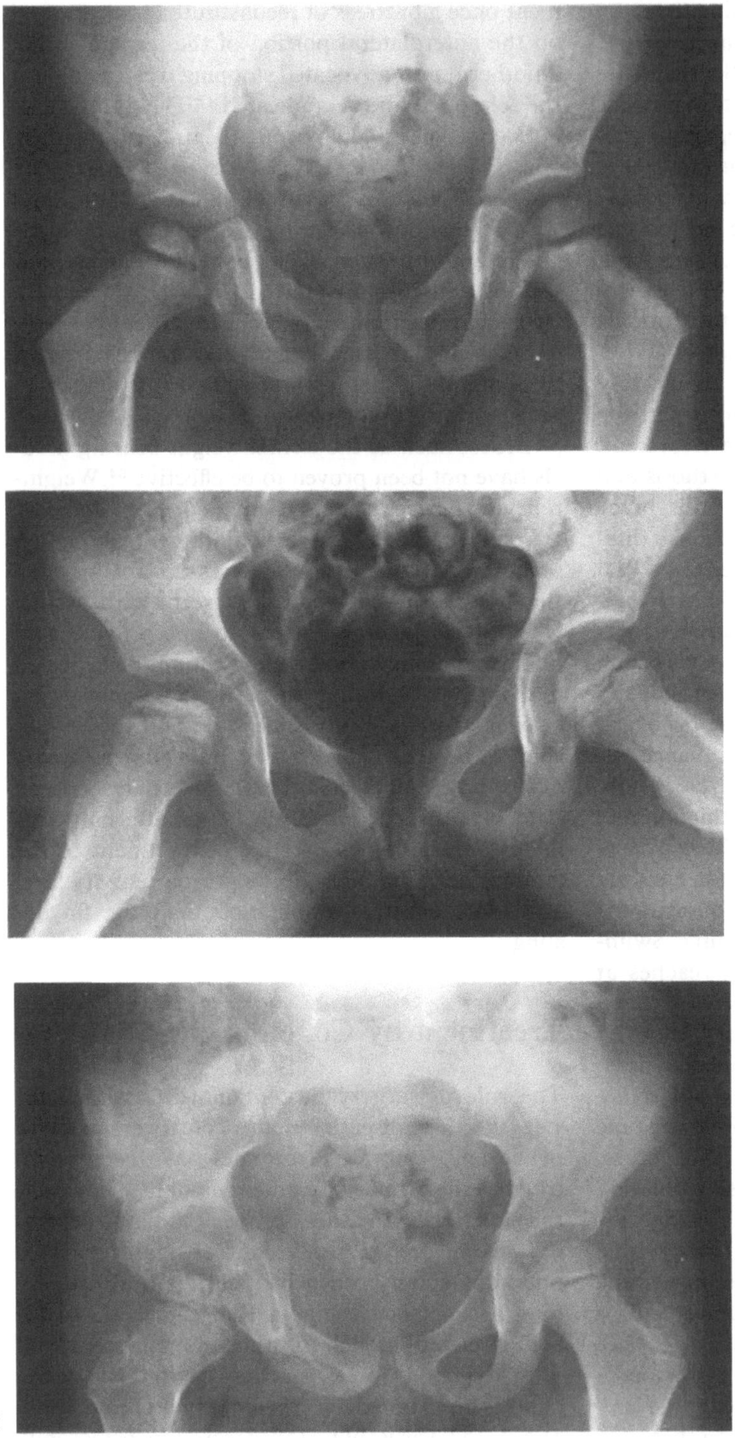

A B C

FIG. 11–10 AP (**A**) and frog-leg (**B**) views of the pelvis of a female, aged 3 years and 8 months, with right Perthes' involvement. For social reasons surgical treatment was used. Photographs courtesy of Dr. Thomas S. Renshaw. **C** AP pelvis, 8 months after innominate osteotomy. (*Cont.*).

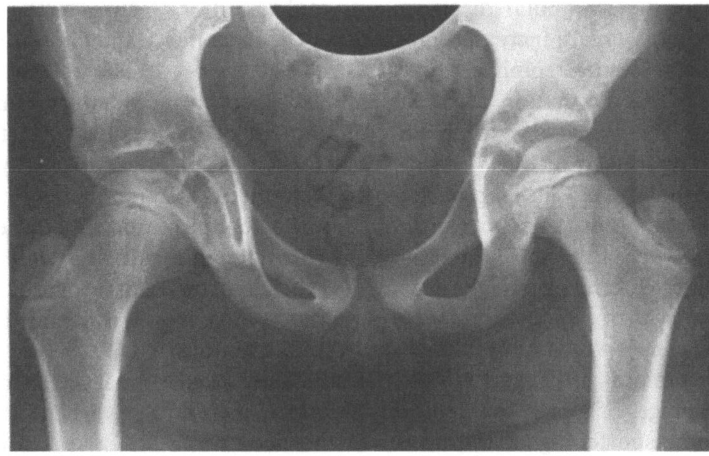

FIG. 11–10 (*Cont.*). **D** AP pelvis, 3 years after surgery, showing good result.

age in proportion to the varus and derotation achieved at surgery. The innominate osteotomy increased anterior coverage by 25° and the lateral coverage varied from a 5° increase at heel strike to 15° at midstance. Both osteotomies altered coverage in one direction at the expense of coverage in the opposite direction. Despite the controversy, surgical treatment needs to be considered when effective containment cannot be obtained by the brace or when psychological or social difficulties make brace wearing impossible.

Experience with pelvic osteotomy in Legg Perthes' disease is primarily with the innominate osteotomy described by Salter.[64] As a primary treatment, innominate osteotomy was advocated for a child more than 6 years of age, for a child with total femoral head involvement or subluxation of the femoral head, and for a child who was unable to cooperate with an abduction brace.[64] A contraindication to the use of innominate osteotomy was preexisting deformity in the femoral head as defined by arthrography. Canale et al.[9] used a modified innominate osteotomy treatment. In their modified osteotomy a quadrangular rather than a triangular graph was used so that better acetabular coverage could be obtained by lateral as well as anterior displacement. Salter [65] reports better results with the innominate osteotomy compared to abduction bracing. In their initial report, the group using the modified innominate osteotomy obtained better results with the pelvic osteotomy; [9] however, a subsequent follow-up report on those patients followed to skeletal maturity demonstrated slightly better results in the control series treated with abduction brace and bed rest.[14]

Although the innominate osteotomy would seem to be a good solution for containment in Legg Perthes' disease, the actual results have not been as pleasing as one would hope. In the author's experience, patients treated by this osteotomy who had met the prerequisites for surgery too often had recurrent synovitis and pain. Recurrent synovitis after an innominate osteotomy may result from inferior displacement of the acetabular rim causing increased pressure on the osteonecrotic anterolateral margin of the femoral epiphysis. This clinical impression has also been confirmed by Kehl and Coleman [39] who reported that containment by nonsurgical techniques or by innominate osteotomy demonstrated similar radiographic results, but the hips treated by osteotomy had decreased functional results with an increased incidence of pain and a decreased range of motion in adult life.

In the author's experience, the only patients who have consistently responded well to containment treatment by the innominate osteotomy are those less than 5 years of age (Fig. 11–10). Of course, this group has the best results under any treatment regimen and now, with the development of the Scottish Rite orthosis, effective ambulation treatment is possible even in this age group. In younger children, the recurrent postoperative synovitis sometimes seen after an innominate osteotomy does not seem to be a problem. Perhaps this is because more effective anterior and lateral displacement of the acetabulum is possible in a younger child when doing a Salter osteotomy. For the child who has subluxation, innominate osteotomy may not be advisable at any age, since in this situation, the acetabular displacement would be more likely to create increased pressure on the osteonecrotic femoral epiphysis.

Varus derotation proximal femoral osteotomy has also been used to obtain containment of the femoral head in Legg-Perthes' disease. A possible advantage of this approach is the better control of containment possible with a femoral osteotomy compared to a pelvic osteotomy. A proximal femoral osteotomy also might decompress the disturbed patterns of venous drainage [73] and venous hypertension [33] which have been observed in the femoral metaphysis in Legg-Perthes' disease. The disadvantages of a proximal femoral osteotomy include some shortening of the limb and the need for a second major procedure to remove internal fixation devices. Another possible disadvantage includes the at least temporary weakening of the hip abductor muscles by the varus positioning of the femoral neck.

Several authors have described the use of proximal femoral osteotomy as an effective treatment for Legg-Perthes' disease.[1,35,44,46] From these reports femoral osteotomy emerges as a possible treatment alternative, but whether the osteotomy is the best treatment cannot be proven because of deficiencies in the studies which include lack of a control series treated by an effective abduction orthosis, inadequate definition of the extent of femoral head necrosis and subluxation, and the lack of objective, reproducible criteria in measuring the results. Despite the persistent questions, the author favors the femoral osteotomy but only when brace therapy is absolutely not possible. The better control in placing the femoral head in the desired position of containment, the possibility of decompressing venous hypertension, the possibility of eliminating hinging of the femoral head on abduction, and the decreased incidence of recurrent synovitis make a femoral osteotomy the preferable surgical alternative in the author's opinion.

Klisic [42] advocates the femoral osteotomy for the child with extrusion, particularly if the child is over 7 years of age. For patients without subluxation, Klisic thought that the possible undesirable sequelae such as joint incongruity and trochanteric elevation made the femoral osteotomy less suitable, but that with subluxation the best treatment was a 15° varus and a 20° derotation femoral osteotomy followed by abduction bracing. This relatively small degree of varization would minimize pressure on the femoral head,[6] shortening of the leg, and undesirable elevation of the greater trochanter. The author would not view extrusion as the primary determinant in selecting femoral osteotomy since some femoral heads with extrusion may be satisfactorily contained with traction followed by abduction bracing. However, some femoral heads, usually those with marked extrusion and some flattening, will show hinging with abduction on the arthrogram study. In this situation, brace treatment may be inadequate and better results may be achieved with the femoral osteotomy as a primary treatment (Fig. 11–11).

When doing a femoral osteotomy for Legg-Perthes' disease, whether as an alternative treatment to bracing or as a means to correct hinging on abduction, the use of arthrography is a definite aid in planning the optimal position of the femoral head. Any areas of femoral head flattening should be positioned to allow full containment without pressure from the acetabular margins. Most authors advocate 15–20° of derotation with the degree of varization ranging from 20 to 30°.[1,35,42,44,46] If excessive varus is required to contain the femoral head, then the use of an abduction orthosis post-surgery may be helpful in allowing one to excise less of a wedge and cause less problems with limb shortening and hip abductor weakening.

The author prefers the Newington plate designed by James Cary [10] for fixation of a femoral osteotomy in Legg-Perthes' disease (Fig. 11–11). This plate can be inserted into the femoral neck with less force than is frequently required with other fixation devices used in children, a feature that may give some protection to the avascular epiphysis. The Newington plate also medially displaces the distal femur, thereby providing mechanical advantage for the hip abductor musculature that has been at least temporarily weakened by varization of the femoral neck. Other advantages of this plate include the fact that when removed, its size minimizes weakening of the femur compared to other devices, and the plate can be used with whatever wedge is desired.

Other fixation devices such as a Coventry plate and screw or the ASIF plate have been utilized with success for proximal femoral osteotomies in children. Probably more important than the type of fixation device chosen is the planning and execution of the osteotomy so that the most effective positioning of the femoral head can be achieved.

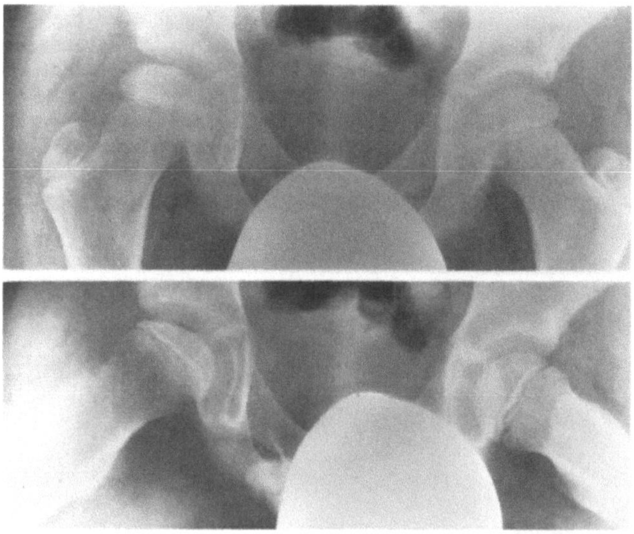

A

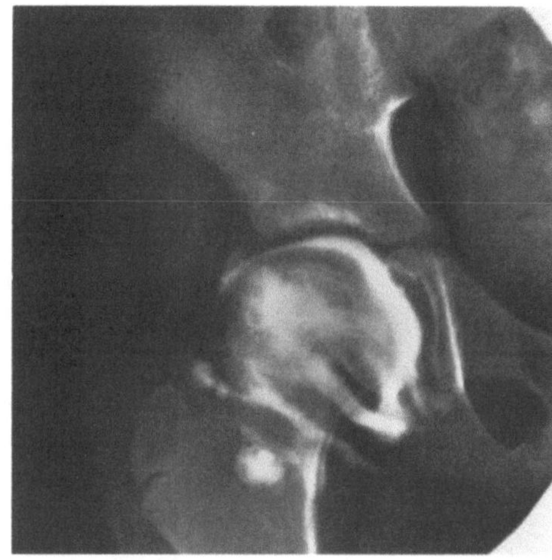

B

FIG. 11–11 **A** AP and lateral (frog-leg) pelvis of a 9-year-old male who presented with poor prognosis due to age, Catterall type III deformity, and epiphyseal extrusion as indicated by an acetabulum–head index of 84. Photographs courtesy of Dr. James M. Cary. **B** Arthrogram shows further evidence of poor prognosis with flattening of the femoral head. Other views showed hinging on abduction. **C** AP pelvis 4 months after varus derotation osteotomy using Newington plate. No postoperative orthosis used. Epiphyseal extrusion has decreased. **D** AP and lateral (frog-leg) pelvis at age 14. Mose circle measurements indicate fair roentgenographic result, but joint congruity probably would be better with osteotomy than brace therapy in this situation.

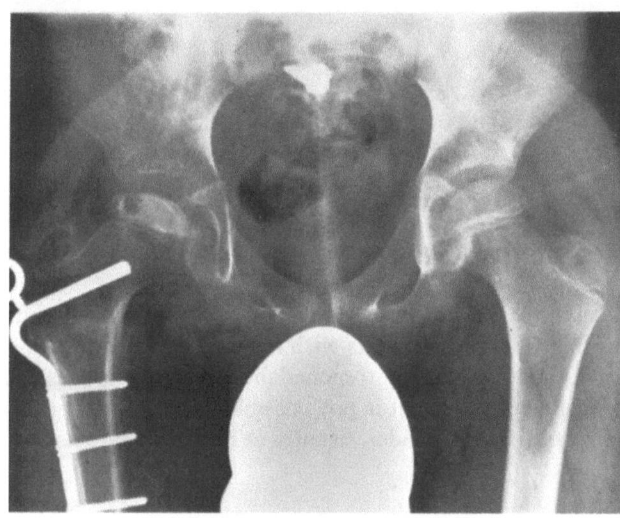

C

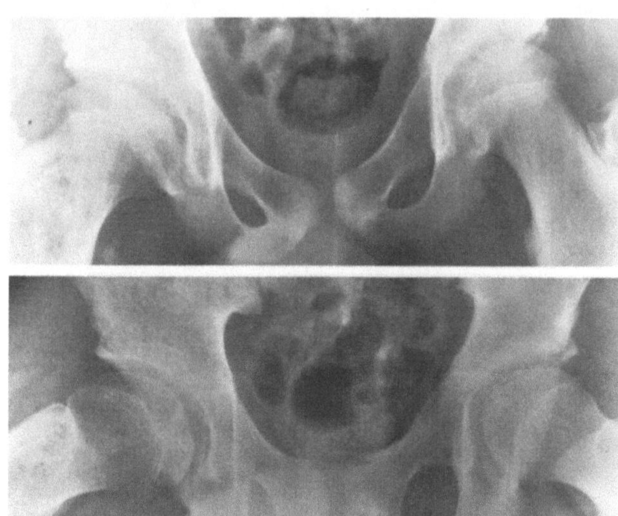

D

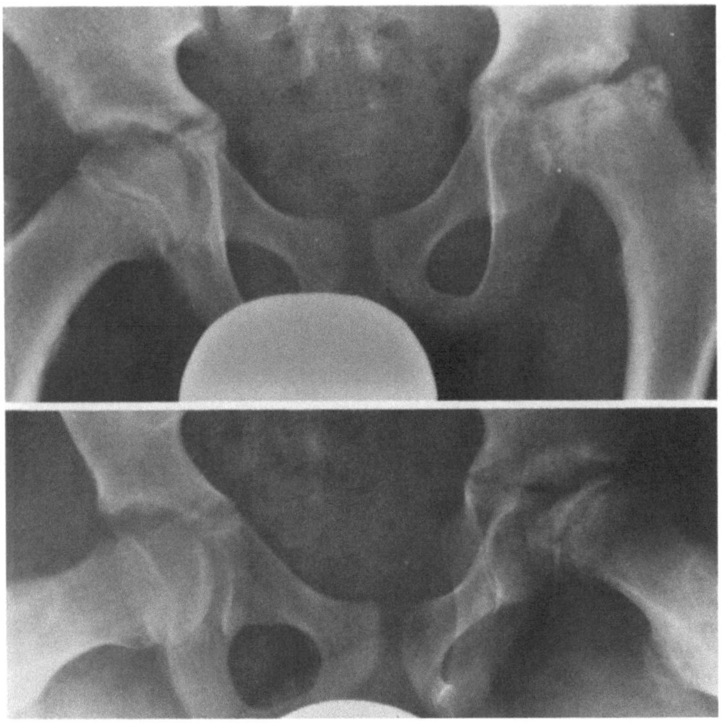

FIG. 11–12 AP and lateral (frog-leg) pelvis of a male, aged 13 years and 11 months, who presented with an 8-month history of left hip pain. Radiographs show saddle-shaped femoral head deformity. Prognosis is poor. Salvage procedure such as partial capitectomy should await resolution of osteonecrosis.

Treatment—Containment Not Possible

For the child who presents with marked extrusion and a saddle hump or trenched head deformity, containment treatment is not possible. These children are frequently older, usually at least 10 years of age. In this situation, trying to force the femoral head into the acetabulum only intensifies crushing and further collapse (Fig. 11–12). The prognosis for a good result is obviously very limited, and salvage treatment is the only alternative. A cheilectomy or partial capitectomy as described by Garceau [26] may remove the bony block which is

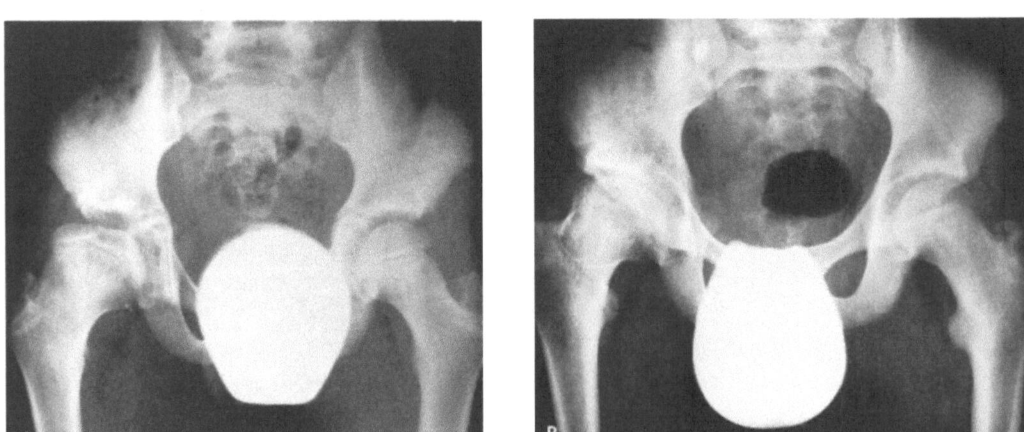

FIG. 11–13 **A** Eleven-year-old male, who had worn a caliper for 1 year, was admitted for pain and limp. **B** Same patient following Garceau procedure of excising bulging part of the head. No pain was encountered in the following 6 years.

markedly limiting hip abduction and internal rotation. If this procedure is done before reossification is complete, further osteonecrosis and synovitis may result.[48,60] The partial capitectomy may improve femoral head congruity, and with a meticulous postoperative plan of traction, exercises, and protective weight bearing, the range of hip motion may be significantly improved (Fig. 11–13). For the patient with painful sequelae of Legg-Perthes' disease in late adolescence or adult life, other salvage treatment such as arthrodesis or Chiari osteotomy may be indicated.

Bibliography

1. Axer, A., Gershuni, D. H., Hendel, D., and Mirovski, Y.: Indications for femoral osteotomy in Legg-Calvé-Perthes disease. Clin. Orthop., 150:78, 1980.
2. Barker, D. J. P., Dixon, E., and Taylor, J. F.: Perthes' disease of the hip in three regions of England. J. Bone Joint Surg., 60B:478, 1978.
3. Blakemore, M. E., and Harrison, M. H. M.: A prospective study of children with untreated Catterall Group 1 Perthes' disease. J. Bone Joint Surg., 61B:329, 1979.
4. Bobechko, W. P., McLaurin, C. A., and Motloch, W.: Toronto orthosis for Legg-Perthes disease. Artif. Limbs, 12:36, 1968.
5. Brotherton, B. J., and McKibbin, B.: Perthes' disease treated by prolonged recumbency and femoral head containment: A long-term appraisal. J. Bone Joint Surg. 59B:8, 1977.
6. Brown, T. D., and Ferguson, A. B.: The development of a computational stress analysis of the femoral head. J. Bone Joint Surg., 60A:619, 1978.
7. Burwell, G., Dangerfield, P. H., Hall, D. J., Vernon, C. L., and Harrison, M. H. M.: Perthes' disease. J. Bone Joint Surg., 60B:461, 1978.
8. Calvé, J.: Sur une forme particuliere de coxalgie greffee sur des deformantions caracteristiques de l'extremité superieure du femur. Rev. Chir., 42:54, 1910.
9. Canale, S. T., D'Anca, A. F., Cotler, J. M., and Snedden, H. E.: Innominate osteotomy in Legg-Calvé-Perthes disease. J. Bone Joint Surg., 54A:25, 1972.
10. Cary, J. M.: Personal communication, 1977.
11. Catterall, A.: The natural history of Perthes' disease. J. Bone Joint Surg., 53B:37, 1971.
12. Chung, S. M. K.: The arterial supply of the developing proximal end of the human femur. J. Bone Joint Surg. 58A:961, 1976.
13. Clarke, T. E., Finnegan, T. L., Fisher, R. L., Bunch, W. H., and Gossling, H. R.: Legg-Perthes' disease in children less than four years old. J. Bone Joint Surg., 60A:166, 1978.
14. Cotler, J. M., and Donahue, J.: Innominate osteotomy in the treatment of Legg-Calvé-Perthes disease. Clin. Orthop., 150:95, 1980.
15. Curtis, B. H.: Personal communication, 1977.
16. Curtis, B. H., Gunther, S. F., Gossling, H. R., and Paul, S. W.: Treatment for Legg-Perthes' disease with the Newington ambulation-abduction brace. J. Bone Joint Surg., 56A:1135, 1974.
17. Danigelis, J. A., Fisher, R. L., Ozonoff, M. B., and Sziklas, J. J.: ^{99m}Tc-Polyphosphate bone imaging in Legg-Perthes' disease. Radiology, 115:407, 1975.
18. Dickens, D. R. V., and Menelaus, M.B.: The assessment of prognosis in Perthes' disease. J. Bone Joint Surg., 60B:189, 1978.
19. Dolman, C. L., Bell, H. M.: The pathology of Legg-Calvé-Perthes disease. J. Bone Joint Surg., 55A:184, 1973.
20. Donovan, M. M., and Urquhart, B. A.: Legg-Calvé-Perthes syndrome. Treatment with ambulatory abduction brace. Orthop. Rev., 8:147, 1979.
21. Ferguson, A. B., and Howorth, M. B.: Coxa plana and related conditions of the hip. J. Bone Joint Surg., 16A:781, 1934.
22. Fisher, R. L.: An epidemiological study of Legg-Perthes' disease. J. Bone Joint Surg., 54A:769, 1972.
23. Fisher, R. L., Roderique, J. W., Brown, D. C., Danigelis, J. A., Ozonoff, M. B., and Sziklas, J. J.: The relationship of isotopic bone imaging findings to prognosis in Legg-Perthes' disease. Clin. Orthop., 150:23, 1980.
24. Gage, H. C.: A possible early sign of Perthes' disease. Br. J. Radiol., 6:295, 1933.
25. Gage, J. R., and Cary, J. M.: The effects of trochanteric epiphyseodesis on growth of the proximal end of the femur following necrosis of the capital femoral epiphysis. J. Bone Joint Surg., 62A:785, 1980.
26. Garceau, G. J.: Surgical treatment of coxa plana. J. Bone Joint Surg., 46B:779, 1964.
27. Gershuni, D. H., Axer, A., and Hendel, D.: Arthrographic findings in Legg-Calvé-Perthes disease and transient synovitis of the hip. J. Bone Joint Surg., 60A:457, 1978.
28. Girdany, B. R., and Osman, M. Z.: Longitudinal growth and skeletal maturation in Perthes' disease. Radiol. Clin. North Am., Vol. 6:245, 1968.
29. Glimcher, M. J., and Kenzora, J. E.: The biology of osteonecrosis of the human femoral head and its clinical implications. I. Tissue biology. Clin. Orthop., 138:284, 1979.
30. Glimcher, M. J., and Kenzora, J. E.: The biology of osteonecrosis of the human femoral head and its clinical implications. II. The pathological

changes in the femoral head as an organ and in the hip joint. Clin. Orthop., 139:283, 1979.
31. Goff, C. W.: Legg-Calvé-Perthes Syndrome and Related Osteochondroses of Youth. Springfield, Ill., Thomas, 1954.
32. Green, N. E., Beauchamp, R. D., and Griffin, P. P.: Epiphyseal extrusion as a prognostic index in Legg-Calvé-Perthes disease. J. Bone Joint Surg., 63A:900, 1981.
33. Green, N. E., and Griffin, P. P.: Intraosseous venous hypertension in Legg-Perthes' disease. Orthop. Trans., 5:407, 1981.
34. Harrison, M. H. M., Turner, M. H., and Jacobs, P.: Skeletal immaturity in Perthes' disease. J. Bone Joint Surg., 58B:37, 1976.
35. Heikkinen, E., and Puranen, J.: Evaluation of femoral osteotomy in the treatment of Legg-Calvé-Perthes disease. Clin. Orthop., 150:60, 1980.
36. Inoue, A., Freeman, M. A. R., Vernon-Roberts, B., and Mizuno, S.: The pathogenesis of Perthes' disease. J. Bone Joint Surg., 58B:453, 1976.
37. Jensen, O. M., and Lauritzen, J.: Legg-Calvé-Perthes' disease. Morphological studies in two cases examined at necropsy. J. Bone Joint Surg., 58B:332, 1976.
38. Kamhi, E., and MacEwen, G. D.: Treatment of Legg-Calvé-Perthes disease. J. Bone Joint Surg., 57A:651, 1975.
39. Kehl, D. K., and Coleman, S. S.: An evaluation of Perthes' disease. Comparison of non-surgical and surgical treatment. Orthop. Trans., 5:407, 1981.
40. Kelly, F. B., Canale, S. T., and Jones, R. R.: Legg-Calvé-Perthes disease. Long-term evaluation of non-containment treatment. J. Bone Joint Surg., 62A:400, 1980.
41. King, E. W., Fisher, R. L., Gage, J. R., and Gossling, H. R.: Ambulation-abduction treatment in Legg-Calvé-Perthes disease. Clin. Orthop., 150:43, 1980.
42. Klisic, P., Blazevic, U., and Seferovic, O.: Approach to treatment of Legg-Calvé-Perthes disease. Clin. Orthop, 150:54, 1980.
43. LaMont, R. L., Muz, J., Heilbronner, D., and Bouwhuis, J. A.: Quantitative assessment of femoral head involvement in Legg-Calvé-Perthes disease. J. Bone Joint Surg., 63A:746, 1981.
44. Laurent, L. E., and Poussa, M.: Intertrochanteric varus osteotomy in the treatment of Perthes' disease. Clin. Orthop., 150:73, 1980.
45. Legg, A. T.: An obscure affectation of the hip joint. Boston Med. J., 162:202, 1910.
46. Lloyd-Roberts, G. C., Catterall, A., and Salamon, P. B.: A controlled study of the indications for and the results of femoral osteotomy in Perthes' disease. J. Bone Joint Surg., 58B:31, 1976.
47. MacEwen, G. D.: Value of prognostic evaluation in Legg-Calvé-Perthes syndrome. Orthop. Rev., 8:173, 1979.
48. McKay, D. W.: Cheilectomy of the hip. Orthop. Clin. North Am., 11:141, 1980.
49. McKibbin, B., and Ralis, Z.: Pathological changes in a case of Perthes' disease. J. Bone Joint Surg., 56B:438, 1974.
50. Molloy, M. K., and MacMahon, B.: Incidence of Legg-Perthes' disease (osteochondritis deformans). N. Engl. J. Med., 275:988, 1966.
51. Mose, K.: Legg-Calvé-Perthes disease, a comparison among three methods of conservative treatment. Arhus, Universitetsforlaget, 1964.
52. Mose, K.: Methods of measuring in Legg-Calvé-Perthes disease with special regard to the prognosis. Clin. Orthop., 150:103, 1980.
53. Mose, K., Hjorth, L., Ulfeldt, M., Christensen, E. R., and Jensen, A.: Legg-Calvé-Perthes disease. The late occurrence of coxarthrosis. Acta Orthop. Scand. (Suppl.) 169:1, 1977.
54. O'Hara, J. P., Davis, N. D., Gage, J. R., Sundberg, A. B., and Winter, R. B.: Long-term follow-up of Perthes' disease treated nonoperatively. Clin. Orthop., 125:49, 1977.
55. Perthes, G.: Uber arthritis deformans juvenilis. Dtsch. Z. Chir., 10:111, 1910.
56. Petrie, J. G., and Bitenc, I.: The abduction weight-bearing treatment in Legg-Perthes' disease. J. Bone Joint Surg., 53B:54, 1971.
57. Purvis, J. M., Dimon, J. H., Meehan, P. L., and Lovell, W. W.: Preliminary experience with the Scottish Rite Hospital abduction orthosis for Legg-Perthes' disease. Clin. Orthop., 150:49, 1980.
58. Rab, G. T.: Containment of the hip: A theoretical comparison of osteotomies. Clin. Orthop., 154:191, 1981.
59. Rab, G. T., DeNatale, J. S., and Herrmann, L. R.: Three-dimensional finite element analysis of Legg-Calvé-Perthes disease. J. Pediatr. Orthop. 1:39, 1982.
60. Roberts, J. M., Meehan, P. L., and Mendez, S.: Partial capitectomy: A salvage procedure for the uncontainable deformity in Legg-Calvé-Perthes disease. Orthop. Trans., 4:333, 1980.
61. Roberts, J. M., and Zink, W. P.: Arthrographic classification in Legg-Perthes' disease. Exhibit, American Academy of Orthopaedic Surgeons Annual Meeting, Las Vegas, 1981.
62. Robichon, J., Desjardins, J. P., Koch, M., and Hooper, C. E.: The femoral neck in Legg-Perthes' disease. J. Bone Joint Surg., 56B:62, 1974.
63. Salter, R. B.: Experimental and clinical aspects of Perthes' disease. J. Bone Joint Surg., 48B:393, 1966.
64. Salter, R. B.: Treatment by innominate osteotomy.

The American Academy of Orthopaedic Surgeons Instructional Course Lectures, Vol. 22. St. Louis, Mosby, 1973, p. 309.
65. Salter, R. B.: Legg-Perthes' disease: The scientific basis for the methods of treatment and their indications. Clin. Orthop., 150:8, 1980.
66. Salter, R. B., and Bell, M.: The pathogenesis of deformity in Legg-Perthes' disease—an experimental investigation. J. Bone Joint Surg., 50B:436, 1968.
67. Salter, R. B., and Thompson, G. H.: Legg-Calvé-Perthes disease: Significance of the subchondral fracture. Orthop. Trans., 4:333, 1980.
68. Sanchis, M., Zahir, A., and Freeman, M. A. R.: The experimental simulation of Perthes' disease by consecutive interruptions of the blood supply to the capital femoral epiphysis in the puppy. J. Bone Joint Surg., 55A:335, 1973.
69. Snyder, C. R.: Legg-Perthes' disease in the young hip—does it necessarily do well? J. Bone Joint Surg., 57A:751, 1975.
70. Spranger, J.: The epiphyseal dysplasias. Clin. Orthop., 114:46, 1976.
71. Stulberg, S. D., Cooperman, D. R., and Wallensten, R.: The natural history of Legg-Calvé-Perthes disease. J. Bone Joint Surg., 63A:1095, 1981.
72. Stulberg, S. D., and Salter, R. B.: The natural course of Legg-Perthes' disease and its relationship to degenerative arthritis of the hip: A long-term follow-up study. Orthop. Trans., 1:105, 1977.
73. Suramo, I., Puranen, J., Heikkinen, E., and Vuorinen, P.: Disturbed patterns of venous drainage of the femoral neck in Perthes' disease. J. Bone Joint Surg., 56B:448, 1974.
74. Sutherland, A. D., Savage, J. P., Paterson, D. C., and Foster, B. K.: The nuclide bone-scan in the diagnosis and management of Perthes' disease. J. Bone Joint Surg., 62B:300, 1980.
75. Thompson, G. H., and Westin, G. W.: Legg-Calvé-Perthes disease—results of discontinuing treatment in the early reossification phase. Presented at the First International Symposium on Legg-Calvé-Perthes disease. Los Angeles, 1977.
76. Trueta, J.: The normal vascular anatomy of the human femoral head during growth. J. Bone Joint Surg., 39B:358, 1957.
77. Van Dam, B. E., Crider, R. J., Noyes, J. D., and Larsen, L. J.: Determination of the Catterall classification in Legg-Calvé-Perthes disease. J. Bone Joint Surg., 63A:906, 1981.
78. Wynne-Davies, R., and Gormley, J.: The aetiology of Perthes' disease. J. Bone Joint Surg., 60B:6, 1978.

CHAPTER 12

Slipped Capital Femoral Epiphysis

DENNIS R. WENGER

Slipped capital femoral epiphysis (SCFE) is a relatively common adolescent disorder whose description predated the radiographic era. Ambrose Pare is credited for the first clinical description in 1572 with methods for surgical treatment appearing in the late nineteenth century.[15,18] According to Howorth,[15] Keetley described a subtrochanteric femoral osteotomy in 1888 and Sturrock described pin fixation of the slipped epiphysis in 1894. The two significant complications associated with SCFE were described by Axhausen [2] in 1922 (avascular necrosis [AVN]) and Waldenstrom [31] in 1930 (chondrolysis).

The irreversibility of the two complications remains today and has led to the current minimalist philosophy of surgical management. The treatment of SCFE evolved through an era of rising surgical expectations, where keen biomechanical theories, new surgical techniques, and better fixation methods were applied in hope that the production of near normal radiographs would be paralleled by concomitant increased hip function. Unfortunately, this well-intended enthusiasm for anatomical correction led, in many cases, to worse rather than improved hip function. More recent long-term follow-up studies [6,25] have verified the superiority of limited surgical intervention, indicating that the most biologically acceptable method for correcting a gradually displacing epiphysis is by in situ fixation with only partial return to normal anatomy via the process of remodeling.

The purpose of this chapter is to describe a current, widely accepted treatment philosophy that provides maximum function with the least risk for the relatively irreversible processes of avascular necrosis and chondrolysis.

Etiology

The etiology of SCFE is unclear; however, certain patterns permit assumptions to be made. The disorder occurs in adolescence, and 80% of patients are male. Bilateral involvement appears in about 25% of children; however, this figure is thought to be higher by some authors who carefully scrutinize contralateral radiographs.[23]

Most slips develop during a period of rapid growth, which is associated with three biomechanical changes. First, the relatively horizontal orientation of the growth plate seen in the juvenile period changes to a more vertical orientation in adolescence; second, adolescence is a period of rapid weight gain; and third, the periosteum and perichondrial ring of the femoral neck and proximal femoral physis thin during adolescence. These factors contribute to greater shear stresses across the growth plate. In addition to the normal rapid increase in body weight at this age, most children who develop SCFE are obese, providing an even greater mechanical stress to the vertically oriented physis.

Because SCFE occurs in adolescence and primarily in males, hormonal factors are thought to be involved. The two classic somatotypes noted in patients with SCFE include an obese, hypogonadal (Freulich) type, whom Harris [13] suggested may have a deficiency of sex hormone (testosterone) for his chronologic age, resulting in a relative increased effect of growth hormone. A less common somatotype is the tall, thin, "marfanoid" adolescent who may have a relative excess of growth hormone as compared to testosterone levels.[13] In both instances, the growth plate would be influenced by the relative excess of growth hormone, which has been demonstrated to decrease the shear strength of the growth plate.[13,26] The final pathway by which the hormonal imbalance produces weakness may be a decrease in collagen formation with a relative increase of intracellular matrix in the physis resulting in physeal weakening.[17] Currently available laboratory methods have not substantiated the proposed hormonal imbalance; thus, no medical treatment is advised (e.g., hormones).

Specific acute trauma as the sole etiologic agent for SCFE is unlikely, even in patients with an acute slip. Children with a true traumatic fracture through the growth plate are often young (birth trauma, child abuse victim) or have received massive trauma (auto accident) with associated severe injuries. Occasionally, an associated metaphyseal fragment (Thurston-Holland sign) identifies the fracture as a Salter–Harris type II. In contrast, acute SCFE occurs in the usual adolescent age group, associated with less severe trauma, involving only the physis and not the metaphysis. The distinction between a true fracture and acute SCFE may be impossible in certain cases. Patients with an acute slip (less than 5% of all SCFE patients) probably have a biomechanical and/or biochemical predisposition to slip with trauma serving only as the final precipitating event. In patients with the more common chronic slip, traumatic episodes are often historically interwoven but probably serve only to precipitate symptoms.

The contribution of endocrine or metabolic disorders to the cause of slips is clearer in patients who have known metabolic or endocrine disorders. Such slips occur at an earlier age (juvenile onset) and are seen in association with renal failure, hypothyroidism, cystinosis, and other systemic diseases. Often the child also has slipping of other physes (e.g., proximal humerus) (Fig. 12–14A and B). Treatment of SCFE in these younger children provides special challenges that will be discussed subsequently.

Valgus slip, which can occur in an otherwise normal child, is rare and probably occurs only in children who already have severe coxa valga.

Diagnostic and Radiographic Patterns

Slipping of the capital femoral epiphysis can be classified both chronologically (chronic, subacute, acute) and anatomically according to the actual degree of slipping as shown radiographically. The chronologic classification describes the duration of hip symptoms prior to presentation (acute, subacute, chronic).

Severity of slip on radiograph may be defined by several classification methods, the simplest being "mild," "moderate," and "severe." Others have divided slip into grades, including grade I (0–33% slip), grade II (33–50% slip), and grade III (greater than 50% slip).[20] Since the grading system requires definition according to percentage of displacement, it seems simpler to use an estimated percentage of slip rather than specific grades.

The often notable difference in percentage of slip on the anteroposterior (AP) versus the lateral radiograph in the same hip further complicates classification. Often the epiphysis migrates primarily posteriorly; thus, only the lateral radiograph provides a good indicator of slip severity. Southwick [30] described a formal method of measuring degree of slip on both the AP and lateral radiographs, using the contralateral normal hip for comparison. These numbers are important in preparing for the corrective subtrochanteric osteotomy that Southwick advises for certain cases. Since corrective osteotomies are rarely needed—as will be discussed—it seems impractical to perform these calculations routinely. Describing the estimated percentage of slip on the view that demonstrates the most severe deformity (usually lateral) seems the most practical method for clinical use.

Routine Radiographs

Both AP and lateral radiographs are mandatory since the AP view often shows little deformity in early cases (Fig. 12–1). The frog-leg view is often used for the lateral film; however, Bonfiglio,[5] who once noted a sudden worsening of the slip when a child was forced into a frog-leg position, advises a cross-table lateral film rather than a frog-leg lateral view. This advice seems reasonable for an acute or subacute slip; however, I have not personally seen slip progression secondary to a child being positioned for a frog-leg view. Another practical problem with the frog-leg view is the symptomatic child's inability to truly position his limb in the frog-leg posture.

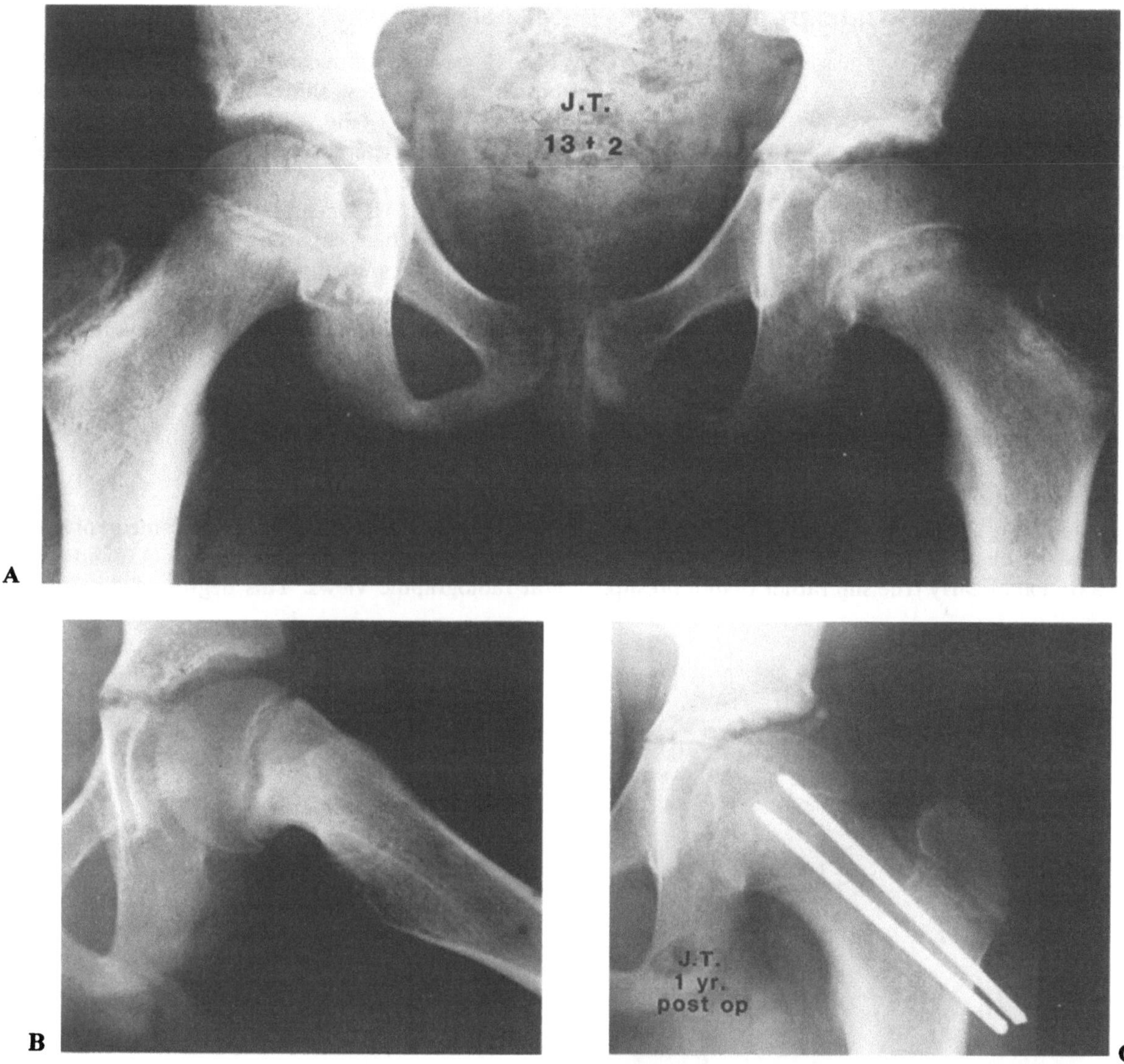

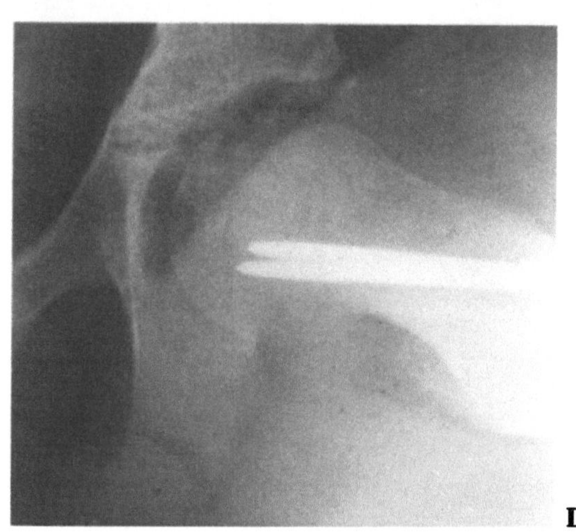

FIG. 12–1 **A** Hip radiographs in an adolescent male with left hip pain. Note the metaphyseal blurring as described by Bloomburg.[4] **B** Lateral view confirms a mild left slip. **C** One year post–in situ pinning with two well-placed pins. Pin position is ideal as the tips are far from the articular surface and the pins diverge. **D** Lateral view demonstrating pin-tip position. The pins cross the physis by about 1 cm.

Chronology and Radiographic Classification

Preslipping Phase

This term is probably a misnomer in that originally the term was used to define widening and irregularity of the physis without true slipping. More recently, Bloomburg,[4] a radiologist, carefully studied the early radiographic characteristics of SCFE and reported that marginal blurring of the proximal metaphysis is a predictable, early radiographic sign. The semilunar crescent of blurring, due to initial posterior displacement of the epiphysis, is commonly seen in early SCFE (Figs. 12–1A and 12–2). Thus, although biochemical changes and abnormal mechanical stresses are present in the preslip phase, the physeal widening previously described as characterizing the preslip phase is a description of early true slip rather than a preslip.

Mild Slipping

The AP view may show only metaphyseal blurring, but the frog-leg view shows clear displacement of the femoral head (Fig. 12–2). Bloomburg,[4] in his radiologic survey, confirmed the value of the step-off on the lateral view as one of the two most dependable factors for early radiographic diagnosis of SCFE, the other being the previously mentioned blurring of the metaphyseal margin. In addition, on the AP view the upper edge of the epiphysis may have dropped below Kline's line, an arbitrary line drawn up the superior edge of the femoral neck (Fig. 12–2).

Severe Slipping

These patients have marked displacement of the femoral head, readily apparent on the AP and lateral radiographic views. This degree of displace-

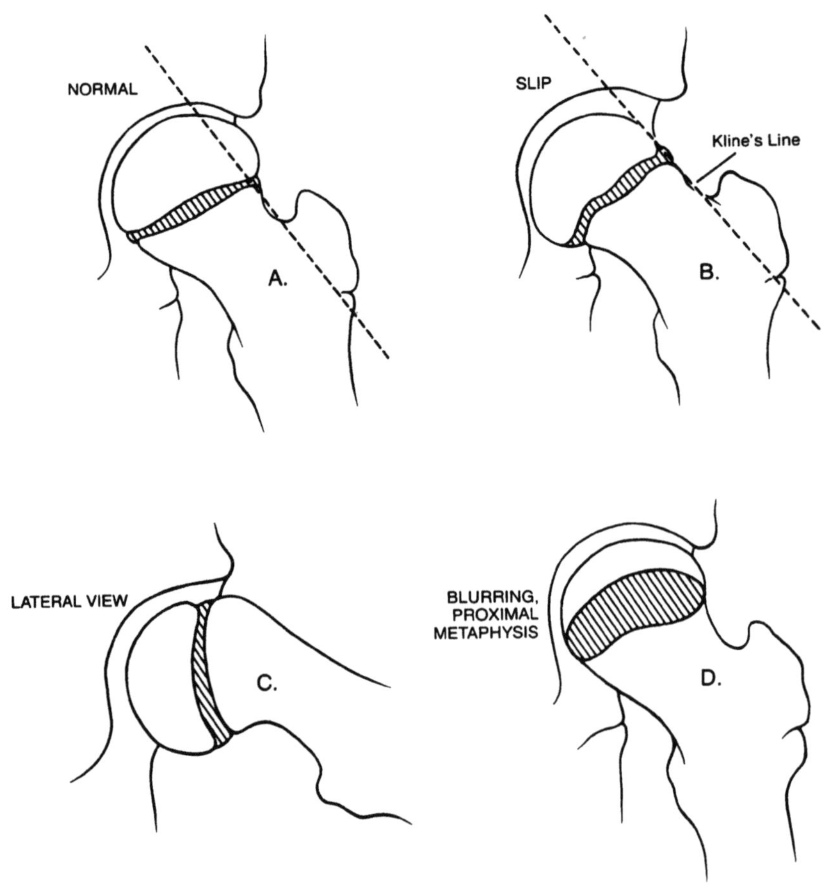

FIG. 12–2 Diagram of radiographic patterns seen in SCFE. **A** Normal hip. **B** SCFE: epiphysis below Kline's line on anteroposterior view. **C** SCFE: posterior displacement on lateral view. **D** SCFE: AP view. Metaphyseal blurring described by Bloomburg.[4]

ment is most commonly seen in patients whose diagnosis has been greatly delayed in a chronic slip or in an acute slip with sudden severe displacement following a traumatic episode.

Establishing Chronicity

As will be discussed later, differentiating between an acute and a chronic slip is of great importance in selecting the correct treatment method. Usually the clinical history and radiographic features must be combined to make an astute decision. Radiographs in an acute slip demonstrate a well-formed femoral head and metaphysis with no "rounding off" of the metaphysis or periosteal new bone. Conversely, chronic slips demonstrate this "rounding off" (remodeling) of the metaphysis and also may have a layering effect due to sequential new bone formation on the posterior metaphyseal margin, noted on the later views. Later, a "hook" formation may be noted as the neck remodels.

Radiographic Perceptual Difficulties in SCFE

Patients with SCFE have externally rotated limbs, yet x-ray films are almost always taken in an AP plane perpendicular to the pelvis. Thus, the so-called AP film of the hip is usually a 45° oblique view of the femoral shaft and neck. Only if the radiographic tube and film cassette are aligned perpendicular to the AP axis of the femur, as determined by flexing the knee to assess the true anteroposterior femoral axis—a so-called Billing's view [1,12]—can an accurate view of the femur be obtained (Fig. 12–3A-C). In many cases, having a distorted AP view does little harm other than producing the misconception that the femoral head in SCFE is commonly displaced medially, whereas a true AP view of the femur will show that in most slips the head displaces posteriorly. The commonly obtained 45° oblique view makes a posterior slip look as though it has a significant medial component. Areas where correct views may matter include preparatory radiographic measurements for the Southwick subtrochanteric osteotomy [30] and in evaluating the effectiveness of traction in reducing acute slips. Occasionally, patients are placed in overnight longitudinal and internal rotation traction after an AP view shows severe medial and posterior slip. Then, a film taken the next day with the femur now internally rotated due to traction forces will show the medial displacement to be "corrected," when in fact only the entire femur plus displaced head has been rotated with no true improvement in the position of the displaced head.

Another radiographic perceptual problem includes assessment of pin-tip position during surgical pinning of SCFE, a subject to be discussed in some detail later. Obtaining clear intraoperative lateral views of the hip in the usually obese adolescent with SCFE continues to be difficult.

Thus, our inability to predictably achieve a clear three-dimensional understanding of both anatomical displacement and intraoperative pin-tip position, because we utilize two-dimensional methods (radiographs) for assessment, is a significant factor in preventing predictable good results in the treatment of SCFE.

Diagnosis and Treatment

Chronic Slipped Capital Femoral Epiphysis

Most children with SCFE will be found to have a chronic slip by the time they see an orthopedist; therefore, this subgroup will be discussed first. The patient complains of a gradual onset of limp and/or pain for several weeks or months prior to the consultation. There may be a recent episode of trauma that exacerbates the pain; however, the slip should be considered chronic if the patient has had symptoms of any type for more than 2 weeks. Although the pain may be localized to the hip or thigh, knee pain is a common complaint, related to referred pain. In some cases, knee pain is the only complaint. Without trauma to the knee, this history should always lead the examiner to suspect hip disease. This classic pattern of hip disease appearing with only knee pain has led to many misdiagnoses when an unwary physician examines and obtains radiographs of only the knee. Because this pattern has been widely understood by orthopedists, until recently few orthopedic surgeons have made this error. The advent of the arthroscope—and the unique sort of tunnel vision that it engenders—is now causing orthopedists to be tricked by the referred pain phenomenon. In the recent past, I have seen three children—two with SCFE and one with Perthes' disease—who had

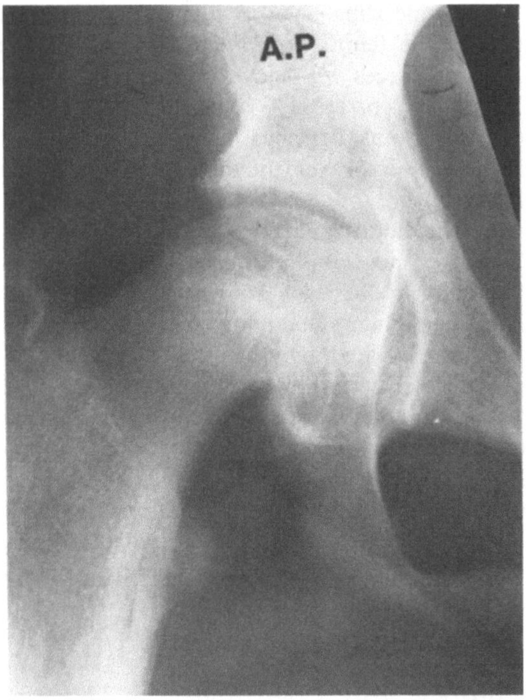

A

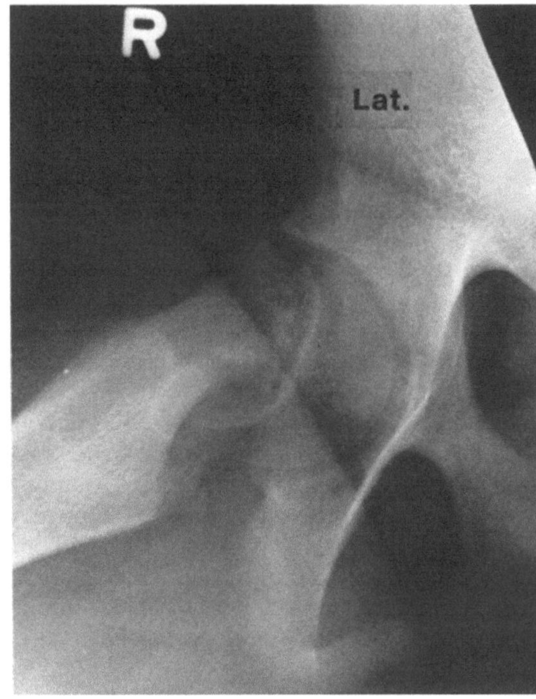

C

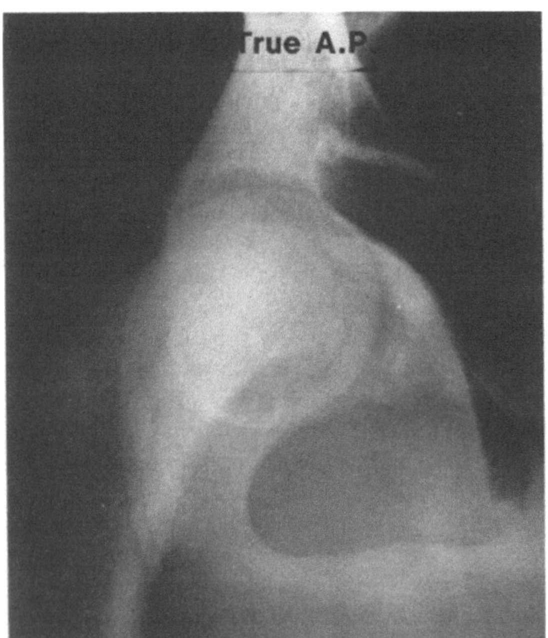

B

FIG. 12–3 **A** So-called AP radiograph of the right hip in a 13-year-old girl with a chronic slip. The slip appears to be at least somewhat medial. Because the girl is holding her limb in external rotation, this is a 40° oblique view, and the slip is actually posterior. **B** A true AP view of the hip taken by elevating the right hip 40° and aligning the radiographic tube and cassette perpendicular to the femur, as determined by flexing the knee 90°. The severe slip is posterior and not medial. **C** Lateral (frog-leg) view, same hip. The patient has an obvious, severe posterior slip.

seen an orthopedist because of knee pain and received only a knee examination (physical and radiographic), followed by hospital admission for arthroscopic examination of the knee. Only subsequently was the true diagnosis of SCFE made by another physician. Orthopedists should heed the age-old advice regarding examination of the hips in a child with knee pain.

The adolescent who has a chronic slip is often obese but occasionally tall and thin with marfanoid features. The affected limb is positioned in external rotation, very much like the limb position of an elderly patient with a femoral neck fracture. The classic diagnostic maneuver involves flexing the hip which automatically tracks into abduction and external rotation. There is little, if any, passive internal rotation of the hip, and in more severe cases, the hip is fixed in external rotation. Patients with chronic slips have only moderate pain with this maneuver, as contrasted to those with acute slips who have severe pain with any motion. The *lateral* radiograph confirms the diagnosis. The radiographs may show evidence of chronicity by exhibiting a "rounding-off" and later a "hook" formation in the proximal metaphysis. Even if the radiograph does not clarify whether the slip is acute or chronic, the history should override the radiographic features. If the child has had symptoms for more than 14 days, the slip is considered to be chronic, although further acute slip may have been superimposed on the chronic component.

Once the diagnosis has been confirmed, plans should be made to surgically stabilize the physis by epiphysiodesis. Patient management during the hours or days between diagnosis and surgical stabilization remains controversial. In general, the hip should be stabilized surgically as soon as possible to avoid further slip. In relatively acute cases, the risk of further slip is greater; thus, immediate hospitalization for skin traction while awaiting surgery is advised. Often the same rather rigid protocol is insisted on for children who have chronic slips with symptoms for months to years. In these patients it seems reasonable to place the child on crutches and allow him to go home, with surgery scheduled on a semiemergency basis during the subsequent several days.

A mandatory 5 to 10 days of preoperative traction to "quiet down the hip" prior to pinning has been advised by some; however, there is no evidence that it benefits a patient with a chronic slip. Preoperative traction for chronic slips, while in situ pinning is planned, seems more a convenient method for limiting patient activity and gaining a spot on the surgery schedule than a treatment method that improves results.

Treatment Choices: Chronic Slip

All patients with SCFE, open physes, and hip symptoms require treatment, no matter how severe the slip. The idea that "it can't really slip much further" is not valid, and symptoms persist until the slip has been stabilized. Although stabilization by epiphysiodesis can be achieved by hip spica immobilization, this method is not advised today. First, maintaining and transporting a massively obese adolescent in a hip spica cast is a severe logistical problem (a pickup truck was required in one case). In addition, epiphysiodesis is not assured by immobilization alone and further slipping may occur during and even after the spica is removed. Moreover, cast immobilization may predispose to chondrolysis in certain instances. Most modern authors advise surgical stabilization which can be achieved by in situ fixation with pins or bone grafts. A second stabilization method includes correction of the deformity by manipulative reduction or corrective osteotomy with pin or plate fixation.

Technique for Operative Pin Fixation

The patient is pinned with a two-plane radiographic control, using either two separate machines or an image intensifier. The patient is placed on a fracture table with moderate longitudinal and internal rotation traction applied to the affected limb without attempting reduction by manipulation or traction. High quality lateral radiographs are mandatory to avoid pin penetration into the articular surface. An alternate method for chronic cases with a relatively stable slip involves the use of a regular operating table with the limb draped free to allow AP and frog-leg lateral positioning of the limb for radiographs taken with a single machine or an image intensifier. Unfortunately, even the latest image intensifier models often have inadequate power to penetrate the pelvis, hip, and so on for clear visualization of the joint in a 200-pound adolescent. Such patients may require traditional two-plane radiography to evaluate the pinning.

Surgical Approach

Through an anterolateral hip approach, pins can be introduced on the anterior surface of the base of the neck, allowing even a severely displaced head to be pinned without exiting and reentering the posterior neck cortex (Fig. 12–4A–D). Learning this near anterior pinning concept is important if severe slips are to be pinned in situ.

Choice of Pins

Cameron et al.[7] have enumerated the difficulties encountered with the many types of internal fixation devices used to stabilize a SCFE. Smith-Petersen nails should not be used because the blunt leading surface may further displace the femoral head. Also, continued physeal growth and further displacement may follow placement of a smooth device across a slipping physis. An acceptable pin should have a sharp tip and threads that will readily engage the displacing head rather than further displacing it.

Pin choice is also determined by need for later pin removal after the physis has fused (1 to 2 years after the original pinning). There are two reasons why many advise pin removal. The first is to avoid a stress riser in the proximal femur that might predispose to a fracture during subsequent sports or trauma; second, despite generally favorable long-term hip function in SCFE patients,[6,25] certain slip patients may require later reconstructive hip surgery that will be more difficult if the pins have not been removed. Thus, removability is an important factor in selecting a fixation device. Pins with threads larger than their smooth shafts (Knowles, Hagie) are difficult to remove several years later, especially if their threads are not designed for reverse cutting. Several manufacturers are developing fixation pins and/or screws that have reverse cutting threads, and these should be considered. A good choice is a large (4.8-mm diameter) completely threaded Steinmann pins with a trochar tip. The diamond tip may cut better at insertion, but the broad flat surface, when covered with strong new bone, may make removal difficult (Fig. 12–5). One should be certain to clearly understand the traditional terminology used to describe pin tips because the pyramid-shaped trochar tip looks more like a diamond than does the so-called diamond tip (Fig. 12–5).

How Many Pins?

Traditional advice has been to place at least three pins deep into the femoral head. I believe that two pins adequately control transitional and rotatory displacement and have not experienced further slip with this method (Fig. 12–1C and D). Certain orthopedists contend that one stout, threaded Steinmann pin is adequate, but I have had no experience with this method and therefore cannot advise it.

Pin-tip Position in the Femoral Head

The pins should cross the physis, directed medially and posteriorly (Fig. 12–4A–D). The area under the superior weight-bearing articular surface should be avoided as this is the first area to collapse if avascular necrosis (AVN) should ensue. A second issue concerns the danger of introducing and actually leaving the pin tips in the joint. Most orthopedists first learned to pin hips via elderly patients with femoral neck fractures. They were taught to place the pin tip deeply for purchase on the subchondral plate because the cancellous bone of an osteoporotic femoral head provides little purchase. Transferring this practice to SCFE is not necessary since children have dense femoral heads. One centimeter penetration beyond the physis (in any one radiographic plane) should be adequate, and in many severely displaced cases the pins may appear not to cross the plate in one of the two radiographic planes (Fig. 12–4B). This position is satisfactory and preferred to risking overpenetration with articular cartilage damage.

The question of joint penetration by the fixation pins is an interesting and changing issue. Traditional teaching suggested that one should avoid even temporary intraoperative penetration (Fig. 12–6), of articular cartilage because the penetration might predispose to chondrolysis, perhaps via an immunological mechanism. Although the immunological theory for etiology of chondrolysis remains intact,[23] few believe that temporary intraoperative pin penetration into the joint has any adverse sequelae, although fortunately even temporary penetration can usually be avoided by using an image intensifier.

The current concern about pins centers on the danger of not only temporarily introducing them into the joint at surgery but actually leaving them permanently in the joint because of failure to ob-

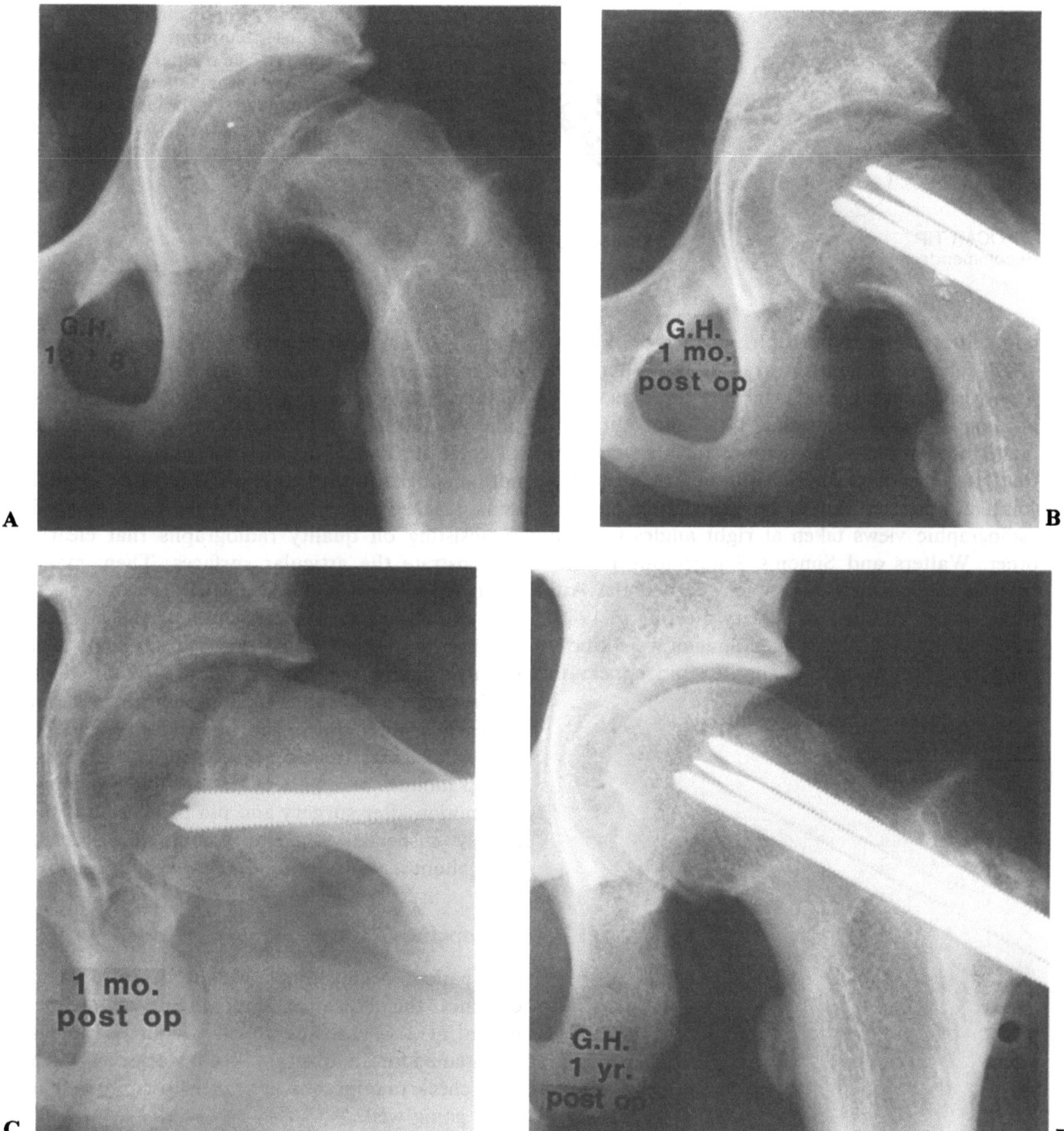

FIG. 12–4 **A** Adolescent with a moderately severe left slip. Note the prominent "bump" on the metaphysis which may limit flexion and internal rotation prior to remodeling. **B** Treatment by in situ pinning. The tips are far from the articular surface and on this AP view appear to barely cross the physis. **C** The lateral view demonstrates excellent pinning technique with the pins entering the anterior cortex of the femoral neck and then piercing the epiphysis without exiting the posterior neck. On this view, the pins cross the physis by 1 cm which is adequate. **D** One year after in situ pinning. Note the remodeling of the superior neck. The patient now has excellent hip motion and has no desire for a corrective osteotomy.

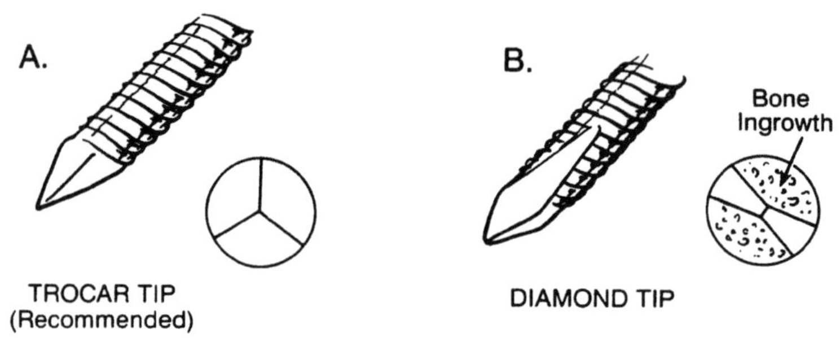

FIG. 12–5 Pin tip choices on heavy, threaded Steinmann pins (4.8-mm diameter). The trochar tip (**A**) is preferred because it is thought to be easier to remove. The broad, flat surface of the diamond tip (**B**), when covered with bone, will be difficult to remove.

tain and interpret radiographs correctly.[32] Figure 12–7A and B demonstrates a cadaveric femoral head with a pin piercing it in the "three-quarter" position to demonstrate the "blind spot" in two-plane radiographs. This demonstrates how a pin that has penetrated several millimeters into a hip joint may appear not to be protruding on two radiographic views taken at right angles to each other. Walters and Simon's [32] ingenious mathematical analysis of this problem earned the Aufranc Award at The Hip Society meeting in 1980. Their illustrations of this phenomenon were kindly submitted for use in this chapter and appear in Fig. 12–8. Their work and the experience of our center and others suggest that in certain cases chondrolysis is the result of permanent pin protrusion into the joint with subsequent damage to the articular surfaces. This minimal penetration may not be noticed until the child has left the hospital and discarded his crutches. This disaster is avoided by insisting on quality radiographs that clearly demonstrate the articular surfaces. Then, maximum penetration is avoided since the only need is to cross the physis. After the final pin position has been accepted, an unscrubbed surgical team member should free the hip from the fracture table so the surgeon can range the hip under anesthesia. When available, the image intensifier should be used to visualize pin-tip position in all variations of hip motion. If a patient has trouble regaining hip motion after surgery and pin protrusion is remotely suspected, the hip should be studied throughout its range of motion under fluoroscopy.

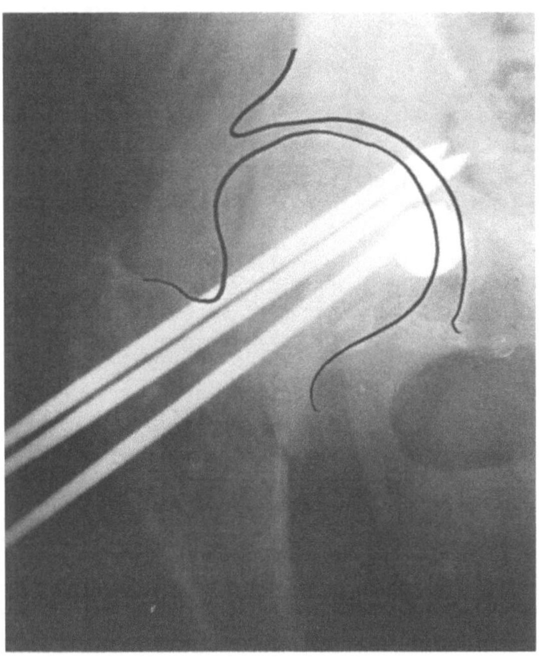

FIG. 12–6 Inadvertent, temporary intraoperative penetration of the hip joint with fixation pins. The pins were immediately withdrawn. This extremely brief type of pin protrusion, although not desired, is not thought to permanently damage the joint.

Postoperative Care

The patient begins touch weight bearing, using crutches, the day after pinning. Sutures are removed at 2 weeks, and touch weight bearing is maintained for an arbitrary 4 to 6 weeks, at which time check radiographs are taken to confirm that all is going well.

The pins are left in until the physis is fused as indicated by radiography, which is usually 1 to 2 years after pinning. Removing the pins any sooner places the hip in jeopardy for further slipping.

Chronic Slip: Treatment by Bone Grafting

Heyman,[14] Howorth,[15] and more recently, Melby et al.[21] have detailed the effectiveness of producing an epiphysiodesis for stabilization of a chronic slip

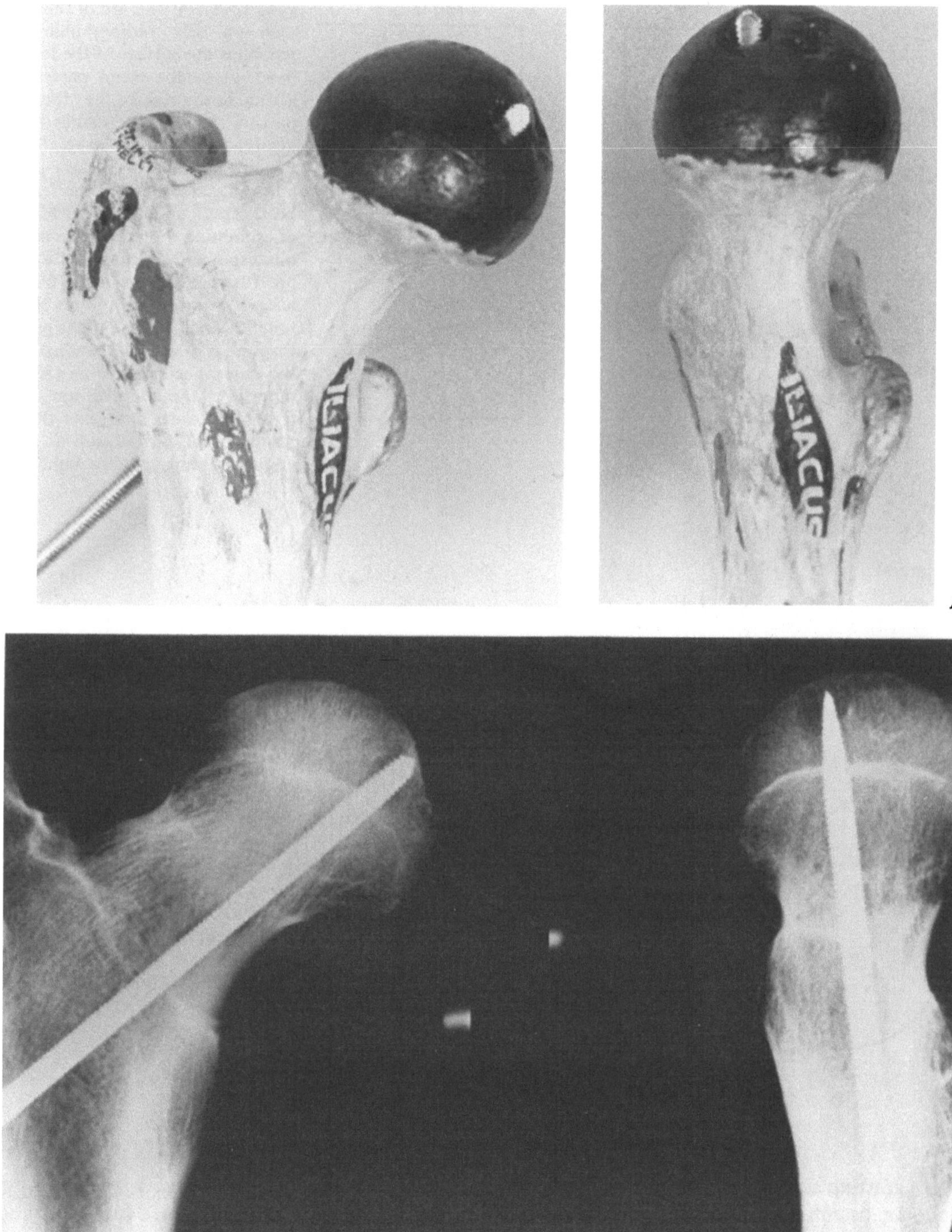

A

B

FIG. 12–7 **A** Cadaveric femoral head with pin protruding several millimeters. **B** Anteroposterior and lateral radiographs of the same specimen demonstrating how the pin tips appear to be safely within the femoral head, although they are protruding several millimeters on the actual specimen.

A

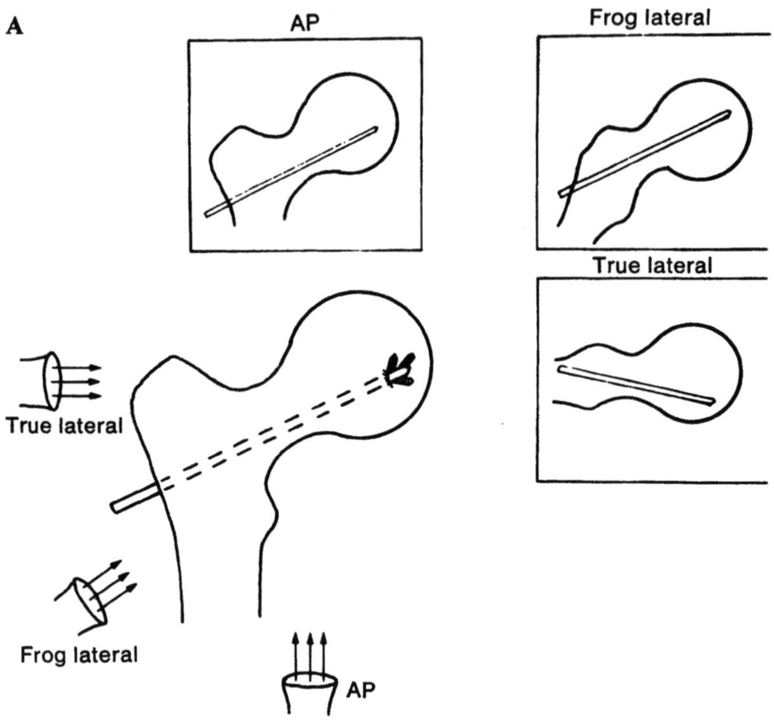

B

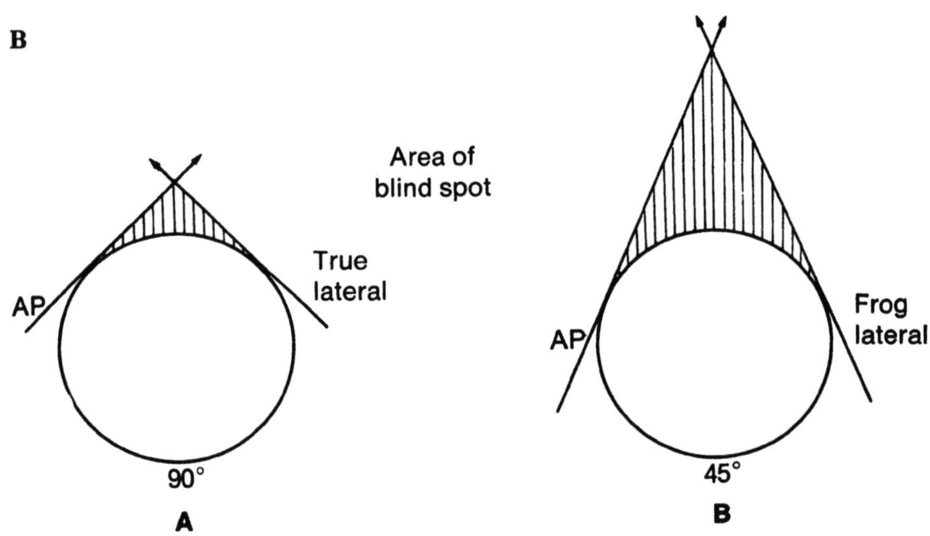

FIG. 12–8 **A** The arc of the circle seen on any radiographic projection is the surface of the femoral head where the beam passes tangential to the surface, i.e., the plane passing through the center of the head perpendicular to the beam. Pin tips not located in these planes and protruded beyond the femoral head can go undetected. **B** Method of estimating the maximum area of blind spot and the magnitude of pin protrusion. Although the frog-leg lateral position (*B*) rotates the femur 90° and creates a plane passing through the head perpendicular to the anteroposterior plane (*A*), the tangent of the lateral beam to the femoral surface intersects the anteroposterior x-ray beam at a 45° angle, creating a large blind spot (*B*).

by bone grafting across the open physis. They also include an osteotomy of the anterolateral metaphyseal "bump" to improve hip motion. Through an anterior approach, corticocancellous bone grafts are taken from the adjacent ilium and impacted through drill holes across the open physis (Fig. 12–9). The recent report from Akron [21] of 289 hips treated by this method reported no necrosis or chondrolysis. Failure due to graft resorption or failure to cross the plate with the graft was noted in only four hips. Hip spica immobilization was not used in most cases. These results are impressive because the traditional, severe, untreatable complications of necrosis and chondrolysis have been avoided. In addition, pin removal was not required since no pins were used.

Because pinning is difficult and has been directly linked to complications in certain cases

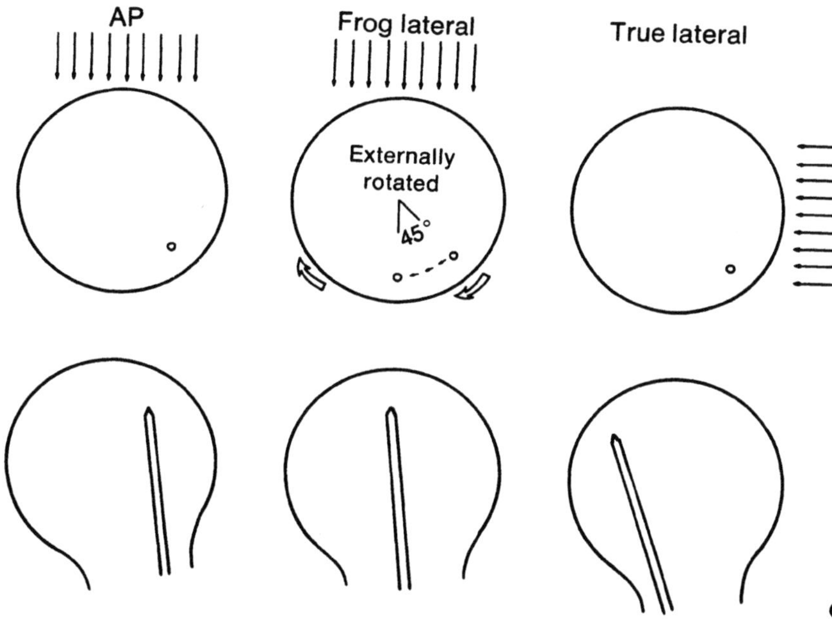

C

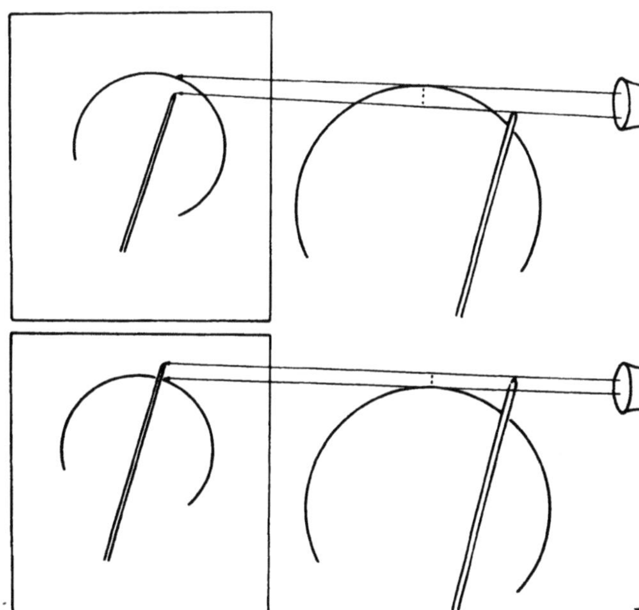

D

FIG. 12–8. (*cont.*) **C** Representative diagram of pin-depth appearance on a single radiograph relative to its actual depth. **D** Representative diagram of pin-depth appearance on a single AP and lateral view given the same actual differences from the surface. From Walters, R., and Simon Sheldon, R.: Joint destruction: a sequel of unrecognized pin penetration in patients with slipped capital femoral epiphyses. In: The Hip Society: The Hip. St. Louis, Mosby, 1980.

(chondrolysis following permanent pin penetration), there is a slow trend toward bone graft epiphysiodesis in North America. As has been stated by sage commentators, once everybody is doing it, any procedure will have complications. Figure 12–10 demonstrates the hip radiographs of a 14-year-old girl treated with bone grafting for a right slipped capital femoral epiphysis in which the corticocancellous graft unknowingly penetrated the articular surface of the femoral head (Fig. 12–10B), requiring repeat surgery 5 days later to extract the graft. The final result was excellent, however.

Acute Slip

Patients with acute slips are rare (less than 5% of all slips) and should be identified because they

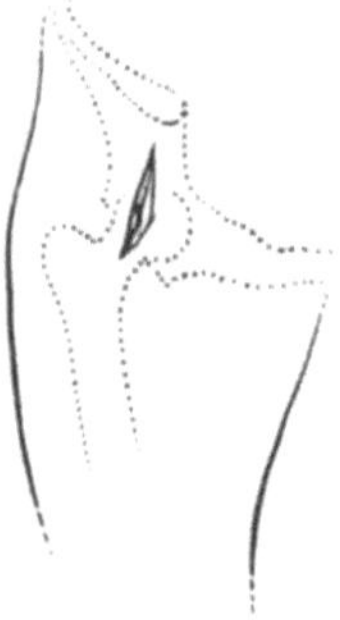

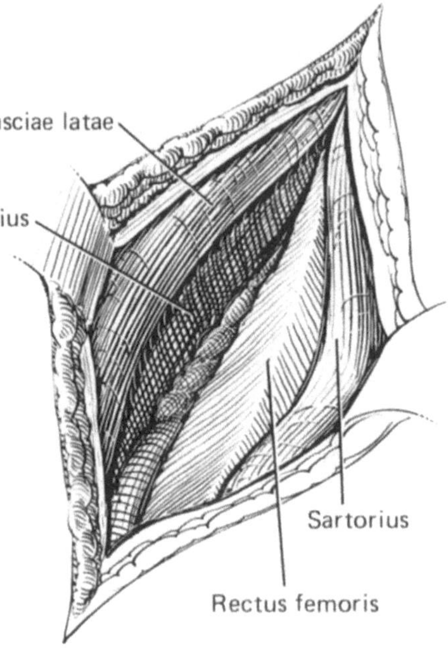

FIG. 12–9 **A** Anterior approach to hip for bone grafting in SCFE. An H-shaped incision is made in the anterior capsule. **B** A reamer and curette are used to open a channel across the physis. **C** Corticocancellous grafts from the adjacent ilium are driven across the physis. **D** Acute SCFE, left hip, in an adolescent. **E** AP view, same patient, 3 years after reduction and bone grafting, left hip. **F** Lateral view, left hip, 3 years after bone grafting. Courtesy of Dr. Dennis Weiner.

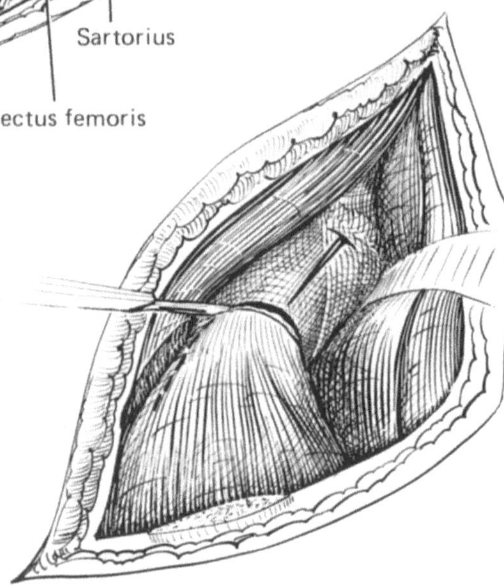

A

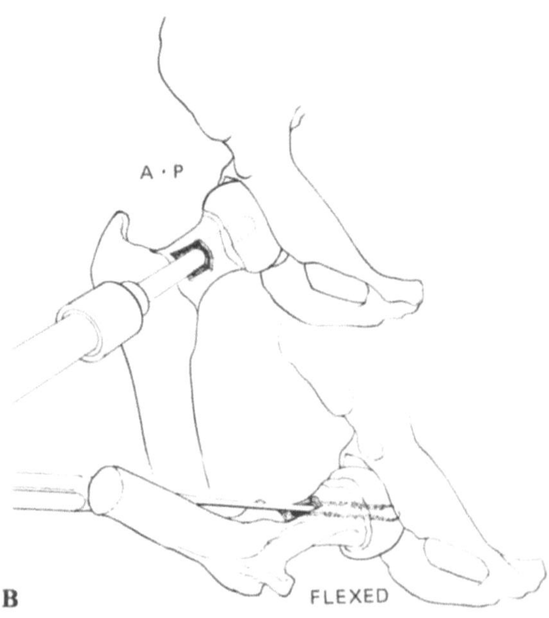

B

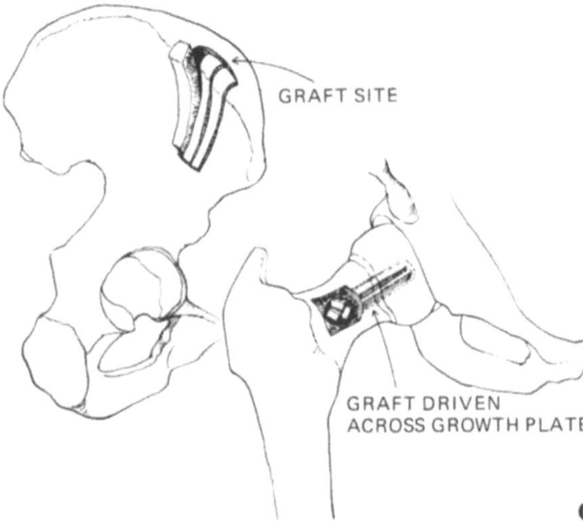

C

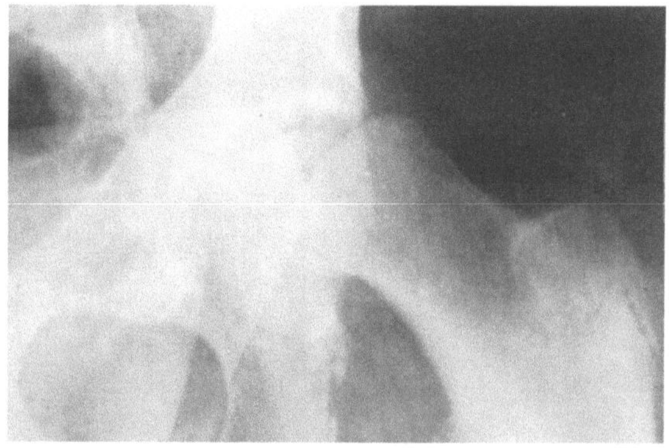

D

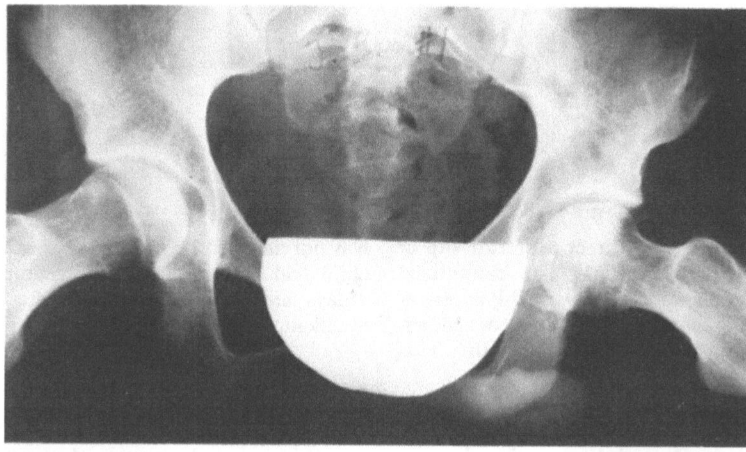

E

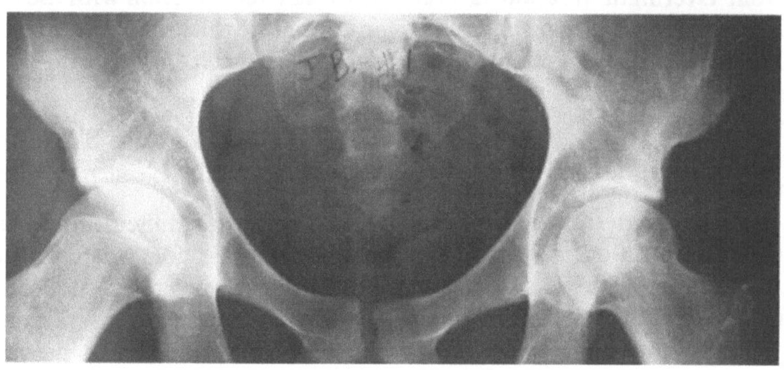

F

are treated differently.[8] Patients with a true acute slip have no prior symptoms and then suffer an injury that produces sudden, severe hip pain. Acute slips are often described as having symptoms for up to 14 days; however, this definition should not be stretched. Treating an acute slip as a chronic slip (by in situ pinning) has few adverse sequelae, whereas treating a chronic slip as though it were acute (with manipulative reduction) often results in disastrous complications (necrosis).

A child with an acute slip has severe pain similar to that seen in an adult with a hip fracture. One boy who came to our hospital in an ambulance after suffering an acute slip vividly recounted every railroad track that the ambulance crossed between his hometown and our hospital.

Range of motion cannot be tested because of acute pain. Radiographs show displacement of the hip (usually severe) with no metaphyseal remodeling (Fig. 12–11A). Treatment of these rare cases includes immediate reduction and pinning, with reduction achieved either by manipulation under

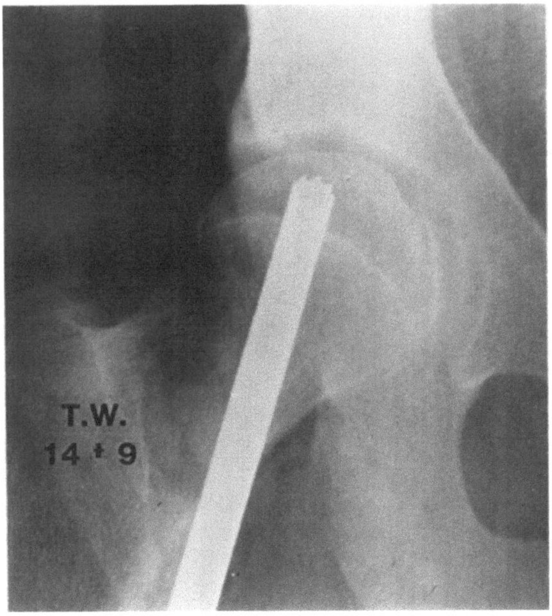

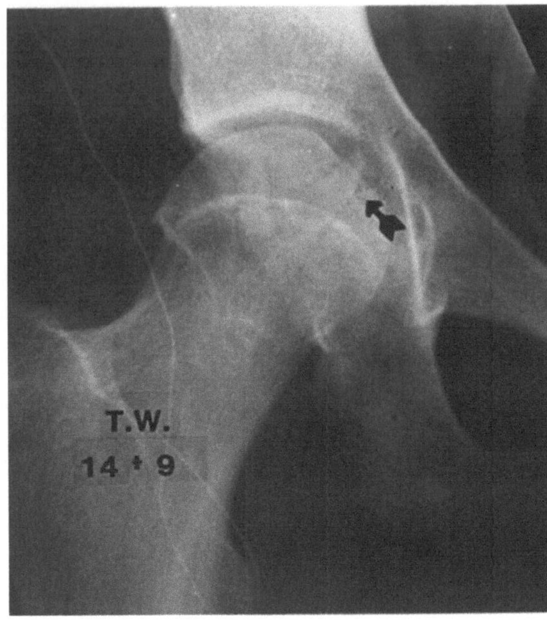

FIG. 12–10 **A** Adolescent with direct posterior slip of right hip, treated by bone grafting. The cannulized reamer is shown directed across the physis. **B** Postoperative radiograph showing that one of the three corticocancellous grafts has been placed across the joint. This was not detected on the intraoperative radiograph. The child had pain with motion, requiring repeat surgery 2 days later to reposition the graft. The final result was excellent, however.

anesthesia in the operating room (Fig. 12–11) or by overnight traction. Overnight traction is preferred because it is less traumatic than manipulative reduction under anesthesia. Reductions in the operating room are always dictated as being "gentle," but in reality seldom are.

Overnight corrective traction, illustrated in Fig. 12–12, includes a stout, threaded distal femoral traction pin left long on the lateral side to allow attachment of an internal rotation traction rope. The patient is then placed in balanced suspension with 8 to 10 pounds of longitudinal traction and 2 to 3 pounds of internal rotation traction applied to the laterally protruding skeletal pin. Within 24 hours the "loose" portion of the displacement will usually be corrected. In an acute slip this may be complete reduction. In an acute upon chronic situation (subacute slip), traction of this magnitude should reduce only the acute component of the slip. Depending on personal preference, internal rotation can also be applied by skin tapes.

The patient is then taken to the operating room, placed on the fracture table, and pinned without attempts to further reduce the hip. Despite these precautions, reducing an acute slip by either manipulative reduction or traction still may result in necrosis (Fig. 12–13D–F). Care should be taken to avoid overreduction with the femoral head tilted into valgus, which has been highly correlated with subsequent necrosis.

Subacute Slip (Acute Slip Superimposed on a Previously Existing Chronic Slip)

This diagnosis is difficult to make accurately. The usual history is for several weeks or months of mild ache, followed by sudden, severe hip pain, usually secondary to a traumatic incident. On examination, the patient has severe pain, with equivocal radiographs (Fig. 12–13A) as regards chronicity. Under these circumstances, the history must be given greatest credence to avoid misdiagnosing this as an acute slip. With a subacute slip, one should attempt reduction of the displaced head back to the position that resulted from the chronic component of the slip prior to the acute episode. With a subacute slip, manipulative reduction under anesthesia is contraindicated. Longitudinal–internal rotation skeletal traction as described for an acute slip (Fig. 12–12) is preferred. The degree of reduction achieved overnight is accepted with primary in situ pinning in that position (Fig. 12–

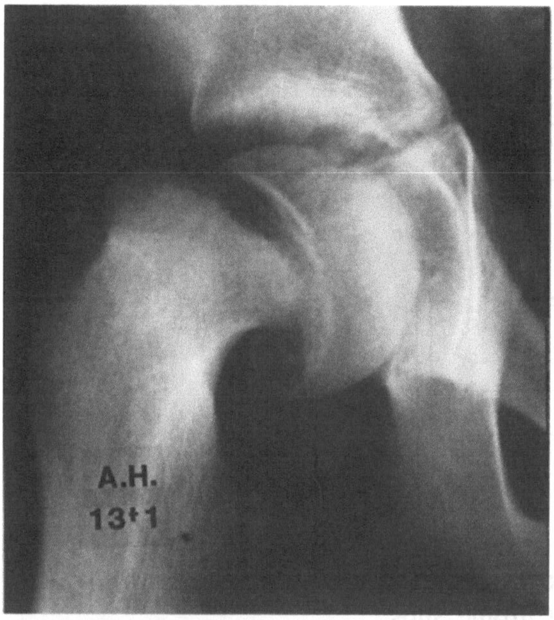

A

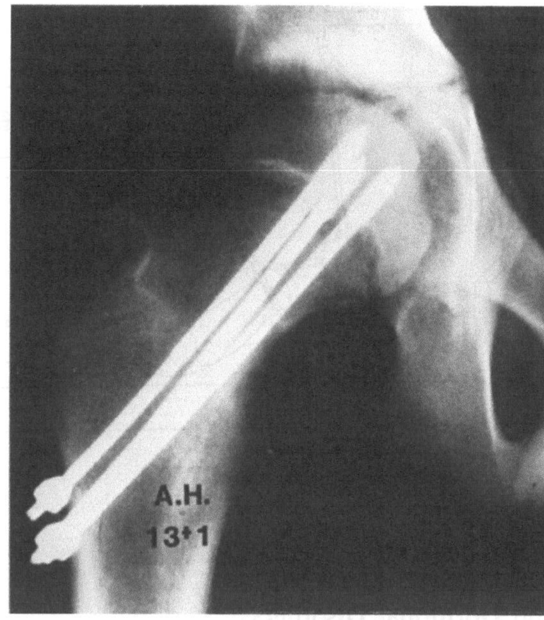

B

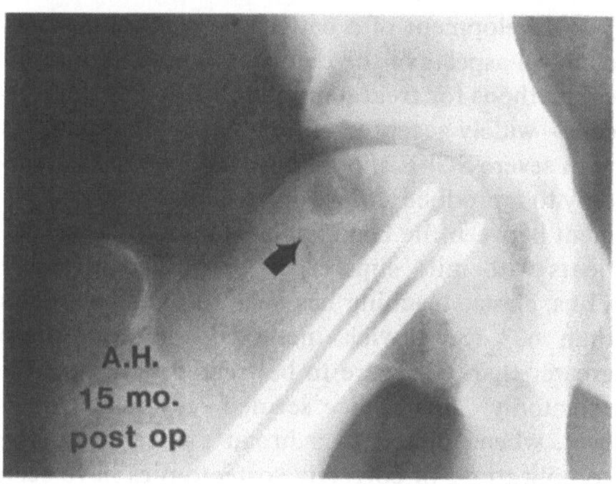

C

FIG. 12–11 **A** Adolescent with an acute slip of the right hip. **B** After manipulative reduction and pinning in situ. **C** AP view taken 15 months after reduction and pinning. Note the focal area of avascular necrosis.

13B and C). The degree of reduction is sometimes overinterpreted because the pretraction films are oblique, and the posttraction films are truly AP. Although reduced in this manner, the patient in Fig. 12–13 developed avascular necrosis, demonstrating the potential danger in reduction attempts of any type in any situation other than a true acute SCFE.

Prophylactic Contralateral Pinning

A frequent past practice was to prophylactically pin the opposite normal hip in any child with SCFE to avoid subsequent slip in the opposite hip, since bilaterality is estimated at 20–25%. Prophylactic pinning of the contralateral hip is not advised because after the first slip children and their parents are aware of presentation patterns (knee pain, limp, and so on) and will recognize them if they appear in the contralateral hip. The physician should review and emphasize these symptoms for the patient. Such a course has proven to be safe and provides a significant economic relief as compared to a policy of unnecessary contralateral pinning in 75% of children with SCFE. In certain unfortunate social, cultural, or geographical circumstances, contralateral pinning of the normal hip may be justified.

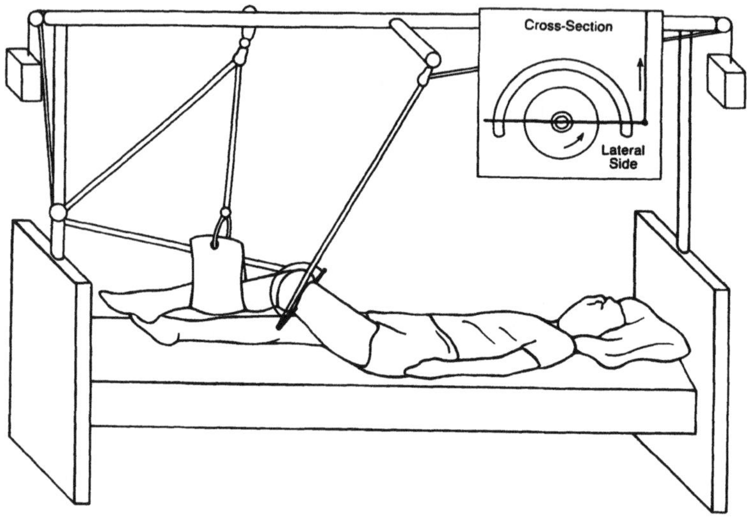

FIG. 12–12 Method for skeletal traction reduction of an acute left SCFE. The distal femoral pin is left long laterally to allow application of 2–3 pounds of internal rotation traction. Longitudinal traction of 10–12 pounds is applied to the same pin.

Treatment in Metabolic and Hormonal Disorders

Patients with metabolic disorders (e.g., renal failure) may develop SCFE, almost always bilateral, at a much earlier age. Figure 12–14 demonstrates an 8-year-old child with renal failure, found to have bilateral SCFE as well as bilateral slipping of the proximal humeral physes—a common association (Fig. 12–14B).

The slip in a metabolic disease is the result of the generalized disorder that weakens the physis; thus, the primary disease should be treated, when possible. Whether or not the primary disorder can be improved, the slip must be stabilized or the deformity will progress. The process is chronic; therefore, treatment by in situ pinning is appropriate (Fig. 12–14C). Occasionally the epiphysis will grow off the end of the pins (Fig. 12–14D), and the pins will have to be advanced. In other cases, the threaded pins will produce closure of the physis at an age that may result in undesired limb shortness, especially in a juvenile with unilateral involvement. In such circumstances, I have modified a normal threaded Steinmann pin by removing the threads from the distal 2–3 cm (Fig. 12–14E); thus, a smooth pin crosses the physis, while the threaded portion engages the lateral cortex to keep the pin from backing off. This allows subsequent physeal growth, although with the risk of further slipping once the epiphysis has grown off the pins. The pins can then be further advanced, however, if they have been left long enough at the initial pinning.

Corrective Osteotomy for Severe, Chronic Slips

The development of a better appreciation for mechanical aspects of the deformity and better surgical methods for treatment of SCFE led to the concept—widely accepted 10 years ago—that patients with severe SCFE should have a corrective osteotomy to reproduce a more normal anatomical alignment between the head and acetabulum, while patients with mild slips could be pinned in situ.[30] Thus, classic teaching has been to pin slips of less than 60° (Southwick method [30]) in situ; those greater than 60° were to be treated by corrective osteotomy. This advice seemed reasonable; however, when applied to a broad clinical base, the complications of corrective osteotomies have been substantial.[11,19,29] Osteotomy through the femoral neck at the growth plate (cuneiform) is clearly dangerous with a high risk for necrosis and therefore has been abandoned. Southwick's subtrochanteric osteotomy has an elegant biomechanical design; however, patients treated by this method have a bothersome incidence of chondrolysis.[11] Osteotomies at the base of the neck (Fig. 12–15) again are based on sound mechanical concepts but may result in an increased incidence of necrosis.

Boyer [6] as well as O'Brien and Fahey [25] have recently demonstrated the profound ability of the hip to remodel in severe chronic SCFE after in situ pinning. These reports and our experience have led to our current practice of in situ pinning for all chronic slips, no matter how severe. Patients are told that if limited motion or limb deformity

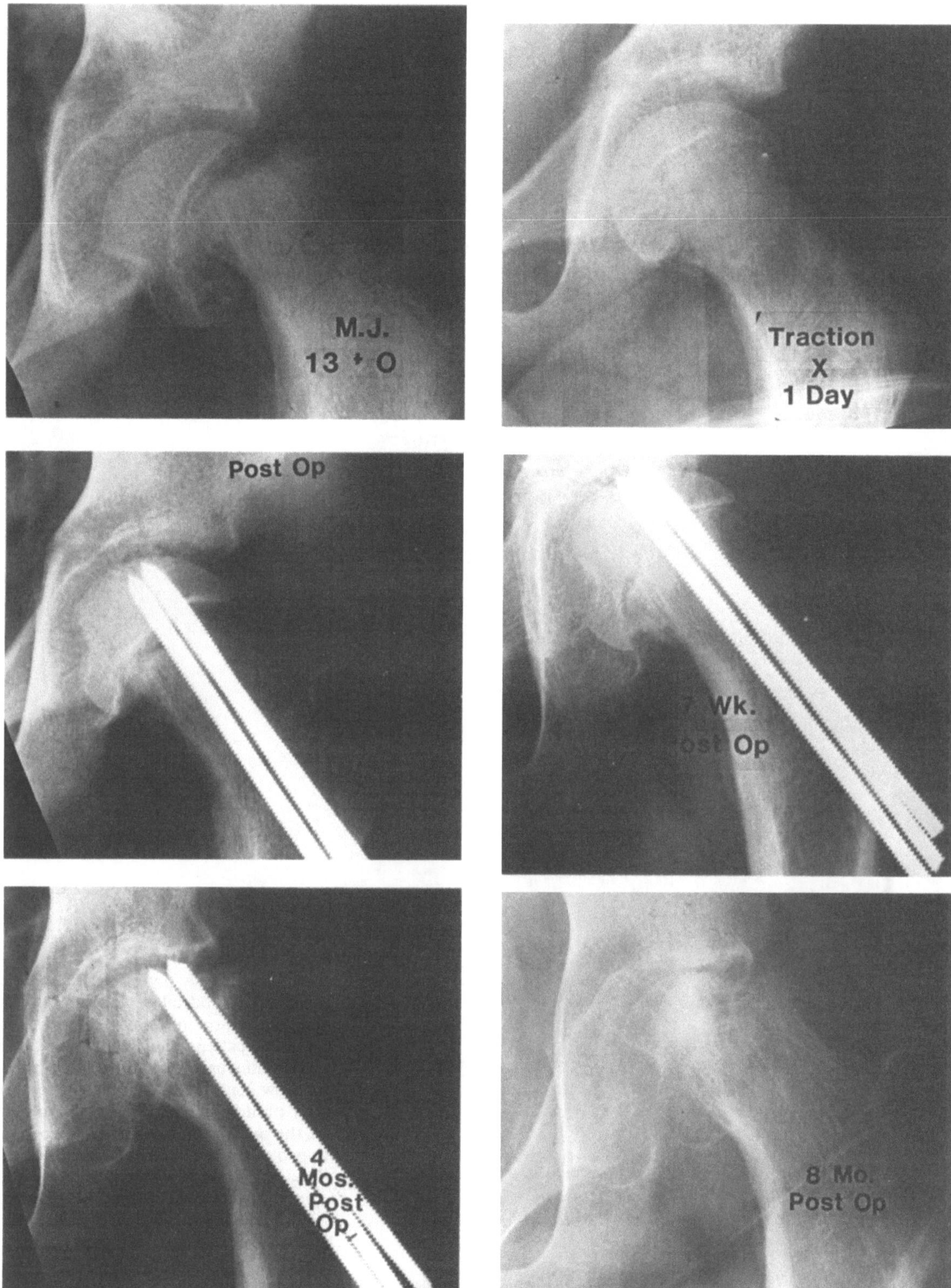

FIG. 12–13 **A** A 13-year-old male with subacute (acute superimposed upon chronic) slip of the right hip. **B** Radiograph after 1 day of longitudinal–internal rotation traction. The slip appears to be markedly improved. **C** AP view after pinning. The pins are too near the articular surface. **D** Seven weeks after pinning. The head has settled, and the pins are protruding into the joint. The pins were then backed off. **E** Four months after pinning. Note AVN with further collapse. The pins again protrude into the joint. **F** Eight months after pinning, further collapse is noted. The pins have been removed and the physis bone grafted to avoid further slip.

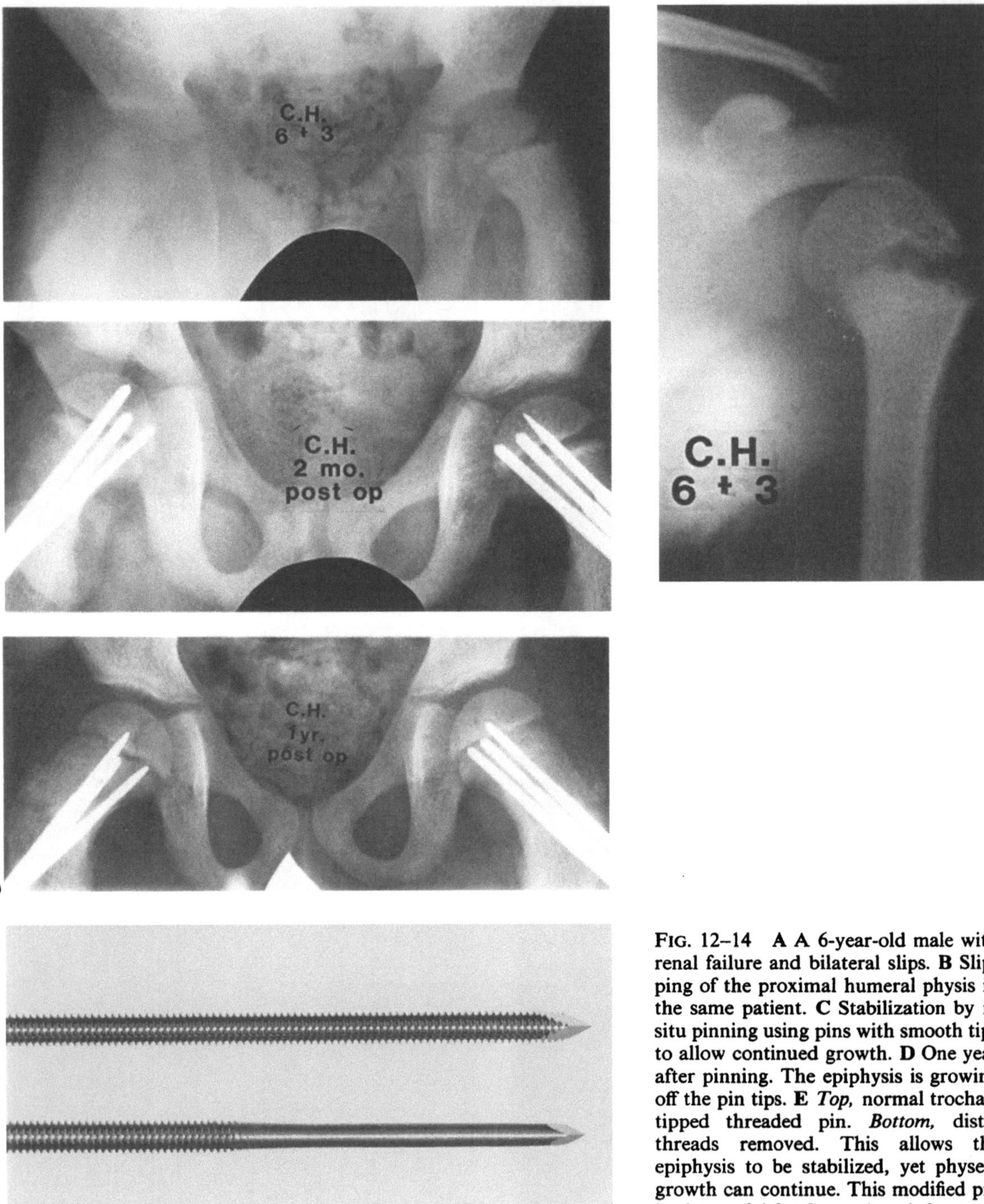

A

B

C

D

E

FIG. 12–14 **A** A 6-year-old male with renal failure and bilateral slips. **B** Slipping of the proximal humeral physis in the same patient. **C** Stabilization by in situ pinning using pins with smooth tips to allow continued growth. **D** One year after pinning. The epiphysis is growing off the pin tips. **E** *Top,* normal trochar-tipped threaded pin. *Bottom,* distal threads removed. This allows the epiphysis to be stabilized, yet physeal growth can continue. This modified pin is also useful for femoral neck fractures in children.

persists at 1 year, follow-up corrective osteotomy can then be considered as a secondary procedure. With this philosophy, corrective osteotomy is rarely required since bony remodeling is followed by improved internal rotation and hip flexion.

Complications

Avascular Necrosis

Segmental collapse due to avascular necrosis (AVN) results from a disruption of blood supply to the epiphysis, often following injudicious reduction of a chronically displaced epiphysis.[22] Once AVN occurs, there is little specific treatment. If the femoral head collapses onto the pin tip (Fig. 12–13D), the pin should be withdrawn to avoid damage to the articular surface. This may risk further slip of the epiphysis, however. In a few cases, I have resorted to bone graft stabilization of the physis with the hope that grafting will hasten revascularization (Fig. 12–13F).

The patient is advised to perform touch weight bearing by crutch walking while the head revascularizes. In mild cases (Fig. 12–11C) the outlook is good. With more severe collapse, the result is often complete destruction of the femoral head, with disabling hip pain. In our hospital these patients (and any normal, active teenager with severely destructive hip disease) are treated by hip fusion. This provides a durable, functional hip suitable for most occupations. We have little faith in the longevity of resurfacing arthroplasty (or other artificial replacement) in a normal, active teenager. A counterargument would be that hip arthroplasty should be tried, resorting to hip fusion when and if the arthroplasty fails.

Chondrolysis

Chondrolysis is a mysterious, devastating complication of SCFE.[16] Since permanent pin protrusion into the joint is one known cause, this category should be eliminated by good pinning technique.

Clearly, pin protrusion is not the only cause, since some patients present with a severe chronic slip and chondrolysis prior to being treated. In most patients with chondrolysis noted prior to treatment, the slip is severe, and diagnosis has been greatly delayed (Fig. 12–16). These cases provide the greatest support for an immunological theory of etiology for chondrolysis.[23] Exposure of bone marrow elements from the denuded metaphysis into the joint may initiate an immunological process that ultimately destroys the articular surfaces. A recent patient with a severe chronic slip and preexisting chondrolysis whom I explored not only had a denuded metaphysis exposed to his joint, but also had multiple bits of bone (fracture callus, injury-and-repair bone) loose in the joint and surrounded by inflamed synovium (Fig. 12–17).

I thus postulate that new bone, which forms as a result of an injury-and-repair response where the epiphysis is sliding off the metaphysis, periodically "fractures off" into the joint, resulting in both mechanical and possibly immunological damage to the articular surfaces. The massive inflammatory response by the synovium would also appear to play a role in the destruction. Since most preexisting chondrolysis occurs in chronic cases, early diagnosis and treatment should reduce the incidence of this problem.

Corrective osteotomies are thought to result in a higher incidence of chondrolysis; [11] therefore, limiting their use should help in reducing the incidence of chondrolysis. The reason for osteotomy producing chondrolysis is unclear; however, forcing a chronically deformed and displaced head back into an acetabulum that it no longer fits may be a factor.

Chondrolysis is difficult to treat. Coleman [9] advised high dose salicylates, heavy skeletal traction, and range of motion exercises with no weight bearing for many months. More recently, constant passive motion machines have been suggested as being helpful. Occasionally, traction or muscle releases, followed by hip spica immobilization in a neutral position for 2 or 3 months, will decrease pain and improve hip position.[10] In many adolescents with chondrolysis, the pain eventually subsides; however, the hip remains stiff, often in an awkward, flexed, abducted, externally rotated position that leaves the patient with an unsightly gait. In these patients I have used traction and/or a hip release, which includes surgical release of the abductors, hip flexors, and often the hip capsule via an anterolateral approach, followed by spica immobilization in the neutral position as described by Duncan.[10] This sequence has relieved pain and improved cosmesis (gait) in several of my patients. In some patients all of these methods fail, and hip fusion is then advised.

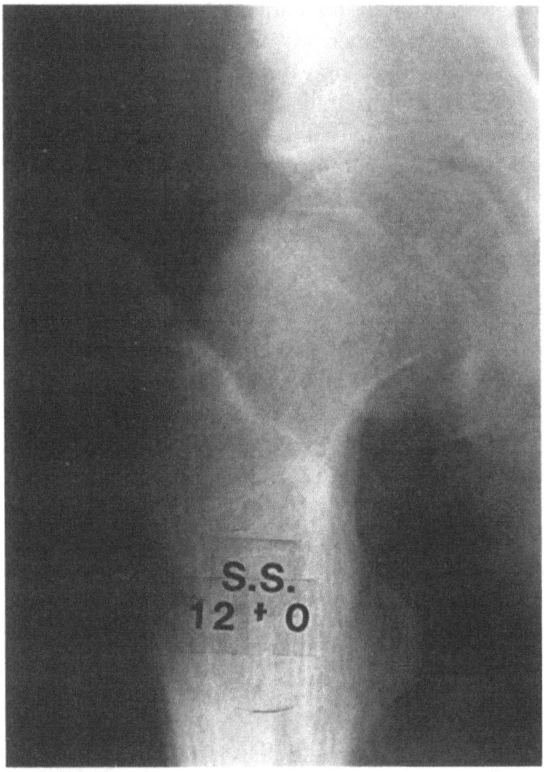

A

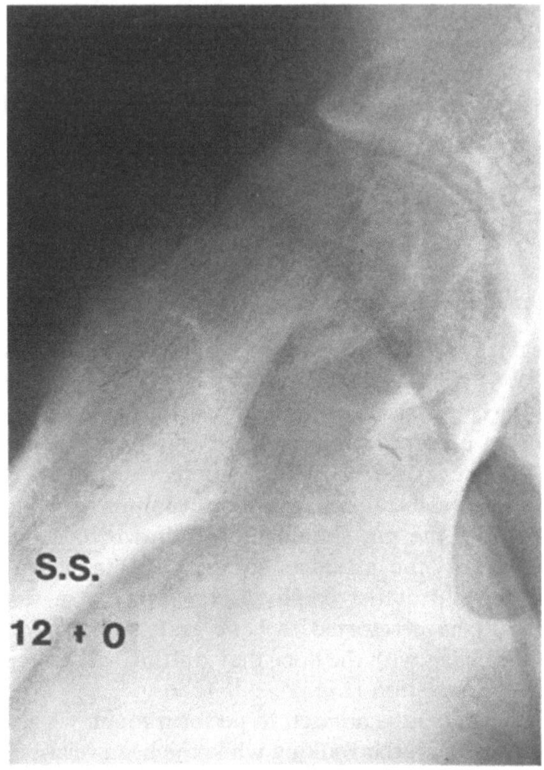

B

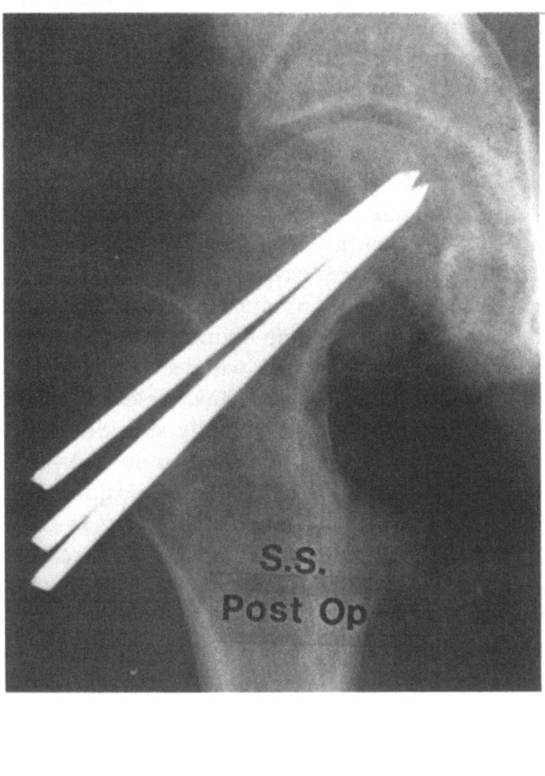

C

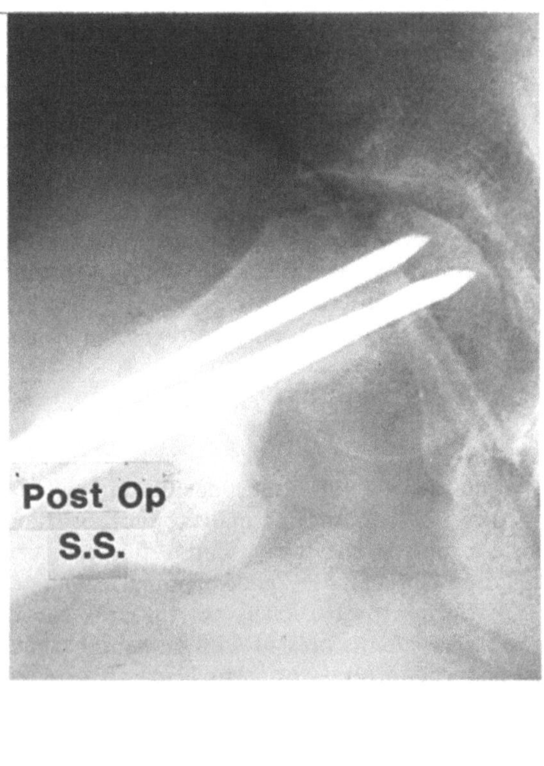

D

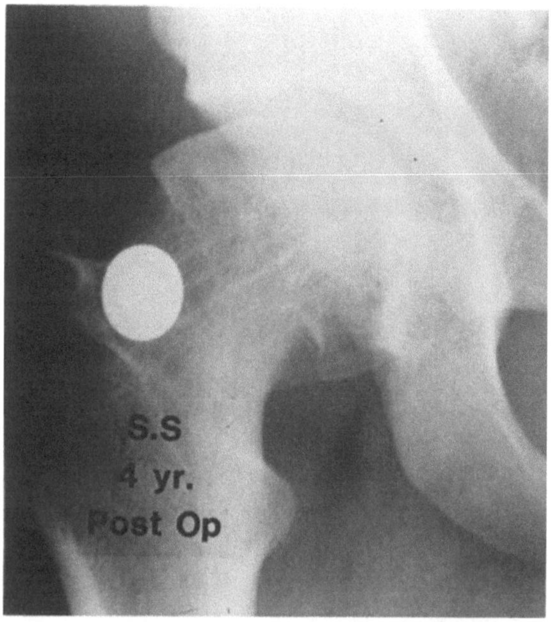

E

FIG. 12–15 **A** and **B** Anteroposterior and lateral views of a 12-year-old girl with a moderately severe right slip. **C** and **D** After corrective osteotomy at the base of the femoral neck and pin fixation. **E** Four years after surgery the patient had no symptoms and excellent hip motion.

Complications in Black Children

The incidence of AVN and chondrolysis has been reported to be higher in black children. Orofino et al.,[27] reported that 55% of a large series of black children with slipped capital femoral epiphysis had unsatisfactory results due to chondrolysis or AVN. More recently, Ingram et al.,[16] reported that 44% of black children treated for SCFE had chondrolysis as compared to an incidence of 14% in whites. In contrast, Bishop et al.[3] reported a chondrolysis incidence of only 6% and an AVN incidence of 7% in a series of black children, while Pierce and Mott [28] reported no difference in the incidence of complications, compared to that noted in white children, in their series of 125 children who had early diagnosis and careful treatment. These studies concluded that the much higher incidence of complications reported in blacks with SCFE is related more to sociological and cultural factors than to biological factors. Patients from poor families tend to have delayed diagnosis (Fig. 12–16), a factor that has clearly been shown to increase the incidence of chondrolysis. Also, once the slip is severe, corrective osteotomy

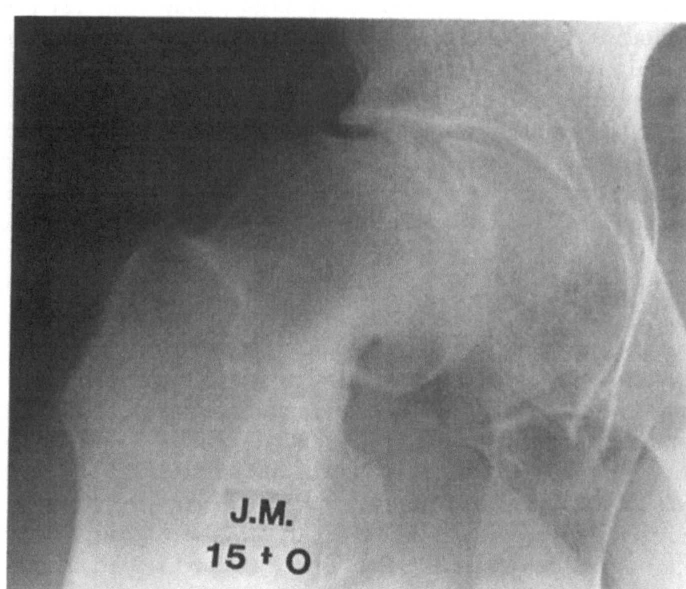

FIG. 12–16 Chondrolysis noted prior to treatment in a 15-year-old black male who presented with a 1-year history of right hip pain.

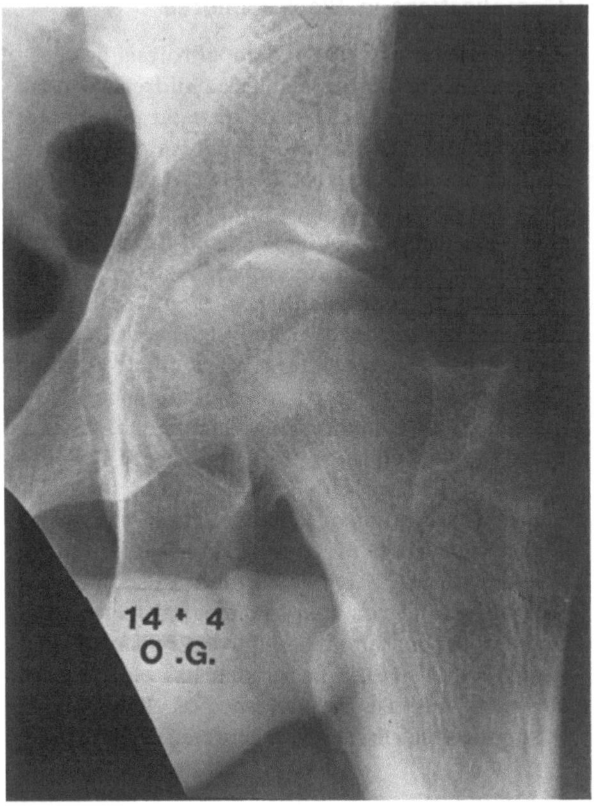

A

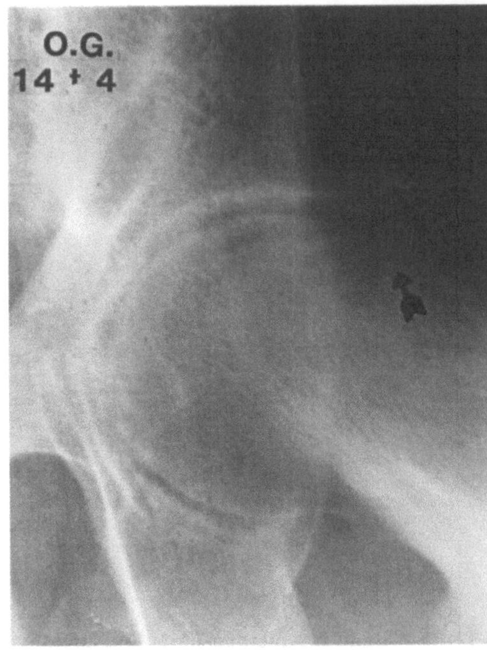

B

FIG. 12–17 **A** Left hip in a boy who presented with a chronic slip and chondrolysis. **B** Lateral view. The arrow points toward fluffy, irregular bone on the superior neck. At exploration, the patient was found to have cancellous bone fragments (injury-and-repair bone) loose in the joint and entrapped in a hypertrophied, inflamed synovium. Severe chondrolysis was confirmed.

may be advised, with its associated morbidity. Because of their economic status, many blacks have been and continue to be treated in large public hospitals by less experienced physicians who may not fully recognize the importance of pin placement, avoiding manipulative reduction, and so on. Bishop [3] concludes by stating that the prognosis following the treatment of SCFE is no different in blacks compared to whites if diagnosis is early and treatment appropriate.

Long-term Prognosis in SCFE

One must carefully analyze studies describing long-term hip function following SCFE since the reports come from two sources. One source comes from long-term follow-up of patients initially treated in a single center and subsequently called back for examination. Examples include O'Brien and Fahey's [25] report and the Iowa City long-term follow-up by Boyer et al.[6] Both studies support the concept of pinning in situ, even for severe slips, since remodeling produced a hip that functioned well for many years. Boyer's study of 149 hips in 121 patients with a mean of 31 years' follow-up demonstrated excellent long-term function in SCFE following in situ pinning. Figure 12–18, kindly provided for this chapter by the Iowa City group, illustrates a patient with a 25-year follow-up who had excellent hip function.

In Boyer's study, only where reduction attempts were made with ensuing AVN were severe problems encountered. Only one of 149 hips required a reconstructive hip arthroplasty at a mean of 31 years' follow-up.

A second, and at first glance seemingly contradictory, source of data comes from large series of adults with degenerative arthritis of the hip who have been retrospectively analyzed in an attempt to determine the etiology of their arthritis. Murray[24] suggests that the "tilt deformity" seen in 40% of hips with degenerative arthritis is due to an undetected subclinical SCFE in adolescence. This second type of statistical report is difficult

FIG. 12–18 **A** Sixteen-year-old male with a left slip, subsequently treated by in situ pinning. **B** Same patient 25 years later. Despite the radiographic abnormality he is employed and has only rare hip symptoms, with an Iowa hip rating of 90. Courtesy of Drs. S. Weinstein and D. Boyer.

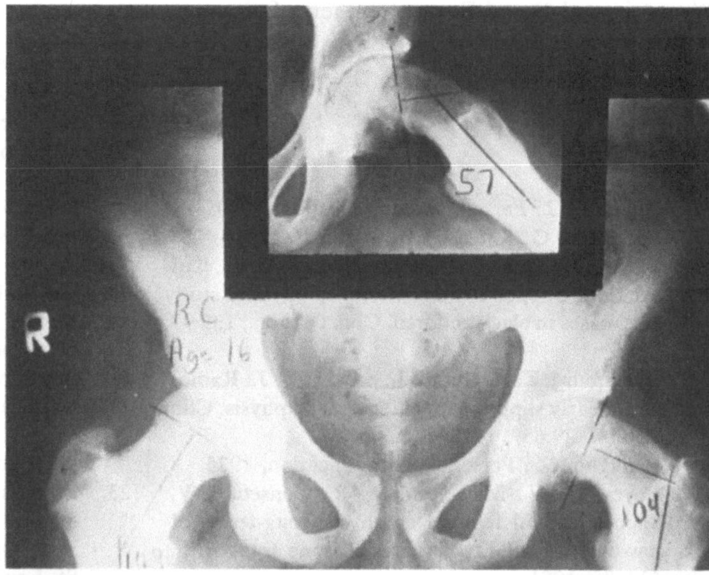

A

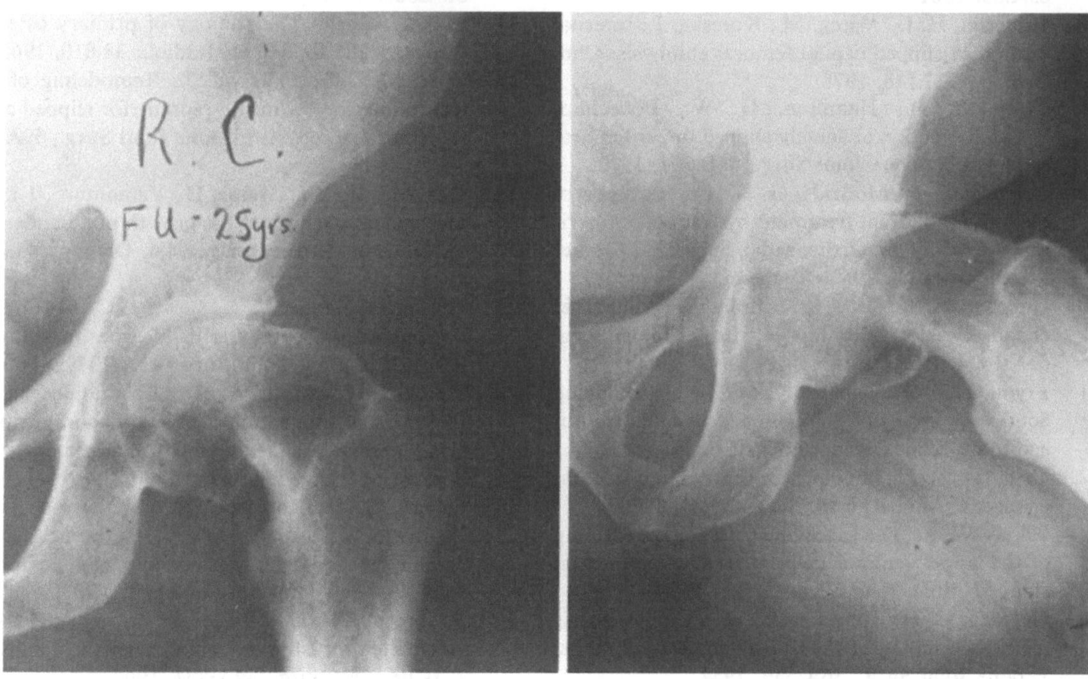

B

to interpret because the patients are drawn from a population of millions, examining only the subset with degenerative arthritis. In addition, the proposed original disease (subclinical, untreated SCFE) is hard to define. Drawing from Boyer's study, it appears that most patients with SCFE will have good long-term hip function if chondrolysis and AVN can be avoided with initial treatment.

Acknowledgements

I wish to give special thanks to the following people who have assisted me in collecting and organizing material for this chapter: Roger Bell and Sandy Carduff, photography; Robert Walters, Pin protrusion data and photographs; Dennis Weiner, pinning in situ—data and photographs; and Stuart

Weinstein and David Boyer, long-term follow-up, Iowa City.

Bibliography

1. Angel, J. C.: Personal communication, 1980.
2. Axhausen, G.: Cited by Howorth, B. H.[15]
3. Bishop, J. O., Oley, T. J., Stephenson, C. T., Tullos, H. S.: Slipped capital femoral epiphysis: a study of 50 cases in black children. Clin. Orthop., 135:93, 1978.
4. Bloomburg, T. J., Nutall, J., Stoker, D. J.: Radiology in early slipped capital femoral epiphysis. Clin. Radiol., 29:657, 1978.
5. Bonfiglio, M.: Personal communication, 1975.
6. Boyer, D. W., Mickelson, M. R., Ponseti, I. V.: Slipped capital femoral epiphysis: long-term follow-up study of 121 patients. J. Bone Joint Surg., 63A:85, 1981.
7. Cameron, H. U., Wang, M., Koreska, J.: Internal fixation of slipped capital femoral epiphysis. Clin. Orthop., 137:148, 1978.
8. Casey, B. H., Hamilton, H. W., Bobechko, W. B.: Reduction of acutely slipped upper femoral epiphysis. J. Bone Joint Surg., 54B:607, 1972.
9. Coleman, S. S., McBride, G. G.: Chondrolysis of the hip in children: treatment by traction. American Academy of Orthopaedic Surgeons Annual Meeting, March, 1983, Anaheim.
10. Duncan, J. W., Nasca, R., Schrantz, J.: Idiopathic chondrolysis of the hip. J. Bone Joint Surg. 61A:1024, 1979.
11. Frymayer, J. W.: Chondrolysis of the hip following Southwick osteotomy for slipped capital femoral epiphysis. Clin. Orthop., 99:120, 1974.
12. Griffith, M. J.: Slipping of the capital femoral epiphysis. Ann. R. Coll. Surg., 58:34, 1976.
13. Harris, W. R.: The endocrine basis for the slipping of the upper femoral epiphysis: an experimental study. J. Bone Joint Surg., 32B:5, 1950.
14. Heyman, C. H., Herndon, C. H.: Epiphyseodesis for early slipping of the upper femoral epiphysis. J. Bone Joint Surg., 36A:539, 1954.
15. Howorth, B. H.: Slipping of the upper femoral epiphysis. Clin. Orthop., 10:148, 1957.
16. Ingram, A. J., Clarke, M. S., Clark, C. S., Marshall, W. R.: Chondrolysis complicating slipped capital femoral epiphysis. Clin. Orthop., 165:99, 1982.
17. Ippoleto, E., Mickelson, M. R., Ponseti, I. V.: A histochemical study of slipped capital femoral epiphysis. J. Bone Joint Surg., 63A:1109, 1981.
18. Key, J. A.: Epiphyseal coxa vara or displacement of capital epiphysis of femur in adolescence. J. Bone Joint Surg., 8:52, 1926.
19. Kramer, W. G., Craig, W. A., Noel, S.: Compensating osteotomy at base of the femoral neck for slipped capital femoral epiphysis. J. Bone Joint Surg., 58A:796, 1976.
20. MacEwen, G. D., Ramsey, D. L.: In Lovell, W. W., Winter, R. B., (eds.): Pediatric Orthopaedics. Philadelphia, Lippincott, 1978, pp. 762–777.
21. Melby, A., Hoyt, W. A., Weiner, D. S.: Treatment of chronic slipped capital femoral epiphysis. J. Bone Joint Surg., 62A:119, 1980.
22. Mickelson, M. R., El-Khoury, G. Y., Cass, J. R., Case, K. J.: Aseptic necrosis following slipped capital femoral epiphysis. Skel. Radiol., 4:129, 1979.
23. Morrissy, R. T.: What's new in slipped capital femoral epiphysis. In: The Hip Proceedings of the Sixth Open Scientific Meeting of the Hip Society. St. Louis, Mosby, 1978.
24. Murray, R. O.: The etiology of primary osteoarthrosis of the hip. Br. J. Radiol., 38:810, 1965.
25. O'Brien, E. T., Fahey, J. J.: Remodeling of the femoral neck after in situ pinning for slipped capital femoral epiphysis. J. Bone Joint Surg., 59A:62, 1977.
26. Oka, M., Miki, T., Hama, H., Yamamuro, T.: The mechanical strength of the growth plate under the influence of sex hormones. Clin. Orthop., 45:264, 1979.
27. Orofino, C., Innis, J. J., Lowrey, C. C.: Slipped capital femoral epiphysis in Negroes: a study of 95 cases. J. Bone Joint Surg., 42A:1079, 1960.
28. Pierce, R. O., Mott, W. H.: Observations on the treatment of slipped upper capital femoral epiphysis. American Academy of Orthopaedic Surgeons Annual Meeting, February, 1980, San Francisco.
29. Salvati, E. A., Robinson, H. J., O'David, T. J.: Southwick osteotomy for severe chronic slipped capital femoral epiphysis: results and complications. J. Bone Joint Surg., 62A:561, 1980.
30. Southwick, W. O.: Osteotomy through the lesser trochanter for slipped capital femoral epiphysis. J. Bone Joint Surg., 49A:807, 1967.
31. Waldenstrom, H.: On necrosis of the joint cartilage by epiphyseolysis capitis femoris. Acta Chir. Scand., 67:936, 1930.
32. Walters, R., Simon, S. S.: Joint destruction: a sequela of unrecognized pin penetration in patients with slipped capital femoral epiphysis. In: The Hip Proceedings of the Eighth Open Scientific Meeting of the Hip Society. St. Louis, Mosby, 1980.

CHAPTER 13

Paralytic Lesions of the Hip

W. JOHN SHARRARD

Paralysis and the deformity arising from it form a substantial proportion of the serious orthopedic conditions in childhood. Paralysis involving the muscles of the hip may develop in poliomyelitis, cerebral palsy, spina bifida, muscular dystrophy, spinal muscular atrophy, or paraplegia arising from injury or disease affecting the spinal column. In adult life, paralytic involvement of the hip is a much less common problem but may require specific attention in the paralysis associated with multiple sclerosis, cerebrovascular disease, cerebral trauma, and traumatic paraplegia.

In childhood, the problems of management are complicated by progressive deformity associated with growth and, in particular, with the liability to dislocation; the latter less often occurs in adults, except in association with sepsis secondary to decubitus ulceration.

Muscles Acting on the Hip

The hip is a polyplanar joint and therefore requires muscles that are capable of producing movement in six directions: flexion, extension, adduction, abduction, medial rotation, and lateral rotation. Because the plane of the joint is oblique, muscle activity and hip movement are seldom direct in any one plane. In order that the thigh may be flexed forward in the plane of the trunk, hip-flexion activity must be accompanied by some rotary action to maintain the line of progress. Thus it is possible only to speak in broad terms of the activity of any individual muscle and the effects that may result from its paralysis.

In walking, the main function associated with hip activity, the action of the muscle is modified depending on whether the lower limb is being moved freely with the trunk as the fixed point or whether the foot is on the ground and trunk movements are being produced by the inverted action of hip musculature. When the foot is on the ground, the function of the hip abductor muscles is to elevate the opposite side of the pelvis by acting from insertion to origin, a function that is much more important in walking than abduction of the hip with the pelvis fixed, the situation usually used to assess abductor action.

Finally, the action of muscles at the hip must be related to the activity of trunk muscles to elevate and rotate the pelvis and of the muscles acting on the knee to produce secondary movement at hip level.

Hip Flexion

The most important hip flexor muscle is the iliopsoas. In the newborn and in early childhood, it is a strong lateral rotator;[22] in later childhood and adult life its lateral rotation component is less strong and is compensated by the vector of medial rotation resulting from the development of the femoral neck. When acting in isolation, the hip is pulled into flexion, lateral rotation, and abduction. The sartorius also flexes and laterally rotates the hip and the pectineus contributes to both flexion and adduction. The rectus femoris and tensor fasciae latae play a part in hip flexion although their main actions are in extension of the knee and abduction of the hip, respectively. The hip flexors are innervated from the first, second, and third lumbar segments.

Hip flexion is one of the two muscle actions very essential for walking. Although it is possible for an individual to walk without hip flexors, as long as he can elevate his pelvis well enough to lift his foot off the ground aided by bracing, the presence of some hip flexor activity makes practical walking possible.

Hip Adduction

The four adductor muscles form a large bulk of muscle of considerable power considering that their action in walking is not as important as the remaining muscle groups acting on the hip. They have quite a strong action as medial rotators when the hip is flexed, which accounts for the flexion-adduction-medial rotation position often seen in cerebral palsy in the presence of spastic hip flexors and adductors. The medial hamstring muscles can also take part secondarily in adduction and may be short when there is severe adduction deformity. The adductor gracilis arises from a thin, vertically disposed tendon, the adductor longus from a combination of a rounded tendon and muscle, and the adductor brevis from an entirely muscular origin, features that must be recognized in the performance of adductor tenotomy. Their innervation is from the second, third, and fourth lumbar vertebrae, mainly through the obturator nerve. The contribution to the supply of the adductor magnus by the sciatic nerve is variable and cannot be relied upon to supply adequate adductor action if the whole obturator nerve is divided surgically.

Weakness of hip adduction does not seem to interfere greatly with ability to walk, unless fixed abduction deformity should develop.

Hip Extension

The principal extensor muscle is the gluteus maximus but the hamstring muscles can act as strong hip extensors if their action in flexion of the knee is prevented by concomitant extension of the knee. The gluteus maximus is innervated mainly from the first and second sacral segments and has the same root supply as the biceps femoris, a feature valuable in the assessment of gluteus maximus activity in infancy.

The gluteus maximus takes very little part in walking on level ground but it does come into action when walking up slopes or stairs. It also has an important function in preventing the trunk from falling forward too far and in restoring the erect position from forward flexion of the trunk.

Paralysis of the gluteus maximus in the presence of activity in other muscles acting on the hip does not prevent walking, but the gait is abnormal and stability is achieved by lateral rotation of the hip so that the posterior fibers of the gluteus medius partially replace the action of the gluteus maximus in maintaining extensor stability.

Hip Abduction

The hip abductors are functionally the most important muscles acting on the hip. They comprise the gluteus medius and gluteus minimus. Their origin is by muscle and the deep fibers of gluteus minimus are closely apposed to the hip joint. In addition to their primary action as abductors, their anterior fibers are medial rotators of the hip. They are innervated mainly from the fifth lumbar and first sacral segments.

In walking, their main function is not so much to abduct the hip actively as to prevent the downward displacement of the opposite side of the pelvis when the opposite limb is lifted from the ground; they achieve this in spite of the fact that their bulk is much less than that of the gluteus maximus muscle. They are assisted in this action by the quadratus lumborum and lateral abdominal muscles of the opposite side. Paralysis of the gluteal abductors therefore results in dropping of the pelvis on the opposite side when the opposite limb is lifted from the ground (Trendelenburg's sign), but it should be remembered that this sign may also be present when there is severe weakness of the lateral trunk muscles on the opposite side. If either or both of this group of muscles is paralyzed, walking can be achieved only by a rolling gait in which the patient leans to the side in order to elevate the pelvis to allow the foot to clear the ground.

Hip Lateral Rotation

Many muscles are concerned in lateral rotation of the hip: obturator internus, obturator externus, quadratus femoris, gemelli, piriformis, gluteus maximus, and sartorius. In childhood, the iliopsoas is also a powerful lateral rotator.

In adult life the joint itself is intrinsically stable, but in childhood the small rotator muscles and the gluteus minimus play an important part in protecting against stress and stretching of the hip capsule. The root supply of the lateral rotators of the hip is extensive and includes the second and third lumbar segments and the first and second sacral segments. Complete paralysis of lateral rotation is therefore uncommon, but overaction may lead to a lateral hip rotation gait.

Medial Rotation of the Hip

Medial rotation of the extended hip is a weak action performed only by the anterior fibers of the gluteus medius and minimus and by the tensor fasciae latae. Medial rotation of the flexed hip is more powerful because it is assisted by the medial hamstrings and adductor muscles. The root innervation of the medial rotators is from the fifth lumbar and first sacral segments.

Paralysis of the gluteal muscles in the presence of a strong hip flexor and lateral rotators results in forceful lateral rotation when the hip is flexed, a factor increasing the liability to stretch the capsule of the hip and predisposing to dislocation in infancy in paralytic spina bifida.

Flail Hip

Complete paralysis of all hip musculature does not necessarily make walking impossible, provided that the trunk muscles are capable of supporting, elevating, and rotating the pelvis and propulsion is aided by strong upper limbs using crutches or activity in other muscles in the lower limbs. In childhood, hip bracing is needed in addition but older children and adults can often achieve balance at the hip in the presence of total paralysis of hip musculature without the need for bracing. Complete paralysis of one hip seldom requires any brace if the opposite limb is strong.

Mechanisms of Paralytic Deformity

Development of deformity is common to all types of paralytic lesions, especially in childhood. An analysis of paralytic deformity in the lower limbs [43] suggested that certain common features are present in all paralytic deformity, whether of lower or upper motor neuron origin. All paralytic deformities commence in the soft tissues, i.e., in tendons, muscles, and tendon sheaths. Alterations in joint capsules and ligaments follow later and deformity of bone does not usually develop until soft-tissue deformity has been present for many months.

Mobile Deformity

Mobile deformity is present when the range of passive movement at a joint is full in all directions. Such deformity is easily recognized in lower motor neuron paralysis such as that due to poliomyelitis when complete paralysis of all muscles associated with the joint may be associated with the posture of a flail and dangling limb (Fig. 13–1), and passive movements are full or even greater than normal. In upper motor neuron lesions, spasticity in some muscles may lead to an abnormal posture suggesting that deformity is present, but pressure applied against the spastic muscles will achieve a full range of movements.

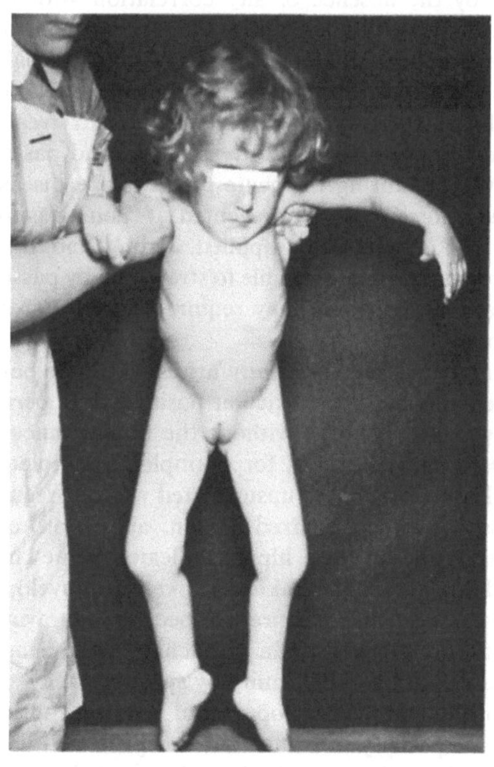

FIG. 13–1 Posture in flail lower limbs. The hips fall into lateral rotation. The range of movements is greater than normal.

Fixed Deformity

Fixed deformity implies that one or more of the arcs of movement of the joint are limited by short tendons, muscles, or their sheaths or by the presence of bony deformity or dislocation. Such limitation is still present in the anesthetized patient. Fixed deformity gives rise to serious consequences in a limb already disabled by limited function arising from paralysis.

Three mechanisms can result in fixed deformity in soft tissues.

Acute inflammatory change in muscle and tendon sheaths with the rapid deposition of collagen with secondary thickening and fibrosis may occur in acute neurological states, notably in the acute stage of poliomyelitis, in pyogenic or tuberculous meningitis, in acute cerebral vascular episodes, or in acute exacerbations of multiple sclerosis. The contracture is characterized by the rapidity of its development and by pain on attempting to stretch the affected tissues, by the characteristic tissues involved which, in the hip, are likely to be the sheath of the tensor fasciae latae and the iliopsoas, and by the absence of any correlation with the distribution of the paralysis. This type of contracture is not found in most types of cerebral palsy in childhood except those developing in association with acute meningitis or encephalitis. If treated carefully but vigorously by splintage and passive movement during the acute phase of the disease, fixed deformity can be prevented. If such measures are not or cannot be applied, strong and thick fibrous tissue not amenable to stretching by passive means develops and may require surgical correction.

Fixed postural deformity arises when the paralyzed limb lies in a particular position for a period of weeks or months without the maintenance of passive movement. If, for example, a completely flail lower limb is left unsupported without regular passive movement, fixed flexion, abduction, and lateral rotation at the hip, fixed flexion at the knee, and equinus at the ankle are likely to develop [34] (Fig. 13–2). This posture is especially aggravated by the prolonged use of a wheelchair. Maintenance of the position of deformity by spasticity may also contribute to the development of postural contracture, especially in adults, but except in flail limbs or limbs with generalized weakness, deformity is more likely to be caused by muscle imbalance. Fixed postural deformity can usually be minimized by regular passive stretching and, if necessary, by the use of night splintage or day bracing. A deformity that has been allowed to become too severe usually requires surgical measures.

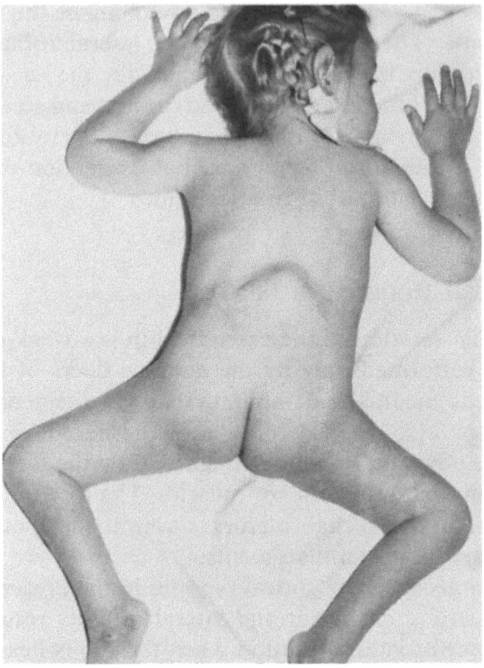

FIG. 13–2 Fixed postural deformity. The lower limbs are flail and have been allowed to develop fixed flexion, abduction, and lateral rotation at the hips, fixed flexion at the knees, and equinus at the ankles.

Deformity arising from unbalanced muscle activity at a joint is the most common and serious cause of fixed deformity. It does not occur in a limb with normal muscles or in limbs in which there is overall weakness affecting each muscle group equally. It does not develop in a completely flail limb and is much more common in children than in adults. It develops slowly, is progressive, and increases at a rate that is related to the rate of growth of the limb. Although regular passive stretching and splintage may delay its progress, increasing deformity develops no matter how vigorous the physiotherapy or how firm the splintage. The distribution of the deformity is directly related to the balance of action of affected muscles. If the hip abductors are weak and the adductors are strong, a gradual limitation of the range of passive abduction develops (Fig. 13–3). The limited abduction is associated with relative shortness of the adductor muscles but macroscopic and microscopic examinations show no fibrosis or true contracture. The muscle is not shorter than it was at the age at which the paralysis developed but it is short relative to the length of the skeleton; it must therefore be concluded that this is due to failure of growth in a muscle that is not receiving the normal tension stimulus of its weaker opponents. In this type of deformity the greater the deformity, the more potent the action of the deforming muscles to cause yet further deformity. This type of deformity always demands measures to restore normal muscle and tendon length and the balance of muscle activity. If the treatment fails to achieve this, the deformity will recur as long as growth continues. Deformity of this type is common in poliomyelitis, cerebral palsy, and spina bifida; in open myelomeningocele, it is responsible for intrauterine deformity and the presence of severe deformities in the lower limbs established at birth. This type of deformity is the prime indication for surgery in paralytic lesions.

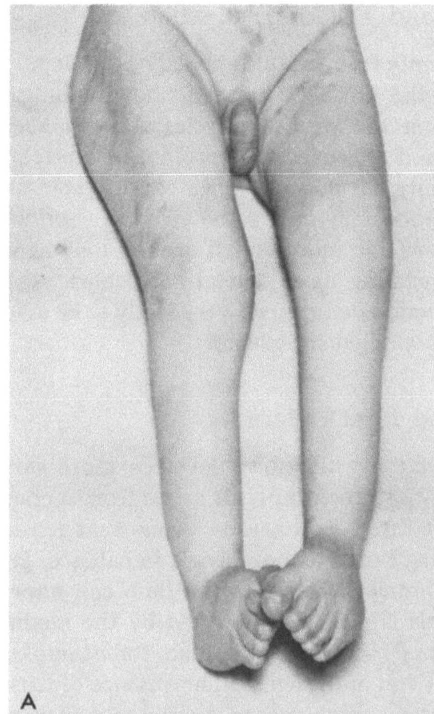

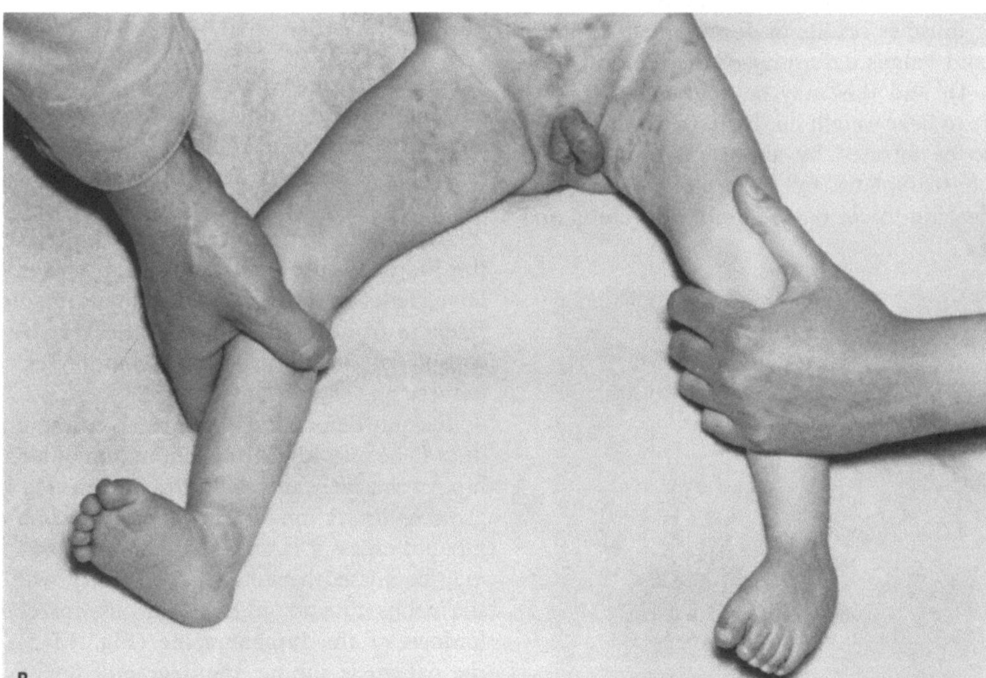

FIG. 13–3 **A** Deformity arising from unbalanced muscle activity. **B** Strong adductor activity in the presence of weak abductors has allowed the development of progressive limitation of the range of passive abduction. Note the tight adductor tendon on the right side which becomes prominent when the hip is forcibly abducted.

Muscle and Tendon Elongation

As deformity from muscle imbalance develops, not only do the stronger muscles show diminished growth but the weaker muscles show increased growth and the effects of prolonged stretching. If deformity has persisted for a considerable time, consideration may have to be given to shortening the tendons and muscles that are too long as well as to elongating those that are too short. At the hip, adduction deformity is very likely to be associated with elongated abductors.

Bone and Joint Deformity

Bone and joint deformity develops more slowly than soft-tissue deformity. It arises from a combination of three mechanisms. Abnormal tensions on growing bones due to muscle imbalance, gravity, or diminished load on the limb can alter its shape; this is well demonstrated by the modified direction of the bony trabeculae, for example, at the upper end of the femur. The absence of tension on the greater trochanter in the presence of paralysis of hip abductors and strongly active flexor and adductor muscles results in development of anteversion and valgus deformity of the femoral neck (Fig. 13–4), and this may be aggravated further by failure to bear weight on the limb. Bone growth may also be affected by abnormal pressures on the epiphyseal plates by abnormal posture and weight-bearing forces on the limb. Stretching and growth elongation of the capsules and ligaments of joints and overgrowth of bone and cartilage that have escaped the confines of the joint add to joint deformity once established.

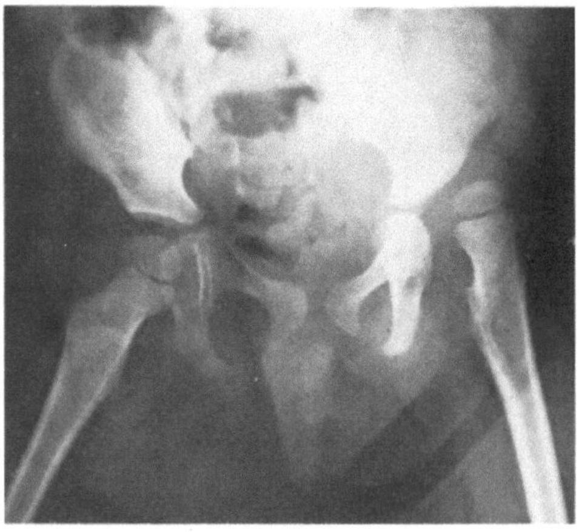

FIG. 13–4 Anteversion and valgus deformity of the femoral neck in abductor paralysis. The right hip is shown in full medial rotation and the left hip in full lateral rotation, to show that both anteversion and valgus deformity are present.

Features of Paralytic Deformity at the Hip

Any combination of deformity can occur if the appropriate paralytic circumstances are present. Instances have been seen with 90° hyperextension deformity at the hip so that the patient sat with the lower limb projecting behind the trunk, but severe deformity in this direction is rare. Because the common distribution of paralysis is toward predominance of flexor activity, this, and prolonged sitting posture, make flexion deformity by far the most common at the hip.

Flexion and Flexion–Lateral Rotation Deformity

Flexion deformity is most likely to be seen in flail hip on which the patient has been allowed to sit for prolonged periods in a wheelchair; it may take 2 or 3 years to develop by this mechanism. It is almost always associated with lordosis of the lumbar spine and, in poliomyelitis, paralysis of the abdominal musculature aggravates the deformity, especially if there is activity in the extensors of the trunk.

All the flexor structures become tight, including the iliopsoas, pectineus, sartorius, tensor fasciae latae, anterior fibers of the gluteus medius, the fascia in front of the hip, and in severe cases, the capsule of the hip and the femoral vessels and nerves.

Flexion deformity is the most common deformity to be missed in the examination of a paralytic hip. In the early stages, it is demonstrated by progressive limitation of range of extension of the hip, but unless it is tested for carefully, this finding may be missed because of the facility with which the pelvis tilts to give a spurious correction by lordosis of the lumbar spine (Fig. 13–5). When the patient is supine, the degree of flexion deformity is often masked by the fact that the hip tends to roll into lateral rotation, making any flexion deformity appear to be abduction deformity. To test for fixed flexion, the affected hip must be brought into neutral rotation and the opposite hip flexed forcibly to insure that all compensatory lor-

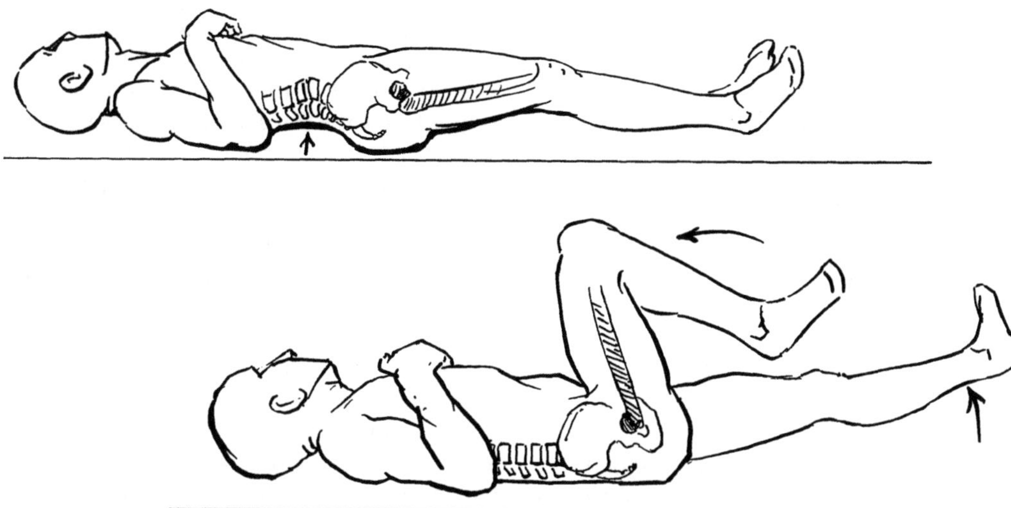

FIG. 13–5 Fixed flexion of the hip concealed by mobile lumbar lordosis. When the lordosis is eliminated by flexing the opposite hip fully and so tilting the pelvis, the true extent of the flexion deformity becomes apparent (Thomas' test).

dosis of the lumbar spine is completely eliminated. When this test is done properly, it will usually be found that the degree of flexion deformity is much greater than at first appeared. It is not easy to perform the test single-handed, especially in an older child or an adult.

Flexion–lateral rotation deformity develops when there is activity in the muscles supplied by the first two lumbar segments, the iliopsoas, sartorius, and pectineus. The lower limbs lie in the frog position. If the thighs are brought up to a position parallel with the trunk and the hips medially rotated, the degree of flexion deformity will become apparent (Fig. 13–6). The fact that the deformity is primarily due to shortness of the iliopsoas and sartorius will be revealed by the fact that lateral rotation of the hip diminishes the degree of deformity. The presence of active flexion in the hip musculature in the presence of paralysis of all other hip musculature confirms the diagnosis as a paralytic growth deformity.

Radiographs may show valgus deformity and anteversion of the femoral neck but dislocation rarely occurs.

Flexion–Abduction Deformity

Flexion–abduction deformity is most commonly seen in poliomyelitis, usually as an immediate sequel of the acute stage, when it is a true contracture. The tissues primarily affected are the sheath of the tensor fasciae latae and the fasciae of the front of the thigh, which are contracted and thickened with the deposition of collagen in them.

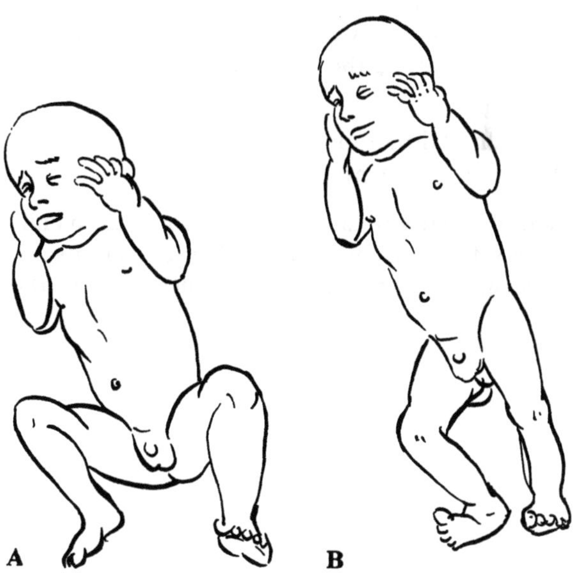

A B

FIG. 13–6 Flexion–lateral rotation deformity due to isolated action in the hip flexor muscles. When the hips are flexed and abducted the deformity can be concealed (A), but when the legs are pulled down and adducted, the deformity becomes obvious as seen in child's right hip (B).

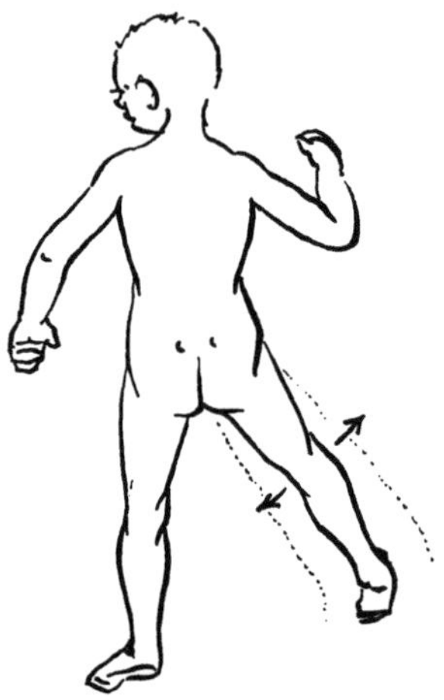

FIG. 13–7 Flexion–abduction deformity. With the patient prone and the hips extended, the affected hip cannot be adducted.

The extent of this deformity is also masked, especially in the supine position. The patient should be turned into the prone position, the hip extended as far as possible in the abducted position, and the range of *adduction* assessed (Fig. 13–7). It is normally possible for the extended hip to be adducted until it crosses behind the opposite limb. In the presence of flexion–abduction deformity, the limb may remain in fixed abduction or approach only to the midline.

Flexion–Adduction–Lateral Rotation Deformity

This deformity is almost entirely confined to children suffering from paralysis due to open myelomeningocele in which there is innervation to the first three or four lumbar segments with paralysis of other musculature. It is one of the most common deformities at the hip in spina bifida and may be present at birth if there has been intrauterine paralysis below the third lumbar neural segment (Fig. 13–8), or later if normal innervation in utero has been converted to complete sacral paralysis.

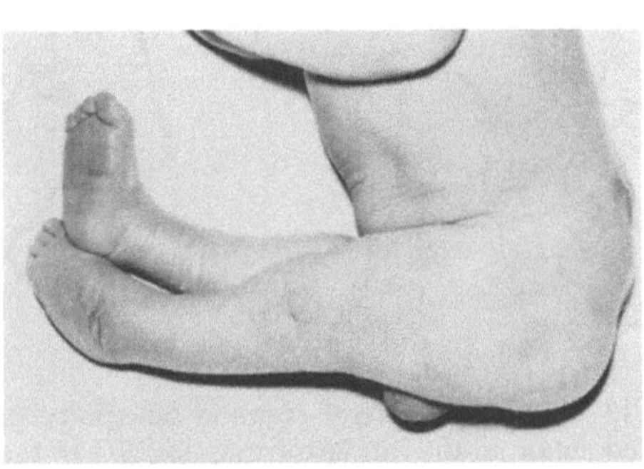

FIG. 13–8 Flexion–adduction–lateral rotation deformity in a child born with spina bifida with paralysis below the third lumbar neural segment.

The hips are flexed, often to 90°, adducted with a range of only 10° of passive abduction, and laterally rotated so the patella faces laterally or even posteriorly. The deformity arises from strong action in the iliopsoas muscle which is always a very strong lateral rotator of the infant hip, together with strong action in the adductor muscles and in the quadriceps. There is complete paralysis of all gluteal musculature and of medial and lateral hamstring muscles. This paralytic pattern of deformity is almost always associated with dislocation of the hip which may be present at birth if the paralysis has been intrauterine or may develop during the first year or two of life.

Lesser degrees of the same deformity may develop more gradually when innervation extends to the fifth lumbar segment, so that there is some activity in the gluteal abductors. There is some limitation of abduction and some fixed flexion at birth which slowly increases during the first two or three years of life and eventually results in dislocation between the second and fifth year.

Flexion–Adduction–Medial Rotation Deformity

This deformity is common in paraplegic or quadriplegic spastic cerebral palsy (Fig. 13–9). It usually develops slowly during the first five or six years of life, first manifesting with gradual limitation of abduction and diminution in the range of extension. It is produced by strong and spastic hip flexor, adductor, and hamstring musculature in the presence of paresis of the gluteal musculature and is associated with progressive subluxation and eventual dislocation of the hip.

In testing for this deformity, spastic posture must be differentiated from fixed deformity. When Thomas' test is performed by flexing the opposite hip, the affected hip tends to rise up into flexion but can be extended gradually by firm pressure to demonstrate the true shortening of the flexor muscles. Abduction should be tested with extended hips and knees. Tightness of the gracilis and hamstring muscles, which are important components in this deformity, may be masked by a flexed position of the knees.

Adduction Deformity

Pure adduction deformity is the most common hip deformity in cerebral palsy. It may appear at any age from the third month of life onward; the common age at which it is noticed to be significant is usually 4 or 5 years. The muscles most commonly affected initially are the adductor longus and gracilis.

With the hips and knees extended, the hips should be abducted slowly to stretch any spasticity in the adductor musculature. At the crucial point at which true shortening is revealed, there is a block to further abduction and the child, if young, will react suddenly against further movement or, if older, will indicate that further abduction is painful. The tight adductor and gracilis tendons of origin are easily visible and palpable. More severe degrees of deformity may show shortening of the adductor brevis, adductor magnus, and the ischial portion of the hamstring musculature.

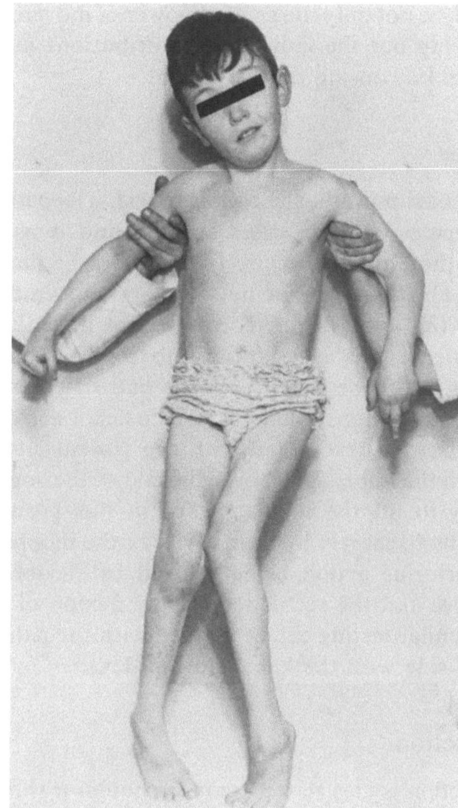

FIG. 13–9 Flexion–adduction–medial rotation deformity due to strong, spastic hip flexor, adductor, and hamstring muscles and paretic gluteal muscles.

Abduction–Extension–Lateral Rotation Deformity

This is an unusual deformity almost unique to patients with paralysis due to open myelomeningocele. It occurs when there is paresis or paralysis of muscles supplied by the lumbar neural segments and spastic activity in the sacral neural segments.

The limbs lie in extension, abduction, and lateral rotation (Fig. 13–10). Occasionally the deformity may appear at birth or in early childhood. The deformity is such that the knees cannot be brought to the midline and there is often severe fixed lateral rotation deformity due to spasticity and shortening of the small lateral rotators of the hip. The gluteus medius and maximus muscles are also short and may be spastic. The knees often show flexion deformity due to shortening of the biceps femoris.

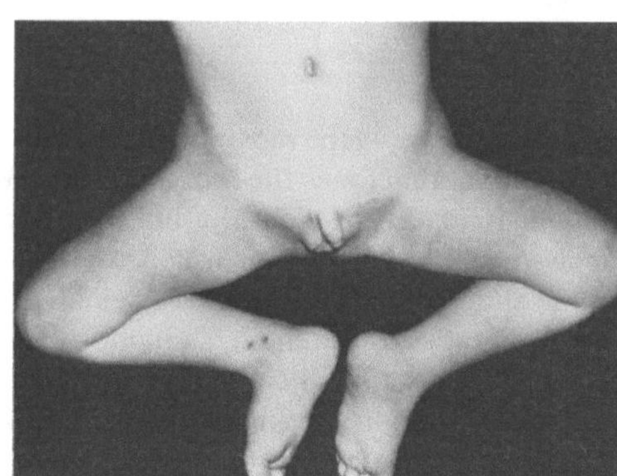

FIG. 13–10 Extension–abduction–lateral rotation deformity in spina bifida with paralysis of the lumbar neural segments and spastic activity in the sacral neural segments.

Assessment of Hip Musculature

The assessment of strength and action in the hip musculature is more difficult than that of any other joint in the lower limb, particularly in infancy and early childhood. An attempt should be made to analyze not only the general power of movement of the hip but the individual contributions made by muscles causing the movement.

Flexion

Hip flexion power is the easiest to test. The patient lies supine with the knees straight and is asked to lift the limb at the hip. In doing so, he makes use of all the hip flexor musculature and grading as fair (3), good (4), or normal is not difficult. If the patient is unable to lift the limb from the couch, flexion should be tested with the patient lying on the side to demonstrate weak (2) hip flexor activity.

Flexion is next tested with the patient sitting up with the knees flexed over the end of the couch. Ability to lift the thigh upward in this position is produced largely by the activity of the iliopsoas, the sartorius action being relaxed by flexion of the knee and the rectus femoris by flexion of the hip. Similar testing can be applied with the patient on his side with the knee and hip flexed.

Adduction

Adduction is also tested easily, although it should be remembered that, to test the action of the adductors against gravity, the patient should lie on the side to be tested and lift the limb upward from the couch. The adductors are a strong group of muscles and this action should easily be possible if the hip adductor power is good or strong.

Abduction

Hip abductor power is the most important activity to assess and is sometimes the most difficult. With the patient lying on the side, the hip is abducted as far as possible. He is then asked to hold the hip in the abducted position without flexing it and he should be able to maintain abduction against the downward force of the examiner's hands. It is particularly important in spastic children to stretch out any spasticity in the adductors before asking the patient to perform this activity.

If the hip drops when it is let go, the abductor power is certainly less than fair (3) and possibly completely absent. Confirmation of gluteal activity can usually be obtained by palpating the gluteal region although sometimes there may be difficulty in young children when there is a heavy deposit of fat in the gluteal fossa.

Ability to abduct the hips with the patient supine can be tested when abduction is weaker than poor (2), although care must be taken to ensure that the movement is not produced by elevation of the pelvis. When testing hip abductor power, the power of the quadratus lumborum and lateral hip flexors of the same side can be assessed by asking the patient to shorten the limb by elevating the pelvis while traction is applied to the extended limb.

Extension

Extension power at the hip is also difficult to estimate. The patient is asked to lie prone on the couch with the lower limbs flexed over the end of the couch. He is then asked to extend the hip at first with the knees extended so that the gluteus maximus and hamstring musculature may both contribute to extensor power, and then with the knee flexed to eliminate the action of the hamstring muscles. The gluteus maximus can be palpated to determine whether it is active.

Rotation

Medial and lateral rotation movements of the hip are best tested with the patient sitting with the knees flexed over the end of the couch to eliminate the action of the iliopsoas and hamstring muscles. The power of medial rotation produced by the anterior fibers of the gluteal muscles and of lateral rotation by the small lateral rotator musculature can be assessed in this position. The grading is not easy since both movements are not strong movements even in normal individuals.

Paralytic Dislocation of the Hip

Dislocation of the hip is a common result of paralytic lesions in childhood.[4] It is most commonly seen in spina bifida, not infrequently in cerebral palsy, and occasionally in poliomyelitis. Watson-Jones [56] was the first to point out that the dislocation was associated with weakness or *paralysis of the hip abductors in the presence of active hip flexor and adductor muscles.* Others [19,30,53] have confirmed this finding for patients with spastic cerebral palsy and Sharrard [41,42] has demonstrated the strong relationship between paralysis of abduction action in the presence of strong adductors and hip flexors in spina bifida and dislocation at birth or its subsequent development. In poliomyelitis dislocation is uncommon, probably because the hip adductors are often paretic,[39] but when weakness of hip abduction is associated with strong hip flexion and adduction dislocation may result.[28]

Paralytic dislocation is frequently, but not invariably, associated with valgus deformity and anteversion of the femoral neck, which some authors [17,20,29,49] believe to be the primary cause of paralytic dislocation. It is true that paralytic dislocation of the hip is almost always associated with such valgus deformity and anteversion but the converse is not true. Many patients with generalized or complete paralysis of all the muscles in the region of the hip, in poliomyelitis, spina bifida, and some forms of infantile spinal atrophy, may have quite marked femoral neck deformity persisting into adult life, but dislocation never occurs (Fig. 13–11). Correction of valgus and anteversion deformity by varus osteotomy reduces the liability to dislocation, but dislocation may recur even after an adequate varus osteotomy if unbalanced action between the adductors and abductors at the hip is not corrected.[18]

The explanation may lie in the effect of muscle pull on the development of the femoral neck. Paresis or paralysis of the gluteal abductors predisposes to the development of valgus deformity and anteversion and results in dislocation of the hip if the adductors and hip flexors are strong. Muscle activity can thus be made to account for the dislocation and the deformity of the femoral neck at the same time. The finding that, following posterolateral iliopsoas transplantation, valgus deformity of the femoral neck disappears and may even be replaced by varus deformity [47] is an additional argument in favor of this explanation.

Paralytic dislocation seldom develops unless there is limitation of hip abduction with short adductor muscles combined with flexion deformity with shortening of the iliopsoas tendon. Adduction contracture alone is less likely to cause dislocation, although it can do so if there is also pelvic obliquity. Flexion deformity alone rarely gives rise to dislocation, but flexion–lateral rotation deformity can do so.

The mechanism of the dislocation has never been completely explained. Observations of the mechanisms of dislocations in cerebral palsy and spina bifida using cineradiography show that, when the hip starts to subluxate, abnormal lateral movement of the head of the femur develops on adduction and abduction (Fig. 13–12). The axis of adduction and abduction of the hip moves from the region of the center of the head of the femur distally to the level of the lesser trochanter at the insertion of the iliopsoas tendon. Repeated movement leads to stretching of the hip capsule and, with increasing adduction deformity, the hip eventually dislocates superolaterally where the capsule is not protected by the strong iliofemoral ligament. In infants and young children, the iliopsoas is also a strong lateral rotator; this increases the liability to dislocation by bringing the head of the femur into contact with the weaker part of the capsule at a younger age than in cerebral palsy, in which there is more likely to be medial rotation deformity.

Dysplasia of the acetabulum is not necessarily present when the hip dislocates either in cerebral palsy [3] or spina bifida [42] (Fig. 13–13). Once the hip has dislocated, the acetabulum may remain relatively normal for periods varying between 6 months and 2 years; eventually dysplasia of the acetabular roof becomes apparent, however, and the changes are comparable with those of an unreduced congenital dislocation of the hip. Acetabular deformity may develop in patients in whom muscle imbalance is not particularly great and subluxation develops slowly so that, for a period of many months, a hip may dislocate in and out of joint on abduction and adduction.

The final proof that paralytic dislocation is primarily due to imbalance of muscle action is demonstrated by the fact that early correction of adductor/abductor imbalance can prevent all but a very few dislocations of the hip,[43,44] and that recurrence of dislocation is rare when balance is obtained by weakening the adductors and strengthening the abductors by tendon transplantation.[28,47] A hip that has been dislocated for several months has a loose capsule that may require reefing; if the deformity has been present for a considerable time, acetabuloplasty or innominate osteotomy may be required to correct obliquity of the acetabular roof. In long-standing dislocation of the hip, the gross shortening of all tissues associated with it may make reduction impossible unless open reduction and tendon transplantation are accompanied by varus osteotomy with excision of a portion of the femoral shaft.[48]

In a hip that has been dislocated for some years, especially with spastic cerebral palsy, degenerative

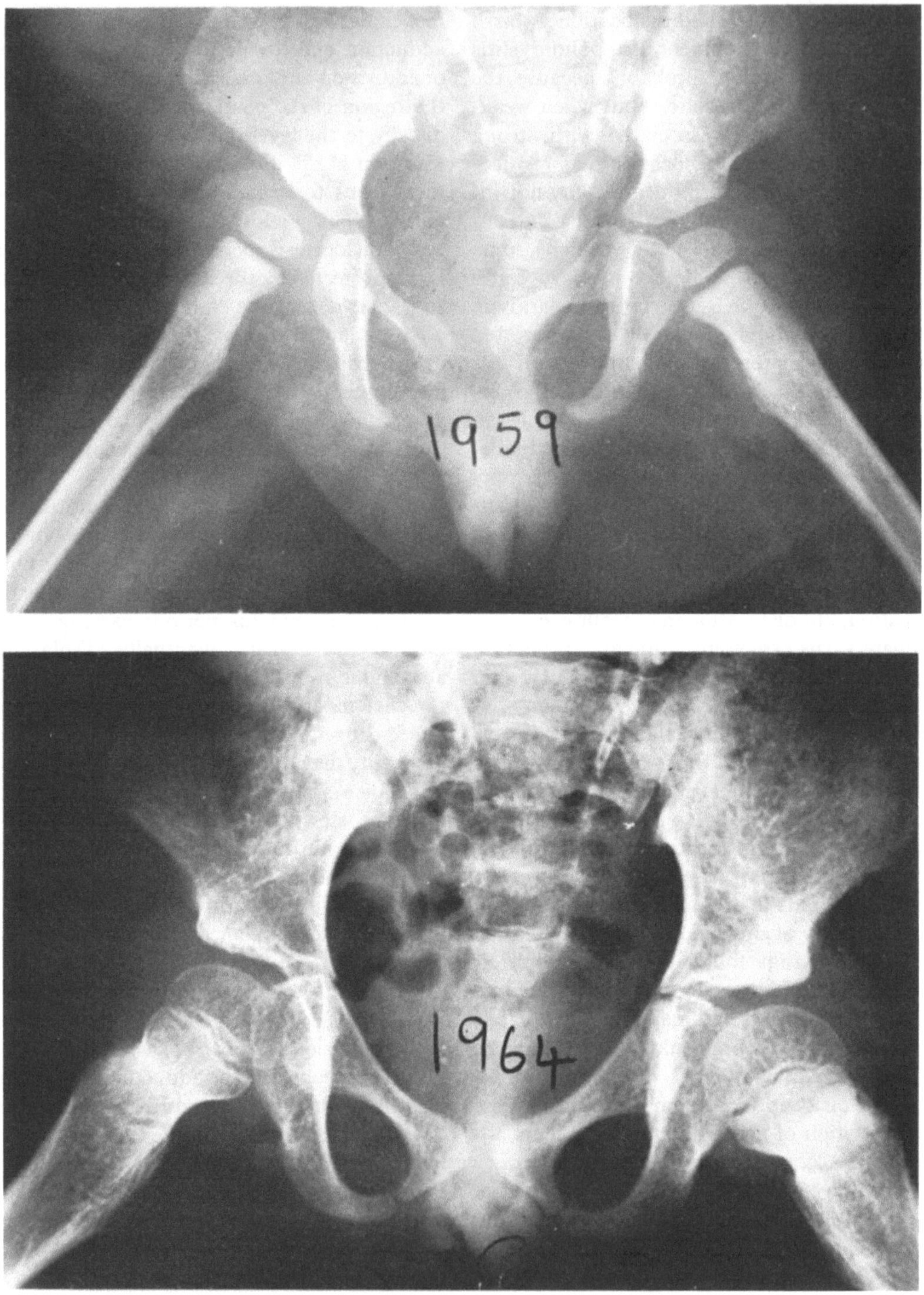

FIG. 13–11 Radiographs of the hips in severe paralysis in spina bifida. In spite of the appearance of subluxation with a sloping acetabulum, the hips subsequently developed normally without any specific treatment. There was no unbalanced muscle activity of the hip muscles.

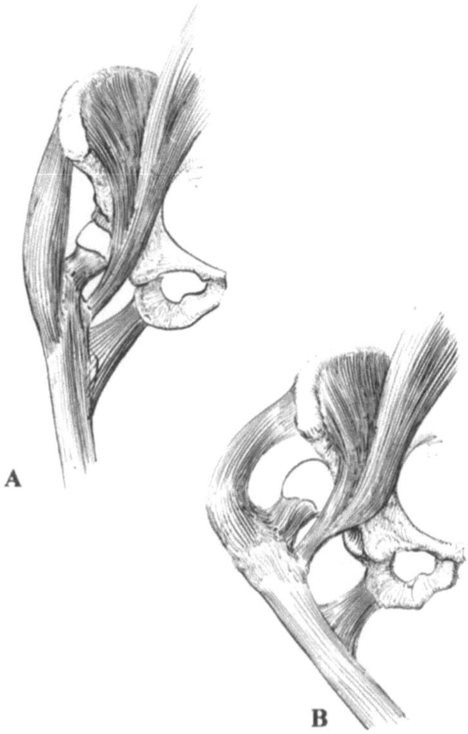

FIG. 13–12 The mechanism of paralytic dislocation of the hip: The short and strong iliopsoas and hip adductor muscles in the presence of weak hip abductors and extensors lead to a shift of the center of movement of the hip from the head of the femur to the level of the lesser trochanter. Anterolateral force is applied to the capsule which stretches and the hip slowly dislocates. **A** Normal balance. **B** Dislocation.

changes in the articular cartilage of the head of the femur develop rapidly and in adolescence the dislocated hip becomes painful. This is in contrast to the situation in congenital dislocation of the hip in which a completely dislocated hip may often remain free of pain for many years. The difference probably arises because, in the spastic hip, the grinding of the head of the femur against the side of the ilium produced by the spastic hip flexor and adductor muscles accelerates degenerative change.

Principles of Management of the Paralytic Hip

Paralysis, whatever the cause, is amenable to five methods of treatment: exercise therapy, passive movements, splintage, bracing, and surgery. Each has its proper place in the management of paralysis but its proper application depends on a knowledge of what it can and cannot achieve.

Exercise Therapy

The development of increased muscle power and prolonged muscle activity by the use of exercise treatment is as well recognized in the athletic world as in medicine. Its use and value in each type of paralysis will be considered in the sections concerned.

Exercise treatment cannot correct unbalanced muscle activity by concentrating on the action of an individual muscle group. If there is weakness of hip abduction in the presence of strong adductors, persistent abduction exercises may, at first, improve the power of the abductors, but in time, the increased activity will also reflect on the power of the adductors which themselves will increase their power yet further, thus maintaining the state of imbalance. Attempts to exercise a severely paretic or completely paralyzed muscle may even make the imbalance worse by increasing the power of the active muscle more satisfactorily than that of the severely paralyzed one.

Splintage and Traction

Splintage (here differentiated from bracing used in ambulation) and traction have their value in attempts to prevent or correct joint deformity. Splints are indicated in conditions in which acute deformity may develop rapidly, e.g., in the acute stage of anterior poliomyelitis or in other acute neurological episodes, when collagen may be laid down in fasciae, tissue planes, and tendon sheaths or when prolonged posture opposed by gravity may, in the presence of edema, result in true fibrous contracture and joint adhesions. Traction may also be used to produce gradual correction of deformities arising in the same way. It is contraindicated in spina bifida by the presence of sensory loss because of the extreme danger of the production of serious pressure sores. In cerebral palsy, it is of occasional value for short periods; the application of splints or traction to spastic muscles tends to cause reflex action to resist the splintage and, in the end, more liability to deformity than was originally present.

A serious disadvantage of prolonged splintage is that the immobilization required causes weakened muscles to become even weaker. Splintage,

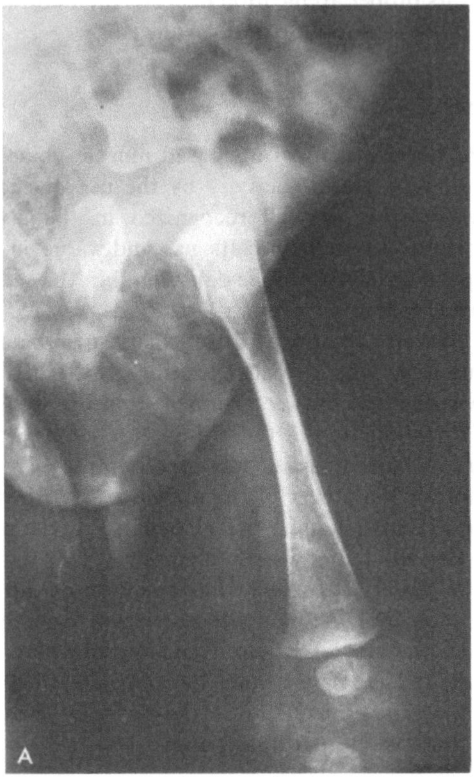

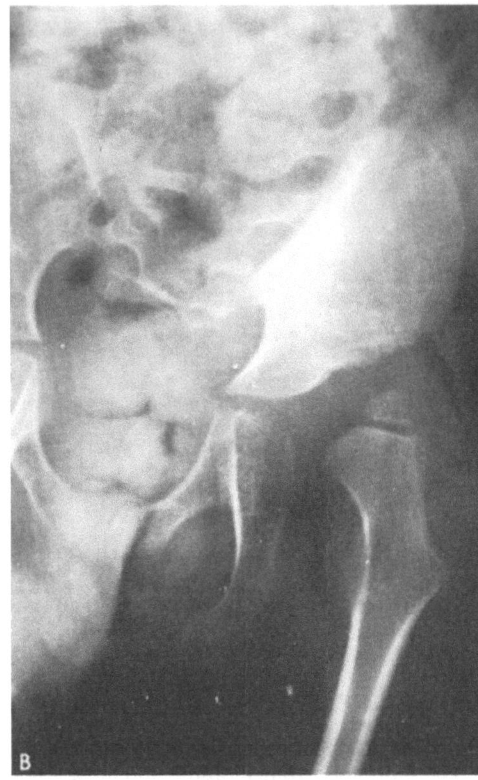

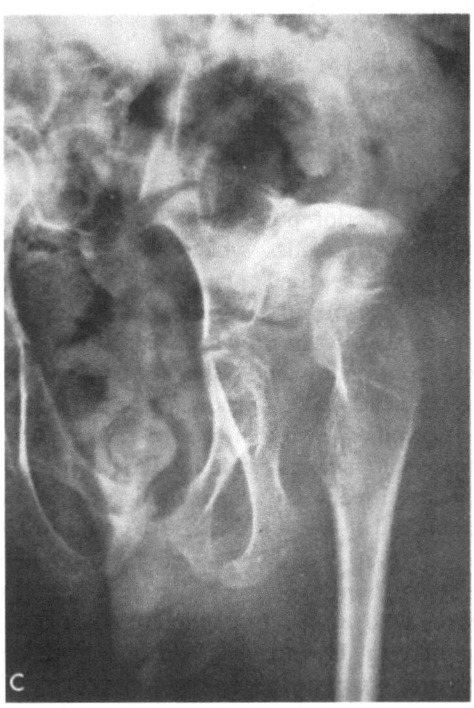

FIG. 13–13 Radiographs of progressive changes in paralytic dislocation of the hip in spina bifida. **A** At birth, the hip was not dislocated. **B** At the age of 3 years, dislocation has occurred. The acetabulum was not dysplastic at the time of dislocation. **C** At the age of 10 years, there was gross acetabular dysplasia. An adequate false acetabulum had developed.

therefore, is of no value in the management of deformity secondary to muscle imbalance. Even if a deformity is partially corrected, the muscle imbalance resulting from immobilization may become greater still.

Passive Movements

Passive joint movements find application in all types of paralysis. Regular manual manipulation of joints to obtain the maximum range of movements possible each day does much to prevent the development of deformity due to posture and may help to diminish the rate of progress of a deformity due to muscle imbalance.

Although such activities are mainly the province of the physiatrist and physiotherapist, parents can be taught to maintain daily passive movements themselves; it must be recognized, however, that many parents are naturally somewhat cautious about the application of excessive force.

Excessive passive movements can cause fractures, notably in spina bifida, and even the best applied regimen of exercise and passive movements will always fail to prevent the gradual development of deformity in the presence of unbalanced muscle activity.

It may be important to ensure that correct passive movements are being made so that muscles and tendons that are tending to contract may be specifically treated. Shortness of the gracilis muscle, for example, requires that the hip be passively abducted with the knee extended and shortness of the sartorius muscle calls for extension and medial rotation of the hip with the knee extended. Serial records should be made by goniometer measurement of the range of passive movement to show whether improvement is being maintained or deterioration is occurring; such measurements may be made monthly, every 3 months or every 6 months, depending on the stage and nature of the paralysis.

Bracing

Bracing is required in two circumstances: to support a joint that is completely flail or paralyzed in such a way that an upright stance is not possible, or to aid in the management of a joint that is not under adequate voluntary control. Bracing should be used with care. It should not be used when other methods of treatment—exercise, tendon transplantation, or surgery—could achieve the same end. If bracing is once applied, the patient may come to rely on the brace and his musculature may diminish in power because the need for muscle activity has been lessened. Bracing may sometimes be used as a temporary measure for a few weeks or months to aid a patient to gain balance and to learn walking, with the object that he may discard the bracing later. If this is done, a planned program of action must be followed so that the need for bracing does not continue indefinitely.

A completely flail hip is an absolute indication for a hip brace in children and in some adults. Gluteal weakness may require the use of a hip brace, but it should not be used if muscles such as the psoas can be transplanted to replace or support gluteal action, even if the gait may not be completely normal.

Hip bracing presents some special difficulties in design and application. The purchase for its support must be taken from the trunk, either by a total trunk support if there is weakness of the lower trunk musculature or through the medium of a pelvic band. The classical hip braces of the past have used a hip hinge with a lock which can be fixed when the patient is walking and released to allow him to sit. If such a lock is used, the patient cannot walk by taking alternate strides in the normal way but needs to rotate his pelvis to move along. If a full trunk support rather than a pelvic band is used, the patient cannot elevate his pelvis to lift the foot from the ground and tends to shuffle rather than walk.

Semimobile hip hinges (Fig. 13–14) that allow 20 to 25° of free flexion or extension and a similar range of free adduction and abduction improve the quality of gait and can be used when the hips are flail.[15] Rose [32] has devised a form of splint for severely paralyzed hips that allows balancing on plates and forward ambulation with a rotary motion of the pelvis. This has the advantage that the upper limbs are unencumbered and there is no need for crutches or sticks but the disadvantage that, as the child gets older, the plates to support the feet and to allow balance must be made increasingly larger. Other types of brace make use of cable attachments to produce extension of the opposite hip when one hip is flexed. Future research may see the development of power-assisted braces for hip paralysis.

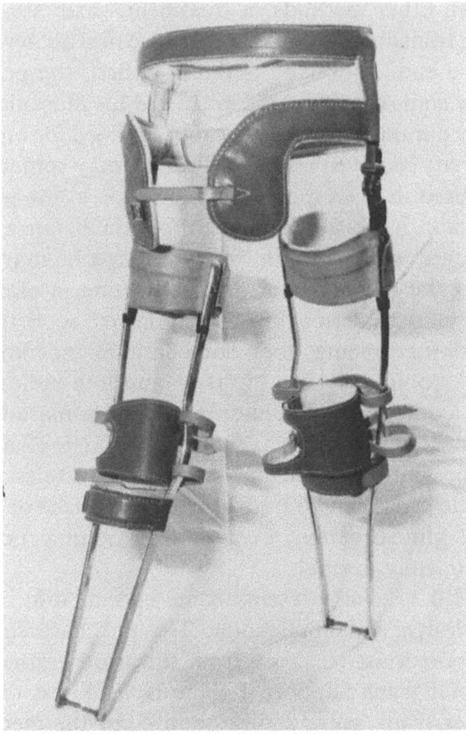

FIG. 13–14 Hip braces with semimobile hip hinges. The hinges allow 20 to 25° of free flexion or extension and a similar range of free adduction and abduction.

Surgical Treatment

Surgery can aid in the treatment of paralysis in three ways: by correcting deformity, by correcting muscle imbalance, and by providing stability at a joint. Initially, deformity in paralytic lesions arises from relatively short muscles and tendons. The lengthening or release of short tendons and muscles is one of the main purposes of surgical treatment. Osteotomy to correct bony deformity may be needed if release of tendons, muscles, and soft tissues fails to give sufficient correction.

Muscle imbalance can be corrected by weakening the stronger muscles by division, lengthening, neurectomy, or a combination of both. Balance can also be achieved by tendon transfer of a strong and deforming muscle to a new site, preferably one in which it may help to maintain correction of the deformity and improve function.

Both methods have an important part to play in the management of a paralytic hip. Surgery to elongate the muscles which are becoming progressively shorter is indicated whenever function is impaired by the deformity or complications such as dislocation of the hip threaten. More than 20° of fixed flexion deformity, less than 30° range of abduction, and fixed medial or lateral rotation deformity are all indications for correction of hip deformity. Progressive subluxation is an urgent indication for surgical treatment, and for dislocation only surgery can succeed in achieving and maintaining reduction.

Occasionally, a severely unstable hip may warrant arthrodesis, especially if only one hip is affected and if the arthrodesis will then allow bracing to be discarded.

The individual indications and techniques of operative procedures for the paralytic hip will be described in subsequent sections.

The Hip and Overall Management of the Paralytic Lower Limb

Whatever the cause of the paralysis, the total management of the patient should never be forgotten, nor should the condition of the hip be considered in isolation. A flexed knee or an equinus deformity of the foot may be more important in the production of flexion deformity of the hip than the hip muscles themselves. Bilateral dislocated hips in a child with flail lower limbs are often better left untouched. Bracing which is so extensive that its weight alone almost precludes walking with weakened or spastic lower limbs is unacceptable when simple, early surgery and good physical therapy can achieve walking without a brace.

In a patient with severely paralyzed lower limbs, a basic decision may have to be made as to whether he should be condemned to a wheelchair for life. If the upper limbs and trunk are strong enough, there is always a value, even if mainly a psychological one, in being able to walk with bracing for a short distance each day, and he should always be given the chance to do so. This is especially true in childhood, when compensation for paralysis has some remarkable potential.

The management of paralytic conditions such as poliomyelitis, cerebral palsy, spina bifida, or muscular dystrophy should be undertaken by a team of individuals interested in and with experience of pediatrics, neurology, and paralytic reconstructive surgery. The occasional surgeon may do more harm than good, particularly if he has not acquired the ability to make regular, serial assessments of function, paralysis, and deformity and is not well cognizant of the effects of the surgery that he may attempt.

The Hip in Paralytic Poliomyelitis

Poliomyelitis affects the neuromuscular and ligamentous tissues in two distinct ways. During the acute stage of the disease, there are pain and spasm in the muscles and a deposition of collagen in the fasciae, tendon sheaths, and fibrous tissues of affected limbs. There is extensive neuronal damage; some of this is permanent, with complete destruction of anterior horn cells, but some is temporary, with potential for recovery of damaged or neurapraxic neurons.

The Acute Stage

During the acute stage of poliomyelitis, if a lower limb is involved, the hip tends to flex, rotate laterally, and abduct. The tissues particularly affected by collagen deposition are the fascia lata of the thigh and the iliopsoas tendon.

During the acute stage of the disease, the limbs should be immobilized to prevent contracture and to ease pain. This is best achieved by simple metal, plastic, or plaster-of-paris splints applied to both lower limbs and linked together to maintain the hip joint in neutral position.[36] Passive movements are directed particularly toward maintenance of extension, adduction, and medial rotation at the hips. As much can be achieved by applying passive movements twice or three times in any one day as by any prolonged repetition of passive stretching. Overforcible passive movements can tear muscles and damage joints, and thus must be avoided. If muscles are painful, as in the acute stage of poliomyelitis, passive movements can be helped by heat in the form of hot packs applied to the surface or radiant heat.

If, in spite of such measures, flexion–abduction deformity develops during the acute stage and is not relieved by attempts to stretch the tensor fasciae latae and hip flexor structures by the end of the fourth or fifth month, surgical division of the tensor fasciae latae and flexor structures of the hip, including, if necessary, elongation of the iliopsoas tendon, may be needed.

The upper lumbar neural segments are frequently affected by poliomyelitis and the hip musculature is often involved. The quadriceps, hip abductors, hamstring muscles, hip adductors, and hip flexors are the six muscle groups most commonly affected by poliomyelitis, but the involvement is usually partial. The hip abductors, adductors, and flexor muscles are much less often completely paralyzed than are the muscles below the knee.[39] When residual muscle activity is present in a severely affected hip it will be usually found that the gluteus maximus and the small lateral rotators of the hip are acting. In children, paralysis at the hip usually affects most of the muscle groups together, so that severe imbalance of activity between, for instance, the hip adductors and hip abductors is much less common in poliomyelitis than in spina bifida or cerebral palsy.

The Recovery Stage

During the stage of recovery of activity in neurons affected by poliomyelitis but not completely destroyed by the virus, the need is for graduated exercises to affected muscles. Most normal individuals utilize less than half the potential power of their muscles in average normal activity. Specific training of muscle action by repeated daily activity against graduated and increasing resistance can increase the power of the same muscle fibers with a given neuromuscular unit supply almost twice, and practice and continuously maintained activity can prolong muscle action without producing fatigue. Power and endurance can both be increased in paretic muscle by techniques well recognized in athletic pursuits, i.e., by daily training; it must be remembered, however, that overexercising does not necessarily improve a muscle by more than a given amount on any particular day and may even result in diminished activity on subsequent days if the muscle is asked to perform activities beyond its maximum capability. About ten contractions of a muscle against the maximum resistance that it is capable of opposing in any one day probably does as much good as any number of contractions greater than this. The increase in power that can be obtained by exercise therapy develops slowly and takes at least 6 months and sometimes longer to reach its maximum. This increase in power is sustained only if the increased strength is utilized regularly in the course of daily activities; a period of immobilization in bed or in plaster may result in loss of power gained by exercise therapy at an earlier date; however, it can usually be restored by an adequate program of exercise therapy in a much shorter time than originally needed.

Exercises may be specific, to increase activity in an individual muscle or muscle group, or associated with function in walking, climbing stairs, getting up and sitting down, or active sporting or athletic pursuits. Exercise therapy has its most important indication in the management of muscles paralyzed by poliomyelitis, at first to help to restore activity in muscles that are innervated from neurons temporarily paralyzed by the infection, and later to increase the activity of residual neuromuscular units to the maximum of which they are capable. If exercise therapy has been properly applied, there is seldom any further improvement to be gained by treatment beyond the end of a year,[40] although improvement in functional ability may continue for longer than this.

At the hip, the particular aims are to develop hip flexion and hip abduction. Exercises directed toward improving the strength of these muscle groups should be done daily and measurements made of improvement in muscle power at monthly intervals. If at all possible, attempts to bear weight should be avoided until the power of hip abduction has become more than sufficient to raise the limb against gravity. However, if such power is not achieved by the eighth or ninth month it is unlikely that it will be achieved, and weight bearing may be essential to allow the patient to start to get about even though the hip abductors are not as adequate as could be wished. During the same period, passive movements to maintain muscle length are carried out.

The Chronic Stage

By the end of a year following the onset of paralysis, almost all recovery of muscle function will have been achieved.[40] If the hip is still severely paralyzed or completely flail, bracing may be needed to allow the patient to walk.

If only one hip is seriously affected, the patient may often learn to balance without the need for any bracing at hip level. If both hips are severely affected, however, walking can be achieved only by the use of a hip brace with or without a trunk support. In poliomyelitis, severe involvement of the musculature of both hips is usually combined with fairly severe involvement of the trunk musculature and some involvement of the muscles of the upper limb, so that ability to walk even with extensive bracing and crutches is necessarily limited.

Partial paralysis of the hip musculature is compatible with walking ability provided that the hip flexor and abductor musculature can act at fair to good levels.

In childhood, particular attention should be paid in the late recovery and chronic stages of poliomyelitis to any imbalance of hip musculature. If the hip abductors are weak but the hip flexors and adductor muscles are also weak, fixed deformity does not develop. Radiographs may show valgus deformity of the neck of the femur but the hip does not subluxate or dislocate. If there is residual weakness of the hip abductors and the hip flexor and adductor muscles are strong, paralytic dislocation is likely to develop at any time from 1 to 4 years after the onset of the acute stage of poliomyelitis, even though adequate physiotherapy, passive movements, and bracing have been used. In this situation, therefore, regular radiographic checks are required every 6 months to determine whether progressive subluxation of the hip is occurring in childhood. In adults, even if there is muscle imbalance, serious deformity and dislocation are extremely unlikely to develop. Parsons and Seddon [28] note that, in their experience, paralytic subluxation was rare if the onset of the paralysis was after the age of 18 months. The author's experience is that subluxation and even dislocation can occur when the onset is in later childhood, although it is progressively less common after the age of 6 or 7 years. Parsons and Seddon also noted that subluxation or dislocation never occurred when there was flexion–abduction deformity, and they concluded, as have many others, that dislocation arose in patients in whom there was imbalance between flexors and adductors relative to extensors and abductors of the hip. Eberle [13] has pointed out that an abduction contracture in one hip with compensatory pelvic obliquity may predispose to dislocation of the opposite hip and that when this condition is present, the abducted hip should be treated first.

Treatment of Hip Disability Following Poliomyelitis

Parsons and Seddon [28] noted that the three conditions of the hip amenable to treatment were contractures, especially flexion–abduction and flexion contractures, subluxation, and dipping gait due to paralysis or weakness of the hip abductors.

Flexion and Flexion–Abduction Contractures

Flexion and flexion–abduction contractures (Fig.

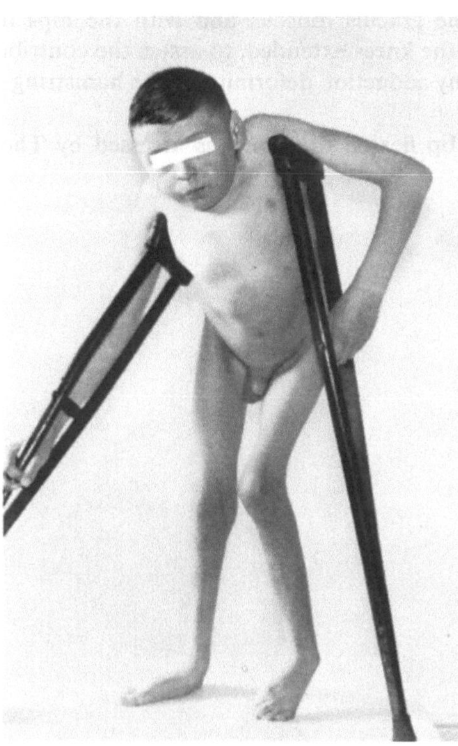

FIG. 13–15 Hip deformity in poliomyelitis. On the right side, there is flexion–abduction deformity due to contracture of the tensor fasciae latae. On the left side, there is flexion–adduction deformity with dislocation of the hip.

13–15) can be treated by soft-tissue operations such as Soutter's muscle slide [50] or multiple subcutaneous fasciotomy. Contracture of the fascia lata, if not severe, can be corrected by Yount's open division of fascia lata and the lateral intermuscular septum.[58] In more severe instances of hip flexion, an extensive soft-tissue release must be performed, including elongation of the iliopsoas tendon and division of the anterior capsule of the hip. Even if such severe measures are required, the hip is not rendered unstable. Flexion deformity greater than 50 or 60° may require that soft-tissue release is followed by subtrochanteric extension osteotomy, usually with removal of a small length of femur to allow complete correction.

Subluxation and Dislocation Subluxation or dislocation of the hip should be treated by open release of the adductors with reduction of the dislocation, followed by anterolateral iliopsoas transplantation if the gluteus maximus is active or posterolateral iliopsoas transplantation [42] if it is not, always provided that the power of the iliopsoas muscle is strong or normal. This procedure alone may suffice, but if the acetabulum has become shallow or dysplastic, the operation may need to be combined with innominate osteotomy.[34] Osteotomy to correct valgus deformity and anteversion fails to prevent subluxation and the valgus deformity recurs. It is able to prevent subluxation only temporarily by virtue of the fact that it slackens the tightness of the iliopsoas and adductor muscles. Arthrodesis is occasionally necessary for longstanding subluxation associated with pain.

Dipping Gait The dipping gait associated with weak but not completely paralyzed hip abductors can be relieved by iliopsoas transplantation, either anterolaterally [25] or posterolaterally,[42] provided that the iliopsoas is at least of good power.[7] An alternative possibility is transfer of the external abdominal oblique muscle to the greater trochanter.[6,54]

The Hip in Cerebral Palsy

Of the various types of cerebral palsy, spastic paralysis is the most likely to produce disability at the hip. Pure athetoid paralysis, with abnormal and involuntary movements of the lower limb as a whole, may give rise to problems of control of abnormal movements at the hips, but fixed deformity requiring surgery is uncommon. Children with a mixture of spastic and athetoid paralysis, however, may show involuntary movements and spasticity with deformity. This state is the most difficult of all to manage.

In the first 6 months of life, there is seldom any abnormality of posture and no fixed deformity. The baby is often a floppy baby, and any abnormal hip posture is due to hypotonia. During this period, spastic paralysis may manifest itself at the hip by the development of spasticity in the adductor muscles and the mother may notice difficulty in applying diapers. In the most severely affected children, true limitation of abduction with relative shortness of the adductor muscles can develop during the first year of life, but in most cerebral-palsied children moderate adductor spasticity is associated with gradual limitation of abduction developing during the first 4 or 5 years.

Examination

In the examination of the hips in cerebral palsy, the aim should be to assess the spasticity and paresis in the hip musculature.

Spasticity most commonly appears in the adductor muscles, less often in the hip flexor muscles, and sometimes in the hip extensors. A measure of the degree of spasticity can be made by comparing the range of abduction obtained by rapidly abducting the hips with the range obtained when passive abduction is attempted slowly. A marked difference between the two ranges of movement suggests the spasticity is considerable.

Paresis of the hip musculature is most likely to be found in the gluteal muscles. In young children, it is not easy to assess the power of active abduction at the hip. Two features may indicate the relative strength of the abductor musculature. When the child is allowed to lie freely on his mother's lap, the posture of the hips (Fig. 13–16), whether in flexion and adduction or in the normal position of slight abduction and flexion, is a useful guide to the tone of the gluteal muscles. Passive adduction of the hips may allow the observer to feel whether gluteal abduction action is present or whether the hips move into adduction easily without much resistance from the glutei. The most useful test of all is to place the child on his side, to abduct the hip to break any spasticity in the adductors, and to let the thigh fall (Fig. 13–17). A normal child or one in whom there is good abductor power will not let the hip fall downward beyond the horizontal. If the limb does fall below the horizontal, the glutei should be regarded as of fair power or less. When the child reaches an age at which he is able to cooperate in producing active abduction of the hip, more accurate testing of the power of abduction and extension can be made.

Examination for shortness of the hip adductor or flexor muscles is a vital part of the examination of cerebral-palsied children. The range of abduction should be examined with the hips and knees extended. The hips are abducted slowly to elicit the minimum amount of adductor spasm until the point is reached at which there is a true bar to further abduction (Fig. 13–18); at this point the child may indicate that the maximum range has been obtained by the fact that it begins to feel pain. The range of hip abduction can also be assessed with the knees flexed to eliminate tightness of the gracilis muscle, and with the hips flexed and the knees extended, to assess the contribution to any adduction deformity by the hamstring muscles.

Hip flexion deformity is assessed by Thomas'

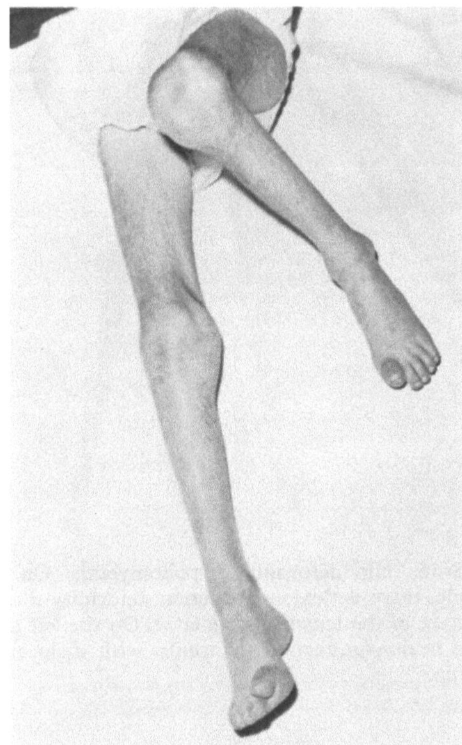

FIG. 13–16 Hip posture in cerebral palsy. When the lower limbs are lying free, the tendency of the thigh to lie flexed and adducted is a measure of the shortness and hypertonicity of the adductors and flexors compared with the abductors and extensors.

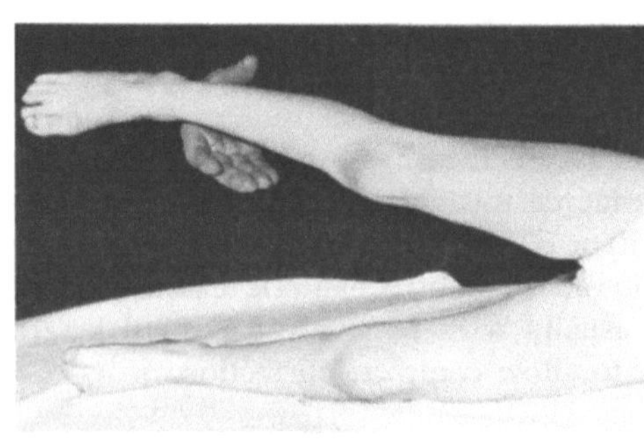

FIG. 13–17 Test for hip abductor power in cerebral palsy. The hip is passively abducted to break any adductor spasticity. In a young child, the limb is allowed to fall; an older child is asked to maintain the hip in the abducted position.

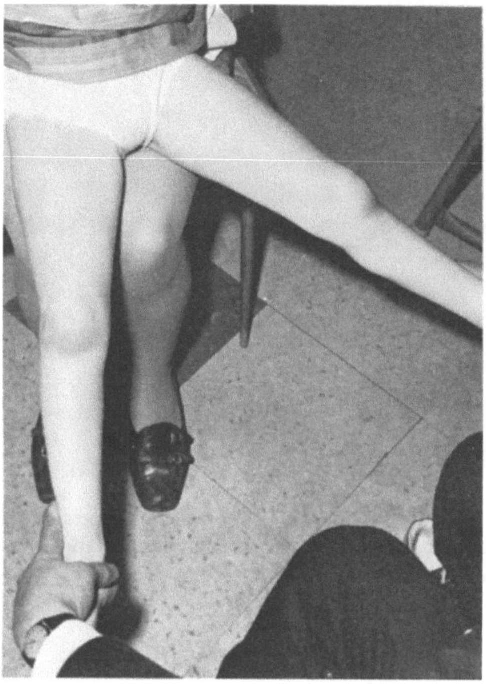

FIG. 13–18 Assessment of passive abduction in the presence of adductor spasm. The hips are abducted slowly to elicit the minimum adductor spasm until the point is reached at which there is a true bar to further abduction.

test, the opposite hip being flexed fully on to the chest to eliminate any lumbar lordosis and the hip under examination being pressed slowly into extension to release any spasm in the flexor muscles. The range of hip rotation is best examined when the hips are extended, since this is the position of function for walking. Flexion–adduction deformity is almost always associated with limited lateral rotation of the extended hip. Limited flexion of the hip due to shortness of the hamstring muscles is assessed by the angle of straight-leg raising.

Assessment of the hip should be made at least every 6 months, and if there is any indication of progressive deformity, every 3 months. Account must be taken of the variations in the normal range of abduction in childhood. In most babies, the range of abduction with the hip extended is at least 80°, but in older children this may normally diminish to 60 or 70°. Some fixed flexion may be present in the early months of life when the normal lumbosacral angle has not yet developed, but after this time any fixed flexion deformity is abnormal. If the range of hip abduction becomes less than 30°, subluxation of the hip is likely to occur; if it is less than 20°, dislocation is impending or may already have occurred. Dislocation does not occur suddenly and is not painful when it develops. Unilateral dislocation is more easily recognized than bilateral, but in cerebral palsy dislocation is very likely to develop in both hips at about the same time. The femoral head can usually be palpated in the buttock; there is marked limitation of abduction or there may be fixed adduction. Fixed flexion deformity may not be so obvious once the hip dislocates because the upward riding of the femoral head slackens the hip flexor musculature.

Radiography

Radiography of the hips should be a routine part of the examination of the child when he is first seen and should be repeated yearly in any patient in whom there is quadriplegic involvement affecting the hip musculature. Progressive limitation of abduction is an indication for an additional radiograph to determine whether there is subluxation. Valgus deformity and anteversion of the femoral neck are present in almost all children with quadriplegic cerebral palsy associated with spasticity of the hip musculature and weakness of the glutei. In itself, this does not imply that the hip is about to dislocate. The earliest sign of subluxation is a break in Shenton's line (Fig. 13–19). This is followed by upward and lateral displacement of the position of the upper femoral epiphysis relative to the acetabulum and progressive uncovering of the femoral head. Eventually, complete dislocation develops. By this time, there may be secondary changes in the acetabulum, the roof of which becomes shallow, and in the femoral head, which becomes distorted with a teardrop appearance of the upper femoral epiphyseal nucleus (Fig. 13–20). In dislocation of long standing, the deformity may become grotesque with the hip grossly flexed and adducted (Fig. 13–21).

Clinical involvement of the hip in cerebral palsy almost never develops in spastic hemiplegia, although radiographs of the hip taken at the end of development show a slight difference between the normal and affected sides (Fig. 13–22). If there is apparent unilateral involvement affecting the hip, the lesion will be found to be an instance of diplegia or quadriplegia with marked asymmetry of involvement.

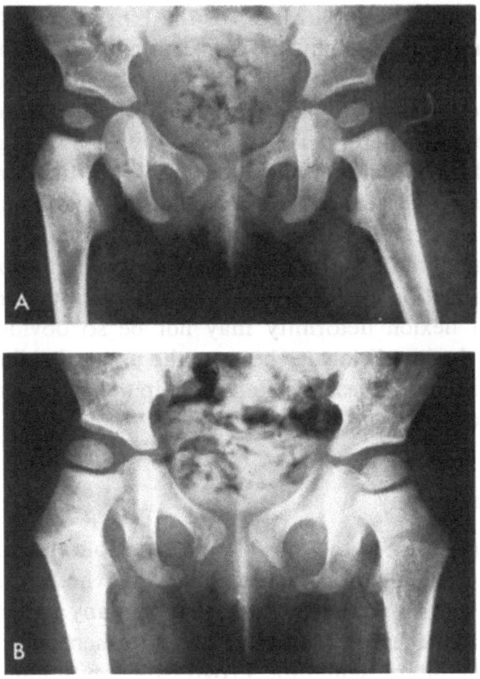

FIG. 13–19 Radiographs of progressive subluxation of the hip in cerebral palsy. **A** The first sign is a break in Shenton's line. **B** One year later, there is progressive upward and lateral displacement of the upper femoral epiphysis and uncovering of the femoral head.

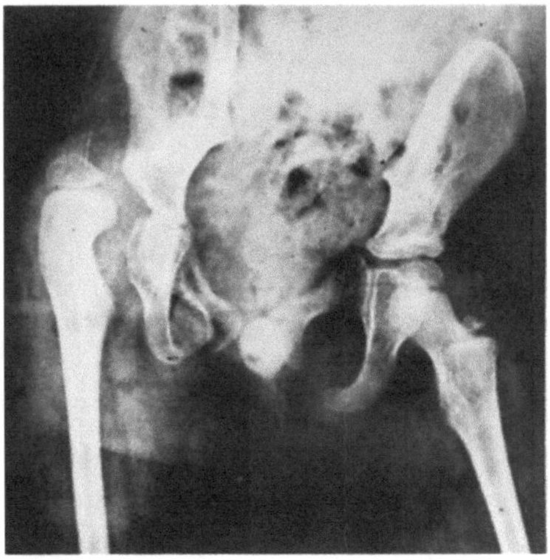

FIG. 13–20 Radiograph of complete dislocation. The acetabular roof shows secondary changes and there is early distortion of the femoral head.

Associated Scoliosis

Any assessment of the hip requires that account be taken of the lumbar spine and the presence of any pelvic obliquity. Pelvic obliquity arises in association with lumbar scoliosis. Scoliosis should be looked for whenever there is asymmetrical quadriplegic involvement affecting the trunk muscles more on one side than the other. It is likely to be seen in patients with mixed spastic and athetoid types of paralysis. Pelvic obliquity increases the liability to dislocation on the elevated side, since it encourages an adducted posture of the hip and adds further to the effective weakness of the hip abductors.

Nonoperative Management

As soon as spastic cerebral palsy of diplegic or quadriplegic distribution is diagnosed, measures should be taken to maintain the range of abduction and extension of the hips by daily passive movements. The parents can usually be instructed in the performance of such movements by a physiotherapist or physical medicine specialist. There are some who advocate the use of splintage in abduction either at night or continuously in early childhood; the author has not found, however, that splintage is any more effective in preventing the development of adduction–flexion deformity than the regular performance of passive movements and there is even a danger that, by inhibiting active movement at the hips, splintage may diminish hip abductor power as much as it maintains adductor length.

The physiotherapeutic measures used to educate lower-limb function toward walking by encouraging normal muscle activity and inhibiting reflex activity in cerebral-palsied children are beyond the scope of this chapter and are, to some extent, independent of the surgical measures that may be required to treat a hip deformity. The gluteal muscles are often paretic in cerebral palsy. Their opponents, the hip flexors and adductors, are often strong and spastic. Exercises designed to improve the power of the abductors must be combined with measures to obtain relaxation of the flexors and adductors, by the use of appropriate posture and combined activity of groups of muscles with the aim of diminishing unwanted reflex activity. This is the basis of many of the methods of physiotherapy in spastic conditions.

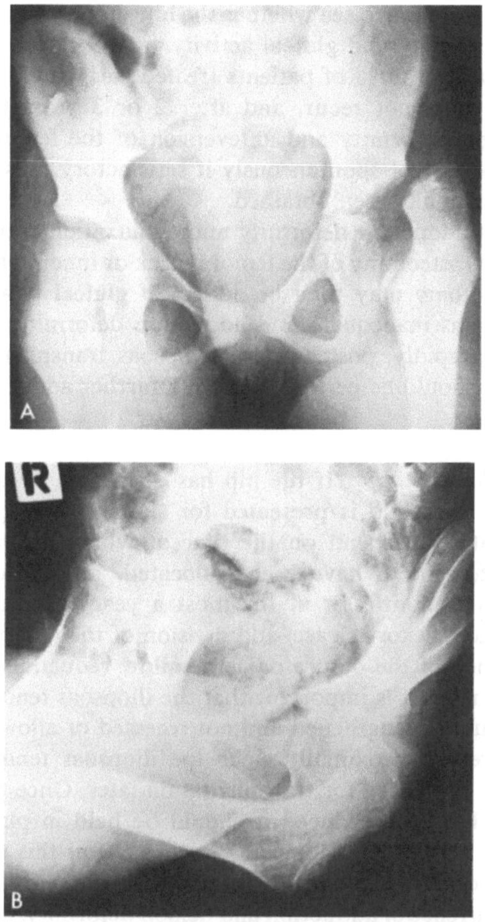

FIG. 13–21 Radiographs of progressive changes following dislocation of the hip in cerebral palsy. **A** The left hip has recently dislocated and the right hip is subluxated. No surgical treatment was given because it was thought that the child's general condition did not warrant it. **B** Five years later, there is dislocation of both hips with gross deformity.

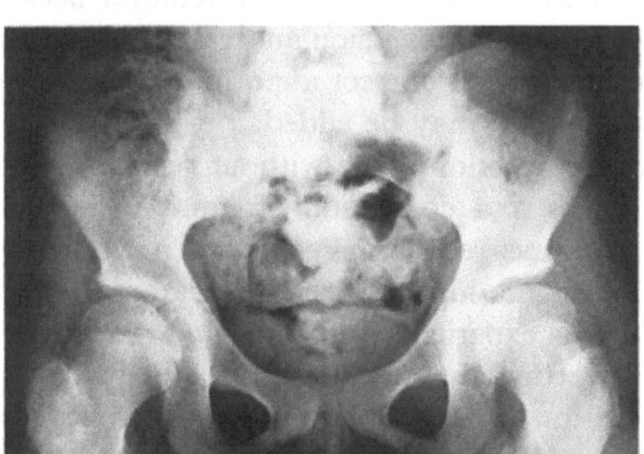

FIG. 13–22 Radiograph of the hips in spastic hemiplegia on the right side. There are minimal differences between the radiological appearances of the two sides. The hip does not dislocate in hemiplegia.

When the child is able to start bearing weight on the limbs, a special watch must be kept for the development of additional hip deformity, not so much because the child is bearing weight on the hips as because the upright position may enhance adductor action at the expense of the abductors, which have to work through an increasingly worsening mechanical advantage.

Surgical Treatment

The primary indication for surgery in spastic cerebral palsy is the correction of developing or established deformity.[35] Deformity develops relatively slowly but inexorably so that measurements, for example, of the range of abduction at 6-month intervals will show the rate at which deformity is increasing. Surgery to correct progressive deformity should never be delayed. Once paralytic deformity starts to develop in spite of adequate conservative treatment, it always progresses unless appropriate and early surgical treatment is given, whatever the age of the child.

Adduction Deformity If the range of abduction decreases to 40° or less and there is evidence of gluteal weakness, surgery is indicated to restore length to the adductors and to correct the imbalance of action between the adductors and abductors.

Adductor division at this time should restore the range of abduction to normal. Subcutaneous tenotomy is not adequate; the operation should be done openly and it will usually be found that the adductor longus and gracilis tendons need to be divided and the adductor brevis stretched. If the gluteal abductors are known to be of only fair or poor power, the anterior branch of the obturator nerve should be divided. The combination of neurectomy and adductor division will reduce the power of the adductors to a fair grade. If there is doubt as to the power of the abductors and they are thought to be fairly good, a simple adductor release suffices. It is always possible to reoperate to divide the anterior branch of the obturator nerve later if necessary. Even if there is thought to be marked weakness of the gluteal abductors, it is still not wise, in childhood, to divide the whole of the obturator nerve. It may be that, after the adductors have been released and exercises given to the abductors, they will recover better power. Intrapelvic obturator neurectomy, which does not allow for any release of tight adductors and which may grossly weaken the adductors, is indicated only in severely neglected hips as a salvage procedure.

Flexion Deformity Flexion deformity often accompanies adduction deformity. If flexion deformity is greater than 20°, adductor release should be combined with elongation of the iliopsoas tendon, which can be done through the same incision in the groin. Flexion deformity of more than 20° may require lengthening of other hip flexors—sartorius, tensor fasciae latae, and rectus femoris—but the iliopsoas is the primary cause of flexion deformity and should always be lengthened or recessed proximally.[5] When flexion and adduction deformity are both considerable, correction should be made through separate incisions in the groin and on the anterior aspect of the thigh.

When there is a combination of flexion and adduction deformity, posterior transplantation of the adductors to the ischium or to the common tendon of origin of the hamstring muscles [31,48,52] is a useful procedure that combines correction of deformity and of adductor/abductor and flexor/extensor imbalance.

These simple operations can be performed at any age, as young as 6 months or as late as 9 years. The indications do not depend on age but on the degree and rapidity of development of deformity. Adductor release and iliopsoas lengthening done sufficiently early will almost always prevent dislocation of the hip.

The value of early surgery in cerebral palsy has been shown by several authors.[9,43,44,55] The only contraindications are the presence of gross lack of head control, lack of balance and equilibrium reaction, or the persistence of strong tonic pathological reflexes. Even in these severely affected children, some measures should be taken to prevent the hip from dislocating by performance of adductor tenotomy. If, in any child, the range of abduction has become less than 20°, adductor tenotomy and anterior branch obturator neurectomy, with or without elongation of the iliopsoas tendon, are urgently indicated. If the hip has not already dislocated, these measures will almost certainly prevent dislocation (Fig. 13–23). Even if valgus deformity and anteversion of the femoral neck and a poor acetabulum are apparent, femoral or innominate osteotomy need not necessarily be performed at this time; it is appropriate to wait for 6 months to see whether the hip shows increasing stability and gluteal activity.

In over 90% of patients treated early subluxation does not recur, and after 2 or 3 years the valgus deformity and anteversion of the femoral neck correct spontaneously if satisfactory muscle balance has been obtained.

If adduction deformity and subluxation recur, varus osteotomy of the femoral neck or innominate osteotomy may then be added. If gluteal power remains inadequate and adduction deformity recurs rapidly, posterolateral iliopsoas transplantation should be performed with a further adductor release.

Dislocated Hip If the hip has dislocated by the time the child is presented for surgery, management will depend on the time at which the hip is thought to have been dislocated. If it is less than 6 months or at the most a year, adductor release, flexor release, and division of the anterior branch of the obturator nerve allow reduction to be made. It is important that the iliopsoas tendon should be lengthened and not recessed or allowed to retract proximally since the iliopsoas tendon may be needed for transplantation later. Once the hip has been reduced it should be held in place in a plaster spica for 6 to 8 weeks. After this the hip can be kept under observation. If there is a recurrence of adduction and flexion deformity, and gluteal power is not restored or proves to be very weak, anterolateral or posterolateral iliopsoas transplantation may be indicated to restore muscle balance. If gluteal power proves to be adequate but the hip continues to be subluxated, but without further progress toward recurrent dislocation, varus derotation osteotomy of the femoral neck to correct femoral anteversion and valgus or innominate osteotomy to correct abnormal alignment of the acetabulum may be added.

Bony correction alone without release of short soft tissues and correction of muscle imbalance almost always results in recurrence (Fig. 13–24). The longer the hip has been dislocated, the more difficulty is experienced in achieving reduction. It is still worthwhile to attempt to reduce a dislocation up to 4 years after it has occurred. When dislocation has been present for more than 1 year, gluteal function has usually become severely diminished. Adductor release usually needs to be extensive and may require all the adductor muscles to be divided from their origins; sometimes the

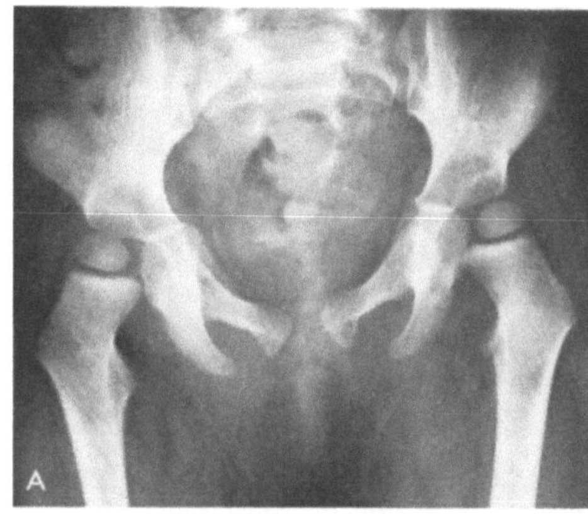

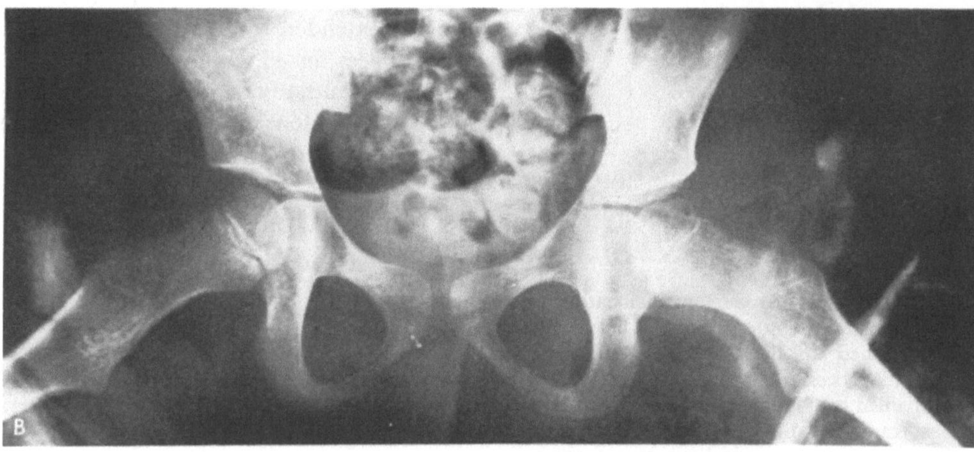

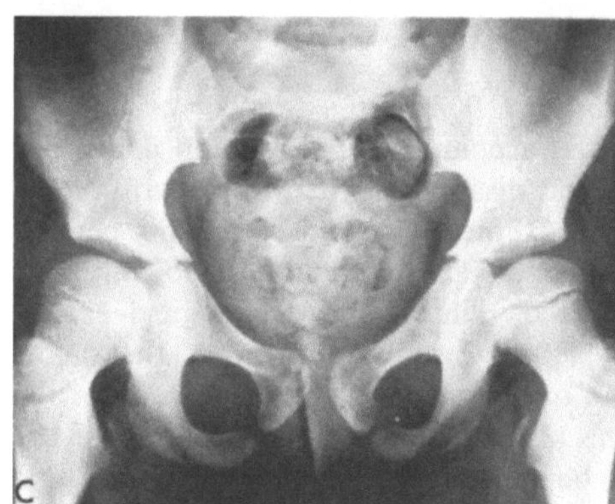

FIG. 13–23 Radiographs of spontaneous correction of hip subluxation following adductor tenotomy. **A** Moderate subluxation of both hips due to weakness of the gluteal abductors and progressive shortness of the adductors. **B** Reduction of the hips following adductor tenotomy. Splintage was needed only for 4 weeks. **C** Three years later, spontaneous correction of the hips.

tendons of the origin of the hamstring muscles must be released from the ischial tuberosity. An adequate adductor release will often allow total or partial reduction of the dislocation with the hip in a flexed position. At a second operation 2 weeks later, flexor release can be performed accompanied by opening of the hip joint to ensure that there is no obstruction to reduction. The iliopsoas tendon should be mobilized down to the lesser trochanter, divided, and transplanted anterolaterally or posterolaterally. If the deformity is predominantly in adduction with not more than 35° of flexion deformity, the transplant should be an anterolateral one. If there is flexion deformity greater than this, the transplant should be a posterolateral one.[38] Finally, 6 weeks later correction can be completed by a subtrochanteric varus derotation osteotomy. By this means, all factors contributing to the dislocation of the hip are corrected.[19] Smith [48] recommends that all parts of the operation be performed at one time, although if this is done the operation is of considerable magnitude. Failure to reduce a dislocated hip, or recurrent dislocation after attempts at reduction, may have to be accepted, but the hip is very likely to become painful in adolescence with secondary degenerative changes. The choice then lies between excision of the femoral head (Fig. 13–24), femoral osteotomy to improve the alignment of the limb, or arthrodesis.

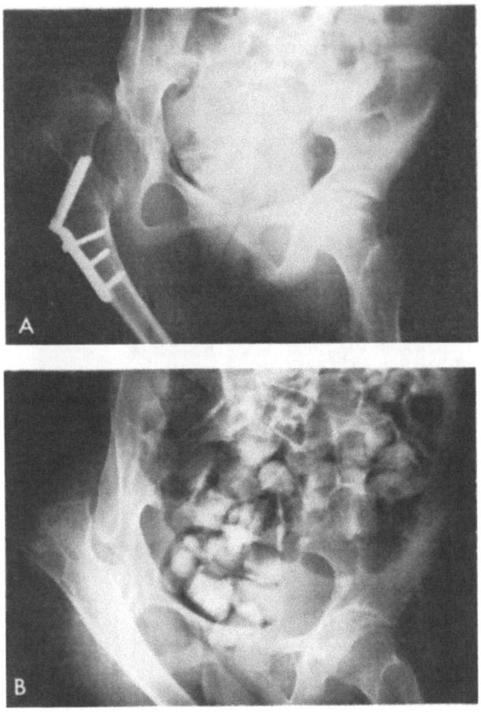

FIG. 13–24 **A** Radiograph of recurrent dislocation of the hip following varus osteotomy. Soft-tissue release had not been performed and the glutei were extremely weak. This could have been avoided if varus osteotomy had been accompanied by adductor release and posterolateral iliopsoas transplantation. **B** The femoral head has been excised in an attempt to relieve pain.

Medial Rotation Deformity Medial rotation deformity often accompanies flexion and adduction deformity and disappears when the deformity has been relieved. If medial rotation deformity persists after the flexion and adduction deformity has been corrected, clinical and radiological examination [12,20,33] will usually show that the deformity arises in association with anteversion of the femoral neck. Lateral rotation osteotomy of the femur can be performed either in a subtrochanteric region or in the lower third of the shaft of the femur, depending on whether valgus deformity of the femoral neck is also present and requires correction at the subtrochanteric level. Baker and Hill [2] advise that one or more of the medial hamstring muscles of the knee should be transplanted posterolaterally to the anterior aspect of the lateral femoral condyle where they may become lateral rotators, but their power in this respect is not unduly great. Steel [51] advocates transfer of the insertion of the gluteus medius and minimus from the greater trochanter to the anterior part of the femur to correct a medial rotation gait.

Hamstring Shortness Shortening of the hamstrings is very common in quadriplegic and paraplegic cerebral palsy and its usual effect is to cause flexion deformity of the knee. Sometimes, when the quadriceps is strong, its main effect is at the hip; this is revealed by marked limitation of straight-leg raising to 30° or less. The patient walks in a characteristic way, with excessive rotation of the pelvis because he is unable to take a full forward stride. He is unable to sit up with the knees extended though he can sit in a chair with the knees flexed without difficulty. This syndrome is substantially relieved by proximal elongation of the tendon of origin of the hamstring muscle.[37]

The Hip in Upper Motor Neuron Lesions in Adults

Hemiplegia arising in adult life may result from cerebral vascular disease, cerebral tumor, or cerebral trauma. In some patients with a good expectation of life, deformity or disability may persist in spite of adequate medical and physiotherapeutic treatment and thus may deserve correction or improvement by surgical means. Hip deformity in traumatic paraplegia or tetraplegia is uncommon if the spinal lesion is well treated and decubitus ulceration or severe urinary tract infection is prevented by good medical management and nursing care. Sometimes difficulties in early management or inadequate treatment may be associated with these complications and, if they are, there is a much greater liability to muscle spasms and sometimes flexion and adduction deformities of the hip. Multiple sclerosis may result in slowly progressing paralysis but its episodic nature may sometimes lead to the patient being bedridden because of extensive contractures although the disease has become quiescent. Surgery may have a part to play in improving the lot of any of these varieties of upper motor neuron lesions.

The main difference from the situation in childhood is that, once the paralytic lesion is stable and any acute episodes have ceased, the deformity is likely to remain unchanged and is not complicated by the progressive effects of growth.

Surgical Treatment

As in childhood, distinction needs to be made between a deformed posture arising from muscle spasticity and fixed deformity due to fibrosis in tendon sheaths. In paraplegia and some other lesions, fixation due to calcification and ossification in musculature in the region of the hip may develop.

If a full range of passive movements can be demonstrated, if necessary while the patient is anesthetized, an abnormal posture, for instance of adduction, may be relieved by neurectomy, either by direct division of branches of the obturator nerve in the groin or intraabdominally or by local injection of alcohol or phenol into the motor points of the nerves. To test the potential effect of neurectomy, local anesthetic is injected into the region of the nerve and will demonstrate the result to be expected by neurectomy.

Fixed deformity of the hip in adduction or flexion or both requires correction by surgical division. A bedridden patient suffering from multiple sclerosis may often have such severe deformity that it is impossible to approach the adductors in the groin until the flexion deformity has first been corrected, using a transabdominal retroperitoneal approach to divide the iliopsoas muscle at the level of the inguinal ligament. Through the same approach, the obturator nerve can be divided intrapelvically. If necessary, a second incision in the groin may be used to divide tight adductor muscles. Ossification in the iliopsoas or adductor muscles may have to be treated by wide excision of the abnormal bone. This should not be done until the bone that has formed is mature or ossification may recur. There is nothing to be lost by radical correction provided that the general condition of the patient is appropriate. At worst, the patient will be able to be nursed more easily and at best he may become able to walk again.

An additional benefit of surgical release of tendons and of neurectomy is an improvement throughout the limb and sometimes throughout the body because of the diminished input to the spinal cord of excessive sensory impulses.[11]

The Hip in Spina Bifida

The paralysis and deformity that may arise in spina bifida produce one of the most complex problems in surgery of paralysis of the limbs. Neonatal closure of the spinal lesion in myelomeningocele and advances in techniques for the treatment of hydrocephalus have resulted in the survival of many more infants born with severe varieties of spina bifida. The management of paralysis and deformity in the lower limbs in these children has received increasing attention during recent years.

More than 60% of babies born with an open myelomeningocele show some primary deformity in the lower limbs at birth. In some the deformity is severe (Fig. 13–8), with dislocated hips showing gross fixed flexion and adduction deformity, recurvatum knees showing fixed hyperextension deformity, and feet with severe varus deformities. In others, the deformity may be minimal, with only clawing of the toes.[45] Clinical and pathological studies of the nature of these deformities indicate that they are unlike deformities such as congenital dislocation of the hip in normal children. The deformities are paralytic, arising as a result of normally innervated hip flexor and adductor muscles in the presence of congenitally paralyzed gluteal musculature acting in utero. When such deformities are present, the sacral segments of the spinal cord have failed to develop, the innervated muscles being those with nerve root supply deriving from the lumbar segments. If by neonatal operation on the spinal lesion the function in these intact lumbar segments is preserved, the innervated muscles can be utilized in the course of reconstructive surgery to correct deformity and to make walking possible. If in this type of case the spinal lesion is treated conservatively, with the strong possibility that the intact neural segments may be destroyed by infection and fibrosis, the normally innervated muscles may become paralyzed. The result is a child with severe congenital deformities and complete paralysis of lower limb musculature.

In babies born with open myelomeningocele without lower limb deformity, the spinal cord, although abnormal in shape and exposed to the body surface, nevertheless has a normal or near-normal neural content. If neonatal surgical closure successfully retains function in these neural segments, innervation in the lower limbs may remain normal and deformity does not develop. Partial failure of primary closure of the spinal lesion, with loss of some neural function, may result in a partial paralysis of the lower limbs which usually affects the sacral segments more than the lumbar segments. In the course of growth and development during the first 2 years, limbs that were undeformed at birth develop deformity related to the residual paralysis. To make things more complex, the paralysis may be purely of lower motor neuron nature or may be a mixture of upper and lower motor neuron affection.

From among the many varieties of paralysis and deformity that may be found at the hip in spina bifida, a number of specific patterns of paralysis and deformity can be defined. The deformity is frequently bilateral and symmetrical. Where there are considerable differences in the deformity and paralysis in the two limbs, the presence of an asymmetrical spinal lesion such as a hemimyelocele may be suspected.

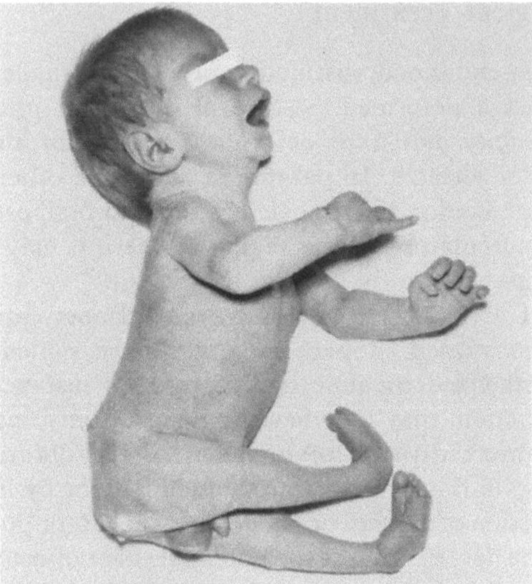

FIG. 13–25 Fixed flexion–adduction–lateral rotation deformity with dislocation at birth in spina bifida with paralysis below the fourth lumbar neural segment.

Patterns of Deformity and Paralysis

L-1,2 Paralysis and Deformity When there is innervation only from the first or first and second lumbar neural segments, the active hip muscles are the iliopsoas, sartorius, pectineus, and possibly some of the adductor muscles. The deformity which develops is of fixed flexion and lateral rotation, the iliopsoas being a strong lateral rotator of the hip in early life. If the hip tends to fall into abduction, dislocation does not occur.

L-3,4 Paralysis and Deformity Innervation from the first three or four lumbar neural segments with paralysis of muscles supplied by the sacral neural segments results in severe hip deformity (Fig. 13–25). There is normal innervation in all hip flexor and adductor muscles. The hip shows fixed flexion, adduction, and lateral rotation deformity. The hip joints are either subluxated or dislocated and, if this level of innervation has been present in utero, the dislocation is present at birth. The radiological features (Fig. 13–26) of this variety of dislocation are quite distinct from those of congenital dislocation of the hip in the normal child. There is evidence that the hip has dislocated several weeks before birth. There is a well-established false acetabulum. The thigh is laterally rotated so that the greater trochanter lies posteriorly or even in the acetabulum. Where this level of innervation arises after birth, dislocation usually develops within the first 12 to 18 months of life.

L-5 Paralysis and Deformity Innervation from all the lumbar neural segments with paralysis of the sacral neural segments results in normal innervation of all the hip flexor and adductor muscles and partial innervation of the gluteal abductors. The gluteus maximus and the small posterior lateral rotators of the hip are paralyzed. Flexion and adduction deformities develop or are present at birth but are not as severe as in L-3,4 paralysis. If this level of innervation has been present in

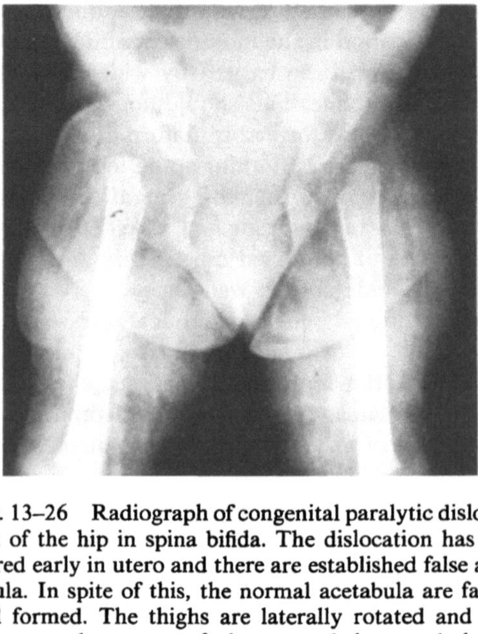

FIG. 13–26 Radiograph of congenital paralytic dislocation of the hip in spina bifida. The dislocation has occurred early in utero and there are established false acetabula. In spite of this, the normal acetabula are fairly well formed. The thighs are laterally rotated and the greater trochanters are facing toward the acetabula.

utero, the hips are subluxated but not dislocated at birth (Fig. 13–27). Without treatment, dislocation develops during the course of the first 2 or 3 years of life. If the L-5 level of innervation develops after birth, hip flexion and adduction deformity develop more slowly but dislocation always occurs eventually, usually by the fifth year of life.

S-1 Paralysis and Deformity Innervation from all the lumbar neural segments and the first sacral neural segment produces normal innervation in all the hip flexors, adductors, and abductors. There is weakness of hip extension by the gluteus maximus but some extension of the hip is produced by the action of the medial hamstrings. Fixed flexion deformity develops slowly during growth. The child has a tendency to walk with lateral rotation to stabilize his hips by using the posterior fibers of the gluteal abductors as hip extensors.

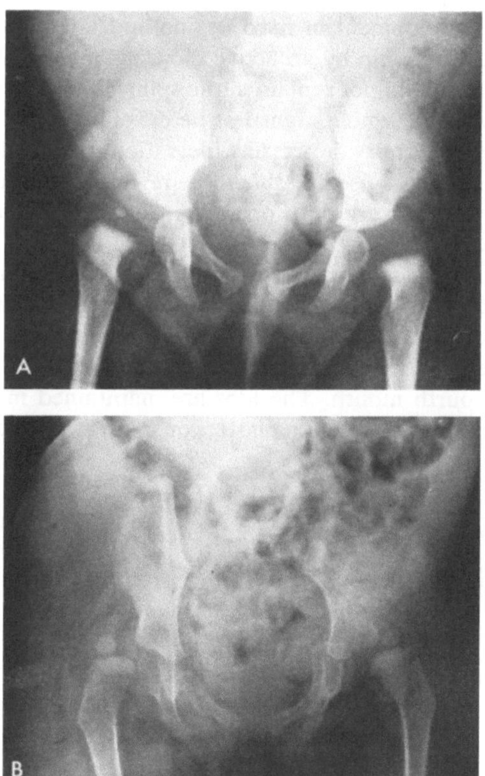

FIG. 13–27 **A** Radiograph of congenital paralytic subluxation of the hips at birth. There was normal innervation down to the fifth lumbar neural segment with paresis of the gluteal abductors and paralysis of the gluteus maximus. **B** In spite of adequate conservative treatment, dislocation occurred by the age of 2 years.

Other Deformities Normal lower motor neuron innervation associated with an upper motor neuron lesion due to abnormality of the spinal cord above the level of the spinal lesion gives rise to spastic paralysis with deformities such as those seen in spastic cerebral palsy. Other deformities may result from mixed neurological patterns of innervation: for instance, when there is normal innervation from the first three lumbar segments, active innervation from the fourth and fifth lumbar neural segments, and reflex innervation from the sacral neural segments. Many varieties of posture and fixed deformity can result from these effects.

In contrast to the situation in poliomyelitis or cerebral palsy, paralysis and deformity in spina bifida are complicated by the presence of sensory loss. This feature makes the orthopedic management of the lower-limb deformities additionally difficult, since any abnormal pressure by splints, braces, or postoperative fixation is likely to give rise to severe pressure ulceration in anesthetic areas. Spontaneous fractures are common features of spina bifida. The more severe the paralysis, the greater the liability to fracture; there is a predilection for fractures to occur in the metaphyseal regions of the long bones, especially after immobilization in a plaster cast.

Principles of Orthopedic Management

The management of paralysis and deformity in children with myelomeningocele requires a completely different approach from the methods used in the management of congenital deformities of other kinds or in the management of deformities arising from paralysis due to poliomyelitis or cerebral palsy, although some of the techniques used in those conditions may be applicable to children with spina bifida.

The disabilities are multiple and a program of orthopedic treatment must be coordinated with the treatment of other abnormalities. Measures to obtain sound healing of the spinal lesion, to control progressive hydrocephalus, and to treat bladder paralysis and secondary renal lesions must usually take priority over orthopedic considerations. It is not appropriate to apply splintage to deformed limbs immediately after birth, since splints may interfere with healing of the back, and it is wise to postpone orthopedic treatment until hydrocephalus has been treated and the neurological situation has become static. Before any orthopedic operation is undertaken, assessment of renal function must be made. For example, if there is progressive hydronephrosis which requires an ileal conduit, this operation should be done first in spite of the fact that the incision for operative treatment at the hip may have to lie close to the conduit orifice.

Since the deformities present are usually paralytic in nature, correction of deformity must be accompanied by restoration of balanced muscle action. In spina bifida, this can usually be achieved by tendon transplantation. Failure to do so always leads to recurrence of deformity, however carefully splints, bracing, physiotherapy, or other measures are applied. Even where there does not, at first sight, appear to be any musculature to cause recurrence of deformity, unrecognized muscle activity of reflex nature which is not revealed by normal clinical testing can be discovered on electrical stimulation or by electromyography.

The aims of orthopedic treatment are to correct deformity, to maintain correction, and to obtain maximum function in the lower limbs.[44] Ideally, the initial orthopedic examination should take place on the first day of life or soon thereafter. Decisions about an orthopedic program of management can usually be made after the third month of life when the definitive paralysis can be established by clinical and electrical studies. Until that time, careful passive movements of the limbs by parents or physiotherapists are all that can be done to minimize deformity.

At the hips, the common deformity is one of fixed flexion, adduction, and lateral rotation. Attempts to correct deformity of this type by traction or forced splintage are dangerous and ineffective. Surgical division of the short soft tissues is the only safe method of treatment. Deformity, once corrected surgically, can be maintained by carefully applied splintage, but wherever possible, permanent splintage should be avoided. Preferably, muscles should be transplanted to equalize the balance of muscle activity so that deformity will not recur. Correction of hip deformity is seldom feasible before the age of 6 months, but correction of all deformities in the limb should be obtained by the time the child is 3 years old so that he is able to walk before he goes to school.

Treatment of the Hip in Infancy

If there is a full range of abduction and no significant flexion deformity at the hip at the neonatal examination, clinical and electrical testing of the muscles controlling the hip usually shows activity in all muscles at the lower motor neuron level and the hips are radiologically normal. No specific orthopedic treatment or splintage is needed but follow-up examination should be made at 3-month intervals to assess the range of abduction and to confirm the state of innervation of the hip musculature. If examination at the third or sixth month suggests that there is weakness of extension or abduction of the hip or both, a careful watch should be kept for progressive limitation and for radiological signs of subluxation.

Progressive Adduction Deformity with Subluxation If limited abduction starts to develop, it is possible to prevent rapid deterioration by the use of an abduction splint (Fig. 13–28). If such a splint is used, it must be carefully applied, well padded, and adjusted to maintain the hips in abduction and extension and medial rotation. Splintage in the frog position is not satisfactory and encourages the development of fixed flexion and lateral rotation of the hip by an active iliopsoas muscle. The child should not remain in the splint for the whole day or the whole night lest he develop secondary fixed deformity or pressure ulceration. If an abduction splint is used, it should be regarded as a temporary measure until operative treatment is feasible.

Progressive limitation of hip abduction, subluxation of the hip, and the development of strong, tight adductor musculature are indications for open adductor division at any time after the third or fourth month. The hips are maintained in abduction by abduction plasters or splints for 3 weeks

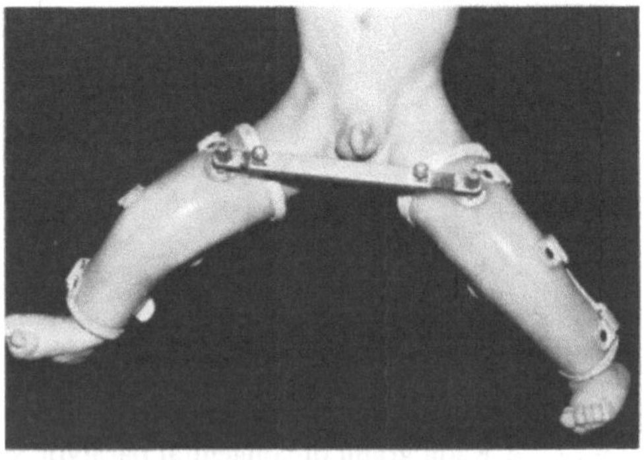

FIG. 13–28 Abduction splints to maintain the hips in abduction and medial rotation. From McKibbon, B.: The action of the iliopsoas muscle in the newborn. J. Bone Joint Surg. 50B:161, 1968.

and a return is then made to the maintenance of passive movements and the partial use of abduction splintage until the child is old enough for a transplantation of muscle. If gluteal abduction and extension remain weak, posterolateral iliopsoas transplantation should be performed, usually between the 9th and 18th month of life, and in any event, before dislocation develops if the hip has not been dislocated at birth.

Progressive Flexion Deformity If at the examination at the sixth month there is evidence of active gluteal abduction but extension of the hip is poor, it is probable that the gluteus maximus muscle is paralyzed or severely paretic. The hip is not likely to dislocate but flexion deformity can develop when the child starts to walk—which he is likely to do with the hips and knees flexed. Fixed flexion of more than 20° or a poor gait would indicate posterior iliopsoas transplantation at the age of 3 or 4 years.

Birth Dislocation The presence of severe flexion and adduction deformity at birth with dislocated hips is almost pathognomonic evidence of congenital paralysis of all the gluteal musculature. Splintage cannot be applied to the limbs, and attempts to correct short, strong hip flexors and adductors by passive stretching are more likely to lead to a fracture of the shaft of the femur or separation of the lower or upper femoral epiphysis than to correction of the deformity.

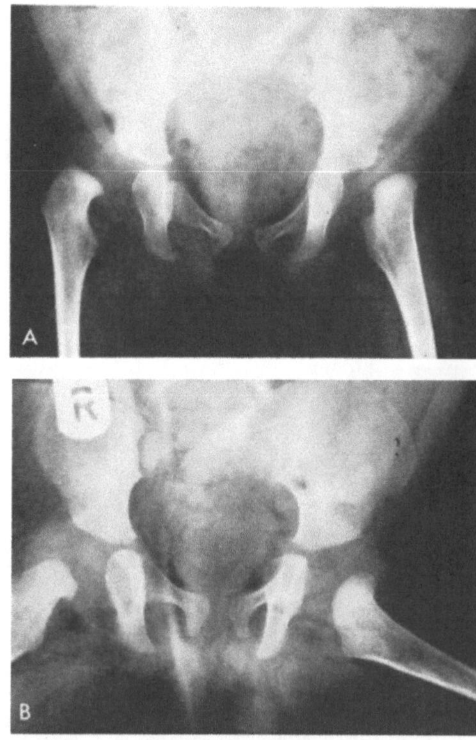

FIG. 13–29 Radiographs of congenital paralytic dislocation of the hip. **A** At the age of 3 months. Note the adequacy of the acetabulum. **B** Reduction of the dislocation following open adductor release. Note that the left hip is still laterally rotated.

Provided that the general condition of the child allows it, radical open adductor release should be made between the third and sixth month of life. In about half of the patients affected by this severe deformity, the dislocation can be reduced at this time (Fig. 13–29). In others, the hip remains dislocated because the iliopsoas blocks the entrance to the acetabulum or maintains the hip laterally rotated. The second operation of posterolateral iliopsoas transplantation should be undertaken, if possible, 2 or 3 weeks after radical adductor tenotomy unless the child's age or his general condition makes it necessary to delay this. After the psoas has been detached, the hip can usually be put into extension and medial rotation and the dislocation can be reduced. If reduction is not obtained, the hip may be opened and any bar to reduction such as a large ligamentum teres or occasionally a limbus can be removed. The capsule of the hip should be reefed. Valgus deformity of the femoral neck or anteversion can be ignored at this time. The hip is maintained in abduction, extension, and medial rotation for a period of 6 weeks following iliopsoas transplantation, after which all fixation is removed (Fig. 13–30). At this point, a careful watch should be kept for the development of spontaneous fractures, especially in the lower third of the thigh; the only manifestation of such fractures may be swelling of the limb. If they occur, the simplest possible treatment should be applied (usually a firm crepe and wool bandage to support the limb) and union occurs very rapidly. The hip should be allowed to mobilize spontaneously. If there is a long delay (more than 3 months) in the restoration of adduction, varus osteotomy may be needed, but in recent years the author has seldom found this to be necessary.

If concentric reduction has been obtained at this time and satisfactory posterolateral iliopsoas transplantation has been achieved, dislocation of

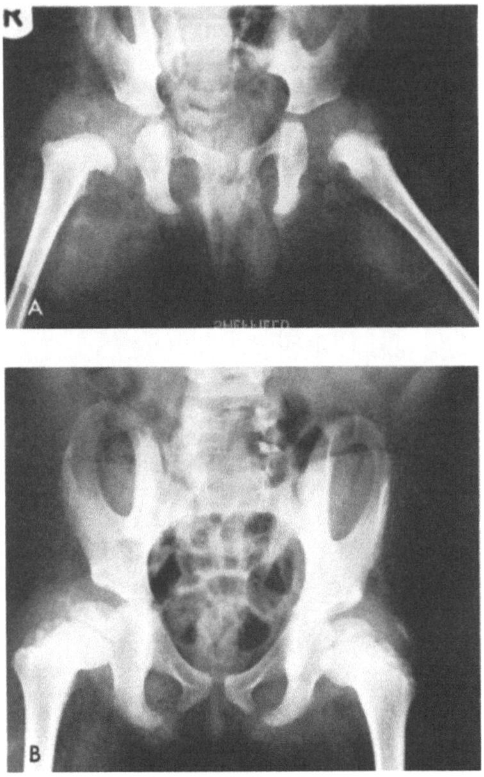

FIG. 13–30 Radiographs of congenital paralytic dislocation of the hip following posterolateral iliopsoas transplantation. **A** Two weeks after transplantation. **B** Five years later. The hips remain concentrically reduced and there has been spontaneous correction of anteversion.

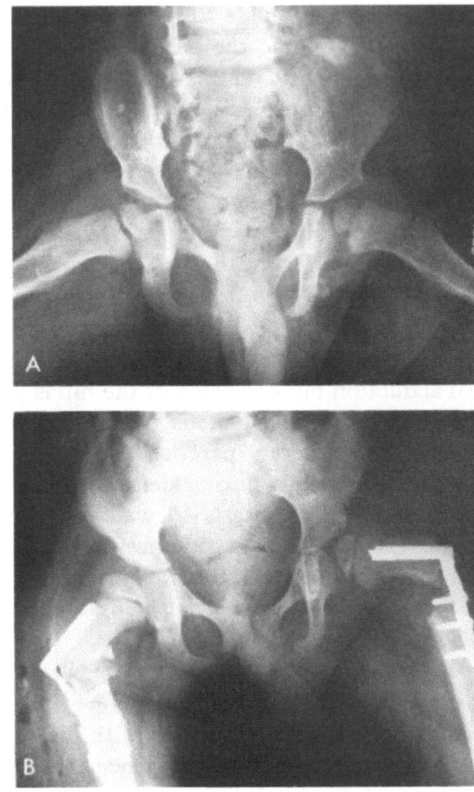

FIG. 13–31 Radiographs of hips in abduction, lateral rotation, extension deformity. **A** Before surgery. **B** Correction after varus–medial rotation osteotomy with nail-plate fixation.

the hip will not recur and the joint will remain stable and radiologically satisfactory in subsequent years.[47]

Flexion–Abduction Deformity Flexion–abduction deformity at birth is uncommon. It occurs only when there has been severe intrauterine paralysis with residual innervation from the first and second lumbar neural segments. There is often a severe spinal lesion with kyphosis of the spine. If fixed flexion deformity increases during the early months of life, and clinical and electrical assessments show that the iliopsoas is the only active muscle at the hip, the iliopsoas tendon should be elongated or, if there is a marked tendency to develop lateral rotation deformity, transplanted to the front of the greater trochanter. Occasionally, fixed flexion, lateral rotation, and abduction deformity with severe valgus deformity of the femoral neck may warrant varus osteotomy of the femoral neck with nail-plate fixation during the first or second year of life (Fig. 13–31).

Abduction–Extension Deformity Abduction–extension deformity at birth is rarely seen and is difficult to treat. It arises from paralysis of the upper lumbar neural segments and the retention of reflex activity in the lower lumbar and sacral segments. The hips lie in abduction, extension, and lateral rotation due to reflex action in the gluteus maximus and short lateral rotators of the hip.

The only method of correction of this deformity is by subtrochanteric adduction and medial rotation osteotomy combined with division of any short abductor and lateral rotator muscles from the greater trochanter.

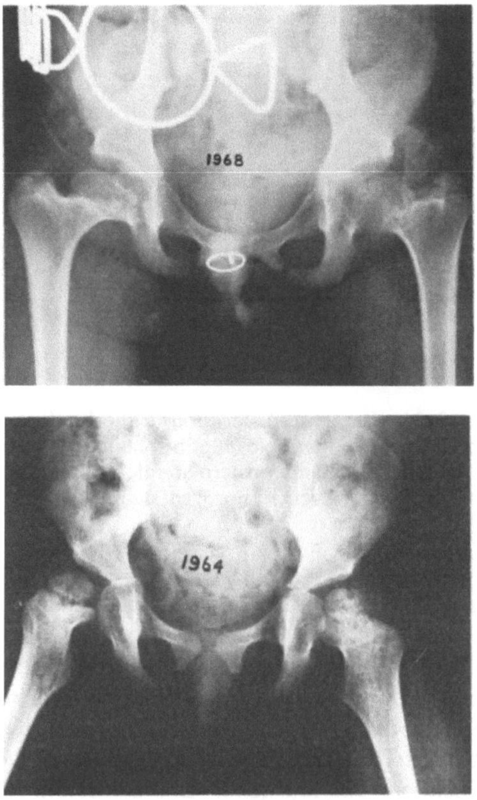

A

B

FIG. 13–32 Radiographs of spontaneous correction of bony deformity, following posterolateral iliopsoas transplantation. **A** Subluxation with valgus and anteversion of the femoral neck with early dysplasia of the acetabulum. There was some activity in the gluteal abductors. **B** Four years after posterolateral iliopsoas transplantation. The combination of residual gluteal power and the action of the transplant has resulted in varus deformity of the femoral neck.

Management of the Hip in Childhood

The principles of correction of deformity in an older child do not differ from those described for the management of the hip in infancy, but with increasing age secondary bony deformity develops.

Subluxation and Dislocation If a child under the age of 5 years shows flexion and adduction deformity of the hip with subluxation or dislocation, adductor division, reduction of the dislocation, and posterolateral iliopsoas transplantation will usually result in a stable hip (Fig. 13–32), even if the acetabulum appears to be dysplastic and the femoral neck is anteverted and in valgus position. The acetabular roof will usually develop well and valgus deformity of the femoral neck recovers spontaneously or may even become deformed into varus position as a result of the action of the iliopsoas upon the greater trochanter.

In a child more than 5 years old, efforts to reduce dislocation are much less rewarding.[16] If the dislocation is bilateral it is better not to attempt reduction of the dislocation but to confine treatment to correction of adduction and flexion deformity by flexor and adductor release sufficient to allow the fitting of calipers. If the dislocation is unilateral, and hip flexion and adduction deformity are not severe, with an acetabulum that still appears to be fairly adequate, it is possible that the dislocation may be reduced (Fig. 13–33). If, following radical open adductor division, the dislocation can be reduced with the hip in flexion, it should be maintained in this position for 2 or 3 weeks until division of the hip flexors and posterolateral iliopsoas transplantation can be performed. If necessary, the operation may be combined with innominate osteotomy of the Chiari or Salter type. Severe deformity of the femoral neck may require varus and derotation osteotomy 2 months after this.

If a child between 5 and 10 years has severe flexion and adduction deformity of the hip with a severely dysplastic acetabulum, it is doubtful whether any attempt should be made to reduce the dislocation (Fig. 13–34). If strong activity has been retained in the hip flexor and adductor muscles, a radical open adductor division, followed 1 or 2 weeks later by release of the hip flexors, possibly with anterolateral or posterolateral iliopsoas transplantation, allows the deformity to be corrected and makes walking possible with or without bracing of the hip. If hip flexion deformity is extreme, correction may be limited by tightness of the femoral nerves and vessels and may have to be completed by a subtrochanteric extension osteotomy.

Flexion–Abduction–Lateral Rotation Deformity Flexion–abduction–lateral rotation deformity develops in older children when there are strong hip flexor muscles acting in isolation or in association with reflex activity in the sacral segments. The lower limbs lie in the extreme frog position. All of the hip flexor muscles, the tensor fasciae latae, the gluteal muscles, and the lateral hip rotators are short. Correction can be obtained by subtrochanteric adduction–medial rotation–extension os-

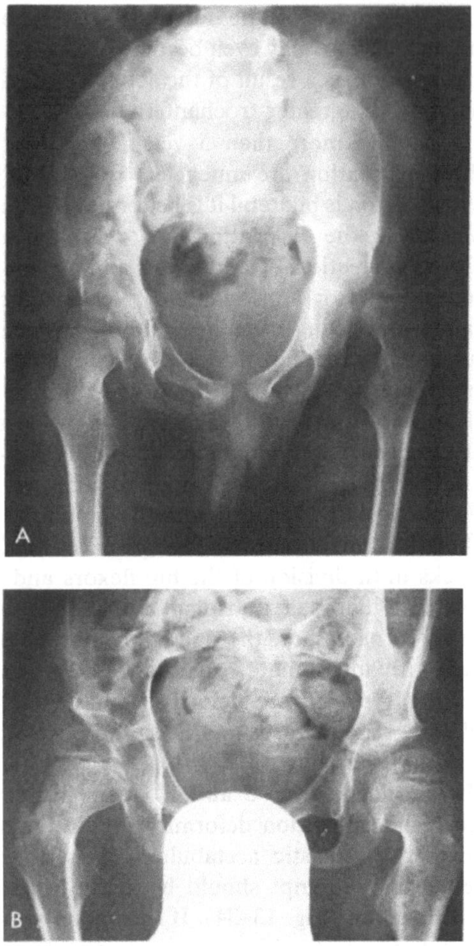

FIG. 13–33 Radiographs of late reduction of paralytic dislocation of the hip. *A* Dislocation of the left hip and subluxation of the right hip in a child aged 5 years. The acetabula are still adequate. *B* Four years after adductor release and posterolateral iliopsoas transplantation. The acetabula and femoral heads are well formed and the hips are stable.

teotomy with removal of 2 to 3 cm of the shaft of the femur. If the lower limbs are brought in line with the trunk, it is then possible, once the osteotomies have united, to apply bracing to the child, who usually has normal upper limb and trunk musculature; he then becomes able to walk for short distances. If there is a tendency for the deformity to recur toward lateral rotation, the iliopsoas tendon should be transferred to the anterior aspect of the greater trochanter to convert it into a medial rotator.

Flail Hip with Deformity If a child at any age shows deformity of the hip but no clinical evidence

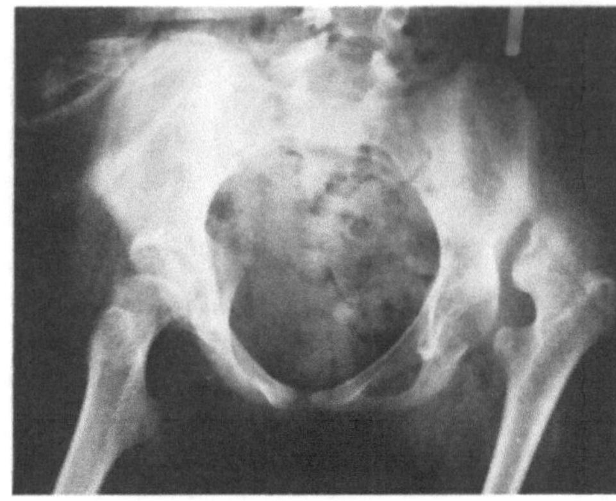

FIG. 13–34 Paralytic dislocation of the hip in a child aged 12 years. Reduction cannot be obtained but correction of deformity and posterolateral iliopsoas transplantation will still give improved stability.

of any activity in any of the hip musculature, and if this is confirmed by electrical stimulation, the aim should be to obtain a stable hip with the deformity corrected sufficiently to allow bracing. If there is bilateral dislocation of the hip, there is nothing to be gained by attempting to reduce the dislocation. The hip flexors and adductors should be divided and a femoral osteotomy performed to correct the deformity. The false acetabulum can be deepened by a shelf operation.[27] If there is unilateral dislocation, an attempt should be made to reduce it to equalize limb length and to make the fitting of braces less difficult.

Lateral Rotation Deformity Sometimes, after satisfactory reduction of a dislocated hip with posterolateral iliopsoas transplantation, the child is able to walk well but flexion of the hip is accompanied by lateral rotation due to the action of the obturator externus and sartorius. If there is no fixed lateral rotation deformity, lateral transplantation of the insertion of the sartorius to the outer side of the knee or medial transplantation of its attachment of origin may help to correct this tendency. If there is fixed lateral or medial rotation following correction of other components of hip deformity, rotation osteotomy through the lower third of the femur should be performed. The presence of valgus deformity, anteversion, or retroversion of the femoral neck is not, in itself, an indication for rotation osteotomy such as might be appropriate in the management of congenital dislocation of the hips.

Other Hip Deformities Flexion–adduction deformity, flexion–abduction–lateral rotation deformity, and simple flexion deformity are the most common defects that arise in spina bifida, but sometimes extraordinary deformities (hyperextension deformity due to isolated action of the gluteus maximus or lateral rotation deformity due to isolated action of the sacrally innervated hip rotators) may develop. Other deformities may arise as a result of a combination of reflex muscle activity and spontaneous fracture. In a few patients, spontaneous dissolution of the femoral neck has developed with upward displacement of the femoral shaft, leaving an intact femoral head in the acetabulum which, surprisingly, may retain a blood supply sufficient to maintain its nutrition. Such unusual deformities may require operative procedures unique to the situation, relying on the principles of correction of deformity to allow fitting of braces and ambulation and correction of imbalanced muscle activity. Superior or inferior gluteal neurectomy, flexion femoral osteotomy, and occasionally arthrodesis, even in a young child, may provide the only solution to a deformity which would otherwise be completely unacceptable cosmetically and functionally. If arthrodesis is required, it is best achieved by ischiofemoral grafting using a tibial cortical graft.

Hip deformity may sometimes be combined with pelvic deformity secondary to fixed lumbar lordosis or lordoscoliosis. Wherever possible, deformities of the hip, especially flexion deformity, should be corrected before attempts are made to correct deformities of the spine, since correction of the spinal deformity may require traction between the skull and femur. An exception to this is subluxation or dislocation of the hip in the presence of severe pelvic obliquity on the elevated side of the hip. In this event, it may be better to correct pelvic obliquity as far as possible by correction and fusion of the spine before deciding about the means of correcting deformity and reducing dislocation of the affected hip.

The Hip in Muscular Dystrophy

In the Duchenne type of pseudohypertrophic muscular dystrophy, the first manifestation of the disease may be an abnormality of gait from gluteal weakness. At about the third year of life, the child, usually a boy, starts to waddle and walk on a wide base with a lordotic lumbar spine. Classically, he becomes unable to get up again in the normal way after falling, because of weakness of hip extension, and he has to climb up his own legs, extending his hips by pushing his arms against his thighs.

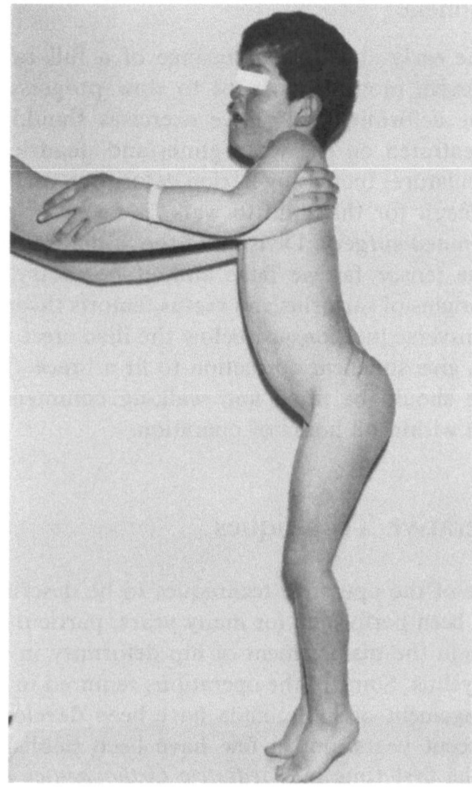

FIG. 13–35 Flexion deformity of the hip in muscular dystrophy.

Clinical examination confirms the weakness in the gluteal musculature and sometimes in the quadriceps muscles. Fixed flexion deformity of the hip (Fig. 13–35) is often missed because of the development of compensatory lumbar lordosis. Thomas' test should be performed with acute flexion of the opposite hip to ensure that any lordosis of the lumbar spine is eliminated.

The mechanism of development of deformity is probably a combination of muscle imbalance, leading to diminished growth in the hip flexor muscles, and fibrosis and abnormality of the flexor muscles themselves. Such a situation is unlike those in other paralytic deformities.

Treatment

In the early stages, maintenance of a full range of passive movements helps to slow progression of the deformity and active exercises should be concentrated on the weak glutei and quadriceps musculature. Increasing flexion deformity, making it difficult for the child to walk, is an indication for limited surgery. Division of the fascial sheaths of the tensor fasciae latae and, if necessary, of the origins of sartorius and rectus femoris through a transverse incision just below the iliac crest will often give sufficient correction to fit a brace. The brace should be fitted and walking commenced again within 48 hours of operation.

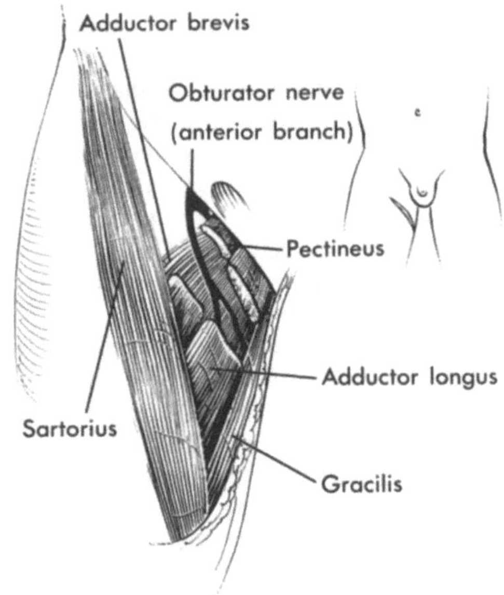

FIG. 13–36 Exposure for adductor release and neurectomy of the anterior branch of the obturator nerve.

Operative Techniques

Some of the operative techniques to be described have been performed for many years, particularly those in the management of hip deformity in poliomyelitis. Some of the operations required in the management of spina bifida have been developed in recent years, and a few have been published for the first time in *Paediatric Orthopaedics and Fractures.*[46] All of the operative procedures described have been performed on many occasions and have been the subject of extensive follow-up for reliability and adequacy.

Soft-tissue Release Operations

Adductor Release Adductor release is indicated whenever there is true shortness of the adductors. The aim is to obtain full passive abduction of the hip if possible, the extent of adductor release required depending on the severity of the condition. It can be done at any age.

Adductor release by subcutaneous tenotomy is rarely adequate in surgery of the paralytic hip and should be used only if it is thought that the adductor longus tendon alone requires division.

In all other instances, the operation should be performed openly, through an incision parallel to the groin crease and 2.5 cm below it, centered over the adductor longus tendon which is always prominent (Fig. 13–36). Skin and subcutaneous tissue are divided and mobilized a little proximally and distally. The fascia overlying the adductor longus is incised longitudinally and bluntly dissected to expose the tendons of the adductor longus and gracilis. These two muscles are almost always short in adductor tightness in cerebral palsy or spina bifida. The tendons are defined close to their attachment to the pelvis and divided. If the division is made 1 cm from the origin, the obturator vessels or nerves will not be damaged. The origin of the adductor longus is primarily from a tendon but there is some muscle attachment as well that must be divided. The gracilis takes its origin from a thin vertical tendon which should be divided completely, particularly at its posterior end. When division is complete, a small vessel almost always needs to be coagulated.

The adductor brevis muscle is then visible. The anterior branches of the obturator nerve are identified running obliquely downward and medially across the anterior aspect of the brevis muscle. These nerves are defined and retracted. The posterior branches of the obturator nerve are defined similarly on the posterior aspect of the muscle. If the adductor brevis muscle is tight it can be divided carefully, but not infrequently it is possible to stretch it by careful passive abduction of the hip. In many instances, this is the total amount of adductor release required.

If adduction deformity is severe, particularly in spina bifida with dislocation of the hip, it may be necessary to divide the whole of the adductor magnus origin and possibly also the pectineus. If abduction is still limited, this may be due to tightness of the medial hamstring muscles. If so, the incision should be extended posteriorly to expose the tendon of origin of the medial hamstring muscle which must be identified carefully from the sciatic nerve before it is divided. The muscles are allowed to retract distally and need not be sutured. At the end of the operation, a full range of abduction should be possible.

If considered appropriate by preoperative indications, the anterior branch of the obturator nerve may also be divided.

The incision is closed in three layers: a vertical layer of fascia defined at the commencement of the operation, a subcutaneous layer, and skin. In older children, suction drainage may have to be used but in young children it is usually unnecessary. Abduction is maintained by plaster casts from groin to toes, separated by two abduction bars.

Some hematoma formation may be anticipated in the wound after operation but it is not usually extensive and can be expected to subside spontaneously after 10 to 14 days. The plaster splintage can be removed after 3 weeks in children under the age of 5 and after 4 weeks in older children. As soon as plaster fixation has been removed, physiotherapy to maintain passive abduction should be instituted and continued daily for 4 to 6 weeks.

In the course of adductor release for dislocation of the hip, the hip may be reduced during the operation. If there is doubt about the completeness of the reduction radiographs can be taken during the course of the operation. If the hip has been dislocated it is usually necessary to perform further operations, such as posterolateral iliopsoas transplantation. This can usually proceed 2 weeks after a bilateral adductor release.

Iliopsoas Tendon Elongation or Release Iliopsoas elongation is indicated whenever there is fixed flexion deformity of the hip. Since flexion deformity often accompanies adduction deformity, the operation can be combined with adductor release in many instances. If so, the iliopsoas tendon can be approached through the incision already described for adductor release, or by that described by Keats and Morgese which is depicted in Figure 4–31, page 111. After the appropriate adductors have been divided, the lesser trochanter is palpated in the depths of the wound, retracting the adductor brevis anteriorly. By dissecting through a layer of fascia, the lesser trochanter can be exposed and the iliopsoas tendon will be found running downward and posteriorly to insert into it. By mobilizing bluntly toward the inguinal ligament and retracting the femoral vessels and nerves anteriorly, 5 to 7 cm of tendon can be exposed. Difficulty may sometimes be encountered in finding the iliopsoas tendon, which lies medially and may be covered by iliacus muscle fibers. The medial femoral circumflex vessels cross the tendon and may have to be ligated to give the exposure necessary for tendon lengthening. The tendon can be lengthened by a Z incision. Before the division is completed, a toothed forceps should be applied to the proximal tendon lest it suddenly disappear up into the pelvis. The tendon ends should be sutured together by two or three strong sutures.

Where there is severe deformity, and particularly in dislocation, the lesser trochanter may be found to lie much more proximally than normal, often level with the ischial tuberosity. It may be impossible to expose sufficient tendon for a formal elongation. In this circumstance, division of the tendon from the lesser trochanter, leaving the iliacus attachment, is a satisfactory alternative. The tendon will not retract too far and will grow to reattach itself to the femur. There is nothing to be gained by suturing the tendon to the anterior aspect of the hip joint where it can serve no useful purpose.

A hip spica is applied to maintain the hips abducted and extended. Alternatively, the position may be maintained by a frame. External fixation should be retained for 4 weeks and active physiotherapy instituted as soon as the hip spica is removed.

If elongation of the iliopsoas tendon alone is indicated (there being no adduction deformity or any adduction deformity having been corrected previously), the tendon can be approached through an alternative incision passing from just below the anterior superior spine along the lateral border of the sartorius muscle for one-quarter of the length of the thigh. After incising subcutaneous tissue and the fascia of the thigh, the sartorius and rectus femoris muscles are defined at their lateral border and retracted forward. Dissection proceeds deep to these two muscles and to the femoral vessels and nerve, which are retracted forward. The lesser trochanter is palpated and its discovery is aided by flexing and laterally rotating the hip. By inserting deep retractors, the iliopsoas tendon can be defined and elongation or division performed as described in the preceding paragraphs. Only deep fascia, subcutaneous tissue, and skin need to be sutured and fixation is obtained by a plaster spica.

Hip Flexor Release Severe flexion deformity of the hip of more than 45° usually requires the release of other flexor muscles and fasciae in addition to the iliopsoas tendon. Among the tight structures that may need to be divided are the tensor fasciae latae and its sheath, the sartorius, pectineus, iliopsoas, and sometimes the anterior capsule of the hip, and the iliofemoral ligaments.

All of these structures can be exposed through an oblique incision along the lateral side of the sartorius in the upper third of the thigh (Fig. 13–37). The skin and subcutaneous tissue are mobilized to expose the inguinal ligament and the femoral triangle medially and the tensor fasciae latae muscle and its covering fasciae laterally. The lateral cutaneous nerve of the thigh should be identified as it emerges from beneath the inguinal ligament about 1 cm medial to the anterior superior spine. This nerve may sometimes be difficult to define and it may emerge medial to its normal site or in two branches. The origin of the sartorius muscle from the inguinal ligament and from the anterior superior iliac spine is defined. The origin is mainly muscular although there are a few tendinous fibers. The sartorius origin should be divided obliquely to allow the possibility of resuture at completion of the operation. The fascia lata on the inner and outer aspects of the tensor fasciae latae muscle are next divided. Beneath the origin of the sartorius, the lateral femoral circumflex vessels may be defined and should either be ligated or carefully retracted. The origin of the rectus femoris muscle is defined, the straight head arising from the anterior inferior iliac spine and the reflected head arising from the acetabular margin. Both heads should be divided obliquely to allow for resuture at the end of the operation. It may not be necessary to divide this muscle if extension of the knee shows that it is not responsible for maintaining flexion deformity at the hip.

The iliacus muscle and the iliopsoas tendon are exposed deep to the femoral nerve and vessels which are retracted medially. The iliopsoas tendon is lengthened or divided as in the preceding paragraphs.

At this point, the extent of correction for a flexion deformity can be assessed. If the hip has been dislocated, an attempt should be made to reduce it. When this has been done, it may be found that the flexor release is not as adequate as was first estimated. However, further attempts to release flexion deformity may then be held up

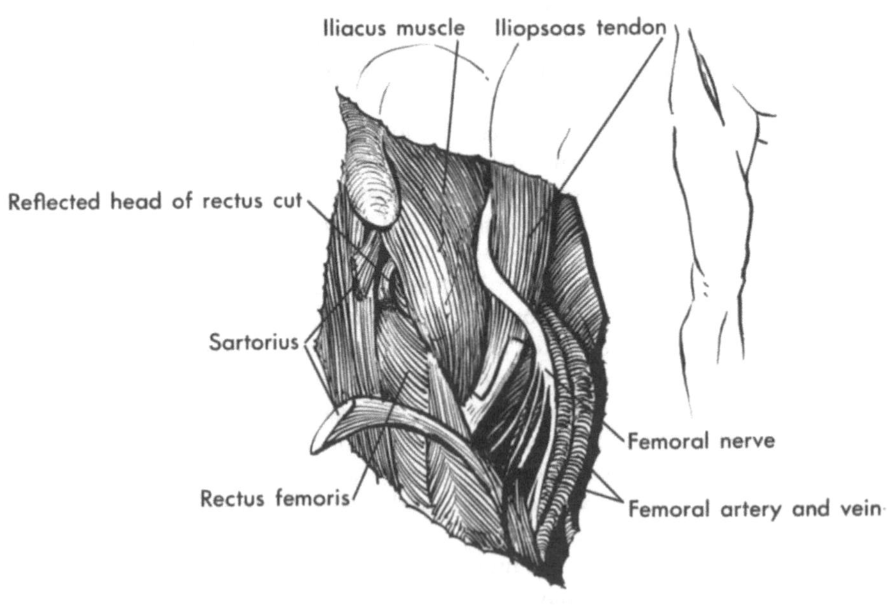

FIG. 13–37 Exposure for hip flexor release.

by tightness of the femoral nerve or femoral vessels or both. If these structures are tight, no further attempt should be made to release the flexion deformity by soft-tissue division. If the vessels and nerve are not tight, and some flexion deformity is still present, the anterior capsule of the hip can be divided at its attachment to the acetabulum. Parsons and Seddon [28] did not find that division of the hip capsule led to instability of the hip joint in such instances.

At the end of the procedure, it may be found that there is an extensive dead space that cannot be sutured without restoring the flexion deformity. This space should be drained by a suction system. A hip spica is applied to give as much correction as possible, although care is taken to avoid excessive stretching of the femoral vessels or nerve. If there is residual fixed flexion deformity, it can be corrected at a later date by extension osteotomy of the femur with removal of a portion of the femoral shaft.

Fixation should usually be maintained for 4 to 6 weeks. After this, passive extension of the hips should be maintained for at least 3 months until scarring has matured. Otherwise the deformity may recur if the deep scar is allowed to contract.

Release of the Tensor Fasciae Latae Isolated release of the tensor fasciae latae may be indicated in flexion–abduction contracture in poliomyelitis or flexion contracture in the early stages of muscular dystrophy. In poliomyelitis, there may also be some contracture of the anterior part of the gluteal musculature.

An incision is made along the outer side of the anterior third of the iliac crest and then vertically downward for 5 cm from the anterior superior iliac spine. The tensor fasciae latae is exposed at its origin from the anterior superior spine and the anterior crest of the ilium. The lateral cutaneous nerve of the thigh is defined and retracted. The fascia lata can be incised at its attachment to the ilium and allowed to mobilize downward. The tensor fasciae latae muscle is mobilized from the ilium by a periosteal elevator, although the dissection should not proceed deep to the periosteum. If there is any contracture of the gluteal musculature, it can also be mobilized from the ilium and allowed to retract distally. Mobilization should continue until full adduction can be obtained with the hip extended as much as possible.

Skin and subcutaneous tissue are sutured. If there is an extensive deep space, suction drains should be inserted. A plaster spica is applied with the affected hip extended and adducted. It is normally possible to operate only upon one hip at a time for correction of flexion–abduction contracture.

In contracture of the tensor fasciae latae in muscular dystrophy, the operation is usually a less extensive one and can be performed through a vertical incision about 5 cm long running downward from the anterior superior iliac spine. The fascia lata is exposed and divided on each side of the tensor fasciae latae muscle. The incision is closed in two layers. No plaster spica is applied but the area is supported with adhesive strapping. The child should be encouraged to get on his feet with supporting calipers on the day following operation. He should be mobilized as quickly as possible so that deterioration in the myopathic musculature is avoided.

Hip Lateral Rotator Release This operation is seldom required except in spina bifida when there is fixed lateral rotation that persists after other lateral rotators such as the iliopsoas and sartorius have been satisfactorily released. Menelaus [24] notes that it is often associated with retroversion of the femoral neck.

The patient lies prone. The short lateral rotator muscles of the hip are exposed through a slightly curved vertical incision posteromedial to the greater trochanter. The fibrous band that forms part of the attachment of the gluteus maximus muscle to the posterior aspect of the greater trochanter is divided to expose the posterior aspect of the greater trochanter. The attachments of the piriformis, obturator internus, gemelli, and quadratus femoris are exposed. Each can be defined and divided.

Through a second anterior incision, it is often appropriate to excise any redundant anterior hip capsule and even reef it. The incisions are both closed in two layers. Fixation is maintained for 3 to 4 weeks by a plaster spica applied with the hip medially rotated as much as possible and flexing the knee by 30° in the spica.

Intrapelvic Iliopsoas Release This operation is most commonly indicated in hip flexion deformity in adults, secondary to spastic paraplegia or multiple sclerosis.

If both sides are to be approached, the operation

can be performed through a suprapubic transverse Pfannenstiel incision or through bilateral pararectal incisions. The abdominal muscles are dissected in gridiron fashion to avoid damage to nerves passing toward the rectus sheath. The peritoneum and bladder are mobilized medially to expose the psoas tendon and iliacus at the level of the inguinal ligament. The external iliac vessels are retracted on the medial side and the femoral nerve mobilized from the iliacus and psoas muscles. The psoas tendon and iliacus muscle are divided at the level of the pectineal line. If necessary, the pectineus muscle is mobilized from its origin. The psoas tendon is allowed to retract freely.

The incision is closed in layers. In adults, the application of a spica is seldom required, the correction being maintained by traction or by daily passive movements.

Proximal Hamstring Release When the hamstrings are short with no flexion deformity at the knee a release is indicated. The operation is performed with the patient prone. An incision is made just lateral to the ischial tuberosity over a distance of about 5 cm (Fig. 13–38). The lower border of the gluteus maximus is defined and retracted upward to expose the tendon of origin of hamstring muscles from the ischial tuberosity. The tendon of origin is divided obliquely and the distal end allowed to retract. The ends of the tendon are sutured with 2 or 3 strong sutures to prevent excessive retraction that could lead to unbalanced weakness of hip extension. The incision is closed in two layers.

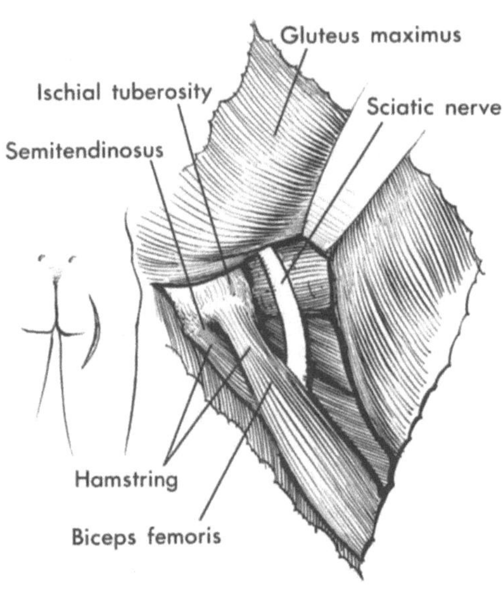

FIG. 13–38 Exposure for proximal hamstring release.

No plaster fixation is indicated or possible. The patient is nursed in the half-sitting position with the knees extended and is gradually encouraged to sit up during the course of the next 2 weeks. Walking can be recommenced after 2 to 3 weeks.[37] The shortness commonly involves both sides and, if so, the operation can be performed bilaterally at one session.

Neurectomies

Obturator Neurectomy—Anterior Branch The anterior branch of the obturator nerve can be divided in an independent procedure when there is severe spasticity of the adductor musculature without shortness. More commonly, neurectomy is performed in association with adductor release.

The approach is the same as for adductor release, through a vertical anteroposterior incision parallel to the groin crease (Fig. 13–36). The anterior branch of the obturator nerve can be found deep to the adductor longus, running on the surface of the adductor brevis, beneath a layer of thin fascia. The nerves should be separated from the obturator vessels which accompany them. If necessary, they should be identified by stimulation with a nerve stimulator. Before the anterior branches of the obturator nerve are divided it is wise to explore the posterior surface of the adductor brevis to ensure that there is a posterior branch; occasionally, the whole of the obturator nerve may pass anteriorly into the adductor brevis and a total obturator neurectomy may inadvertently be performed if this is not recognized.

If the posterior branch of the obturator nerve is present, the anterior branches should be isolated and divided with resection of at least 1 cm of nerve. There are usually two branches to be divided. If the obturator vessels are accidentally divided also, this is of no serious consequence provided the vessels are ligated or coagulated.

Occasionally, in the presence of severe adductor spasticity, there may be an indication for crushing the posterior branches of the obturator nerve at the same time, but it is unwise to divide both branches of the obturator nerve in childhood.

If adductor release has not been performed plaster fixation is not necessary, but there may be some increase in general spasticity in the limb for 2 or 3 weeks in a cerebral-palsied child following obturator neurectomy; this usually can be controlled by appropriate drug therapy.

Intrapelvic Obturator Neurectomy Complete division of the obturator nerve through an intrapelvic approach is most often indicated in adults with severe adductor spasticity associated with traumatic paraplegia or multiple sclerosis; it is frequently done in association with division of the iliopsoas. The approach is the same as for intrapelvic iliopsoas division. The obturator nerve is divided by blunt dissection and palpation at the point where it passes into the obturator foramen. The nerve should be visualized and the obturator vessel carefully mobilized from it before the nerve is divided. Care must be taken to ensure that no damage is caused to anomalous obturator vessels or communicating vessels.

Other Neurectomies Rarely, neurectomy may be required of specific nerves such as the nerve to the rectus femoris or branches of the superior gluteal nerve or of the inferior gluteal nerve in instances of severe spasticity affecting the rectus femoris, the gluteus medius or minimus, or gluteus maximus. The nerve to the rectus femoris can be identified by an incision passing from just below the inguinal ligament along the medial side of the sartorius. The sartorius is retracted to expose the medial border of the rectus femoris into which a branch from the femoral nerve passes, and the nerve can be identified and divided. Care should be taken to ensure that branches of the lateral femoral circumflex vessels are not damaged.

The superior or inferior gluteal nerves are best exposed through an oblique incision passing from just below the posterior superior iliac spine toward the tip of the greater trochanter. The fibers of the gluteus maximus muscle are exposed and dissection may be made between the fibers to define the posterior aspect of the hip joint and the greater sciatic notch. The inferior gluteal nerve can be identified as a long nerve passing into the deep surface of the gluteus maximus. The superior gluteal nerve may be more difficult to find; it emerges through the upper part of the greater sciatic notch in close company with the superior gluteal vessels which must be carefully defined. It is seldom advisable or necessary to divide all of the branches of the superior gluteal nerve, but up to 50% of the fibers can be divided when there is severe abductor spasticity. The incision is closed in two layers.

Tendon Transplantations

Posterolateral Iliopsoas Transplantation Posterolateral iliopsoas transplantation is indicated as part of the management of paralytic subluxation or dislocation of the hip when there is loss of abduction and extension power in the presence of strong hip flexion and adduction.[42] It is most commonly needed in paralytic dislocation of the hip in spina bifida and less often in cerebral palsy or poliomyelitis. Preceding the operation, an adequate adductor release should have been performed to ensure that there is a full range of abduction. If the hip is subluxated but not dislocated, it is possible to combine adductor release with posterior iliopsoas transplantation.

The mean blood loss can be expected to be 100 ml in a child aged 1 to 4 years. The patient lies supine with a sandbag beneath the affected buttock.

The skin is incised along the anterior two-thirds of the iliac crest (Fig. 13–39), passing just lateral to the anterior superior spine and along the medial side of the sartorius, to a point halfway between the anterior superior spine and the medial femoral condyle. The skin and subcutaneous tissue are mobilized to expose the inguinal ligament, the femoral triangle in the thigh, the anterior two-thirds of the gluteal region, the tensor fasciae latae, and the gluteal fascia on the outer side of the thigh. By a combination of blunt and sharp dissection, the outer side of the iliac crest is defined. The muscles of the abdominal wall are often found to overhang the iliac crest and must be mobilized upward.

The gluteal fascia is incised carefully at its attachment to the iliac crest, care being taken to avoid incising the underlying periosteum. The gluteal muscles are mobilized from the periosteum covering the ilium to expose the posterior half of the outer surface of the ilium. The wound is packed while the dissection continues in the thigh.

The deep fascia covering the sartorius is divided in line with the medial border of the muscle, care being taken to avoid division of the branches of the femoral nerves that supply the sartorius. The sartorius muscle is usually well innervated and the quality of the innervation corresponds to that of the iliopsoas muscle. The sartorius is mobilized

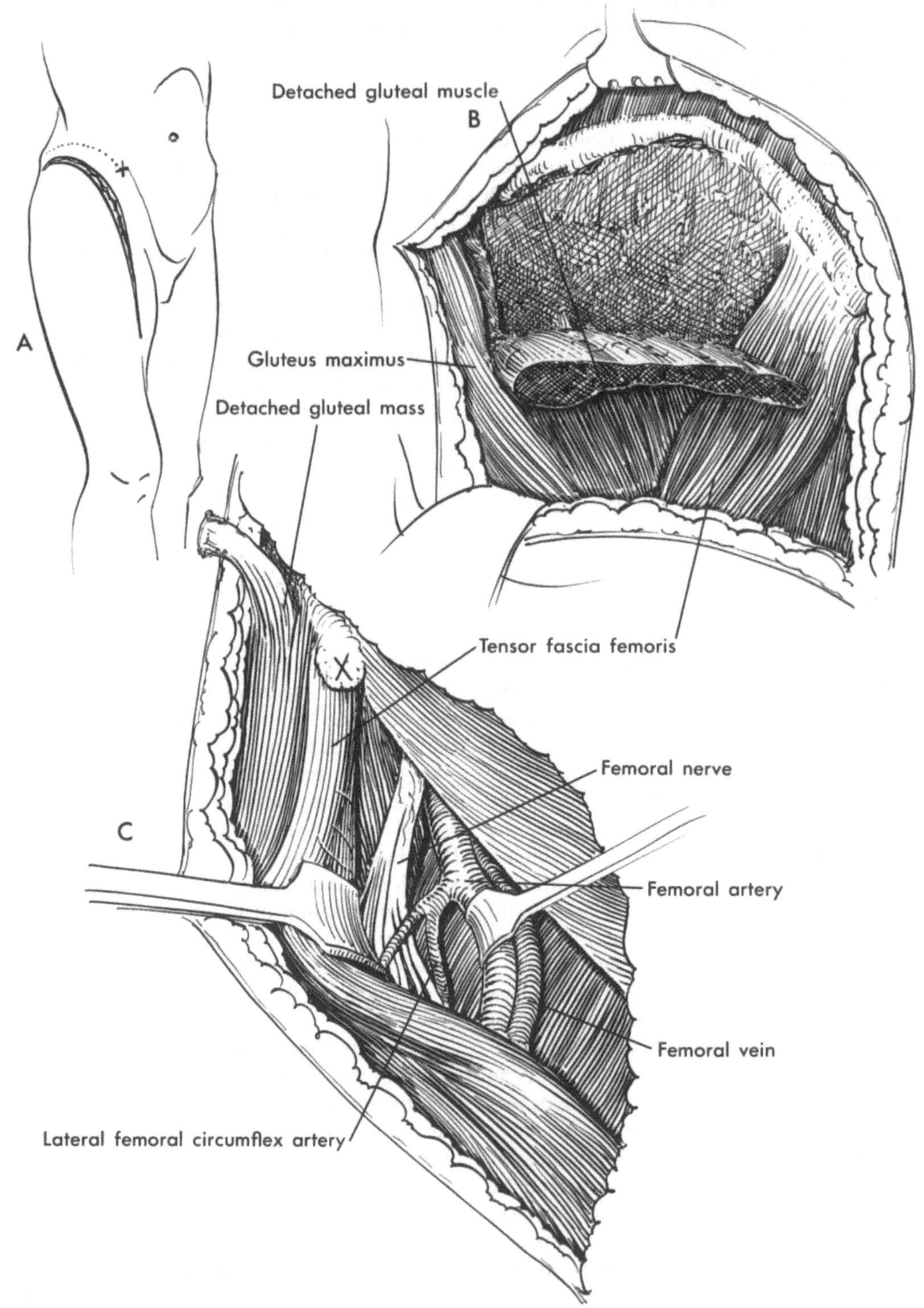

FIG. 13–39 Posterolateral iliopsoas transplantation. **A** Incision. **B** Exposure of outer side of ilium. **C** Exposure of deep structures.

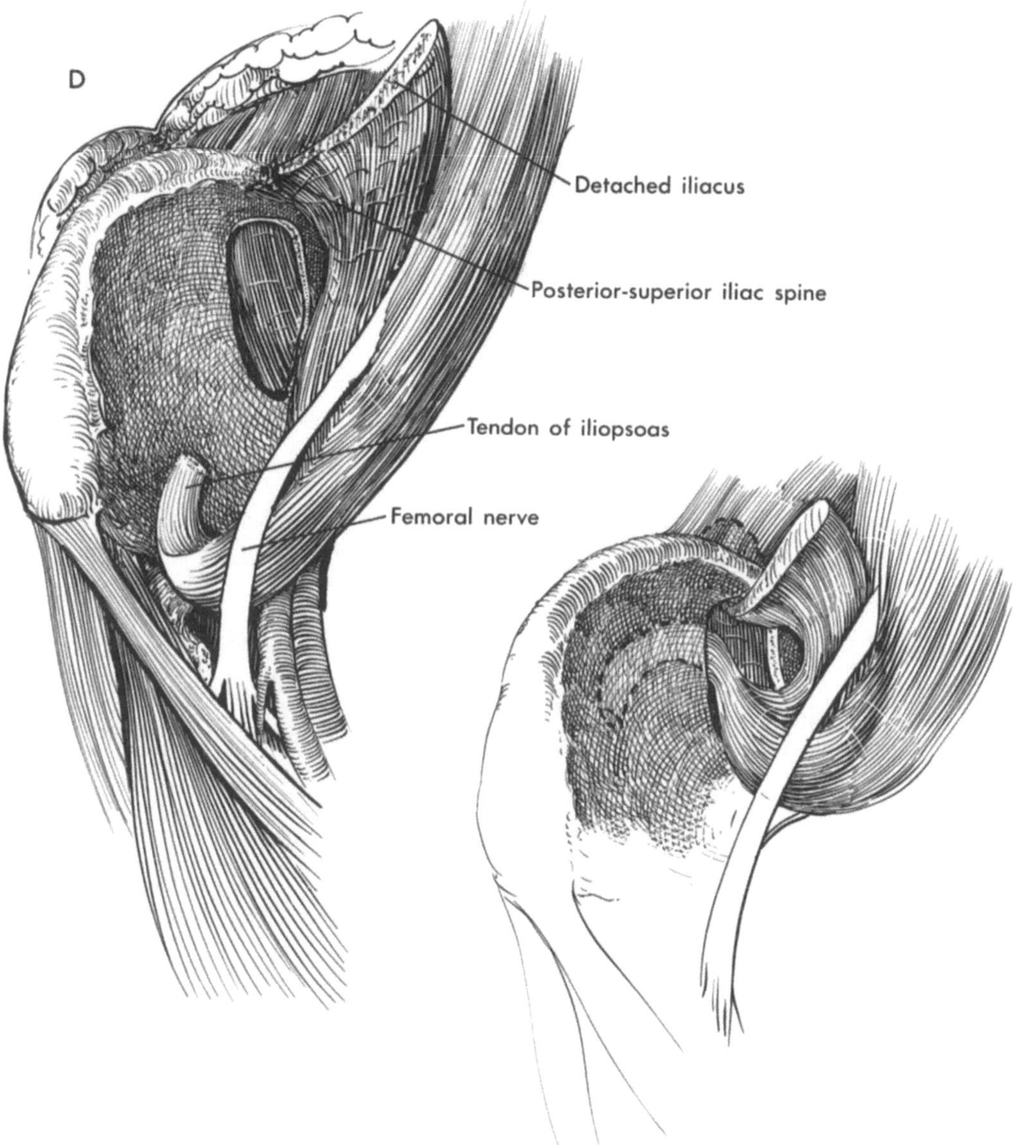

FIG. 13–39 (CON'T.) **D** Dissection of iliacus and formation of foramen in the ilium.

laterally distal to its attachment to the inguinal ligament to expose a thin layer of fascia overlying the femoral nerve. The femoral nerve is exposed by blunt dissection as it emerges from beneath the inguinal ligament. Its most medial branches are defined and carefully mobilized laterally to allow the nerve to be retracted from the femoral vessels. The most medial branch of the femoral nerve is the saphenous nerve, which is exposed by blunt dissection to the point where it comes to lie on the anterior aspect of the femoral vessels. Blunt dissection continues to expose the femoral artery and vein in the femoral triangle.

Medial retraction of the femoral vessels will be prevented by the lateral femoral circumflex artery and vein. The artery is usually a branch of the femoral artery; the vein usually enters the profunda vein or may join the femoral vein separately from the profunda. The lateral femoral circumflex vessels must be defined by very careful blunt dissection; hemostats are applied and the vessels are divided. They should always be ligated, even in

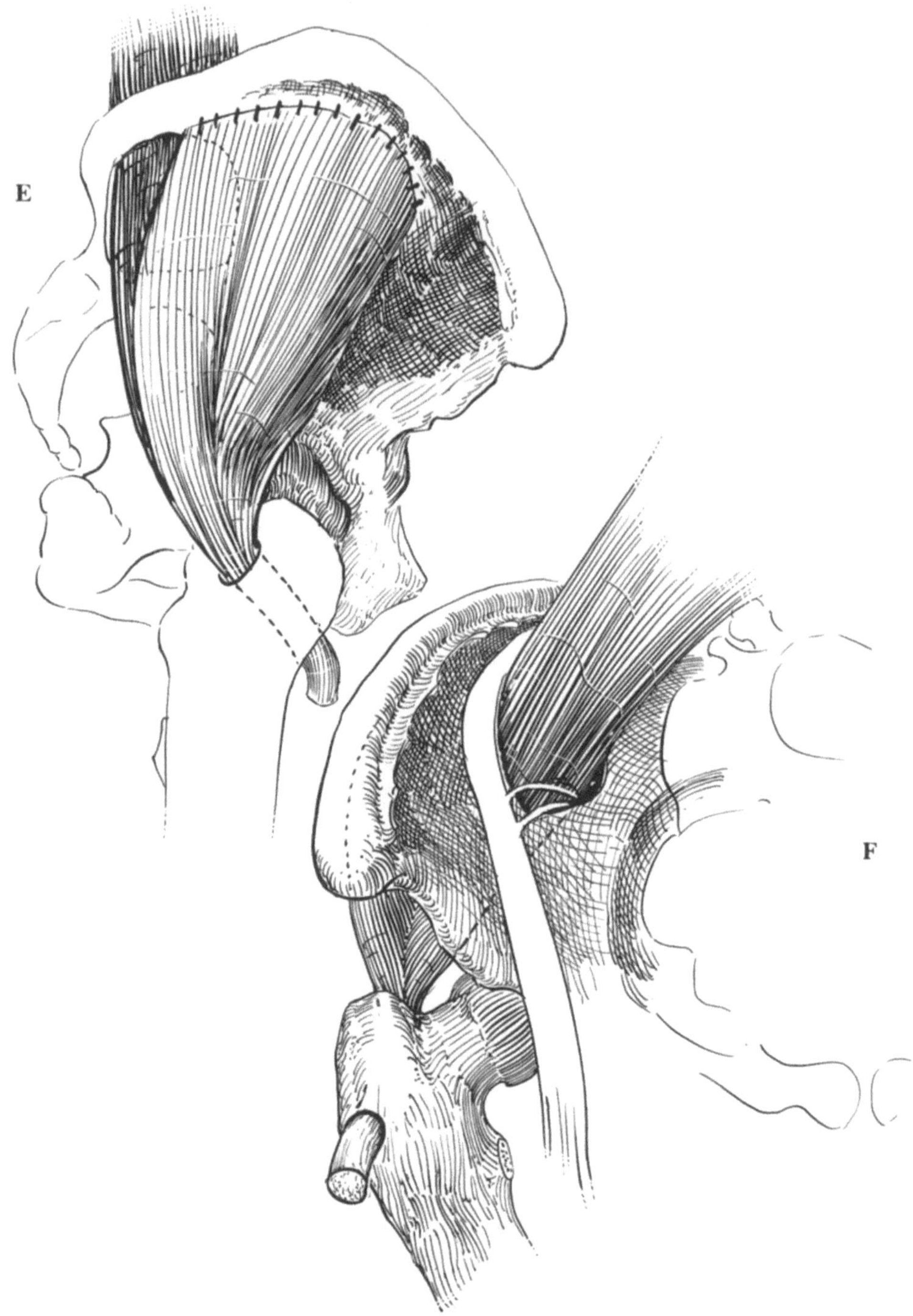

FIG. 13–39 (CON'T.) **E** Fixation of tendon to greater trochanter and reattachment of iliacus to outer wall of pelvis, lateral view. **F** Fixation of tendon to greater trochanter with hip extended and abducted 45°.

small children. When this has been done, the femoral vessels can be retracted medially while the femoral nerve and its branches are retracted laterally to expose the iliacus and the iliopsoas tendon beneath a thin layer of fascia. The object of this approach is to expose the lesser trochanter which should always be visualized clearly. It can first be palpated to identify it and brought into the wound by flexing and laterally rotating the hip. The combined iliopsoas tendon is defined on its medial and lateral sides with detachment of a few fibers of the iliacus muscle that are inserted into it at this level. The tendon is detached with a small piece of cartilage of the lesser trochanter using a Smillie meniscus knife in children below the age of 4 or an osteotome in older children. The iliopsoas tendon is mobilized proximally with division of any remaining tendon attachments and of fibrous tissue forming the walls of the subpsoas bursa.

The false pelvis is next entered by defining the inguinal ligament and detaching it and the abdominal musculature from the anterior two-thirds of the iliac crest. In a young child, this is most easily achieved by incising the cartilaginous border of the iliac crest. The pelvis is entered superficial to the iliacus to expose the whole of the iliacus and intrapelvic portion of the femoral nerve. The femoral nerve is mobilized gently from the surface of the iliacus, and the nerve supply to the iliacus muscle which usually arises in two branches is preserved. The iliopsoas tendon with the iliacus attached is passed deep and lateral to the femoral nerve. Before the iliopsoas can be mobilized proximally into the pelvis, some fibers of the iliacus which pass independently down to the femoral shaft must be divided at the level of the pectineal line. The iliacus then mobilizes easily from the inner surface of the ilium to which it is attached only along the iliac crest; it should be dissected extraperiosteally. The attachment of origin of the iliacus should be mobilized completely on the whole of the pelvic rim to the posterior superior iliac spine. On its deep surface, the nutrient vessels of the ilium may be found and may have to be coagulated or ligated in older children. When the iliacus muscle has been completely detached at both ends, the whole of the ilium in the false pelvis is exposed and the fibers of the anterior ligaments of the sacroiliac joint can be seen.

With an angled osteotome, an oval hole is made in the ilium immediately lateral to the sacroiliac joint, its width being approximately two-fifths of the greatest width of the false pelvis—large enough easily to accommodate the iliopsoas muscle. The iliopsoas tendon with the attached iliacus is passed through the hole, the origin of the iliacus being passed first into the gluteal region. The nerve supply to the iliacus is preserved so that, when the iliacus lies on the outer side of the pelvis in the gluteal region, the nerves to the iliacus pass from the femoral nerve through the bony foramen into the deep surface of the iliacus muscle. The femoral nerve should lie comfortably without undue tension or kinking.

The dissection now proceeds to the outer side of the thigh, where the fascia lata is incised vertically to define the anterior aspect of the greater trochanter. An anteroposterior tunnel is made in the greater trochanter by bone burrs (0.25-inch "rose bud"), the line of the tunnel passing a little upward and medially. A curved tendon cannula is passed through the tunnel so that its tip is in the gluteal region.

The end of the iliopsoas tendon and its attached piece of lesser trochanter are trimmed to a size appropriate to traverse the hole that has been made in the greater trochanter. A length of strong silk is attached to the tip of the iliopsoas tendon by a clove-hitch stitch. This stitch is pulled through a tendon cannula to apply the tip of the tendon to the end of the cannula. Tendon and cannula are then withdrawn together to guide the iliopsoas tendon through the tunnel in the greater trochanter from behind forward. It is usually possible to deliver the fragment of the lesser trochanter at the tip of the tendon to well in front of the greater trochanter; while this is being done, the hip should be abducted and extended.

At this point, if the hip has been dislocated, its reduction should be assured. If need be, the hip joint can be exposed on the lateral side to open it to remove any obstruction to reduction. The capsule of the hip may have to be reefed, and this should be done before the iliopsoas tendon is sutured to the greater trochanter.

The transplanted tendon should be made as tight as possible with the hip extended and abducted (35 to 45°). It is sutured to the greater trochanter using a Mayo trochar-pointed needle capable of passing through cartilage and employing strong silk or other nonabsorbable sutures. The firmness of the attachment of the tendon should be tested by flexing and adducting the hip.

The wound is closed by sutures passed through the cartilage of the iliac crest and the gluteal fascia, the upper end of the iliacus muscle being included in the sutures. The space between the inguinal ligament and the pectineal line resulting from the removal of the psoas and iliacus is obliterated by one or two sutures. The remainder of the wound is closed in two layers. In children over the age of 4 years, one or two suction drains may be needed to prevent postoperative hematoma. A plaster hip spica is applied to the toes on the operated side and to the knee on the other limb with the hip in full abduction and extension.

After operation, intravenous infusion with glucose-saline is continued until adequate fluid intake has been assured and the possibility of paralytic ileus has passed. In children with spina bifida, the plaster should be trimmed so that bladder expression can be performed. Electrolyte balance and urine production must be monitored during the first 2 or 3 days.

Fixation is retained for 3.5 to 4 weeks in children below the age of 3, and for an extra 1 to 2 weeks in older children. If the hip has been dislocated, fixation should be retained for an extra 1 or 2 weeks; fixation for longer periods than 2 months should be avoided, however, as the hip becomes fixed in extension and abduction. After removal of the plaster, the hip is allowed to lie free and to mobilize spontaneously. Parents and physiotherapists should be warned against forced passive movements during the first 2 or 3 weeks after the child comes out of the plaster. There is considerable liability to spontaneous fracture of the upper or lower end of the femur after the plaster has been removed because of the combined effects of paralysis, porosis of bone, and immobilization.

In a young child, mobilization of the hip and activity in the transplant develop within 6 or 8 weeks of removal of the plaster. In an older child, a period of specific reeducation may be necessary.

Reeducation of children for walking after the posterior iliopsoas transplantation is fully discussed by Martin.[23] If the hips remain abducted and do not mobilize spontaneously toward adduction within 2 or 3 months, subtrochanteric varus osteotomy may sometimes be needed. An unacceptable amount of medial or lateral rotation of the thigh may benefit from femoral rotation osteotomy.

In older children, iliopsoas transplantation can be combined with acetabuloplasty [14] or innominate osteotomy.[1,34] If innominate osteotomy is performed, the acetabulum should not be made to face posteriorly or the hip is liable to dislocate posteriorly on medial rotation.

If there is marked fixed flexion deformity at the commencement of the operation, posterolateral iliopsoas transplantation may be combined with hip flexor release, but the sartorius and rectus femoris should be resutured with elongation.

The residual power of hip flexion by the sartorius, rectus femoris, and pectineus muscles is usually fair. If there has been complete paralysis of the gluteal abductors before operation, active abduction by the transplant seldom reaches a power greater than fair and active extension seldom reaches a grade of more than poor.[47] In some patients no voluntary activity may be observed, but stability in extension and abduction is almost always achieved by a muscular tenodesis and bracing at hip level can usually be discarded. Standing and walking, if a patient can do so, can be allowed at any time after 6 to 8 weeks following tendon transplantation, even if the hip has been dislocated. A satisfactory transplant will maintain the reduction of a dislocated hip.

Electromyographic studies of the transplanted iliopsoas muscle show that it is active in walking during the stance phase. Fears that the transplanted iliacus may be too severely deprived of blood supply to survive with good activity have proved to be unfounded.[46] Electromyography and muscle biopsy have shown that the muscle usually survives and retains normal activity.

If bilateral transplantation is needed, it is seldom advisable for both operations to be done at the same time. The second transplantation should be performed not less than 2 weeks and not longer than 4 weeks after the first transplant.

Posterior Iliopsoas Transplantation Posterior iliopsoas transplantation is indicated when there is adequate action in the hip abductor muscles but paresis or paralysis of the hip extensors. The technique is the same as for posterolateral iliopsoas transplantation except that the iliopsoas tendon is inserted into the shaft of the femur at its junction with the greater trochanter rather than into the tip of the greater trochanter (Fig. 13–40). When this is done, the transplanted iliopsoas acts mainly as an extensor and its insertion is close to that of the site of insertion of the gluteus maximus.[46]

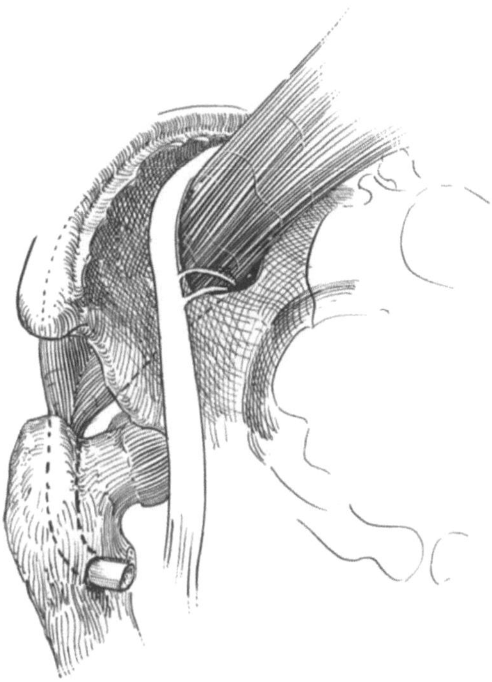

FIG. 13–40 Posterior iliopsoas transplantation. The same general technique is followed for a posterolateral transplantation except here the iliopsoas tendon is passed into the *shaft* of the femur at its junction with the greater trochanter.

Anterolateral Iliopsoas Transplantation Anterolateral iliopsoas transplantation is indicated for weakness of hip abduction, with or without subluxation of the hip. It was first described by Mustard,[25,26] primarily for the treatment of paralytic poliomyelitis. In his first paper, Mustard [25] indicated that hip extension should be adequate; this prerequisite is important because, in this transplant, the iliopsoas remains anterior to the hip joint and is still capable of some flexor activity.

A full range of abduction should first be restored by open adductor release. The patient lies supine with a sandbag beneath the affected hip. The incision is similar to that used for posterolateral iliopsoas transplantation (Fig. 13–41), except that it extends only along the anterior half of the iliac crest. The iliopsoas tendon is reached by dissection between the femoral nerve and vessels in the same way and the tendon is detached with a small piece of lesser trochanter. The pelvis is opened by dividing the lateral attachment of the inguinal ligament and the abdominal muscles from the anterior part of the iliac crest to allow the iliopsoas muscle to be mobilized proximally. A notch is cut from the anterior part of the iliac wing to allow the iliopsoas muscle to be transplanted laterally and attached to the tip of the greater trochanter in the region of the gluteal insertion. If possible, the tendon should be anchored in a bony tunnel. The transplanted muscle should be sutured under a fair degree of tension with the hip abducted. The sartorius is reattached to its origin. The incision is closed and a suction drain applied in an older child. A plaster hip spica is applied to the toes on the affected side and to the knee on the opposite side. Fixation is retained for 3 to 4 weeks if the hip has not been subluxated or dislocated, and for 1 to 2 weeks longer if there has been hip instability.

In addition to its value in preventing progressive subluxation and dislocation, the transplant improves a dipping gait caused by abductor weakness.

In both posterolateral and anterolateral iliopsoas transplantation, the power of the iliopsoas muscle and of the other hip flexors should be normal or strong. Reeducation occurs rapidly with the help of normal physiotherapy.

Lateral Iliopsoas Transplantation Lateral iliopsoas transplantation is most often indicated when there is severe paralysis in the region of the hip with activity present only in the hip flexor muscles. The lateral rotator action of the iliopsoas and of other flexor muscles of the hip leads to persistent flexion and lateral rotation deformity, which may recur even after adequate medial rotation osteotomy of the femur. The transplant is also of value when there is paralysis or severe paresis of medial rotation of the hip.

The iliopsoas tendon is approached through the same incision as for iliopsoas lengthening, passing beneath the sartorius and the femoral nerve and vessels. The tendon is detached from the lesser trochanter with a small piece of cartilage and mobilized laterally beneath the femoral nerve and vessels to the anterior aspect of the greater trochanter. It is anchored, by firm nonabsorbable sutures passed through the end of the tendon and the small piece of cartilage of the lesser trochanter, to the cartilage or periosteum of the anterior aspect of the greater trochanter.

It is not usually possible to put the tendon through a bony tunnel. With moderate flexion and lateral rotation deformity, release of the iliopsoas

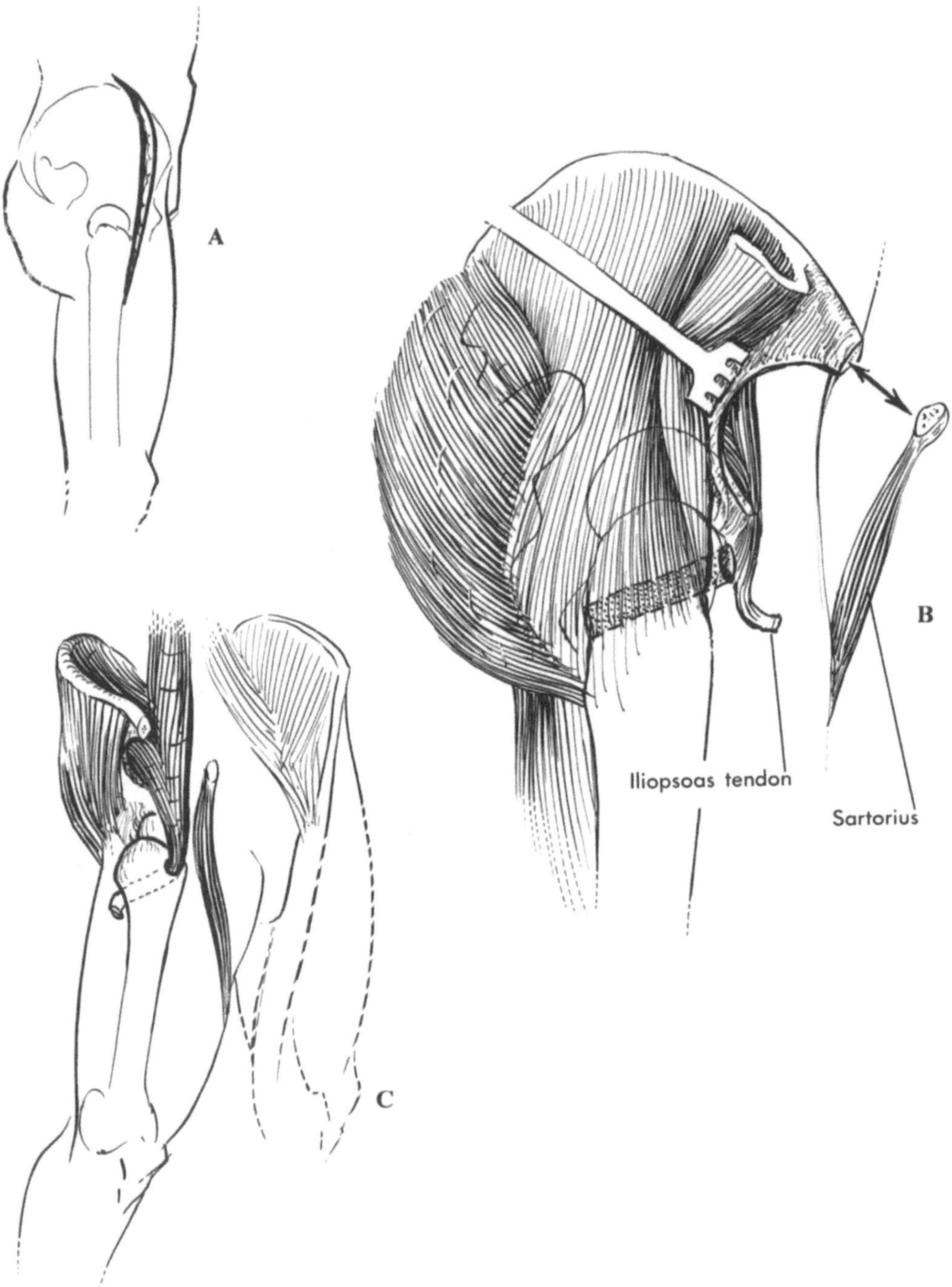

FIG. 13–41 Anterolateral iliopsoas transplantation. **A** Skin incision. **B** Anterior resection of ilium. **C** Attachment of the iliopsoas tendon into the greater trochanter under tension with the hip abducted 45°.

tendon will usually give good correction. The hip is immobilized in neutral extension and medial rotation in a plaster spica for 3 to 4 weeks. The operation is not a major procedure and it can be performed bilaterally without risk. Blood loss is very small and blood transfusion is seldom necessary.

External Oblique Transplantation Transplantation of the external oblique abdominal muscle is a good alternative to anterolateral transplantation of the iliopsoas when that muscle is needed to maintain hip flexion in poliomyelitis,[6,54] and can also be used in myelomeningocele patients to restore abduction in the presence of paralysis of gluteus medius and minimus when combined with posterior transfer of the adductors to the ischium.[21,57] An incision is made from the pubic tubercle along the crest of the ilium to end at the costal margin at the posterior axillary line. A strip of the aponeurosis of the external oblique muscle is made from the tissue just above the inguinal ligament. The main mass of the external oblique muscle is detached from the remainder of its aponeurosis up to the level of the costal margin. It is mobilized laterally. A separate incision is made over the outer side of the greater trochanter and the tendon formed from the strip of aponeurosis is passed subcutaneously to be attached to the greater trochanter through a bony tunnel. A plaster spica is applied with the hip in abduction for 4 weeks.

Sartorius Transplantation Transplantation of the origin of the sartorius is sometimes needed for paralysis or paresis of medial rotation, especially after posterior iliopsoas transplantation. The action of the sartorius as a lateral rotator of the hip arises from the fact that its origin lies lateral to the vertical axis of the hip joint and its insertion lies medial to it.

Its action as a lateral rotator can be neutralized by detaching it at its origin from the anterior superior spine and the lateral part of the inguinal ligament and mobilizing it medially to be attached to the medial part of the inguinal ligament.

If it is intended to try to obtain some active medial rotation, the more extensive procedure of transplantation of the insertion of the sartorius to the outer side of the knee can be undertaken. An incision is made along the distal two-thirds of the sartorius muscle. The muscle is mobilized from the roof of the femoral canal to its tendinous attachment to the tibia, from which it is divided. The nerve supply of the sartorius enters in its upper half, so that the muscle and tendon of insertion can be mobilized proximal to the middle thigh. A second incision is made over the outer side of the knee and the sartorius is transferred subcutaneously to the outer side of the knee where it can conveniently be sutured to the lateral ligament.

Whichever operation is used, fixation is obtained by a plaster spica with the hip in extension and medial rotation; it is maintained for 3 to 4 weeks.

Adductor Transplantation to the Ischium Smith,[48] in discussing the treatment of hip dislocation in cerebral palsy, mentions adductor transplant to the ischium as an alternative to adductor release; he attributes the credit for the idea to Nickel. Through a vertical incision parallel to the groin crease, the adductor muscles are approached in the same way as for adductor release. The adductor magnus and longus and gracilis are divided close to their origin and transferred posteriorly to be attached to the ischium or to the common tendon of origin of the medial hamstring muscles. It is felt that in this way the adductors can contribute some power of extension to the hip.

The disadvantage of the procedure is that, to obtain an adequate suture of the adductors, there may be a temptation to elongate them adequately so that some adduction deformity remains; this complication must be avoided. A hip spica applied with the hip extended and abducted is required until the adductor tendons have become soundly united after 3 to 4 weeks.

Medial Hamstring Transplantation to the Adductors This operation is seldom required, but it has a specific indication in a patient in whom too extensive an obturator neurectomy has been performed in the presence of fair or strong hip abductor power. The hip passes into fixed abduction. If allowed to persist, abduction deformity can become intractable and may recur even after adequate varus osteotomy of the femur.

The operation is performed through an incision in the groin. The common tendon of origin of the medial hamstring muscles is defined, care being taken to identify and retract the sciatic nerve. The tendon is divided close to the ischium and mobilized forward to be attached in the adductor region at the attachment of the adductor longus tendon to which it is sutured. If there is fixed abduction, it should be corrected through a second incision along the iliac crest by mobilizing the fascia lata and gluteal muscles from the ilium. The wound is closed in layers and the hip maintained in adduction by a hip spica for 3 to 4 weeks.

Lateral Transplantation of Semitendinosus This operation is indicated for persistent medial rotation deformity, usually in cerebral palsy but occasionally in spina bifida or poliomyelitis. Any fixed flexion and adduction deformity should have first been corrected by flexor and adductor release. If fixed medial rotation deformity remains, or if the hip tends to rotate medially because of weakness of lateral rotators, lateral transplantation of the insertion of the semitendinosus is indicated.[2] With fixed medial rotation deformity, the operation may be combined with lateral rotation osteotomy of the femur to the lower third of the shaft of the femur (Fig. 13–42).

The insertion of the semitendinosus tendon is approached through a posteromedial incision. The tendon is detached as far distally as possible and mobilized proximally to the lower third of the thigh. A second incision is made on the outer side of the lower third of the femur. The fascia lata of the thigh is divided to expose the femoral shaft. The semitendinosus tendon is transplanted posterolaterally to the lateral incision to be attached to the lateral or anterolateral aspect of the lateral femoral condyle, where it can be sutured through a bony tunnel or to a strong subperiosteal strap. The incision on the outer side of the femur can also be used to perform rotation osteotomy with application of a plate. The transplanted tendon should not be sutured until the osteotomy has been performed. The limb is immobilized in a unilateral spica with the hip laterally rotated.

It is difficult to assess the action of the semitendinosus as a lateral rotator in this situation but it is evident at operation that, when the transplanted muscle is sutured tightly, the tendon comes under tension when the hip is medially rotated. Fixation is maintained for 3 to 4 weeks.

Distal Transplantation of the Gluteal Insertion This operation is indicated when there has been longstanding adduction deformity at the hip with subluxation or dislocation. After hip flexor and adductor release to allow the hip to be abducted, the gluteal abductors are slack. In a young child, growth will take up the slack; in a child over the age of 8 or 9 years, however, this will not occur within a reasonable time.

An incision is made over the outer side of the greater trochanter. The gluteal insertion is identified and the excessive slackness of the gluteal muscles confirmed. The insertion of the gluteus medius by a wide flat tendon to the outer side of the upper third of the greater trochanter is defined by identifying the subgluteal bursa. The tendon is detached at its insertion and mobilized distally, putting it under as much tension as possible with the hip fully abducted. The tendon is attached in its new site on the lateral side of the shaft of the femur by a combination of suture to the periosteum and surrounding soft tissue and application of a staple. The wound is closed in two layers and a hip spica applied with the hip abducted as far as possible.

Osteotomies

Femoral or pelvic osteotomy is indicated for paralytic hip deformity when there is residual deformity after soft tissues have been released, or when valgus deformity of the femoral neck or rotational deformity of the femur needs to be corrected. Osteotomy at the junction of the shaft with the trochanter can be used to correct any hip deformity, but where only rotation needs attention, it is simpler to perform the operation in the lower third of the shaft of the femur.

Varus Osteotomy Varus osteotomy is indicated for fixed abduction deformity of the hip or for valgus deformity of the femoral neck. Some authors, believing that valgus of the femoral neck in itself is the primary cause of paralytic subluxation, have advocated varus osteotomy for the treatment of paralytic dislocation of the hip.[17] Jones[18] indicated that varus osteotomy was not always successful in stabilizing a dislocated hip, a finding confirmed by Parsons and Seddon.[28] If adequate soft-tissue release and muscle balancing operations have been performed, varus osteotomy is not often needed and, with growth, a normal angle of the femoral neck may be restored spontaneously.

If, after reduction of the dislocated hip, the valgus deformity of the femoral neck is so marked that the hip remains abducted after removal of the plaster, varus osteotomy may be needed to bring the limbs in position for walking. In a child over the age of 7 or 8, varus osteotomy may also be needed to speed up the process of mobilization.

The operation (Fig. 13–43) is performed through a lateral approach over the greater trochanter in the upper third of the shaft of the femur. Dissection proceeds through the fascia lata of the thigh with separation of the fibers of the vastus lateralis to expose the femoral shaft. The periosteum is incised vertically and mobilized anteriorly and posteriorly. The periosteum should be detached from the intertrochanteric line so that the anterior and medial aspects of the base of the femoral neck and uppermost femoral shaft can be seen.

If valgus deformity only must be corrected, this can be achieved by removing a wedge based medially at the junction of the neck and the shaft of the femur using an end-cutting saw. The lateral cortex of the femur is retained intact to allow a greenstick osteotomy to be performed. The position should be retained by a nail plate. For children younger than 18 months, subminiature nail plates are available; for older children, special nail plates can be found.

Additional fixation by a hip spica is advisable for the first 3 weeks in a child below the age of 3 and for 4 weeks in an older child. After this, the hip can be allowed free but weight bearing should not be allowed until the osteotomy has united (6 to 8 weeks).

Rotation Osteotomy Rotation osteotomy of the femur can be performed either at subtrochanteric level or at the lower end of the shaft. If combined varus and lateral or medial rotation osteotomy is needed, it must be done at the intertrochanteric level (Fig. 13–43). The approach is the same as for varus osteotomy but the shaft must be divided completely to allow the distal fragment to be rotated. Before the bone is divided, marker pins should be applied above and below the level of the proposed osteotomy to estimate the degree of rotation to be obtained. Fixation with a nail plate is essential in young children; in older children, fixation can be either by nail plate or by thin Steinmann's pins applied through the upper and lower fragments and incorporated in a plaster spica.

Extension Osteotomy Severe fixed flexion deformity of 80 to 90° can seldom be corrected by flexor release alone. An adequate flexor release will gain 40 or 45° of correction, but further correction is prevented by tightness of the femoral vessels and nerve; the correction can be completed only by osteotomy.

The upper third of the femoral shaft is approached from the lateral aspect, as for varus osteotomy. The femoral shaft is exposed and divided at the junction of the shaft with the greater trochanter by a transverse osteotomy (Fig. 13–44). The two fragments are separated completely from each other and 1 or 2 cm of shaft are removed obliquely from the distal fragment. This allows the femoral shaft to be extended and its end placed on the posterior aspect of the greater trochanter, which is cleaned of soft tissues and scarified to provide a bleeding surface for contact. If this is done, the proximal fragment is left flexed but excellent correction of flexion deformity is obtained. The fragments are not easy to maintain in position either by a plaster spica or by internal fixation, but a combination of the two is usually adequate. A 4-hole plate applied to the greater trochanter proximally and the femoral shaft distally maintains apposition of the fragments. After skin closure, a plaster spica maintaining the hips in extension and neutral rotation completes fixation. The osteotomy usually unites within 6 to 8 weeks.

Rotation Osteotomy of the Femoral Shaft Pure medial or lateral rotation deformity at the hip can be corrected easily by rotation osteotomy in the lower third of the femoral shaft (Fig. 13–42). The shaft is approached through a lateral incision. The fascia lata of the thigh is divided and the vastus lateralis mobilized from the outer side of the shaft of the femur. The periosteum is incised and similarly mobilized. Before osteotomy is performed, marker pins are applied above and below the proposed site. Ideally, the pins are applied at an angle to each other so that, when the fragments are rotated, the pins protrude parallel to each other and a 4- or 6-hole plate can be passed over the pins which conveniently hold it in place while screws are being applied. The wound is closed in three layers and fixation completed by the application of a plaster spica. Union is usually sound after 6 weeks.

Innominate Osteotomy Innominate osteotomies of the Salter [34] or Chiari [7] types are described in Chapter 8. Innominate osteotomy can be combined with open reduction of the dislocated hip or with anterolateral or posterolateral iliopsoas transplan-

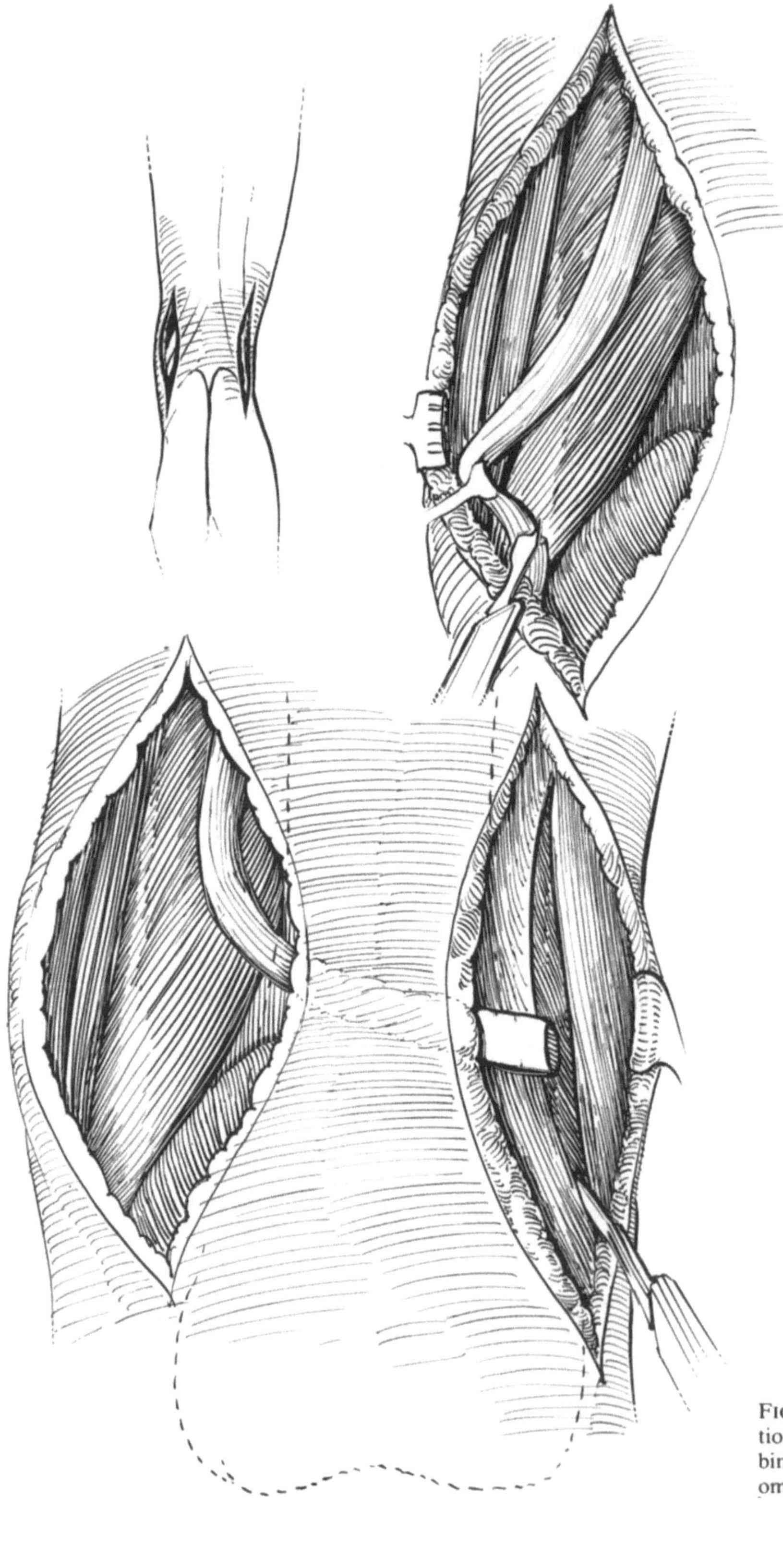

FIG. 13–42 Lateral transplantation of the semitendinosus combined with lateral rotation osteotomy of the femur.

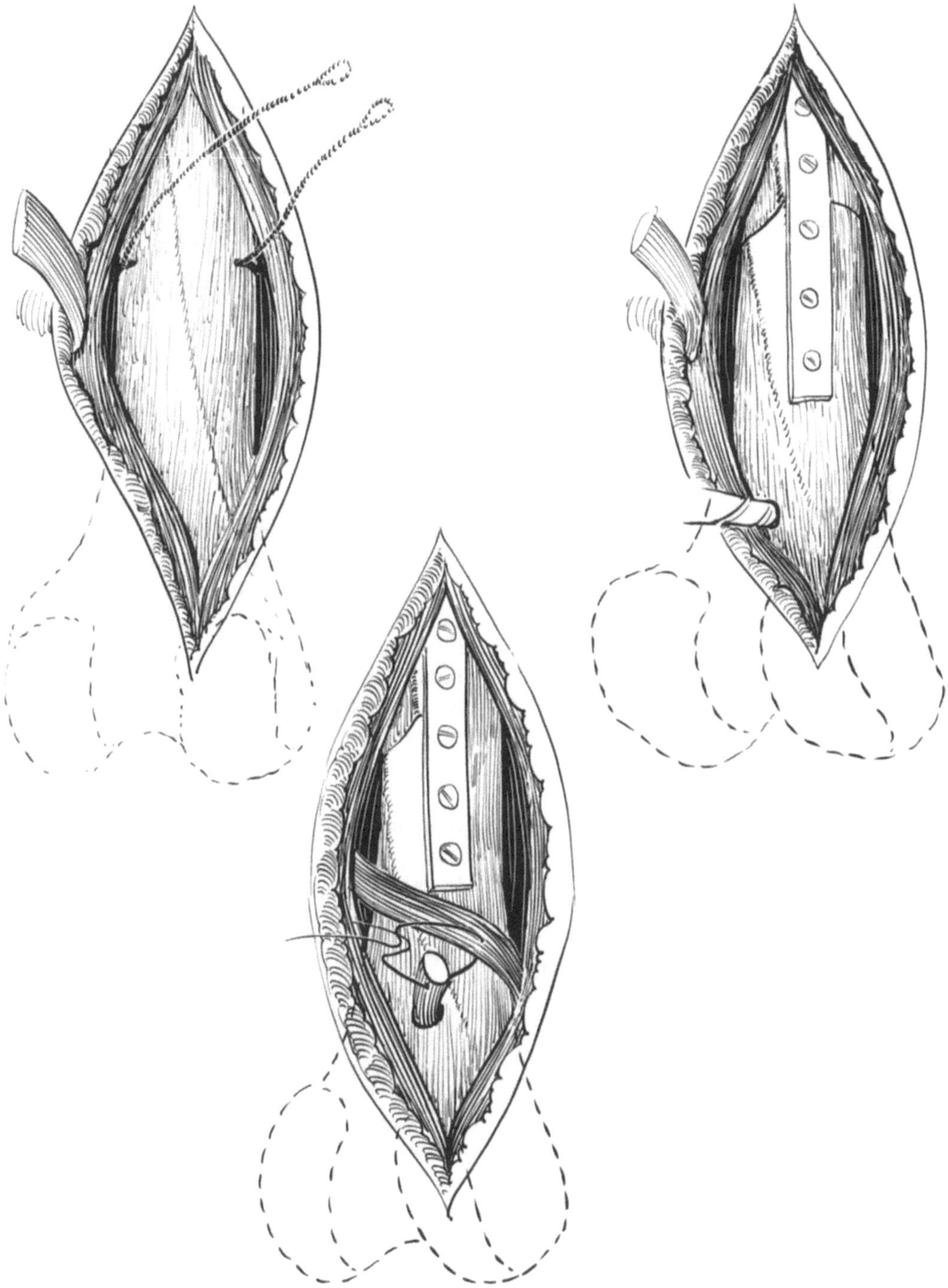

FIG. 13–42 (CON'T.) The femoral shaft is exposed through the lateral incision.

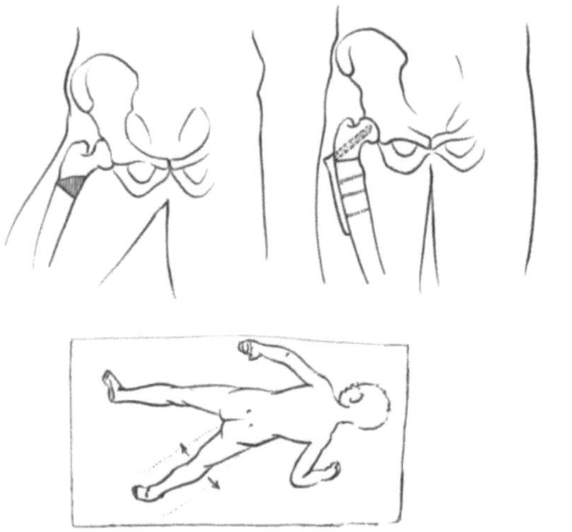

FIG. 13–43 Intertrochanteric femoral varus or varus and rotation osteotomy.

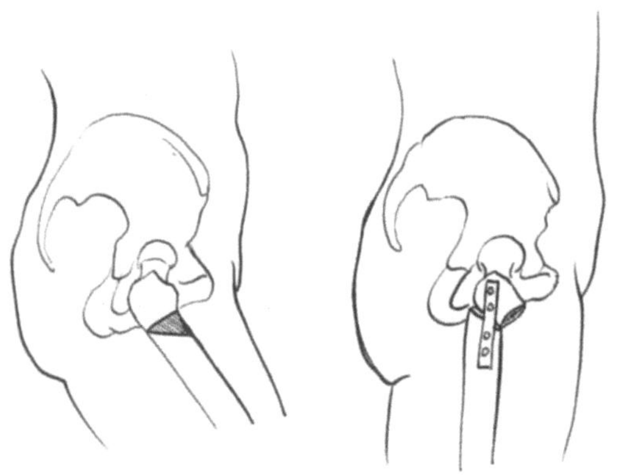

FIG. 13–44. Subtrochanteric femoral extension osteotomy for severe flexion deformity.

tation, since the main part of the approach is the same.

Combined Operations

Neglected paralytic dislocation of the hip or severe hip deformity may have to be corrected by a combination of several operations. Smith[48] has described how adductor release, psoas release and posterolateral transplantation, open reduction of the dislocation, and subtrochanteric osteotomy of the femur can be combined in one operation to achieve correction of deformity and balanced muscle activity. Whether this is feasible in a young child depends on his general state and the severity of the deformities. It is always possible to complete some of the stages of the operation and to await healing of these before proceeding with the further stages if the general condition of the patient requires it.

Dega et al.[10] have described a one-stage procedure for the treatment of congenital dislocation of the hip in older children by extensive soft-tissue release of the hip flexors and adductors, capsular arthroplasty according to the principles described by Colonna,[8] varus and derotation osteotomy, and shortening of the femoral shaft. A similar procedure can be undertaken in longstanding paralytic dislocation in older children, combining it with posterolateral iliopsoas transplantation and distal transplantation of the gluteal insertion to correct all factors responsible for maintenance of the dislocation.

In these difficult cases it is only by radical measures that stability can be obtained, and stiffness of the hip and avascular necrosis of the femoral head are not infrequent complications. Such possibilities have to be set against the gross deformity, disability, and pain that may develop in longstanding paralytic dislocation in poliomyelitis, cerebral palsy, or spina bifida.

Bibliography

1. Allan, J. A.: The challenge of spina bifida cystica. In: *Current Practice in Orthopaedic Surgery, 1963* (Adams, J. P., ed.). St. Louis, Mosby, 1963.
2. Baker, L. D., and Hill, L. M.: Foot alignment in the cerebral palsy patient. J. Bone Joint Surg., 46A:1, 1964.
3. Banks, H. H., and Panagakos, P.: Orthopedic evaluation of the lower extremity in cerebral palsy. Clin. Orthop., 47:117, 1966.
4. Bazih, J., and Gross, R. H.: Hip surgery in the lumbar level myelomeningocele patient. J. Pediat. Orthop., 1:405, 1981.
5. Bleck, E. E.: Postural and gait abnormalities caused by flexion deformity in spastic cerebral palsy. Treatment in iliopsoas recession. J. Bone Joint Surg., 53A:1468, 1971.
6. Cabaud, H. E., Westin, G. W., and Connelly, S. J.: Tendon transfers on the paralytic hip. J. Bone Joint Surg., 61A:1035, 1979.
7. Chiari, K.: Ergebnisse mit der Beckenosteotomie als Pfannendachplastik. Z. Orthop., 87:14, 1955.
8. Colonna, P. C.: Capsular arthroplasty for congenital dislocation of the hip: Indications and technique. J. Bone Joint Surg., 47A:437, 1966.

9. Craig, J. J.: Cerebral palsy. In: *Modern Trends in Orthopaedics* (Graham, W. D., ed.). London, Butterworths, 1967.
10. Dega, W., Krol, J., and Polakowski, L.: Surgical treatment of congenital dislocation of the hip in children. A one-stage procedure. J. Bone Joint Surg., 41A:920, 1959.
11. Dillon, V. M., Solovieff, E. N., and Treanor, W. J.: Orthopaedic surgery in adult spastic hemiplegia. J. Bone Joint Surg., 40A:727, 1958.
12. Dunlap, K., et al.: A new method for determination of torsion of the femur. J. Bone Joint Surg., 35A:289, 1953.
13. Eberle, C. F.: Pelvic obliquity and the unstable hip after poliomyelitis. J. Bone Joint Surg., 64B:300, 1982.
14. Hayes, J. T., Gross, H. P., and Dow, S.: Surgery for paralytic defects secondary to myelomeningocele and myelodysplasia. J. Bone Joint Surg., 46A:1577, 1964.
15. Herzog, E. G., and Sharrard, W. J. W.: Calipers and brace with double hip locks. Clin. Orthop., 46:239, 1966.
16. Jackson, R. D., Padgett, T. S., and Donovan, M. M.: Posterior iliopsoas muscle transfer in myelodysplasia. J. Bone Joint Surg., 61A:40, 1979.
17. Jones, G. B.: Paralytic dislocation of the hip. J. Bone Joint Surg., 36B:375, 1954.
18. Jones, G. B.: Paralytic dislocation of the hip. J. Bone Joint Surg., 44B:573, 1962.
19. Lamb, D. W., and Pollock, G. A.: Hip deformities in cerebral palsy and their treatment. Develop. Med. Child Neurol., 4:488, 1962.
20. Lewis, F. R., Samilson, R. R., and Lucas, D. B.: Femoral torsion and coxa valga in cerebral palsy. A preliminary report. Develop. Med. Child Neurol., 6:591, 1964.
21. McKay, D. W.: McKay hip stabilization in myelomeningocele. Orthop. Trans., 1:87, 1977.
22. McKibbin, B.: The action of the iliopsoas muscle in the newborn. J. Bone Joint Surg., 50B:161, 1968.
23. Martin, M. C.: Physiotherapy in relation to myelomeningocele. Physiotherapy, 50:50, 1964.
24. Menelaus, M. B.: Dislocation and deformity of the hip in children with spina bifida cystica. J. Bone Joint Surg., 51B:238, 1969.
25. Mustard, W. T.: Iliopsoas transfer for weakness of the hip abductors. J. Bone Joint Surg., 34A:647, 1952.
26. Mustard, W. T.: A follow-up study of iliopsoas transfer for hip instability. J. Bone Joint Surg., 41B:289, 1959.
27. Norton, P. L., and Foley, J. J.: Paraplegia in children. J. Bone Joint Surg., 41A:1291, 1959.
28. Parsons, D. W., and Seddon, H. J.: The results of operations for disorders of the hip caused by poliomyelitis. J. Bone Joint Surg., 50B:266, 1968.
29. Phelps, W. M.: Prevention of acquired dislocation of the hip in cerebral palsy. J. Bone Joint Surg., 41A:440, 1959.
30. Pollock, G. A., and Sharrard, W. J. W.: Orthopaedic surgery in the treatment of cerebral palsy. In: *Recent Advances in Cerebral Palsy* (Illingsworth, R. S., ed.). London, Churchill, 1958.
31. Root, L., and Spero, C. R.: Hip adductor transfer compared with adductor tenotomy in cerebral palsy. J. Bone Joint Surg., 63A:767, 1981.
32. Rose, G. K.: Splintage for severe spina bifida cystica. J. Bone Joint Surg., 52B:178, 1970.
33. Ryder, C. T., and Crane, L.: Measuring femoral anteversion: The problem and a method. J. Bone Joint Surg., 35A:321, 1953.
34. Salter, R. B.: Innominate osteotomy in the treatment of congenital dislocation and subluxation of the hip. J. Bone Joint Surg., 43B:518, 1961.
35. Samilson, R. L., et al: Dislocation and subluxation of the hip in cerebral palsy. Pathogenesis, natural history and management. J. Bone Joint Surg., 54A:863, 1972.
36. Seddon, H. J.: Poliomyelitis. II. Treatment of poliomyelitis. In: *British Surgical Practice, Surgical Progress 1954* (Carling, E. R., and Ross, J. P., eds.). London, Butterworths, 1954.
37. Seymour, N., and Sharrard, W. J. W.: Bilateral proximal release of the hamstrings in cerebral palsy. J. Bone Joint Surg., 50B:274, 1968.
38. Sharrard, W. J. W.: Paralytic dislocation of the hip in cerebral palsy and the place of iliopsoas transplantation. J. Bone Joint Surg., 62B:278, 1980.
39. Sharrard, W. J. W.: The distribution of permanent paralysis in the lower limb in poliomyelitis. A clinical and pathological study. J. Bone Joint Surg., 37B:540, 1955.
40. Sharrard, W. J. W.: Muscle recovery in poliomyelitis. J. Bone Joint Surg., 37B:63, 1955.
41. Sharrard, W. J. W.: The mechanism of paralytic deformity in spina bifida. Develop. Med. Child Neurol., 4:310, 1962.
42. Sharrard, W. J. W.: Posterior iliopsoas transplantation in the treatment of paralytic dislocation of the hip. J. Bone Joint Surg., 46B:426, 1964.
43. Sharrard, W. J. W.: Paralytic deformity in the lower limb. J. Bone Joint Surg., 49B:731, 1967.
44. Sharrard, W. J. W.: The orthopaedic surgery of cerebral palsy and spina bifida. In: *Recent Advances in Orthopaedics* (Apley, A. G., ed.). London, Churchill, 1969.
45. Sharrard, W. J. W.: Newer aspects of myelomeningocele. In: *Recent Advances in Paediatric Surgery* (Wilkinson, A. W., ed.). London, Churchill, 1969.
46. Sharrard, W. J. W.: *Paediatric Orthopaedics and Fractures.* Oxford, Blackwell Scientific, 1971.
47. Sharrard, W. J. W., and Carroll, N.: A long-term

follow-up of posterior iliopsoas transplantation for paralytic dislocation of the hip. Fifth Combined Orthopaedic Meeting, Sydney, 1970.
48. Smith, E. P.: Hip dislocation in cerebral palsy. Develop. Med. Child Neurol., 11:291, 1969.
49. Somerville, E. W.: Paralytic dislocation of the hip. J. Bone Joint Surg., 41B:279, 1959.
50. Soutter, R.: A new operation for hip contractures in poliomyelitis. Boston Med. Surg. J., 170:380, 1914.
51. Steel, H. H.: Gluteus medius and minimus insertion advancement for correction of internal rotation gait in spastic cerebral palsy. J. Bone Joint Surg., 62A:919, 1980.
52. Stephenson, C. T., and Donovan, M. M.: Transfer of hip adductor origins to the ischium in spastic cerebral palsy. In: Proceedings of the American Academy of Orthopaedic Surgeons. J. Bone Joint Surg., 51A:1040, 1969.
53. Tachdjian, M. O., and Minear, W. L.: Hip dislocation in cerebral palsy. J. Bone Joint Surg., 38A:1358, 1956.
54. Thomas, L. I., Thompson, T. C., and Straub, L. R.: Transplantation of the external oblique muscle for abductor paralysis. J. Bone Joint Surg., 32A:202, 1950.
55. Thompson, S. B.: Indications for surgery in the lower limbs of the cerebral palsied child. Develop. Med. Child Neurol., 8:437, 1966.
56. Watson-Jones, R.: Spontaneous dislocation of the hip. Brit. J. Surg., 14:36, 1926.
57. Yngve, D. A., and Lindseth, R. E.: Effectiveness of muscle transfers in myelomeningocele hip measured by radiographic indices. J. Paediat. Orthop., 2:121, 1982.
58. Yount, C. C.: The role of the tensor fasciae femoris in certain deformities of the lower extremities. J. Bone Joint Surg., 8:171, 1926.

CHAPTER 14

Congenital Hip Dysplasia: Treatment from Infancy to Skeletal Maturity

MICHAEL B. MILLIS

The goal of treatment in the patient with idiopathic congenital hip dysplasia (CDH) is to have a lifetime of normal hip function. Treatment of the dysplastic hip at any age must consider not only immediate results, but also long-term consequences. The dysplastic hip damaged during treatment may become painful many years earlier than if left totally untreated. The risks of this iatrogenic morbidity must be appreciated, particularly since disturbances of the fragile growth processes about the hip are not amenable to direct treatment.

This chapter describes a variety of surgical treatment programs for the dysplastic hip. Surgery rarely should be necessary in the patient born with a dysplastic hip if the early application of appropriate treatment were universal. A main thrust of orthopedic effort in the area of congenital hip disease should continue to involve early diagnosis and the institution of safe, effective treatment in the "golden period" soon after birth.[3,55]

Correlation between degenerative joint disease and even small degrees of persisting hip deformity after congenital dislocation seems ever more clear. Increasingly sophisticated surgical techniques seem capable of altering pathoanatomy sufficiently to achieve a normal prognosis in the malaligned but biologically plastic hip. All too often, though, frankly palliative conditions exist, and qualitatively different surgical techniques, i.e., "salvage programs," must be applied.

An underlying theme in this chapter is the concept that prevention of secondary deformity is preferable to the most elegant hip reconstruction. In the foreseeable future, however, there will continue to be "problem hips" which demand surgical attention. In such situations, to which this chapter is specifically addressed, the orthopedist should always try to heed Heinz Wagner's credo: "Try to match the lifetime of the operation to the lifetime of the patient." [96]

Infancy

At birth CDH represents a spectrum of clinical abnormality that ranges from subluxability to teratologic dislocation with established contracture and irreducibility. Dunn [17] convincingly considers typical congenital hip dysplasia a "congenital deformation," a gradual alteration in initially normal hip anatomy. Abnormal intrauterine mechanical stresses seem to produce hip pathology which initially is that of capsular and ligamentous laxity alone. Time spent in the non–concentrically articulated relationship, however, soon results in secondary progressive maldevelopment of femur and acetabulum.

Diagnosis of every dysplastic hip ideally should take place soon after birth. This can only occur through universal infant screening. Following diagnosis, the early atraumatic achievement and maintenance of concentric reduction, with consequent development of normal anatomy and function, represents the ultimate in treatment.

The role of surgery in the treatment of hip instability in infancy is very small; the role of early diagnosis and nonoperative splinting is large. In the first several months of life, careful use of atraumatic dynamic abduction techniques, such as the Pavlik harness [59,66] or Spreizhosen,[4] should yield an extremely high percentage of excellent results with a minimal risk of ischemic damage to the hip. These dynamic orthoses are useful for maintaining unstable hips in a position of safe stabilization. Such orthoses also encourage gentle stretching by the patient himself to eliminate any secondary contractures, often resulting in the gradual atraumatic reduction of the hip that at the institution of dynamic treatment was irreducible.

Dynamic abduction devices require care in their use if complications are to be avoided.[51,66,90] Radiographic monitoring is necessary to ensure that concentric reduction does occur. One should rule out persisting posterior femoral head displacement with both clinical examination and oblique views (beam directed cephalad), since such malpositioning can be missed easily on the anteroposterior radiograph. One should avoid extreme positioning, since ischemic damage can occur even in these devices. Leg position must be within the "safe zone," [66] as detailed in the section on closed reduction.

If reduction has not occurred in 2 to 3 weeks in a well-applied abduction device, consideration should be given to traction and adductor tenotomy as adjuncts to achieving gentle reduction. In children over 6 months of age at diagnosis, we usually proceed directly to traction and tenotomy unless the hip is particularly supple.

Closed Reduction

Formal closed reduction after congenital hip dislocation has a limited place in the armamentarium of some pediatric orthopedic surgeons and no place at all in the hands of others.[96] It is generally agreed that indications for closed reduction are becoming ever more restricted. Sometime during the second year of life, careful open reduction, usually with some bony realignment above or below the joint, yields a higher percentage of satisfactory long-term results than does closed treatment.[90]

If closed reduction is to be performed at all, it should be done only after any contractures are eliminated. This may involve prior traction, because any increased pressure across the joint after reduction may damage the proximal femoral growth centers.

Our routine for closed reduction employs a period of Bryant's traction, first in minimal abduction and 90° of flexion, with just enough weight applied to the legs so that the child's buttocks are off the bed. Abduction is gradually introduced over a period of days. We employ traction in this attitude because it approximates our usual position of immobilization after reduction (the so-called "human" position),[69] with flexion of more than 90° and rarely more than 100° of combined abduction, in approximately neutral rotation. Some authors prefer prereduction traction in less flexion and employ radiographic control to help decide the timing of reduction.[9,24,97] Each morning, while the child sleeps, gentle passive reduction is attempted by the Ortolani maneuver.[57] If the hip can thereby be felt to reduce, the patient is scheduled for a general anesthetic. We have not found radiography in Bryant's traction useful.

In the operating room, under general anesthesia, a simple positioning of the hip in a flexed and moderately abducted position is carried out. The "safe zone" [66] between maximum abduction and the point of redislocation is determined. Flexion is usually 90° or more, since this relaxes the psoas and probably reduces the pressure across the joint. The desired amount of abduction is in the midposition of the safe zone. Adductor tenotomy routinely is done to enlarge the safe zone, rendering the maintenance of reduction more secure, and most importantly, further reducing the pressure on the reduced femoral head.

Adductor Tenotomy

Adductor tenotomy is useful in eliminating the adduction contracture that is an early secondary deformity in the congenitally dislocated hip, thus expanding the so-called safe zone. Ramsey et al.[66] define the safe zone as "the arc between the angle of abduction that can be comfortably attained and the angle which allows redislocation (Fig. 14–1)." At the time of diagnosis, there may be no safe zone at all, since abduction may be so limited as to prevent reduction, even in the attitude of more than 90° of flexion (human position) that Salter [69] and others emphasize as being essential for safe closed treatment with minimal risk of ischemic damage.

Technique The perineum is walled off with a plastic drape and the groin is prepped and draped. The hip is flexed and gently abducted until the tight adductor tendons are palpable just distal to their pubic origins (Fig. 14–2). A fine tenotome is inserted into the skin just posterior to the tendons, just distal to their origins. The tenotome is advanced slightly underneath the adductor

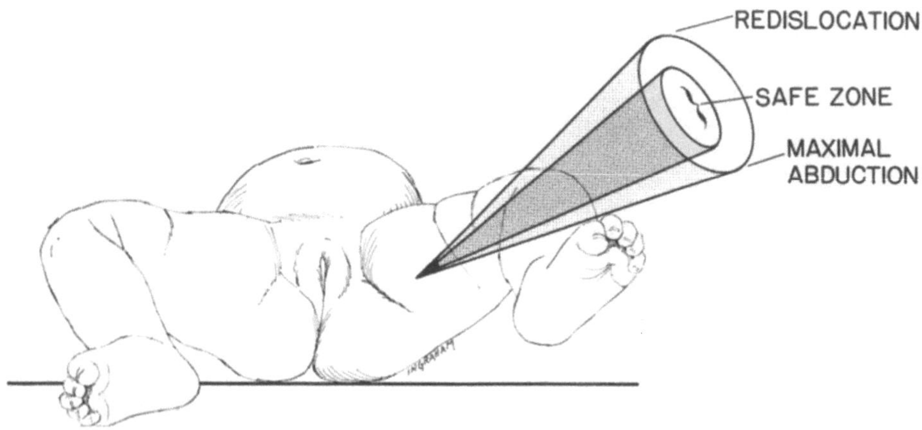

FIG. 14–1 The *safe zone* is the arc between the angle of abduction that can be attained without undue risk of ischemic damage and the angle that allows redislocation. Eilert [17b] has broadened the concept to a "safe cone" which includes the flexion–extension arc of safety and stability. Adductor tenotomy may enlarge the safe zone considerably.

longus tendon. The surgeon's nondominant index finger is placed on the skin over the adductor longus tendon, while the dominant finger lifts the tenotome blade anteriorly against the taut tendon. The tenotome should divide the tendon, which gives way audibly and palpably, but should stop short of the skin. Any remaining palpable bands are divided with similar care. The hip is then extended about 45° and the process repeated. Thirty or more degrees of increased abduction may be apparent immediately. Pressure is held on the small puncture wound briefly and a small dressing is applied. Supplementary treatment is then instituted as indicated. (Open tenotomy may be carried out if preferred, usually through a longitudinal medial incision.)

After adductor tenotomy, the stability of the hip is reassessed. If the hip is quite stable, an abduction orthosis may be used. If not, a spica cast is applied. In any case, the quality of the reduction should be determined radiographically. If there is any persisting question of the quality of the reduction, arthrography [26] or CAT scan [8,61] should be done. If the reduction is imperfect, open reduction is the surest way to eliminate the obstacles to reduction without force.

If a spica cast is to be applied, the initial cast is usually made of plaster rather than fiberglass,

FIG. 14–2 Technique for percutaneous adductor tenotomy involves abducting the reduced hip until the adductor longus tendon is palpable just distal to the groin crease. The area is prepped, and a small tenotome is introduced deep to the tendon, just distal to its pubic origin. The blade is gently lifted toward the tendon, which is stabilized by the surgeon's nondominant index finger lying on the skin. With small excursions of the blade, the palpable bands are divided, first with the hip flexed 90°, and then in about 45° flexion. The skin need not be transgressed except for the original small stab wound. Pressure is held on the wound for about 1 minute and a sterile dressing is applied.

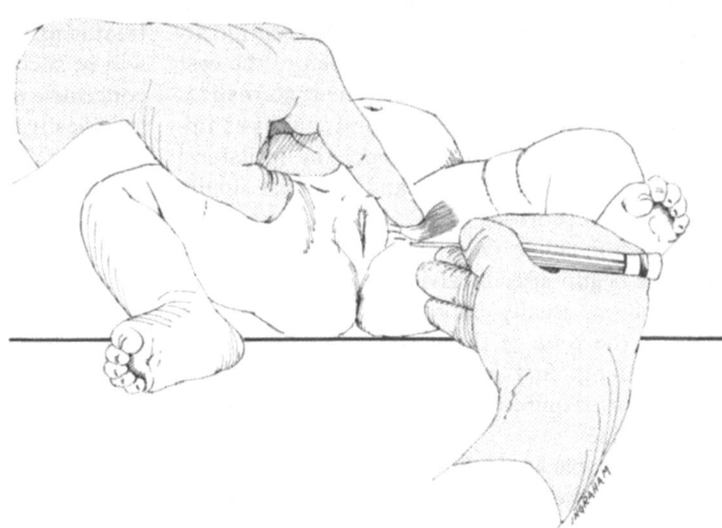

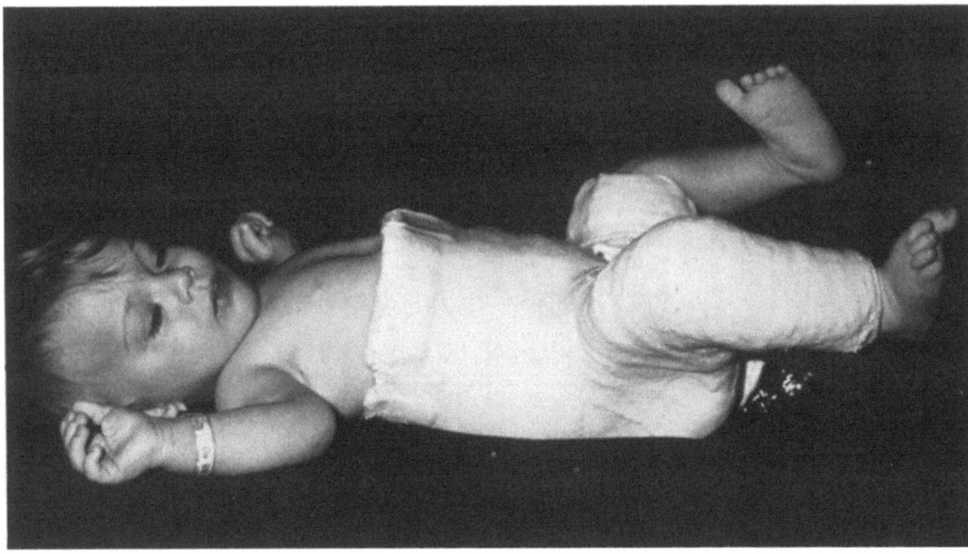

FIG. 14–3 The initial spica cast used to stabilize a closed reduction should extend from about the nipple line proximally to at least the ankle on the unstable side. The cast should maintain the position chosen at the time of closed reduction to maximize both hip stability and safety from ischemic damage. A careful mold over the greater trochanter pushing in a medial and anterior direction usually is helpful in stabilizing the hip, as are molds above the iliac crests and over the pubis anteriorly.

because of plaster's superior moldability. Careful molding over the posterolateral aspect of the greater trochanter is important (Fig. 14–3), as is molding over the pubis and above the iliac crests. A plain radiograph, or if necessary a tomogram of the hip, is made in the cast before the patient is awakened following reduction (Fig. 14–4). Cast change is done at 4- to 6-week intervals, always under general anesthesia, with one radiograph taken after the cast is removed to confirm the maintenance of reduction. The legs are maintained in the human position throughout. No routine attempt is made to test the stability before the cast is replaced. As acetabular development normalizes and the size of the capital femoral epiphysis approaches that of the normal side, the ipsilateral lower leg may be left free and the cast finally changed to a short-leg bivalved fiberglass type or an abduction splint. Gentle range of motion exercises are begun after bivalving. The period of immobilization usually approaches the age of the child at the time of the initial reduction (i.e., a dislocated hip first reduced at age 4 months is expected to require about 4 months of treatment to normalize).

The drawback of closed reduction treatment programs is the considerable risk of ischemic necrosis in the proximal femur, ranging from 8 to 50% in those series with careful long-term follow-up and critical assessment of even subtle signs of vascular insult.[9,83,84,90,92,99] The more frequent recent use of open reduction in ever younger children reflects the effort of orthopedists to reduce this risk of ischemic damage.

Open Reduction

The older the child when a dislocated hip is discovered, the less likely it is that simple positioning treatment, which is the basis of safe closed therapy, will be successful in achieving the goal of a stable concentric reduction without vascular insult. More specifically, the child who presents with a dislocated hip after walking age is very likely to demonstrate one or more of the indications for open reduction.[14] These include (1) stable but nonconcentric reduction; (2) any reduction requiring extreme positioning or any force for either stability or concentricity; (3) gross instability; and (4) frank irreducibility.

Skillful open reduction is far less dangerous to the fragile young hip than closed reduction requiring any force. Surgical reduction should allow exposure and direct treatment of those lesions interfering with gentle concentric reduction, such as capsular constrictions, iliopsoas contracture, in-

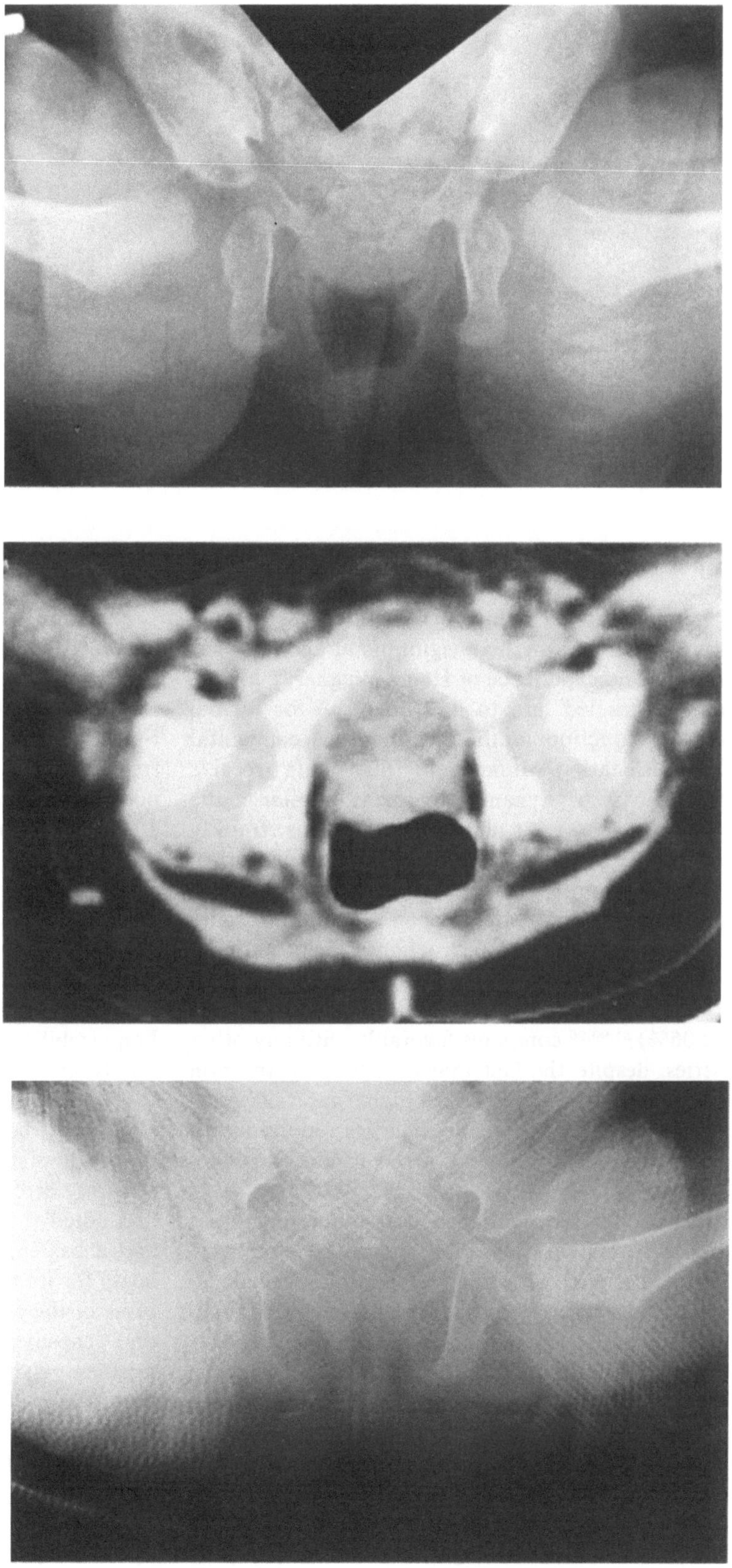

A

B

C

FIG. 14–4 CAT scan is useful in evaluating the questionable reduction. **A** Position of hips following closed reduction of bilateral dislocation in a 4-month-old child was difficult to assess by plain radiography. **B** CAT scan demonstrates satisfactory reductions bilaterally. **C** Plain radiograph in plaster of 14-month-old child is difficult to assess following attempted closed reduction.

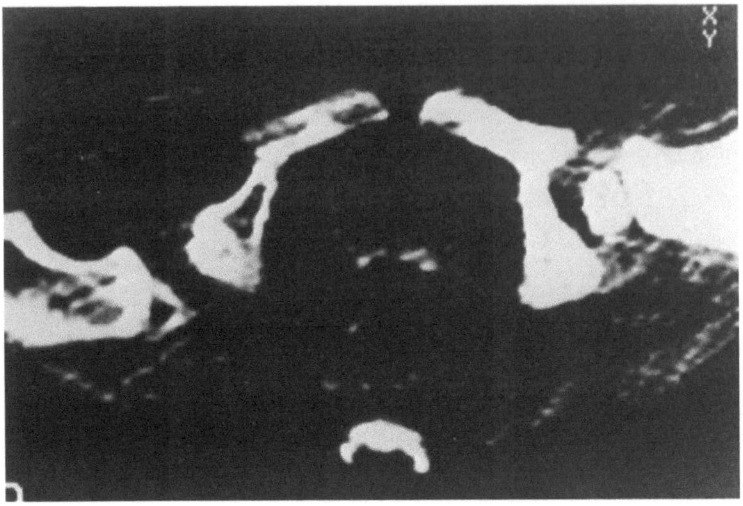

FIG. 14-4 (*cont.*) **D** CAT scan clearly demonstrates persisting posterior dislocation.

folded labrum, or taut transverse acetabular ligament.

Some centers employ open reduction as the primary treatment method beginning at about 1 year of age. The experience of Heinz Wagner,[96] for example, has led him to find no place for formal closed reduction in the treatment of congenital hip dislocation. Infants in his clinic receive Spreizhosen [4,90] dynamic treatment (similar to the Pavlik harness). At about 1 year of age, frankly dislocated hips or unstable hips not showing progressive improvement, whether under previous treatment or not, undergo open reduction, usually followed by femoral intertrochanteric derotational varization osteotomy. His reported rate of ischemic damage for previously untreated hips (2.06%) [81,90,96] compares favorably with any other series, despite the fact that preoperative traction is not used by Wagner. Much higher rates of proximal femoral growth disturbance are reported with every long-term follow-up series of closed reduction.

It should be mentioned that in certain cases no reduction of dislocation should be attempted at all. Patients with bilateral teratologic dislocations, as in arthrogryposis, are unlikely to be functionally improved by reduction. Similarly, high bilateral dislocations in patients over age 6 are so likely to lead to a poor result on at least one side, despite femoral shortening, that we suggest withholding primary treatment. Even in adulthood, such untreated patients rarely have pain, before middle age, although they complain of their limp. Arthroplasty in middle age is difficult but probably preferable to bilateral attempts at late open reduction in childhood.

In summary, an untreated congenital hip dislocation warrants reduction treatment at almost any age before puberty. There is a wider indication for treatment of the unilateral case for two reasons. First, the postural imbalance associated with untreated CDH is considerable. Second, a fair or poor result of treatment for CDH is better tolerated opposite a normal contralateral hip.[37]

Medial Approach The medial approach [20-22,46,47,67,71,75,98] to open reduction of CDH has a restricted indication. It has severe anatomical limitations and is useful only in eliminating obstacles to reduction, not in achieving either capsular or bony stabilization. The child must be young, preferably under 1 year of age, or up to 2 years if the acetabular index is under 40°.[67,71] The hip should not be highly displaced, should have had no previous surgery, and preferably not even prior splinting or casting.[22]

Ludloff [46] first reported this approach in 1908, and it has enjoyed subsequent intermittent popularity for its relative ease in dealing with contractures of the adductor and psoas tendons, the medial capsule, and the transverse acetabular ligament. All proponents of this approach agree that postoperative immobilization must be used for superior capsular laxity to be eliminated.

The medial approach is contraindicated if capsulorrhaphy, acetabuloplasty, or femoral osteotomy is needed. The medial approach is also contraindicated in any high-riding, stiff, or teratologic dislocation, in which peeling adherent capsule off the lateral aspect of the ilium is necessary.

Coleman,[14] among others, also excludes any previously operated hip joint (Ferguson reports 30% avascular necrosis after medial approach open reduction in his own series of previously treated patients [22]) and any patient over 2 years of age from consideration for the medial approach. An anterior approach offers better visualization of the joint, is more versatile, and should be chosen whenever there is doubt of which approach to use.

Several authors have noted the considerable incidence of ischemic damage associated with the medial approach.[71,75,98] Although preliminary traction may, as suggested by Staheli,[75] reduce this incidence, long-term corroborating results are lacking still in the English literature. Ferguson's series of 125 cases (all without prior treatment) is often cited for its reported lack of incidence of avascular necrosis, without the use of preliminary traction, but only 25% of his patients were reported as being over 5 years old at the latest follow-up.[22]

An important anatomical consideration seems to be carrying the plane of dissection posterior to the adductor brevis in approaching the capsule (so-called posteromedial approach),[20-22] thus avoiding branches of the medial femoral circumflex artery. Series employing this posteromedial approach report a lower incidence of ischemic damage than those series using anteromedial approaches, anterior to the adductor brevis (Fig. 14–5).[71]

TECHNIQUE With the legs abducted, a medial thigh incision is made distal to the inguinal fold and deepened between the adductor longus and gracilis tendons, which may be released if desired. (Ferguson approaches the psoas tendon behind the adductor brevis, whereas others dissect anterior to both longus and brevis.[22]) Blunt dissection is carried out to the lesser trochanter behind the adductor brevis, between the brevis and the adductor longus.

The psoas tendon insertion is divided and the tendon peeled off the medial capsule in a proximal direction. The medial capsule is opened longitudinally down to and including the transverse acetabular ligament. The pulvinar and hypertrophied ligamentum teres may be excised if necessary.

The femoral head should then reduce easily, protruding slightly through the medial capsular incision. The capsule is left open, and the hip position of greatest stability is then determined. The reduction is confirmed by x-ray. A carefully molded spica cast is then applied. Any position between the "functional position" of 30° abduction and 30° flexion and the human position is permissible. Following surgery, about 3 or 4 months of casting is recommended, with abduction bracing thereafter as indicated.

Anterior Approach The routine utility approach for open reduction of congenital hip dislocation is anterior,[68,71,72] with the deep dissection following the method of Smith-Petersen [72] (Fig. 14–6). The versatility of the anterior approach is unmatched by any other, with its good access to the acetabulum, the entire capsule, and intracapsular structures.

The role of preoperative traction before carrying out open reduction is controversial. Contracture must somehow be eliminated either preoperatively or intraoperatively, and most authors recommend the routine use of preoperative traction in patients over the age of 18 months.[68] From 18 months to about 3 years of age, skin traction in an attitude of slight flexion and abduction is usually effective in bringing the femoral head down to the level of the true acetabulum. It is usually helpful to elevate the foot of the bed and use the child's body weight for countertraction. Skeletal traction through a distal femoral pin may occasionally be useful. An arbitrary period of 2 weeks of preoperative traction is suggested by some.

Some authors prefer supplemental femoral varization osteotomy, with or without additional femoral shortening, to preoperative traction.[2,14,37,96]

TECHNIQUE The patient may be positioned supine or in a semilateral attitude (Fig. 14–6). Preliminary adductor tenotomy is carried out if needed. The skin incision can be varied. Our standard incision is after the method of Salter,[68] running obliquely from just distal to the iliac crest posteriorly to pass anteriorly over the level of the anterior inferior iliac spine, and on medially to about the midinguinal point. This incision heals in a more predictably cosmetic manner than the usual Smith-Petersen skin incision. If femoral osteotomy is to be performed simultaneously with open reduction, we prefer an extended Watson-Jones–type skin incision, which runs from posterior and proximal to the anterior superior iliac spine to the greater trochanter, and then distally along the

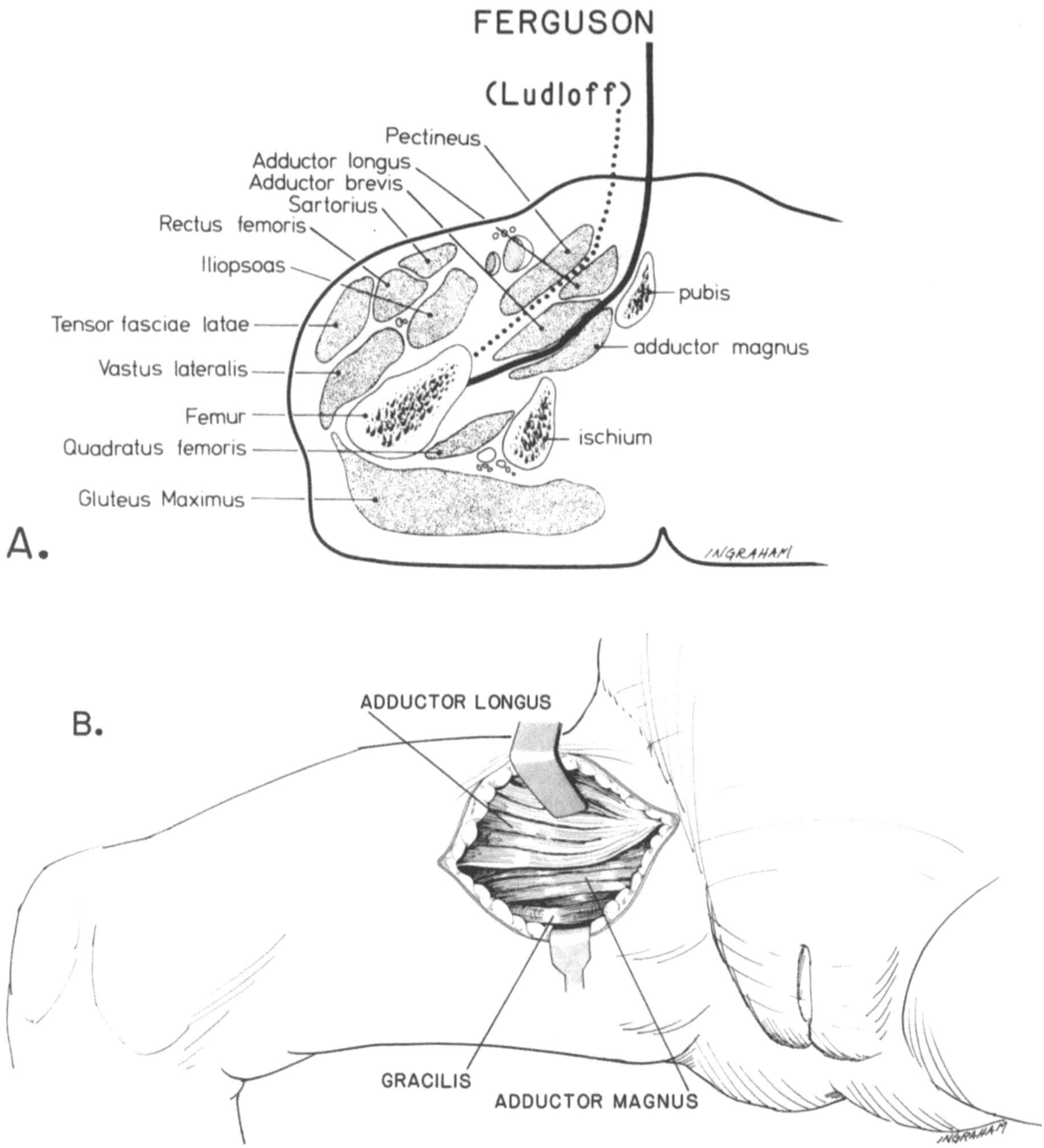

FIG. 14–5 Medial approach for open reduction. **A** The preferred posteromedial approach (Ferguson) is carried out by dissecting between adductor longus and gracilis and then behind adductor brevis to expose the iliopsoas tendon and hip capsule. **B** The dissection is deepened by retracting adductor longus, adductor brevis, and pectineus forward.

lateral aspect of the proximal thigh (two separate incisions are an alternative).

The interval between the sartorius and tensor fasciae latac muscles is located and entered, preferably just within the medial fascial envelope of the tensor.[96] This minimizes the risk to the lateral femoral cutaneous nerve which enters the interval just medial to the anterior superior iliac spine. Ascending branches of the lateral femoral circumflex artery traverse the interval distally. This distal extent

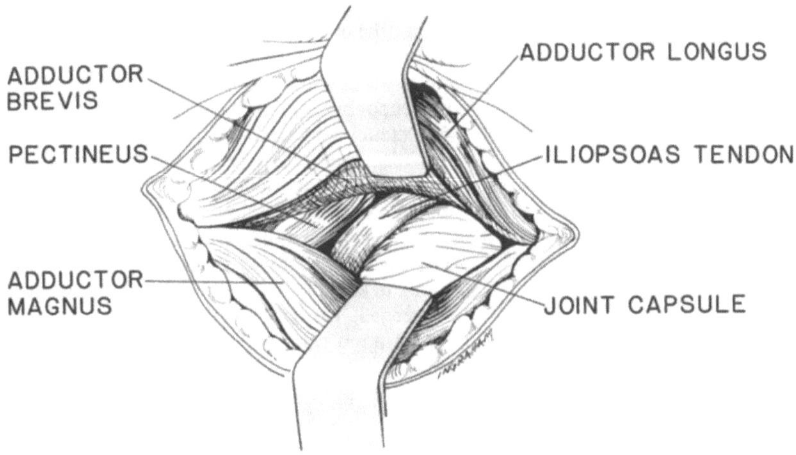

C.

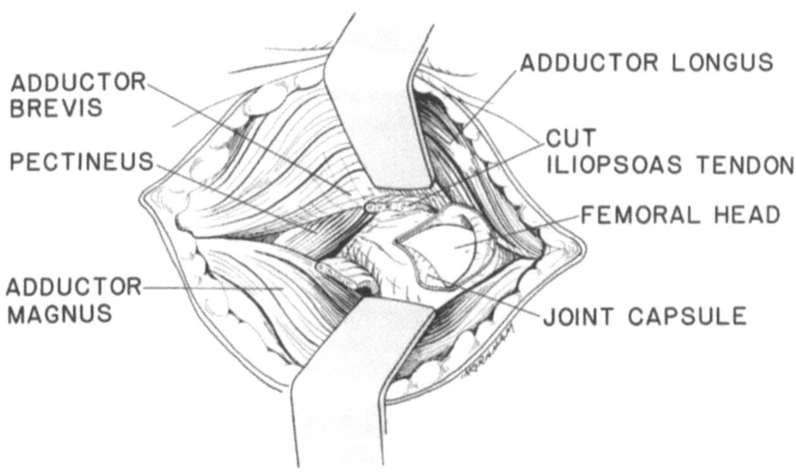

D.

FIG. 14–5 (*cont.*) **C** Adductor magnus is retracted posteriorly to expose the iliopsoas tendon lying on the medial hip capsule. **D** The iliopsoas tendon is divided and peeled proximally (adductors may also be divided if necessary). A longitudinal capsulotomy is performed under direct vision, allowing reduction. The bulging capsulotomy is left open. Wound closure and casting follow.

of the exposure is crucial for adequate visualization later in the procedure. The anterior dissection is deepened by incising the periosteum precisely along the bony prow between the anterior superior and anterior inferior iliac spines. The tensor and abductor muscle mass is then reflected subperiosteally off the lateral ilium. We prefer splitting the apophysis carefully with a scalpel to assist in this reflection of the abductors, and we find a small Cobb elevator or raspatory helpful in the subperiosteal dissection, which extends posteriorly enough to visualize the dorsal capsule. (Alternatively the apophysis may be left intact and the subperiosteal reflection of the abductors is begun just distal to the crest.)

The reflected head of the rectus femoris is divided at the anterosuperior edge of the capsule. The origin of the direct head of the rectus is divided, and its tendon tagged and peeled distally off the capsule. The psoas tendon is dissected off the medial capsule, and if lengthening is necessary, division of the tendinous portion alone may be done at the level of the pelvic brim. Fibers of the capsular iliacus must be reflected medially, and fibers of the capsular minimus are reflected posteriorly to expose the capsule. The capsule must

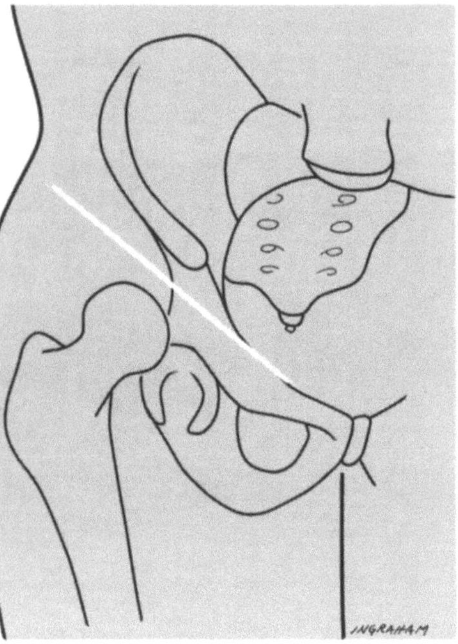

A.

FIG. 14–6 Anterior approach for open reduction. **A** Preferred oblique skin incision (Salter) minimizes scarring. **B** Interval between the tensor and sartorius is entered from within the medial fascia of tensor. Lateral femoral cutaneous nerve is carried medially. Dissection is carried distally as far as the ascending branch of the medial circumflex artery. Iliac apophysis is split with the scalpel. **C** Anterior iliac periosteum is incised along prow between superior and inferior iliac spines. Lateral and anteromedial aspects of ilium are exposed subperiosteally. **D** Heads of rectus are reflected distally. Capsular minimus and iliacus are peeled off capsule. Tendinous portion of psoas is divided at pelvic brim. A wide T-shaped capsulotomy is made. **E** Ligamentum teres is followed to base of true acetabulum. True acetabulum is cleared as needed. Head is gently reduced by flexion, abduction, and internal rotation. Reduction is confirmed radiographically.

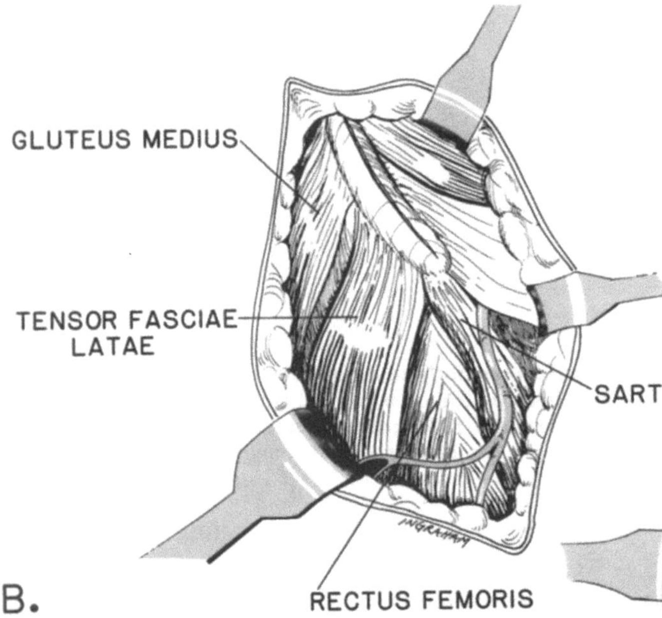

B.

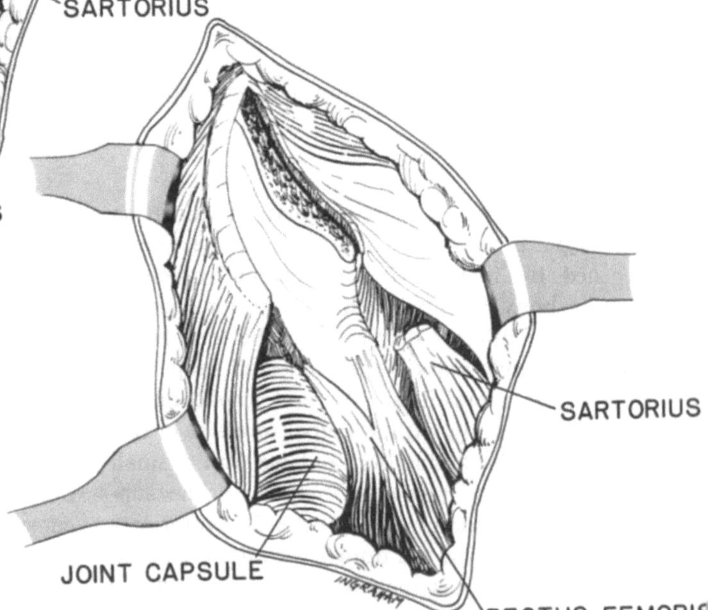

C.

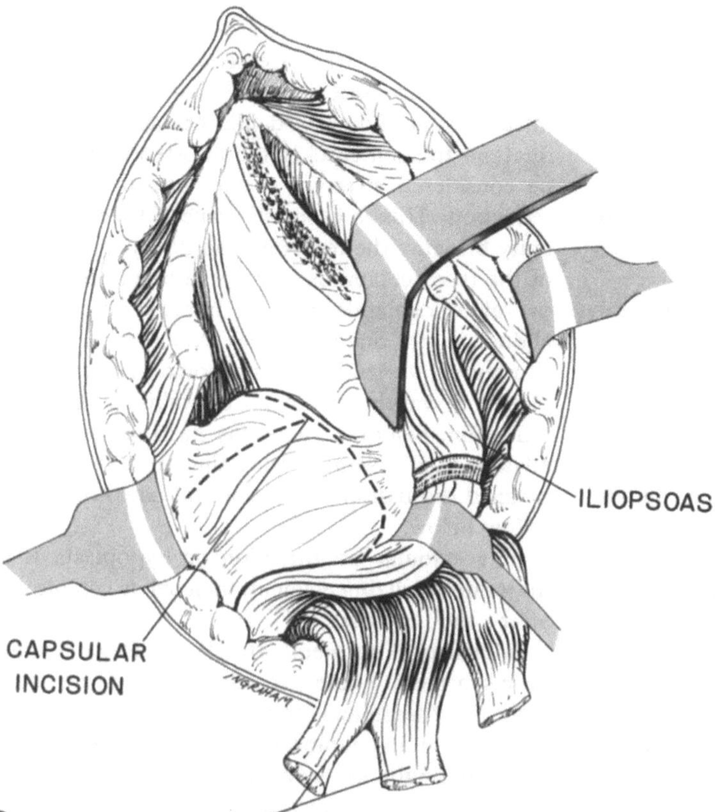

D.

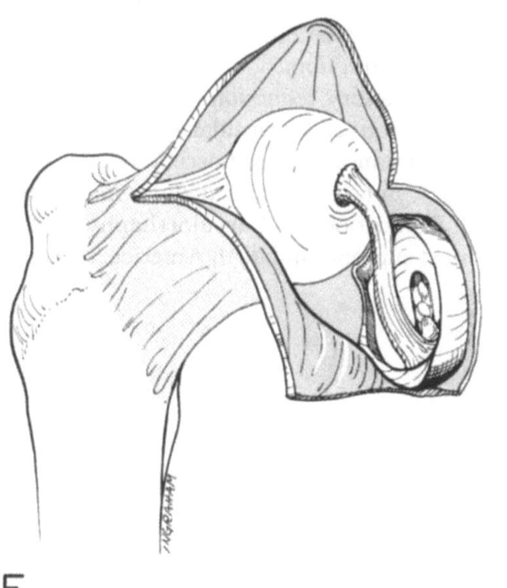

E.

be exposed enough anteriorly and posteriorly to define its extent clearly. The superior capsule is then dissected off the ilium in a distal direction as necessary until the prominence of the true acetabular rim and labrum are located. Small Hohmann retractors are helpful in this exposure and for the ensuing capsulotomy. Care must be taken not to disturb the critical medial circumflex vessels outside the inferomedial capsule, just medial and posterior to the psoas tendon at the base of the capsule.

A wide capsulotomy is essential for adequate visualization of the depths of the acetabulum. If capsulorrhaphy is to be done later, then the placement of the capsulotomy is crucial. A T-shaped capsular incision is recommended,[68] with the transverse limb paralleling the rim of the true acetabulum and lying a few millimeters away. The longitudinal rim of the T splits the superior capsule and is directed toward the tip of the greater trochanter, stopping short of the vessels in the trochanteric sulcus.

As the capsulotomy is begun, slight traction

on the leg will prevent cutting into the articular cartilage of the dislocated femoral head. After the capsulotomy is completed, external rotation and adduction displaces the head laterally and helps to expose the acetabulum. The ligamentum teres should be followed to its origin at the transverse acetabular ligament. This confirms the location of the true acetabulum, a *crucial* step in the procedure.

In order to allow the femoral head to seat deeply into the true acetabulum, the following steps are often necessary: The ligamentum teres can be resected if hypertrophic, the transverse ligament divided, and the pulvinar fat removed with a pituitary rongeur. If an inverted limbus prevents deep reduction, the limbus should be lifted up and turned out over the reduced femoral head, rather than being resected. Making one or two radial cuts into the limbus may facilitate its eversion with a nerve hook. Subsequent suturing of the capsular flap to the limbus will help maintain the limbus in a stabilizing everted position.

At this point in the procedure, the quality of the reduction should be confirmed radiographically. With the leg held in a position of moderate flexion, abduction, and internal rotation, the ossific nucleus of the reduced femoral head should lie below the level of the triradiate cartilage and medial to Perkins' line (Fig. 14–7). If the ossific nucleus has not yet appeared, Tachdjian [85] suggests carefully interposing fine mesh tantulum gauze between the acetabulum and reduced femoral head to aid in radiographically visualizing the reduction. Alternatively, the radiopaque string from a marked gauze sponge may temporarily be laid between the semilunar cartilage of the acetabulum and the femoral head.

In an older child, a teratologic dislocation, or any previously treated case, reduction may be difficult to achieve and maintain despite clearing all intraarticular and periarticular obstacles to the reduction. In such cases, femoral osteotomy should be considered strongly at the time of the open reduction. This is especially true if there is difficulty bringing the femoral head down to the level of the true acetabulum, or if extreme anteversion or valgus demands extreme internal rotation or abduction to maintain the reduction. Femoral shortening, varization, and derotation can be employed in varying amounts to stabilize the open reduction. Femoral osteotomy has the theoretical advantage of decompressing the femoral head. A detailed discussion of the femoral osteotomy will follow below.

If acetabular maldirection or hypoplasia is a major destabilizing element, then pelvic osteotomy after the method of Salter [68] or the acetabuloplasty [37] of Pemberton [60] or Dega [16] may be performed. These procedures above the joint have the theoretical drawback of increasing the pressure on the femoral head and therefore are used sparingly by some surgeons. Chiari osteotomy [12,13] rarely may be indicated along with open reduction; [37] however, its basic nature as a salvage procedure makes a lifetime of normal postoperative hip function unlikely. We have only once found Chiari osteotomy necessary in association with open reduction.

Once a satisfactory reduction is achieved, consideration next is given to capsular reconstruction. Some surgeons consider capsulorrhaphy not only not necessary but contraindicated in idiopathic congenital dislocations.[96] Capsulorrhaphy is favored by most surgeons in North America, though,

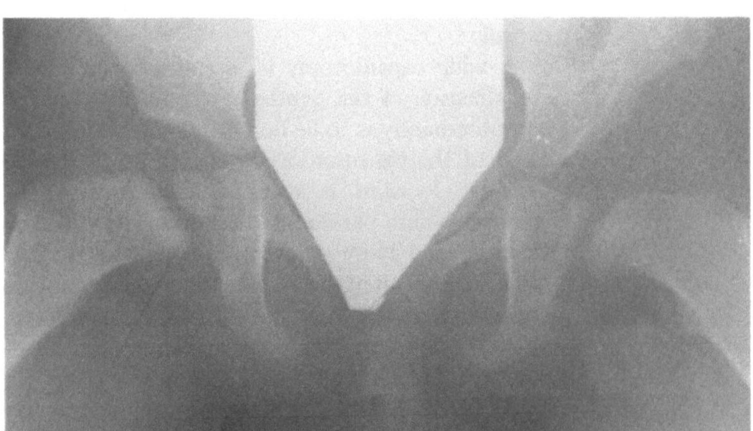

FIG. 14–7 Radiographic confirmation of a deep concentric reduction should show the ossific nucleus of the femoral head to lie below the level of the triradiate cartilage and medial to Perkins' line.

with considerable attention usually given to its details.

Capsulorrhaphy The previously mentioned T-shaped capsulorrhaphy lends itself to stable reconstruction (Fig. 14–8). The hip is held in a reduced position from the time capsulorrhaphy is begun until after the postoperative spica cast is completed. It is best that one assistant give undivided attention to the task of maintaining the hip gently reduced by holding the leg in the position of stability. The desired position of stability is no more extreme than 30° each of abduction, flexion, and internal rotation. If more extreme positioning is necessary, we employ stabilizing osteotomy routinely, although sometimes it is performed at a second sitting.

We prefer the method of Salter in performing capsulorrhaphy. The corner of the anterolateral flap is pulled anteriorly and medially to be sutured to the most anterior edge of the capsulotomy with nonabsorbable material. The second suture is then placed through the superolateral capsule at the base of the limb of the T-shaped capsulotomy closest to the greater trochanter. This suture is pulled medially and anteriorly, and is tied down to the anteromedial capsular edge. At this point, most of the posterolateral flap of the capsule is redundant and may be removed. Further nonabsorbable sutures are employed to close any remaining gaps in the capsulotomy, and further reinforcing sutures are inserted as felt necessary. In this manner, maintenance of reduction is facilitated by giving the hip a slight internal rotation contracture, and the redundant superior capsule fold is eliminated.

An alternative capsulorrhaphy is described by Tachdjian.[85] He recommends the same capsulotomy but suggests suturing the corner of the superolateral flap to the anterior labrum after it is advanced forward. The anteromedial capsular flap is then pulled superolaterally over the first flap as a reinforcement, and is sutured through the superior capsule to the labrum. Last, the everted medial rim of the capsule next to the acetabulum is sutured over the two other flaps (Fig. 14–8).

The postoperative spica should be carefully molded over the greater trochanter and iliac crests to prevent excessive hip motion. Most authors suggest a minimum of 4 to 6 weeks of spica immobilization, with almost all favoring an additional 6 to 8 weeks of gradual mobilization either in broomstick plasters, bivalved spica, or abduction brace.

Osteotomy carried out in association with open reduction may modify the nature and extent of postoperative immobilization. Weight bearing is allowed as range of motion, strength, and control return.

Osteotomies in Association with Open Reduction

There is considerable controversy over how often, how much, and how quickly the secondary deformities of the proximal femur and acetabulum will resolve spontaneously following reduction.[30,31,45,48] Most authors accept that the usual patient older than 15 to 18 months who requires open reduction has enough bony deformity to require realignment above or below the joint. Nonetheless, each patient must be assessed critically regarding position of greatest stability after concentricity has been achieved at open reduction, *before* capsulorrhaphy is performed. Patients relatively free from secondary deformity will demonstrate hip stability in the so-called "functional position" of 30° each of flexion, abduction, and internal rotation. Such patients may be spared immediate supplemental osteotomy and followed expectantly as long as progressive radiographic normalization of the acetabular angle, acetabular contour, and femoral head is occurring.

Any patient whose hip requires extreme positioning for stability at the time of open reduction should be treated with supplemental osteotomy. Such bony realignment not only assists in short-term stabilization, but also reduces the risks of ischemic necrosis associated with extreme positioning. In addition, normalization of the side of the joint not osteotomized is usually promoted.

Some surgeons, notably Salter,[69] favor acetabular realignment. Others, including Lloyd-Roberts,[45] Somerville,[75] and Wagner,[94,96] employ femoral osteotomy more or less routinely following open reduction. Klisic [37] has popularized the use of one-stage open reduction, femoral varization-derotation shortening osteotomy, and pelvic osteotomy to treat late-diagnosed congenital hip dislocations at age 8 or more.

The best approach in deciding where to carry out supplemental osteotomy after open reduction is to correct the most deformed side of the joint, whether acetabular or femoral. If soft tissue tension is great, however, this argues for including femoral shortening as a component of the program.

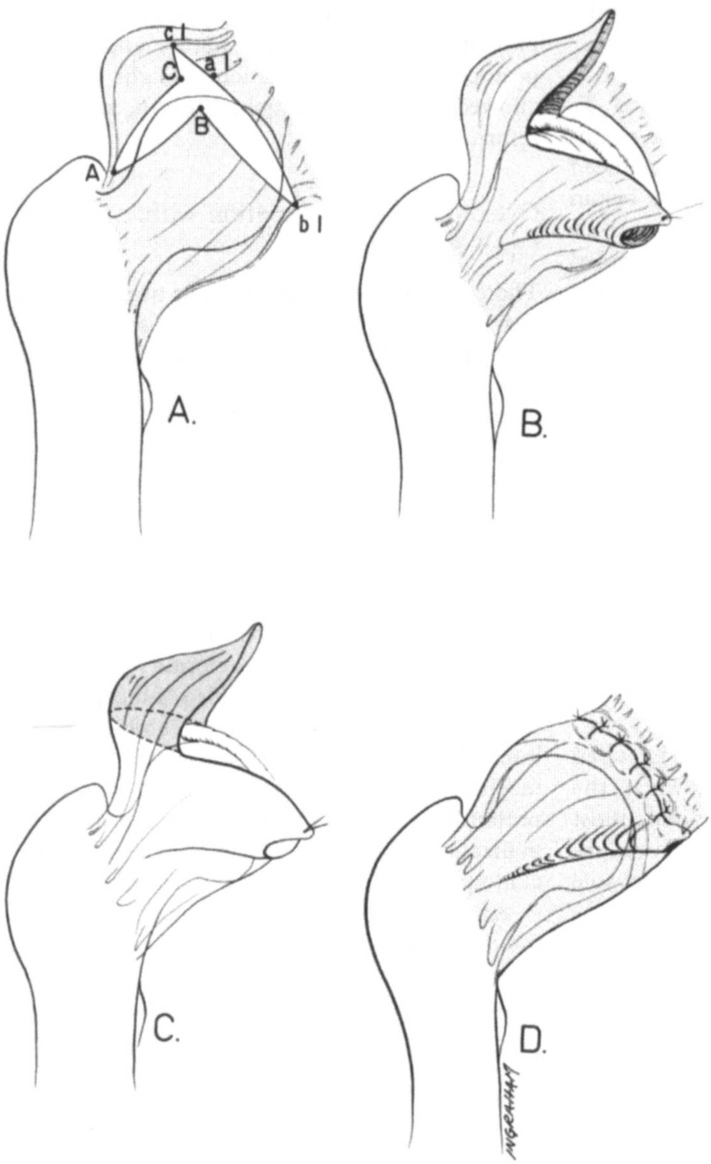

FIG. 14–8 Capsulorrhaphy after open reduction via anterior approach (Salter). **A** The transverse limb of the T-shaped capsulotomy parallels the true acetabular rim, lying a few millimeters from it. This portion of the capsulotomy extends far anteromedially. The longitudinal limb of the T bisects the transverse limb and is directed toward the greater trochanter, stopping short of the vessels at its base. Ultimately, point *A* will be secured to point *a*, and point *B* will be secured to point *b*. Point *C* will lie in the redundant superior flap. **B** Point *B*, at the free corner of the anteromedial flap, is pulled anteromedially to be sutured to point *b*, at the extreme anteromedial corner of the capsulotomy. **C** The redundant superior flap is trimmed. Point *A*, at the base of the T, is pulled medially and sutured to the thin medial capsular rim just above the labrum. **D** Further sutures are placed to stabilize the capsular repair.

It is rarely necessary to realign both sides of the joint to stabilize an open reduction in a previously untreated child under 3 or 4 years of age. Our usual primary procedure in the previously untreated dislocation between age 18 and 30 months is single-stage open reduction with psoas tenotomy and innominate osteotomy,[69] although others [14] have noted occasional stiffness following this procedure. Open reduction with either simultaneous or delayed femoral varization-derotation osteotomy is done if femoral deformity predominates or the dislocation is high. In our experience, patients who have had open reduction performed alone after more than 15 months of age usually require subsequent bony stabilizing procedures. Consequently, open reduction rarely is performed in our institution in the patient older than 15 months without supplemental osteotomy.

The most important concept to emphasize in connection with osteotomy performed in association with open reduction is the *absolute requirement* that the reduction be perfect before any bony procedure is done. If deep concentric seating of the femoral head cannot be demonstrated by simple appropriate positioning of the leg, then the open reduction must be revised prior to any osteotomy.

Femoral Osteotomy in Association with Open Reduction In some centers, femoral osteotomy is indicated almost routinely following open reduction. Wagner [96] usually carries out a varization intertrochanteric osteotomy, with derotation as indicated, 2 or 3 weeks after open reduction. Others employ femoral osteotomy simultaneously with reduction if shortening is felt necessary or if extreme internal rotation is needed to maintain reduction. General indications for femoral osteotomy include pathological femoral anteversion (greater than 30°), coxa valga (neck–shaft angle greater than 130°), and residual soft tissue contracture that favors shortening of the femur. Femoral osteotomy should reduce the neck–shaft angle to about 115° and anteversion to about 15°.

If femoral osteotomy is done simultaneously with open reduction, we prefer a single curved anterolateral and lateral skin incision (Watson-Jones type for the skin only), and for the deep tissues both an anterior approach proximally and a lateral approach to the proximal femur through the distal portion of the incision (Fig. 14–9). Whether done with open reduction or separately, the femoral exposure, osteotomy, and osteosynthesis are the same.

A meticulous atraumatic reflection of the vastus lateralis in an anterior and distal direction is essential. After the fascia lata is incised, the vastus origin is divided from anterior to posterior, down to bone. The trochanteric apophysis is avoided. The vastus fascia then is opened longitudinally anterior to the lateral intermuscular septum, and the vastus fibers are carefully peeled off the septum. The fibers insert on the septum in a proximal and posterior direction, making dissection of these fibers in a proximal direction more efficient. As the muscle fibers are reflected, the perforating vessels are visualized and electrocoagulated. The periosteum is then incised longitudinally just anterior to the intermuscular septum. As the subperiosteal flap is reflected anteriorly and distally, the placement of a small Hohmann retractor under the anterior periosteum assists in the exposure while the dissection is continued distally. At the intertrochanteric level, the subperiosteal exposure posteriorly is facilitated by Wagner's technique [96] of tapping on a small periosteal elevator with a mallet, to lightly decorticate the femur. This greatly reduces bleeding.

If femoral shortening is to be done, one may estimate preoperatively the length of the segment to be removed by measuring radiographically the distance between the level of the dislocated femoral head and its desired level after reduction.

We prefer the method of Wagner in executing both the intertrochanteric osteotomy and its osteosynthesis (Figs. 14–9 and 14–10).[94] With the patient supine, the leg is positioned in abduction sufficient to seat the head well and in enough internal rotation to eliminate the anteversion. Under image intensifier control, a positioning Kirschner wire is drilled through the lateral femoral cortex just distal to the trochanteric apophysis, directed perpendicular to the long axis of the table and parallel to the floor. The wire should be within the femoral neck, with its tip just distal to the medial end of the physis. (Returning this wire to its attitude perpendicular to the axis of the table and parallel to the floor will at any subsequent point in the procedure reproduce the desired reduction of the femoral head.) Hohmann retractors are positioned under the posterior and anterior periosteum at the intertrochanteric level. The osteotomy is then executed with a slowly oscillating saw, directed parallel to the positioning wire to end medially just proximal to the lesser trochanter at the base of the femoral neck. A small periosteal elevator is inserted into and around the osteotomy to gently mobilize the fragments from the periosteum. The distal fragment is then adducted and externally rotated to open the osteotomy cleft. Manipulation of the proximal fragment and its positioning pin is minimized to avoid fracture or pin dislodgement. The proximal-medial corner of the distal fragment proximal to the lesser trochanter may be trimmed to facilitate bony coaptation. If femoral shortening is to be done, the measured amount of bone is removed from within the periosteal envelope of the distal fragment with the oscillating saw. The distal fragment is then displaced about 50% medially on the proximal fragment, as the proximal fragment is maintained in correct position. The distal fragment is aligned in a neutral attitude. An Altdorf hip clamp of appropriate size is selected. The prongs of the bifurcated plate may be trimmed if too long, and the angle changed by bending, as necessary.

The hip clamp is mounted on its holder and the prongs are firmly seated at an appropriate angle

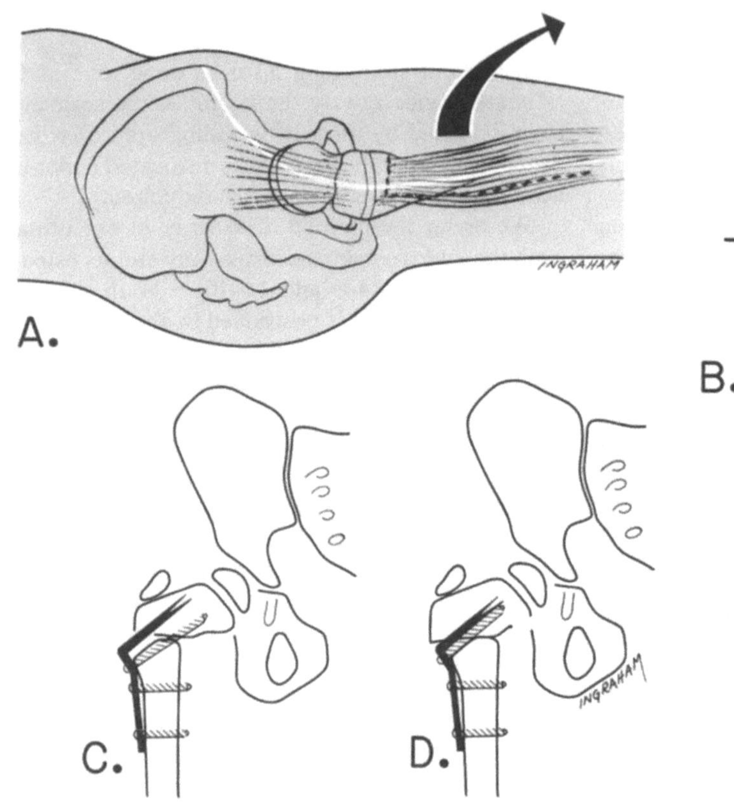

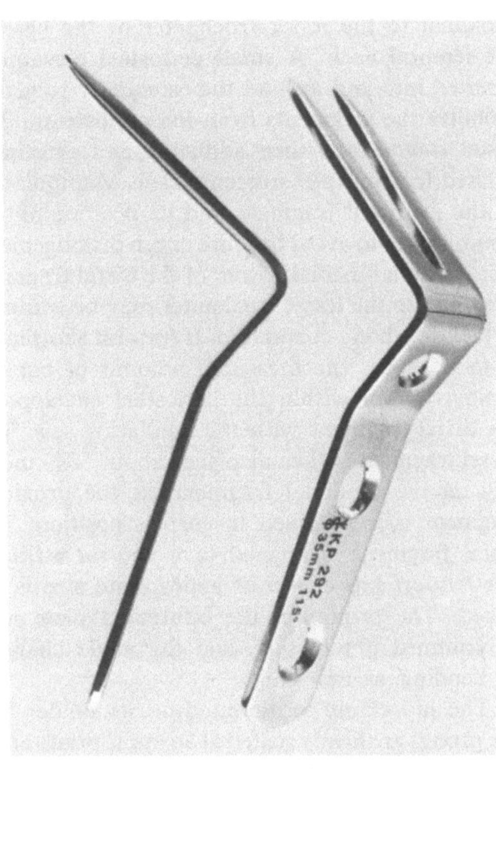

FIG. 14–9 Proximal femoral osteotomy in association with open reduction. **A** Approach to both hip joint and proximal femur is made through a curved incision from the area of the anterior superior iliac spine passing over the greater trochanter and extending distally. The alternative approach is through two incisions: oblique Salter incision proximally and straight incision laterally. Deep approach to the femur is through atraumatic reflection of vastus lateralis in an anterior and distal direction. **B** Proximal femur is brought into desired relationship with acetabulum. Kirschner wire is inserted into neck, parallel to floor and perpendicular to long axis of patient. Osteotomy is made distal and parallel to guide wire, to end medially at base of neck just proximal to lesser trochanter. **C** Position of proximal fragment is maintained by reference to guide wire. Distal fragment is trimmed as needed for coaptation or shortening. Distal fragment is brought to neutral and medially translocated. Prongs of Altdorf hip clamp are impacted into osteotomy surface on proximal fragment, followed by insertion of proximal lag screw. Rotational correction is confirmed before distal screws secure distal fragment to plate. **D** Tightening of proximal lag screw increases interfragmentary compression, increases medial translocation of distal fragment, and slightly increases varus of proximal fragment. **E** Altdorf hip clamp (Aesculap). Adapted with permission from Wagner, H.: Acetabular Dysplasias, Skeletal Dysplasias in Childhood. Heidelberg, Springer-Verlag, 1978, p. 91.

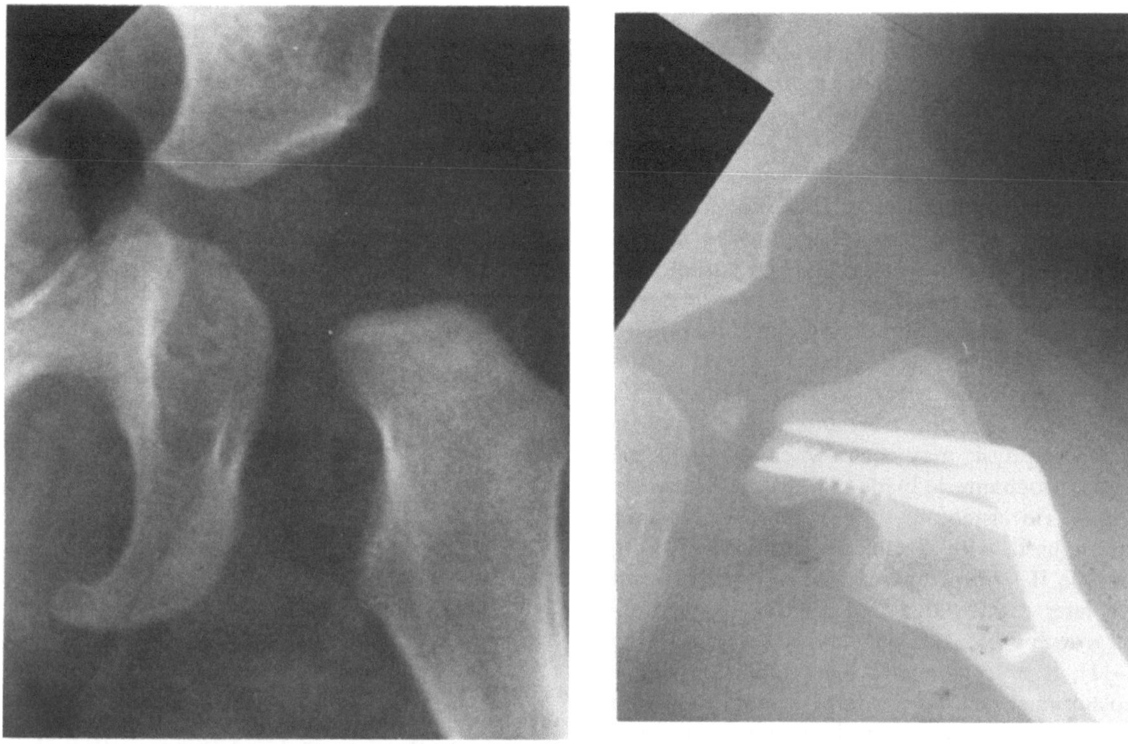

A B

FIG. 14–10 The Altdorf hip clamp provides stable fixation of derotation–varization intertrochanteric osteotomy in the young child. **A** Dysplastic proximal femur is shown prior to osteotomy. **B** Normalized proximal femur is shown following intertrochanteric osteotomy with implant in place.

within the femoral neck by driving them through the osteotomy surface of the proximal fragment. The plate should be oriented so as to lie along the femoral shaft in its corrected position. The prongs should be seated medially enough in the proximal fragment to maintain the desired medial displacement. Next, a small fragment screw is inserted in the proximal hole of the plate, directed to a point between the prongs, to supplement fixation of the proximal fragment.

The distal fragment is then abducted very slightly, so its proximal end is slightly overdisplaced medially, and there is a 1-mm gap at the osteotomy site medially. The distal end of the plate should still lie against the femoral shaft. The distal hole in the plate is then drilled, tapped, and screwed. As the remaining next screw is tightened, interfragmentary compression is achieved, and the desired varization is restored. Light impaction of the blade, plus retightening of all screws, should then be carried out.

The vastus origin is then reconstructed by a running Dexon suture to the abductor insertion on the trochanter. This provides a dynamic tension band effect that further promotes healing of the osteotomy. Suction drains are placed, the superficial layers closed, and the skin approximated with a running subcutaneous suture. A one-and-one-half long-leg spica is applied in the functional position of slight abduction and flexion.

Within 6 weeks, the osteotomy should be strong enough for functional exercises to begin. Soft tissue considerations related to the open reduction may dictate the rapidity of weaning from plaster. The plate may be removed after 4 to 6 months.

This particular osteosynthesis is elegant in several respects. It allows precise control of varization and derotation, as well as allowing for the medial displacement, without harming the fragile and important apophysis of the greater trochanter. The medial displacement of the femoral shaft is important, as in any varus osteotomy, to optimize conditions for rapid bony healing at the osteotomy by converting interfragmentary forces to compression type and virtually eliminating bending stress by the extra medial support. It is equally important to locate the osteotomy at the intertrochanteric level, for several reasons. The bony surfaces here are broad, encouraging coaptation, and the blood supply to the bone is excellent. In addition, locating the osteotomy above the greater trochanter allows anterior transposition of the psoas insertion as the femur is derotated. This encourages the psoas to act more physiologically, as an internal rotator of the hip, instead of having a pathological external rotatory component (as it does in severe anteversion). In the very young child, the greater trochanteric growth plate forms the lateral portion of the single chondroepiphysis for the proximal femur. Damage to this trochanteric portion of the chondroepiphysis may occur when the children's size AO trochanteric blade plate is used for intertrochanteric osteotomy, or when percutaneous pins are used, with serious consequences. An Ogden type II [11] form of ischemic injury can result with later caput valga and relative trochanteric overgrowth with proximal femoral deformity (Fig. 14–11). If a trochanteric blade plate or similar implant must be used, for some reason, in fixation of varus osteotomy in a patient under the age of 5, the trochanteric apophysis can be spared only by making the osteotomy at the undesirable subtrochanteric level. The Altdorf hip clamp or similar device provides a better solution until age 4 or 5. Thereafter the trochanteric apophysis is high enough so that a small trochanteric blade plate may be used safely.

Pelvic Osteotomy with Open Reduction If at the time of open reduction, proximal femoral deformity seems mild compared to the acetabular dysplasia, and if the soft tissues are supple, then supplemental bony stabilization of the reduction probably should be done at the acetabular level. More exact guidelines are difficult to define.

Besides noting that the acetabulum is shallow, with a deficient anterolateral lip (in most cases of congenital hip dislocation that come to open reduction), as one considers surgery about the acetabulum, one should also attempt to distinguish between abnormality of acetabular contour and of acetabular direction.

If acetabular maldirection,[69] or excessive anteversion,[45] seems to be the principal lesion, then acetabular redirection is indicated, of which the innominate osteotomy of Salter is the prototype. If, on the other hand, deformity of acetabular contour is more striking, and the acetabular cavity is capacious, then an acetabuloplasty that deepens the reduction by lowering the anterolateral acetabular roof, and reduces the acetabular volume, may be chosen. Procedures described by Dega,[16] Pemberton,[60] and Hughes [33] are the prototypes (Fig. 14–12).

A modification that includes elements of both acetabular redirection and changing acetabular contour, the so-called Pem-Sal procedure, has been described by Marafioti and Westin.[48] This may be useful in intermediate cases.

Innominate Osteotomy Since Salter performed his first innominate osteotomy in 1957,[69] the concept of acetabular maldirection in the attitude of persisting excessive anterior and lateral version as one of the basic secondary deformities in CDH has become well known.

A complete iliac osteotomy from sciatic notch to anterior inferior iliac spine allows the distal fragment plus the acetabulum to be rotated anterolaterally about an axis along a line between the posterior edge of the osteotomy and the pubic symphysis as the osteotomy is kept closed posteriorly. A triangular bone graft is taken from about the anterior superior iliac spine and interposed in the open osteotomy cleft anteriorly to maintain the acetabular redirection.

Salter [68] has clearly enumerated the prerequisites for the success of his procedure. He notes that (1) the femoral head must come easily to the level of the true acetabulum; (2) any contractures of the iliopsoas and adductor muscles must be released before the osteotomy; (3) the reduction must be complete and "reasonably congruous"; and (4) the range of motion must be good. He considers the procedure indicated in the treatment of frank dislocation between the ages of 18 months and 6 years. He considers performing a bilateral innominate osteotomy during a single operative session to be contraindicated due to mechanical inefficiency in displacing the second side.

TECHNIQUE The anterior approach through the sartorius–tensor fascia lata interval is standard, using the oblique incision previously described (Fig. 14–13). If open reduction and innominate osteotomy are being carried out simultaneously, it is best to perform the innominate osteotomy after the joint has been opened and deep reduction made possible, but before capsulorrhaphy. It is useful to know at this point in what position the hip will dislocate with the capsule open.

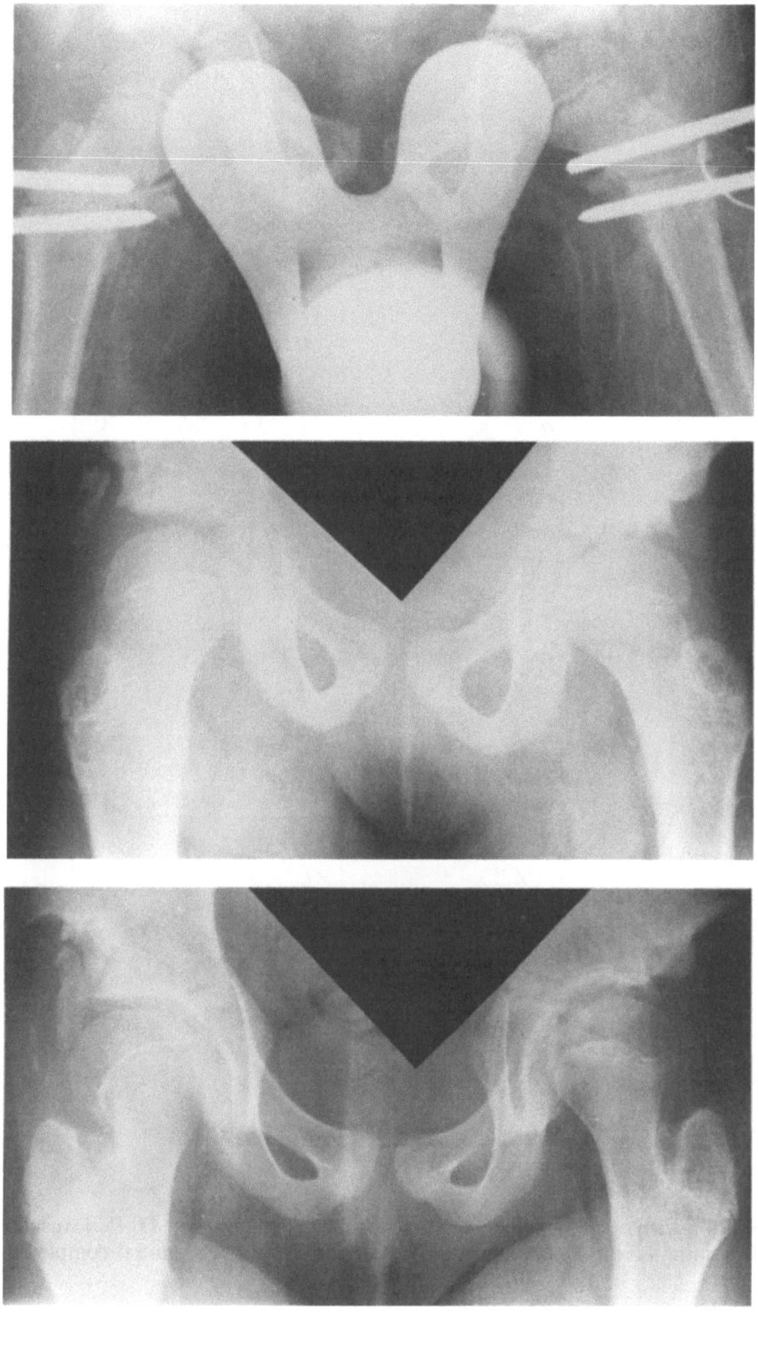

A

B

C

FIG. 14–11 Improper implants may cause ischemic damage to the young child's hip, the commonest injury leading to the Ogden type II lateral growth arrest. **A** Bilateral derotational intertrochanteric osteotomy was done, with fixation by percutaneously inserted Steinmann pins, which transgressed the trochanteric growth plate. **B** Early valgization of the head is apparent 18 months later. **C** Four years after osteotomy, severe bilateral deformity is present, with femoral neck valgus and trochanteric hypoplasia on the left side, and the same deformities plus eversion of the articular surface on the right side. These deformities are preventable. Courtesy of Dr. J. E. Hall.

The medial periosteum and iliacus are dissected off the medial aspect of the ilium along with the straight head of the rectus femoris. The sciatic notch is exposed and packed with gauze sponges both medially and laterally. It is important to remember the anatomical fact that the sciatic notch is located posterior to the hip capsule and only very slightly proximal to it. The osteotomy line between the sciatic notch and the anterior inferior iliac spine should run just proximal to the true acetabulum.

At this point, the mandatory tenotomy of the tendinous portion of the iliopsoas should be carried out, preferably at the level of the pelvic brim, so

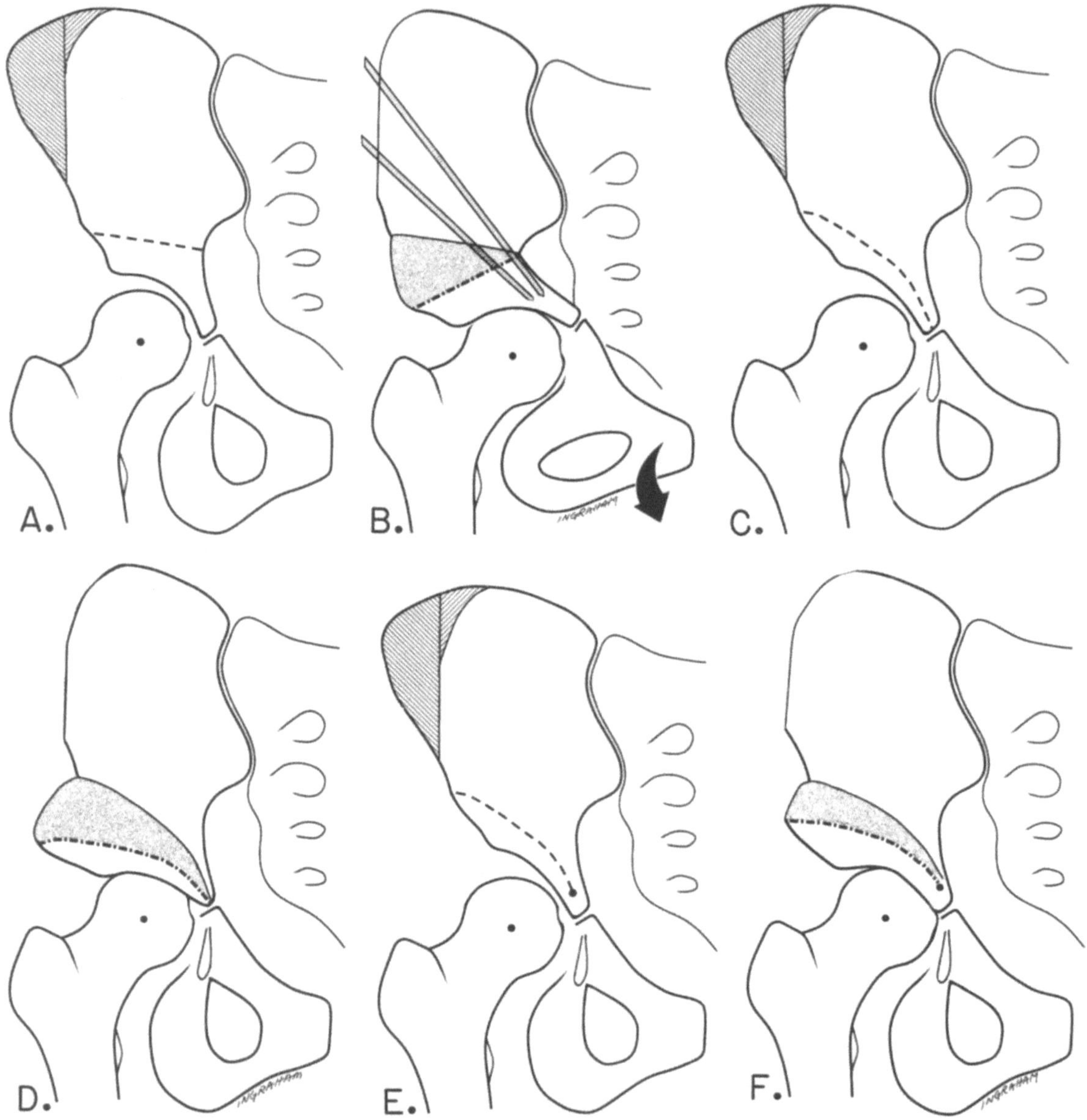

FIG. 14–12 Pelvic osteotomies in association with open reduction. **A** Innominate (Salter). **B** Innominate completed. **C** Pericapsular (Pemberton). **D** Pericapsular completed. **E** Pem-Sal (Westin). **F** Pem-Sal completed.

that the muscular portion remains in continuity with the distal tendon. The iliopsoas is located most easily at this level by incising the medial iliac periosteum longitudinally, with the musculotendinous unit thereupon bulging through the incision of the periosteum. Blunt dissection is then carried out anterior and medial to the psoas, to allow its retraction in a lateral direction while the neurovascular bundle is gently protected medially. As the hip is flexed and externally rotated, the iliopsoas is lifted up and rotated over a scissors or Kelly clamp before the tendinous portion is divided. As the hip is extended and internally rotated, the intact muscular portion should slide on the divided tendon, providing the desired lengthening for joint decompression. It should be noted that the tendinous portion usually lies posteromedially within the musculotendinous unit.

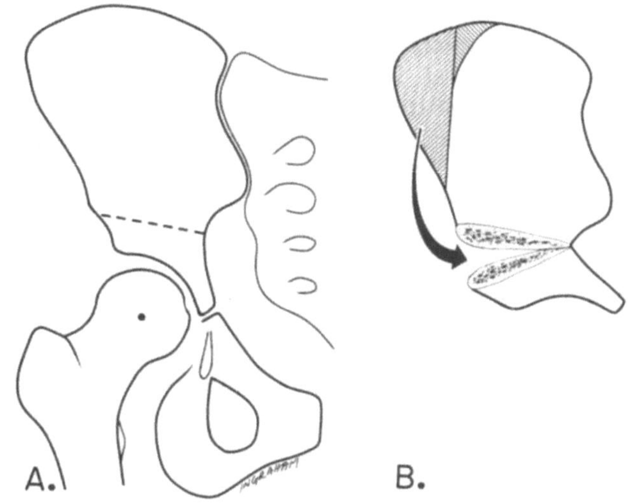

FIG. 14–13 Technique of innominate osteotomy. **A** The osteotomy with Gigli saw exits anteriorly precisely at anterior inferior iliac spine. **B** Interposition graft is cut from anterosuperior ilium and iliac corner is trimmed. **C** The acetabulum is redirected by anterolateral rotation about an axis of rotation between the sciatic notch and symphysis. The towel clamp gripping the distal fragment is rotated anterolaterally, ensuring that the osteotomy remains apposed posteriorly and there is no posterior displacement of the distal fragment. **D** Two threaded Kirschner wires are drilled to pass posterior to the acetabulum to transfix both osteotomy fragments and the interposed graft. The distal hemipelvis and acetabulum thus are secured in an anterolaterally redirected attitude.

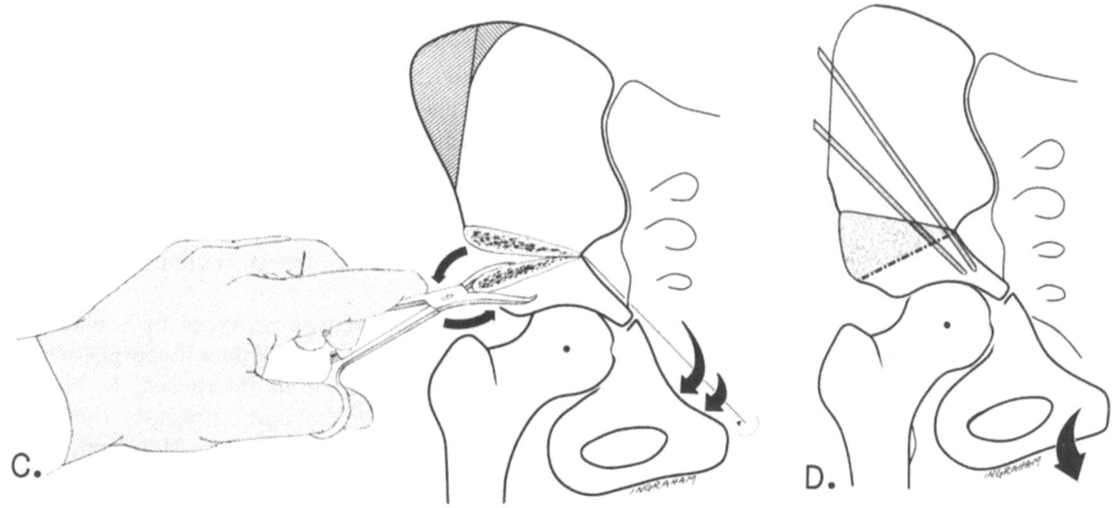

Lane bone levers or Hohmann retractors are inserted into the sciatic notch from each side. A right-angled forceps then is passed through the notch superficial to the retractors. One looped end of a Gigli saw is passed over one jaw of the forceps, which is closed and then rotated 90° to further stabilize its grasp on the saw as it is withdrawn through the notch. The saw is advanced on one side as it is withdrawn on the other side. Soft tissues are carefully retracted as the osteotomy is made from the sciatic notch to the anterior inferior iliac spine. One must guard against the tendency for the osteotomy to exit anteriorly above the anterior inferior iliac spine. With a bone cutter, the iliac bone graft for interposition is then cut, beginning at a point two-thirds down the anterior iliac prow from the anterior superior iliac spine to the anterior inferior iliac spine, and directed posterosuperiorly. The triangular graft is appropriately shaped to fit into the osteotomy anteriorly. The sharp corner left on the superior ilium is then rounded off with a rongeur. To displace the osteotomy, a large towel clamp grips the distal osteotomy fragment, pulls it slightly forward, and rotates it anterolaterally. This rotation must maintain the fragments approximated posteriorly and separated anteriorly. The distal fragment should not be allowed to slide posteromedially, because this reduces acetabular redirection. The graft is then inserted and held with a clamp into the triangular osteotomy cleft. The distal iliac fragment and the interposed graft are held stabilized while two threaded Kirschner wires are drilled through both osteotomy fragments and the posterior half of the graft with a power drill. The two wires should pass just posterior to the hip joint. A third wire may be inserted anteriorly if necessary, although there are only a few millimeters of ilium above the acetabulum anteriorly in the distal fragment. With the joint open, the acetabulum should be inspected to rule out joint penetration. The stability of the fixation is checked, as well as the position of the fragments and graft. No posterior or medial translation of the distal fragment is permissible, nor is any posterior gap in the osteotomy, since each of these situations reduces the potential acetabular redirection achieved.

The hip should then be reduced gently by traction, abduction, and internal rotation, and the point at which it dislocates should be noted. Only slight flexion, abduction, and internal rotation should be necessary to maintain reduction. If the reduction remains quite unstable, both intraarticular and extraarticular causes of instability should be sought, including residual tightness of the adductors, iliopsoas, and hamstrings. Hamstring tightness may be dealt with by simple knee flexion, but any residual psoas or adductor tightness must be eliminated before closure. Capsulorrhaphy is carried out as desired. The apophysis and muscle layers are reapproximated and sutured over small suction drains. The Kirschner wires are clipped long enough so their ends protrude several millimeters above the iliac apophysis into the superficial fat. Subcuticular skin closure is employed and a spica is applied in a functional position of slight abduction, flexion, and internal rotation. Before closure the adequacy of the reduction should have been confirmed radiographically.

Six weeks of spica immobilization allows the osteotomy to heal enough so that the pins may be removed under a brief anesthetic. An additional several weeks of less restrictive immobilization in either a short-leg spica or broomstick abduction plasters usually is desirable to allow satisfactory soft tissue stability to be achieved, and yet not risk permanent stiffness.

The threaded pins should be removed as soon as the osteotomy is healed to minimize the risk of premature closure of the triradiate physis.

Pericapsular Acetabuloplasty If a major destabilizing element after reduction is the pathologically large capacity of the acetabulum with a steep anterolateral roof, an acetabuloplasty may be indicated.[33] Acetabuloplasty reduces the acetabular volume and changes its contour by lowering the anterolateral acetabular roof. A certain incongruence between femoral head and acetabulum is indeed an indication here, i.e., the presence of a larger radius of curvature for the acetabulum than for the femoral head. The main indication is a deep reduction, but with instability in the weight-bearing position, just as is the case with acetabular redirection.

Acetabuloplasty presupposes a certain plasticity of the acetabular roof, allowing this incomplete iliac osteotomy just above and behind the roof to be opened anterolaterally and a bone graft inserted without fracture of the roof. An open triradiate cartilage is a prerequisite, whether or not this type of osteotomy actually enters the triradiate cartilage itself. Even by late childhood, the hip joint may not tolerate the abrupt change in contour effected by acetabuloplasty, even though the apparent change is in the direction of increased congruence between the head and acetabulum. Acetabuloplasty is, therefore, best limited to the patient under 6 years of age. The occasional older child with a capacious acetabulum may also benefit from the procedure, although results are less reliable.

There are at least three types of acetabuloplasty,[16,33,60] each being a distinct incomplete iliac osteotomy with bone graft interposed. In North America, probably the best known is that described originally by Pemberton,[60] which is a curved osteotomy from the anterior inferior iliac spine into the region of the triradiate cartilage.

TECHNIQUE OF PEMBERTON OSTEOTOMY An anterior approach is employed identical to that used for innominate osteotomy. With a narrow, curved osteotome, a curvilinear cut is made through the lateral iliac cortex beginning anteriorly just proximal to the anterior inferior iliac spine to end at the ilioischial rim of the triradiate cartilage at its mid point (Fig. 14–14). Retractors should be inserted into the sciatic notch medially and laterally to ensure that the curved osteotomies remain well anterior to the sciatic notch in their posterior extent.

Using the same osteotome, a corresponding cut is made in the medial cortex of the ilium, roughly parallel to the lateral cut. If more lateral coverage than anterior coverage is desired, the medial cut

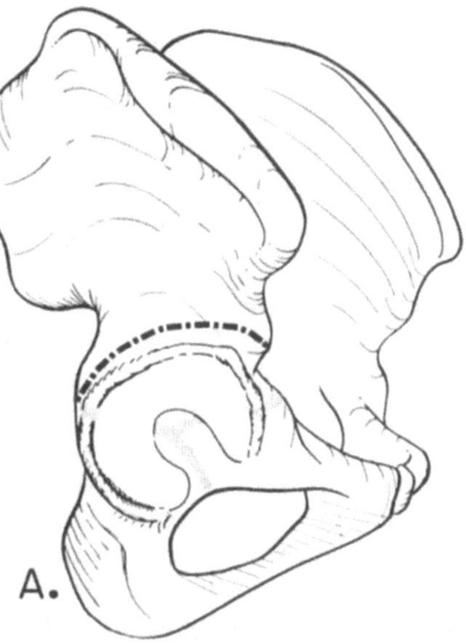

FIG. 14–14 Technique of Pemberton pericapsular osteotomy. **A** The lateral portion of the Pemberton osteotomy extends along the lateral iliac cortex from the anterior inferior iliac spine posteriorly to the ilioischial limb of the triradiate cartilage. The medial inclination of the osteotomy and the degree of penetration of the osteotomy through the medial iliac cortex depend on whether more lateral correction or more anterior correction of acetabular obliquity is desired. **B** The osteotomy cut is performed carefully with a curved osteotome. The curved osteotome then is used to slowly and gently bend the acetabular roof down into the desired corrected position. Full-thickness iliac bone graft is then taken from the area of the anterior superior iliac spine and is appropriately shaped before being interposed in the iliac osteotomy. The incomplete osteotomy usually retains the bone graft in a stable position, although smooth Kirschner wires may be used to fix the bone graft in position if desired.

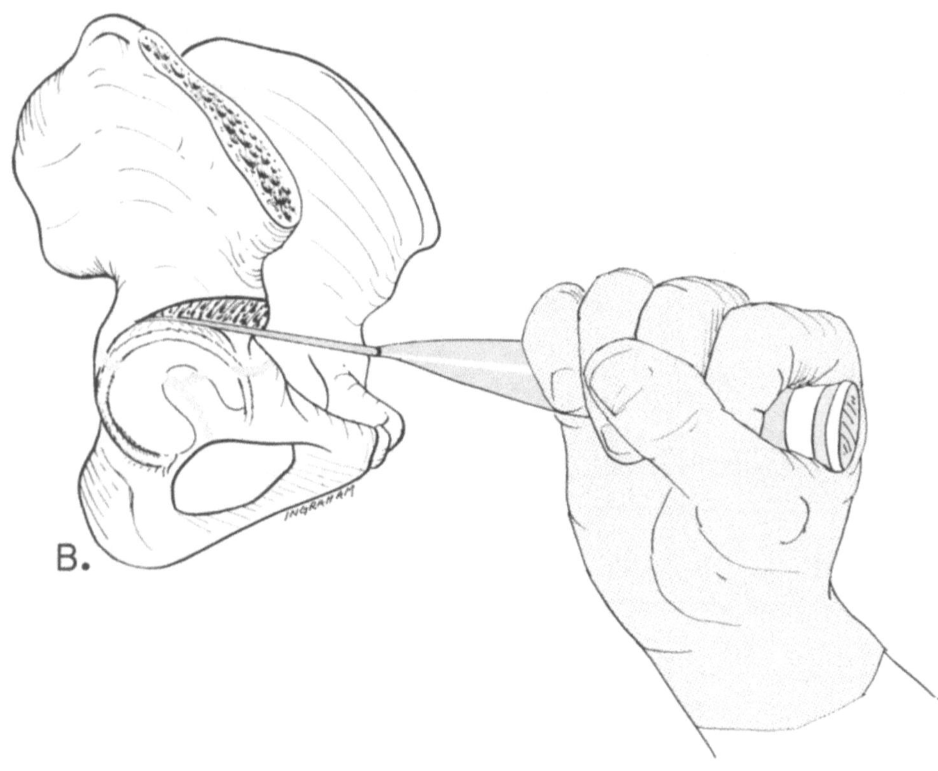

should be positioned slightly lower than the lateral cut. If more anterior coverage is desired, the medial and lateral cuts should be positioned at the same level.

After the osteotomy of the two cortices is complete, a wide, curved osteotome should be gently inserted deep into the osteotomy and the distal fragment should be levered gently in a distal direction until the desired change of acetabular contour has been achieved. Patience and gentleness are to be emphasized during this step, to avoid either fracture of the relatively thin distal fragment or extending the osteotomy into the triradiate cartilage and damaging it. Radiographic confirmation of the correction should be carried out at this point. Next, bone graft should be taken from the superior ilium and inserted into the osteotomy. Internal fixation with pins may be used if desired. A spica is usually used for 2 months following surgery.

OTHER ACETABULOPLASTIES Other relatively similar acetabuloplasties are described by Dega[16] and Hughes.[33] Westin and Marafioti have described the so-called Pem-Sal acetabuloplasty (Fig. 14–15).[48] This procedure involves a curved incomplete osteotomy from just above the anterior inferior iliac spine to the posterior iliac fossa anterior to the sciatic notch. The curve of the osteotomy is not so sharp posteriorly, nor is the triradiate cartilage approached so closely as in the Pemberton type of acetabuloplasty. The osteotomy does stop short of the notch, unlike the Salter procedure, and it is more curvilinear in contour than the Salter procedure. Some acetabular redirection and some change in acetabular contour can be achieved if the posterior cortex remains intact as the osteotomy is gently levered open anteriorly. An interposing bone graft from the superior ilium maintains the correction. Tenotomy of the tendinous portion of the iliopsoas is indicated, because of the lengthening effect on the hemipelvis. Internal fixation may not be necessary. Postoperative plaster immobilization is suggested.

Mid-childhood

Between the ages of 1.5 and 3 years the prognosis after treatment of late-diagnosed congenital hip dislocation changes markedly. The amount of incongruence that usually has developed by age 3 or 4 may exceed the remodeling capability of the joint, even if no iatrogenic growth disturbance occurs. In addition, it must be remembered that an untreated complete dislocation may remain free of hip symptoms until late middle age or beyond. This situation creates a difficult decision for the orthopedist. By carrying out even the most skillful

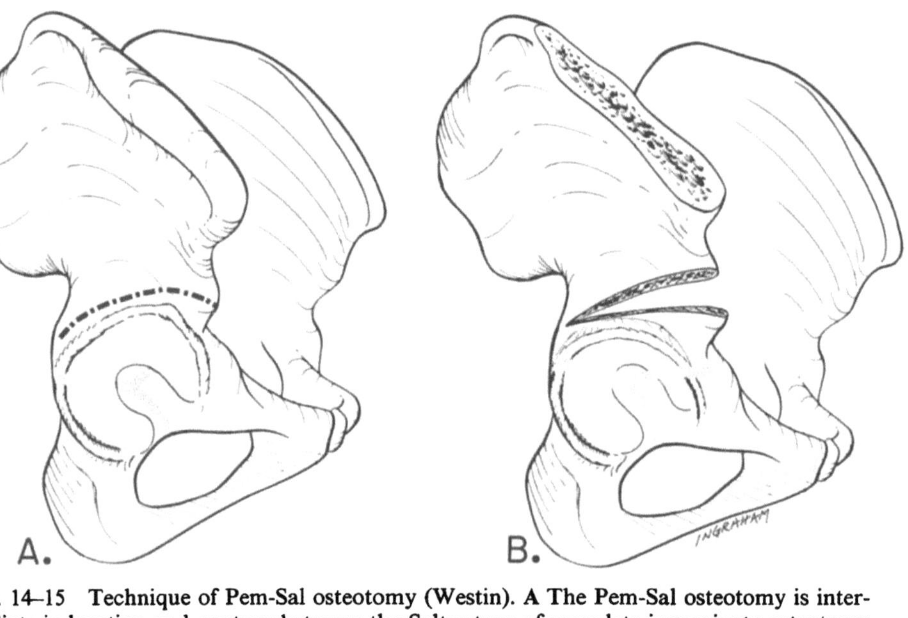

FIG. 14–15 Technique of Pem-Sal osteotomy (Westin). **A** The Pem-Sal osteotomy is intermediate in location and contour between the Salter type of complete innominate osteotomy and the Pemberton osteotomy. The cut extends from the anterior inferior iliac spine to the posterior iliac cortex, anterior to the sciatic notch but superior to the triradiate cartilage. **B** The gently curved osteotomy is performed most easily with a slightly curved osteotome. The osteotomy may be opened gently and slowly with either the osteotome or a bone spreader. Correction involves both some tilting downward of the iliac sector of the acetabulum as well as some additional redirection of the entire acetabulum. Bone graft is interposed as with Pemberton's procedure.

open reduction supplemented by appropriate soft tissue release and bony stabilization, the orthopedist may, even if no short-term complication occurs, create a hip with normal short-term function but a limited prognosis. The price of such normalization of hip function for late childhood and adolescence may be osteoarthritis with an earlier onset in adulthood than if no treatment had been instituted.

Klisic [37] reported a huge experience of 115 cases of open reduction in children between 7 and 15 years of age, with an even larger experience in younger children well above walking age (Figs. 14–16 and 14–17)

He distinguishes between high complete dislocations unsupported by false acetabula and dislocations supported by false acetabula, noting as mentioned above that untreated high complete dislocations have a relatively good prognosis, with limp being the major complaint. Klisic suggests withholding treatment from bilateral supported dislocations above age 10 and bilateral unsupported dislocations above age 8. However, his longest reported follow-up is only 12.5 years, and longer follow-up may change his indications.

Klisic [37] notes importantly that "the patient is extremely handicapped when both hips are poor or even fair in result." There is of course considera-

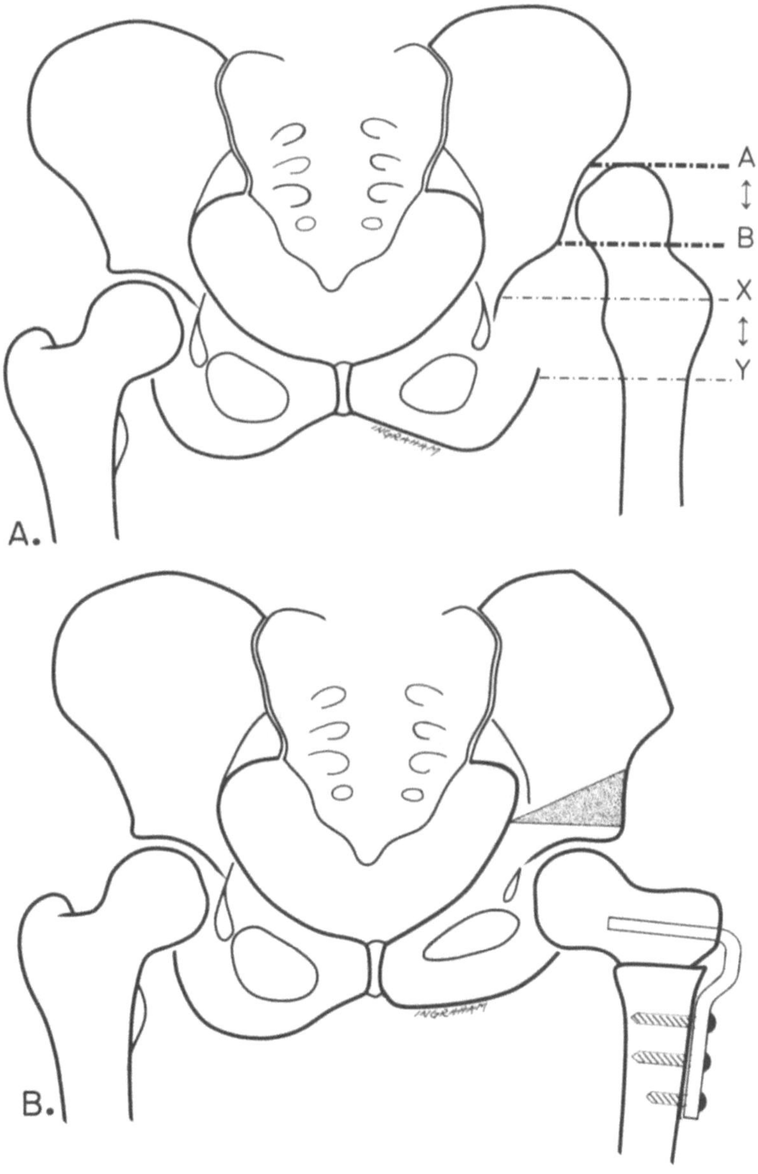

FIG. 14–16 Klisic procedure: combined open reduction, femoral shortening, and pelvic osteotomy. **A** In the older child, it is useful to measure the amount of proximal femoral displacement on the dislocated side (*A–B*). Carrying out this amount of intraoperative femoral shortening helps to achieve reduction without excessive soft tissue tension, even without preoperative traction. **B** Femoral shortening by the amount *X–Y* (*X–Y* = *A–B*) is a component of varus derotational osteotomy. Pelvic osteotomy and capsulorrhaphy allow complete hip joint stabilization in one stage, without excessive soft tissue tension.

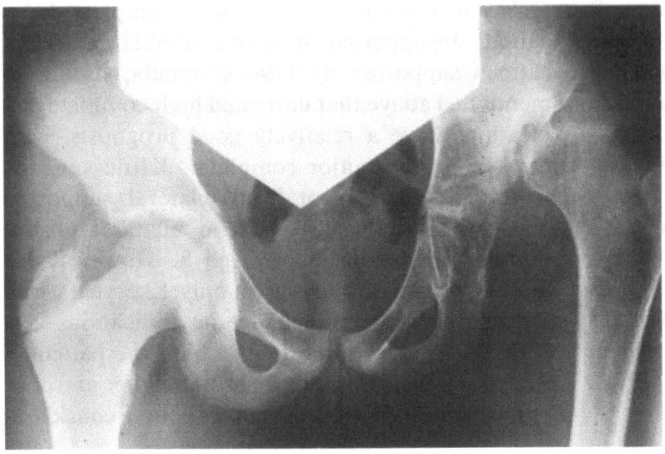

A

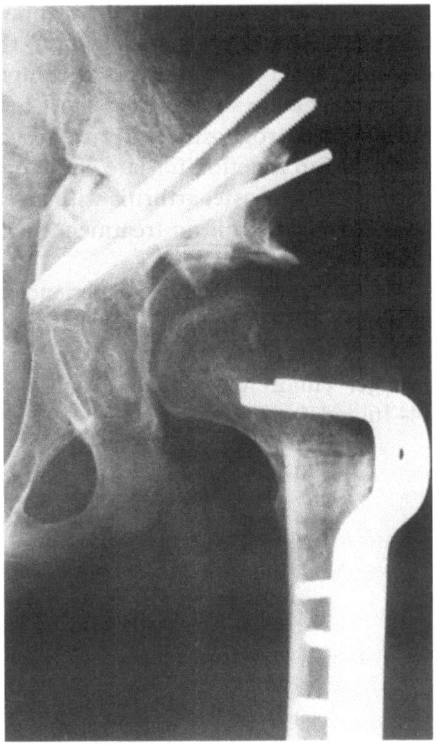

B

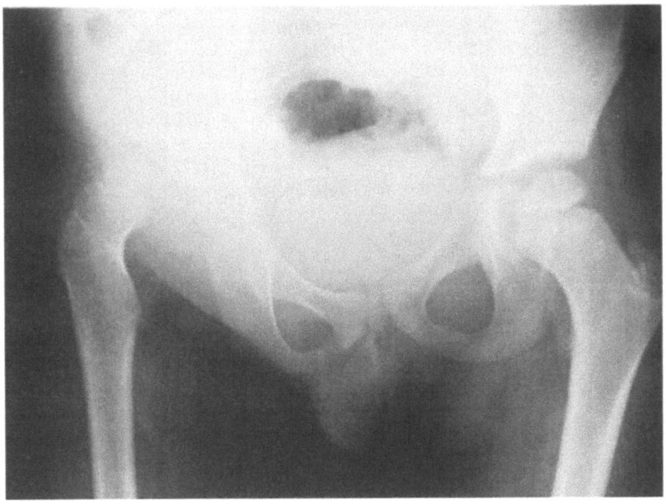

C

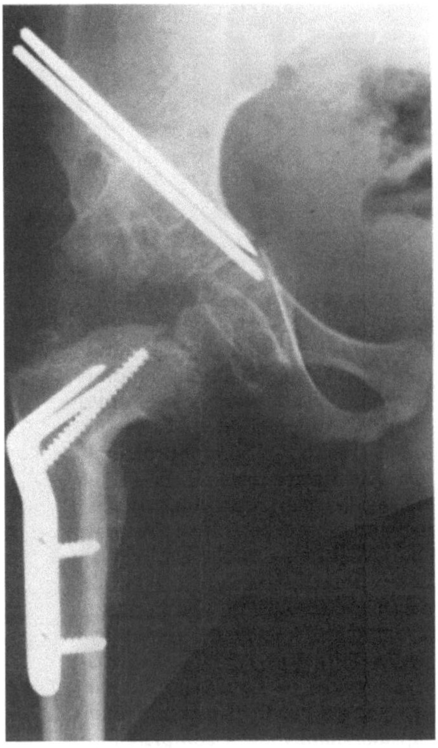

D

FIG. 14–17 Klisic procedure. This 12-year-old white female had undergone several previous attempts at open reduction and bony stabilization and yet remained dislocated. Her disease was unilateral and her ipsilateral femoral head remained relatively round. **A** Preoperative radiograph. **B** Postoperative radiograph, following femoral shortening–derotational osteotomy and Chiari osteotomy. **C** Preoperative radiograph of 8-year-old male with previously untreated congenital hip dislocation. **D** Nine months following combined open reduction, femoral shortening–derotation–varus osteotomy, and innominate osteotomy, hip is stable.

ble risk of a fair or poor result in both hips even early on, when the reduction is achieved late. This should make the age at which one would withhold primary treatment for bilateral congenital hip dislocation younger than that for unilateral cases.

In general, a unilateral dislocation should be considered for treatment at almost any age during childhood. A first reason is the existence of considerable pelvic asymmetry and secondary stresses placed on the lower back in a unilateral dislocation, in contrast to bilateral cases. In bilateral cases there is usually increased lumbar lordosis, but no lateral tilt. Secondly, a poor result in one hip can be tolerated relatively well if the contralateral hip is entirely normal. In addition, the salvage of a poor unilateral result is much less complex than the bilateral situation.

The art of arthroplasty in the salvage of the poor result of treatment of CDH is ever improving, as are the techniques for late primary treatment. Nonetheless, we still urge recognition of biological limitations of late primary treatment and the definite wisdom of withholding treatment in the occasional case.

The Hip with Residual Deformity in the Older Child and Adolescent

When a state of incomplete reduction exists, the femoral head is partially supported by the true acetabulum. Short-term function may be normal, but the long-term prognosis is terrible unless normalization of the pathoanatomy can be achieved before irreversible cartilage damage has occurred. The onset of osteoarthritis in uncorrected subluxation is much earlier than in complete dislocation, often in the third decade of life. Diagnosis and treatment of subluxation is therefore important. Such subluxation often is a sequela of either insufficient primary treatment for CDH or of proximal femoral growth disturbance secondary to treatment. Rarely, though, a patient with no early history will present in late childhood or adolescence with a dysplastic hip.

The treatment of residual deformity necessitates recognition of two categories of surgical therapy: reconstruction and salvage. Distinguishing between these theoretically mutually exclusive situations is essential (Table 14–1). Reconstructive methods aim to achieve a normal prognosis for the hip joint, specifically for a lifetime of normal symptom-free function. This is possible only if certain conditions exist: (1) irreversible articular cartilage damage has not occurred; (2) macroscopic deformity of acetabulum and proximal femur can be eliminated; and (3) the articular cartilaginous surfaces retain enough biological plasticity to adjust to the reorientation imposed on them by the reconstructive surgery.

Any candidate for reconstructive surgery by this definition should at the time of evaluation still be virtually free from pain and no older than 18 to 20 years of age. *The range of motion should be nearly normal.* Radiography should reveal smooth congruent articular surfaces, or in the child, surfaces capable of remodeling to spherical congruency. There should be no subchondral sclerosis nor cartilage space narrowing. In short, the function must be quite good but the prognosis poor, by virtue of surgically correctable malalignment.

Present concepts of the etiology of degenerative joint disease after congenital dislocation of the hip suggest that an important factor is the long-term generation of physiologically normal loads across a hip joint whose components are anatomically malaligned. The existence of anterolateral acetabular insufficiency, for example, creates abnormally large pressures on both femoral and acetabular articular surfaces because of the *reduced load-bearing area.* The radiographic correlate of this situation is the enlarged sourcil [58] (eyebrow) in the subchondral bone above the superolateral corner of the insufficient acetabulum. This type of subchondral sclerosis is physiological and reversible as long as the function within the joint (of which the sourcil is a sensitive indicator) is able to be normalized (Fig. 14–18).

Abnormally large pressures also can be caused in a similar manner by proximal femoral malalignment into valgus and anteversion. It should be mentioned that overcorrection of the proximal femur into an abnormal varus attitude will not compensate for persisting acetabular insufficiency. Although joint pressures are initially even lower than with a normal neck–shaft angle, eventually further subluxation of the proximal femur will occur, even in coxa vara, out of the insufficient acetabulum, drastically reducing the weight-bearing area and leading to degenerative joint disease.[7]

TABLE 14–1 Reconstruction vs. Salvage

	Reconstruction	Salvage
Age	≤20–25 years (some biological plasticity remains)	Any age
Symptoms	Minimal	Moderate to severe
Motion	Near normal	≥60° of flexion
Function	Good to normal	Fair to poor
Pathoanatomy	No irreversible changes	Irreversible changes
Radiology	Smooth but malaligned surfaces	Cartilage space narrowing and incongruity
Prognosis	Poor	Poor
Therapeutic goal	Restoration of normal prognosis; maintenance of normal present function	Improvement of present function; least possible compromise of future treatment options
Character of surgical therapy	Normalizing orientation of hyaline cartilage and bony joint components	Reduce joint pressures in presence of incongruity; increase weight-bearing areas; reduce muscle forces
Surgical procedures	Normalizing acetabular or femoral reorientation—innominate osteotomy and variations; acetabular osteotomy; femoral osteotomy	Chiari or other shelf osteotomy; valgus intertrochanteric osteotomy (rare: varus osteotomy)

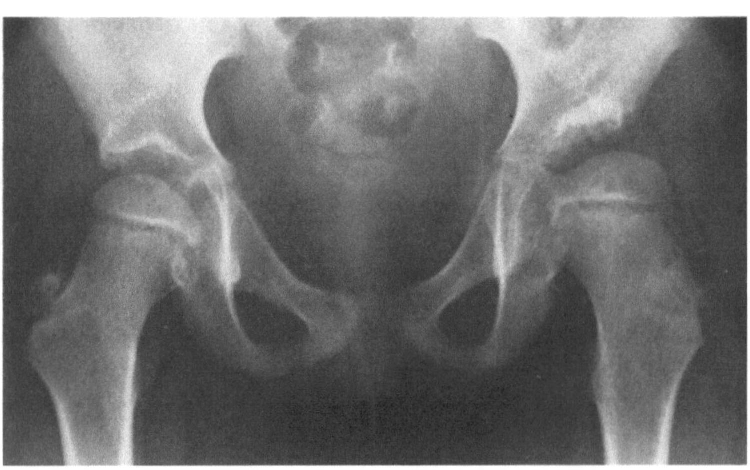

FIG. 14–18 Radiographs usually reflect sensitively the state of intraarticular function. An abnormal concentration of forces on the superolateral portion of the acetabulum is reflected by abnormal subchondral sclerosis. This area of subchondral bony acetabular condensation is called the *sourcil* (French, eyebrow). The difference between a sourcil of normal character (right hip) and abnormal character (left hip) is seen.

Evaluation of the Dysplastic Hip

Residual deformity in the dysplastic hip may be either acetabular, femoral, or both. Implicit in the concept of reconstruction is restoration of normal anatomy, with preservation or improvement of the already quite good function. This is accomplished by repositioning of the hyaline cartilage joint surfaces. Specifically, preoperative roentgenographic evaluation must confirm that a certain position of the hip (usually abduction, perhaps with some lesser elements of flexion or internal rotation) will produce a normal relationship of the femoral head to the acetabulum. If normalization can be demonstrated radiographically, then the task of reconstruction is to establish surgically this relationship with the limb in the weight-bearing situation; i.e., with the entire hip joint oriented normally to the line of weight bearing across it, as in stance.

The deviations from normal in the residually dysplastic hip must be characterized precisely if surgical correction is to be successful. This presupposes knowledge of the anatomical and functional parameters of the normal hip (Table 14–2).

The normal proximal femur at birth has a neck–shaft angle of approximately 135° and anteversion of approximately 30°, with each of these angles being reduced by about 10° by skeletal maturity.[40] The tip of the greater trochanter should at maturity lie at the level of the middle of the femoral head, and lateral to it by a distance of 2–2.5 times the radius of the head.[40,94] In addition, the epiphysis should be oriented with the capital C-G angle from 0 to +15°, so that femoral articular cartilage is aligned optimally to receive the transarticular loads for which it is designed.[58,94]

Proximal femoral reconstruction presupposes that although malalignment exists, the femoral articular surface is smooth and either round or capable of remodeling to be round. With severe proximal femoral growth disturbance, the greater trochanter and femoral head may seem fused together with no recognizable femoral neck. Not only in this complex situation, but also whenever any proximal femoral osteotomy is planned, the most complete assessment possible of the proximal femoral pathoanatomy should be carried out before any decision (and certainly any incision) is made. This may be done conveniently with an image intensifier with memory tape, involving minimal radiation.

First, a position of the leg must be found which creates the desired relationship between the femoral head and acetabulum. A good range of motion is presumed. (The subsequent operative procedure serves merely to maintain the femoral head in this position while bringing the legs to their neutral weight-bearing position in stance.) An essential view is in the anteroposterior plane, with the leg rotated enough to eliminate any version of the femoral neck. This throws the head, neck, and trochanters into profile to eliminate radiographic superposition. It is often only from such a view that an accurate line drawing of the proposed osteotomy can be made. This type of evaluation aids greatly in planning both osteotomy and osteosynthesis.

It must be emphasized again that the most important consideration in planning a proximal femoral reconstruction is the determination of the desired postoperative orientation of the femoral articular surface. This is not trivial, because in certain cases, as in Ogdon type II ischemic damage to the proximal femoral growth centers (lateral

TABLE 14–2 Radiographic Parameters of the Mature Hip

Parameter	Normal	Dysplastic
Acetabular angle	25–41°	≥42°
Acetabular depth	14–27 mm	<15 mm (M) <14 mm (F)
Acetabular roof slope	0° (downward slope)	≤ 0°
Center-edge angle	24–46°	≤20°

Adapted from Stulberg.[82]

physeal growth retardation), the articular surface and physis may be inclined into much more valgus than the neck itself. Only after the character of the desired reorientation of the femoral head itself is determined can one consider what supplemental realignment should be done to normalize the remaining proximal femoral anatomy.

The Varus Intertrochanteric Osteotomy

The best indication for a varus osteotomy (Figs. 14–19 and 14–20) is a valgus orientation of the entire proximal femur (including greater trochanter), with lateralization of the femoral head which corrects in abduction.

Simple varus osteotomy in the older child or adolescent should follow the basic principles outlined by the AO.[53] The osteotomy is best done in the intertrochanteric region. This not only facilitates healing but also avoids pathological retroversion of the iliopsoas insertion if derotational reduction and anteversion is planned. Medialization of the distal fragment is usually indicated and good medial interfragmentary compression is essential. Some over-correction may be desirable if further growth and spontaneous revalgization is anticipated.

A few points in the lateral approach to the proximal femur are to be emphasized. The vastus lateralis should be elevated atraumatically in a distal and anterior direction to avoid damage to the trochanteric apophysis and the vastus itself. After the osteosynthesis, the vastus should be resutured carefully to its origin at the base of the trochanter to promote a dynamic lateral tension band effect opposite the osteotomy, promoting good early function and early bony healing. Suction drainage should be routine for the first 1 or 2 postoperative

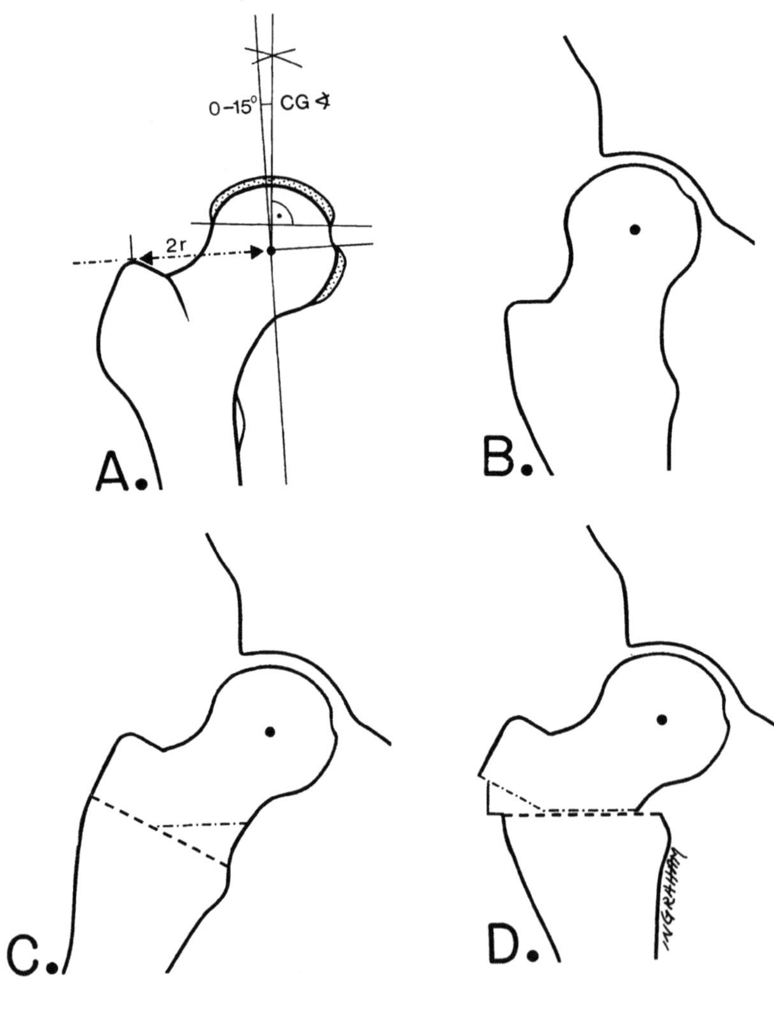

FIG. 14–19 Indications for varus intertrochanteric osteotomy. **A** The normal proximal femur has slight medial inclination of its articular surface (C-G angle, 0–15°). The tip of the greater trochanter lies at the level of the center of the femoral head and lateral to the center of the head by a distance of about two times the femoral head radius. There should be congruence between the head and acetabulum in the weight-bearing position. **B** Ideal indication for varization exists with a valgus attitude of both the femoral articular surface and the subcapital anatomy, with improved congruence in abduction. **C** The degree of abduction which normalizes both the joint congruence and proximal femoral relationships is the amount of varization desired. **D** Ideal varization maintains the proximal femur in corrected position while realigning the shaft to weight-bearing position. Medial displacement of the shaft usually is indicated to prevent varization of the distal limb axis. Fig. 14–19A adapted with permission from Wagner H: Acetabular Dysplasias, Skeletal Dysplasias in Children. Heidelberg, Springer-Verlag, 1978, p. 134.

days. We prefer the trochanteric blade plate for the osteosynthesis unless proximity of the greater trochanteric apophysis precludes its use. In such cases (rare over age 4 or 5) a device whose blade enters the proximal osteotomy surface is preferable (e.g., Altdorf hip clamp).

Varization effectively shortens the limb through the intertrochanteric region and thus theoretically reduces the pressures across the joint.

Valgus Osteotomy

True coxa vara is relatively rare as a residual deformity after congenital hip dislocation. Ogdon type III or type IV growth disturbance [11] could result in such deformity and valgization of the proximal femur would be indicated (Figs. 14–21 and 14–22). Valgization effectively lengthens the intertrochanteric region and thereby increases the pressures across the joint. If lengthening is not desirable, then at the time of valgization osteotomy, an appropriate femoral shortening should be done by a transverse osteotomy through the proximal end of the distal fragment, with preservation of the iliopsoas insertion.

It should also be noted that valgization tends to reorient the distal limb more directly under the hip joint. This may tend to overload the lateral compartment of the knee and subject the knee to valgus stresses, and consideration should be given to a slight lateralization of the distal fragment when carrying out a valgus osteotomy. If a lengthening effect is desired beyond what the valgization itself will produce, the intertrochanteric osteotomy line may be made to ascend medially. This creates additional effective lengthening

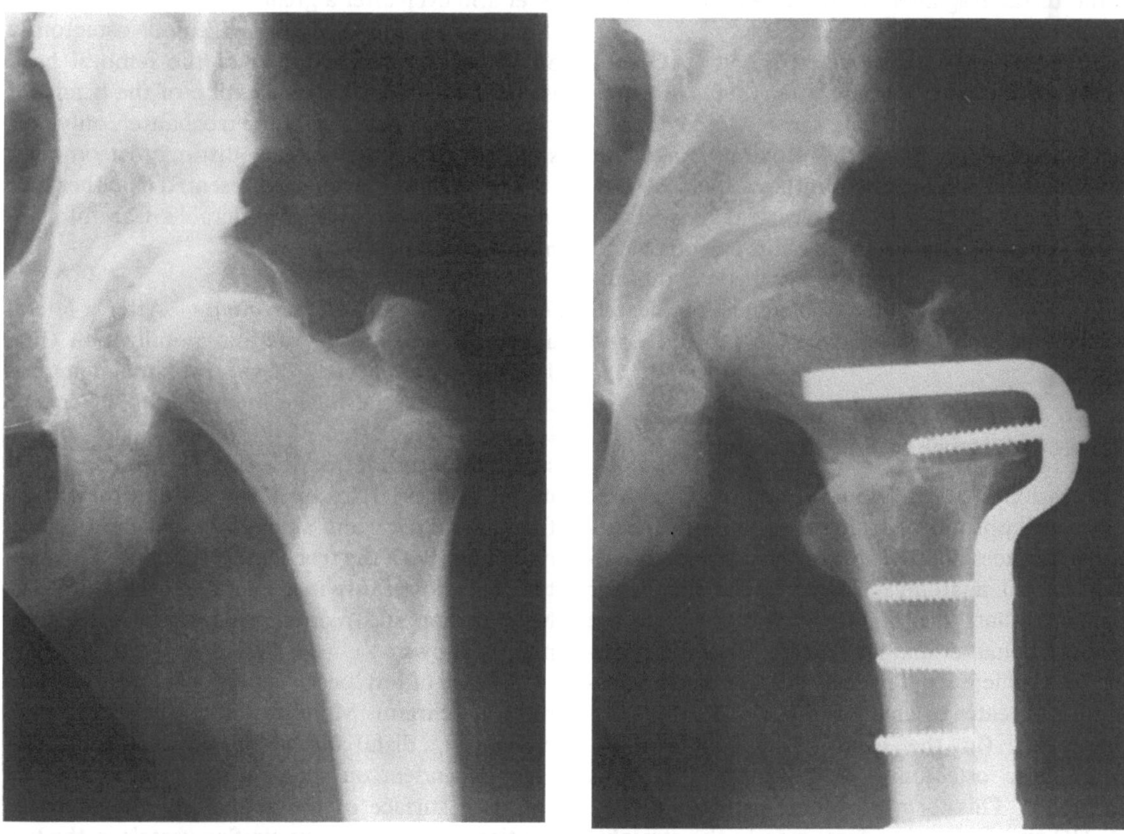

A B

FIG. 14–20 **A** Varus osteotomy in the adolescent or young adult is best accomplished by making an initial transverse cut just proximal to the lesser trochanter, followed by removal of an appropriate wedge of bone from the distal and medial corner of the proximal fragment. Both slight medialization of the distal fragment and good interfragmentary compression can be achieved efficiently using the AO intertrochanteric blade plate **(B)**. The adult-size implant allows insertion of a supplementary screw in the proximal fragment just distal to the blade.

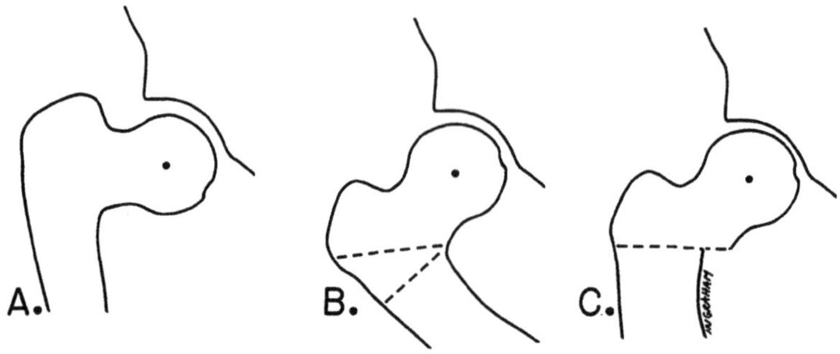

FIG. 14–21 Indications for valgus intertrochanteric osteotomy. **A** Ideal indication for valgization exists with a varus attitude of both the femoral articular surface and subcapital anatomy, with improved congruence in adduction. **B** Degree of adduction which normalizes both joint congruence and proximal femoral relationships is the amount of valgization desired. **C** Ideal valgization maintains the proximal femur in corrected position while realigning the shaft to weight-bearing position. Lateral displacement of the shaft usually is indicated to prevent valgization of the distal limb axis.

as the distal fragment is lateralized at the time of osteotomy (Fig. 14–22A and B).

In mature patients, we prefer the 95° AO condylar plate for osteosynthesis after valgus intertrochanteric osteotomy. A long screw should supplement the blade in fixing the proximal fragment. In children, a special osteosynthesis must be created (Fig. 14–22C and D). A careful reconstruction of the vastus lateralis is again essential, and proximal advancement of its origin onto the lateral surface of the greater trochanter is indicated to maintain the desired dynamic tension band effect.

Double Intertrochanteric Osteotomy

On occasion, a single femoral osteotomy may not suffice for appropriate realignment of both the articular surfaces and the rest of the complex proximal femoral anatomy. Wagner [94] has noted, for example, that varization always elevates the greater trochanter and may create a secondary abductor insufficiency. This may suggest distal transfer of the greater trochanter to be done either simultaneously (in the form of a double intertrochanteric osteotomy) or following the varus osteotomy. This form of double osteotomy (Fig. 14–23C and D) is, therefore, merely the straightforward combination of varus osteotomy with trochanteric transfer.

A different, more complex form of double osteotomy [94] seems the unique solution when the femoral neck is too short to function as an effective lever arm even after a greater trochanteric transfer (Fig. 14–23A and B). In this ingenious osteotomy, any necessary reorientation of the femoral head is supplemented by medialization of the head and neck and lateralization of the trochanter, only possible by two simultaneous distinct osteotomies.

The technical challenge presented by either type of double osteotomy is considerable. Careful planning is critical.

Technique for Double Osteotomy After a lateral approach with vastus lateralis mobilization (Fig. 14–24), a profile view of the proximal femur is obtained with the image intensifier to determine the exact orientation of the femoral neck and to select the attitude for the two osteotomies. It is useful to insert Kirschner wires along the axis of the femoral neck and along both proposed osteotomy lines. Both the trochanteric and intertrochanteric osteotomies are made with an oscillating saw. Mobilization and reorientation of the three fragments follows.

Release of any periarticular scar must be complete yet careful. Mobilization of the greater trochanter in a distal and lateral direction is particularly dependent on such release of adhesions on the deep surface of the abductors. One must be cautious to avoid the circumflex vessels in the trochanteric fossa (see discussion of technique for trochanter transfer). The head–neck fragment is then reoriented as desired (usually into valgus) and its lateral and distal corner is impacted into the proximal and medial corner of the shaft frag-

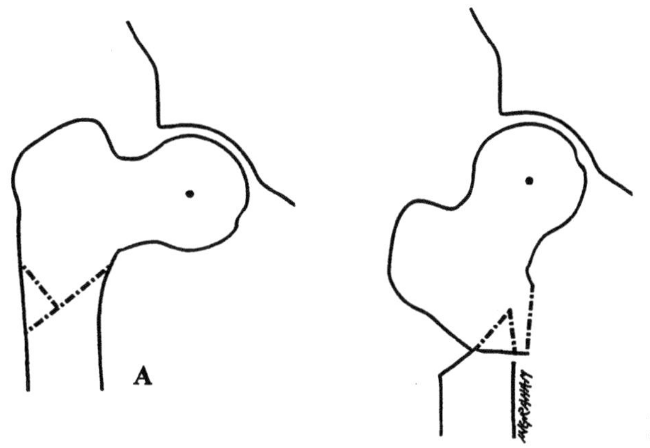

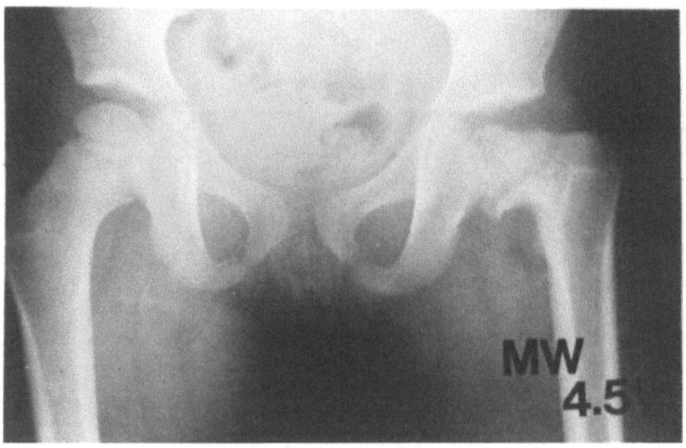

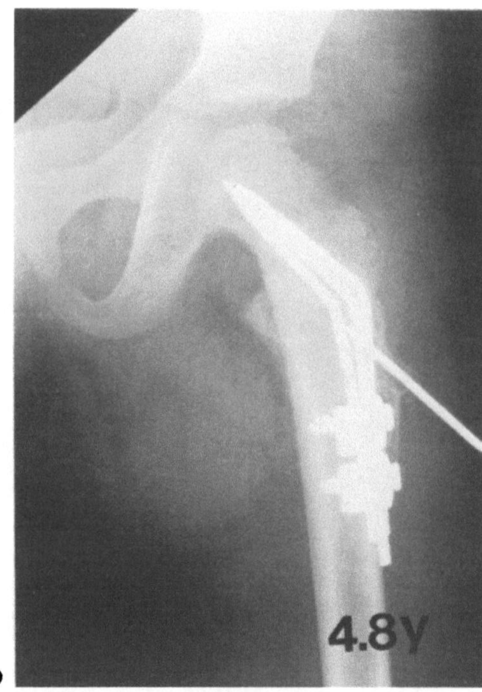

FIG. 14–22 Examples of valgus osteotomy. **A** and **B** An additional lengthening effect may be achieved beyond what the valgization itself will produce. The intertrochanteric osteotomy lines must in this situation be made to ascend medially. With displacement of the distal fragment laterally and valgization of the proximal fragment, the extra lengthening effect is achieved. **C** This 4-year-old child suffered ischemic damage to the proximal femoral growth plate in conjunction with closed reduction. She had retroversion as well as varus deformity. **D** By flexion and valgization, the proximal femur was appropriately realigned. A special osteosynthesis was created by appropriately bent Kirschner wires, held to the lateral surface of the proximal femoral shaft by small contoured plates.

ment. Provisional fixation of these two fragments is carried out with a Kirschner wire. The greater trochanter is then displaced laterally and then distally, and it is also provisionally fixed with a Kirschner wire.

Position of the fragments should be confirmed at this time with the image intensifier, and any adjustments in position made. A good medial buttress must be present.

A creative osteosynthesis must next be carried out. A trochanteric blade plate may be used, although there is some risk of fracturing either the trochanteric or head–neck fragments. Wagner prefers to avoid such massive internal fixation,[94,96] yet he achieves enough stability with an ingenious osteosynthesis to avoid any necessity for prolonged immobilization or relief from weight bearing.

Usual Wagner's osteosynthesis after double osteotomy consists of a long, specially fashioned hooked plate applied to the lateral surface of the greater trochanter and the shaft fragment to function as a tension band. Multiple interfragmentary cancellous and cortical screws are used. Supplemental pins are sometimes necessary to maintain the medial buttress.

If this osteosynthesis is carried out effectively,

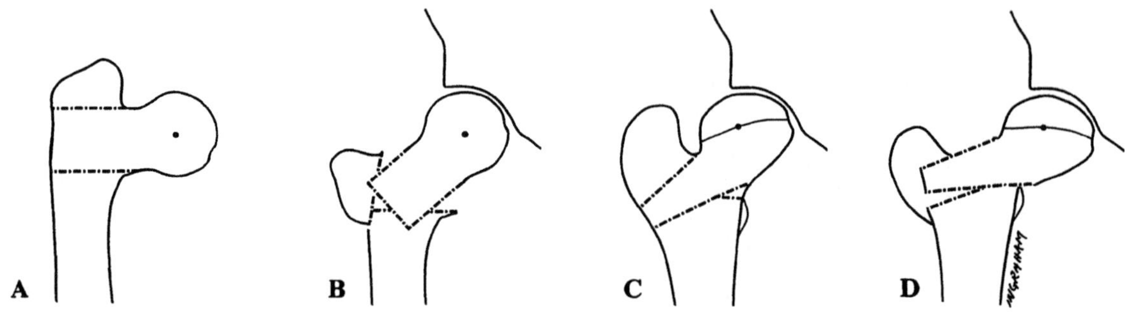

FIG. 14–23 Double intertrochanteric osteotomy. **A** True coxa vara with short femoral neck requires two separate osteotomies to both normalize articular surfaces and restore abductor efficiency. **B** Valgization, lengthening of femoral neck, and trochanteric realignment achieved. **C** Caput valga and breva also requires two separate osteotomies for complete normalization. **D** Varization, lengthening of femoral neck, and trochanteric realignment achieved.

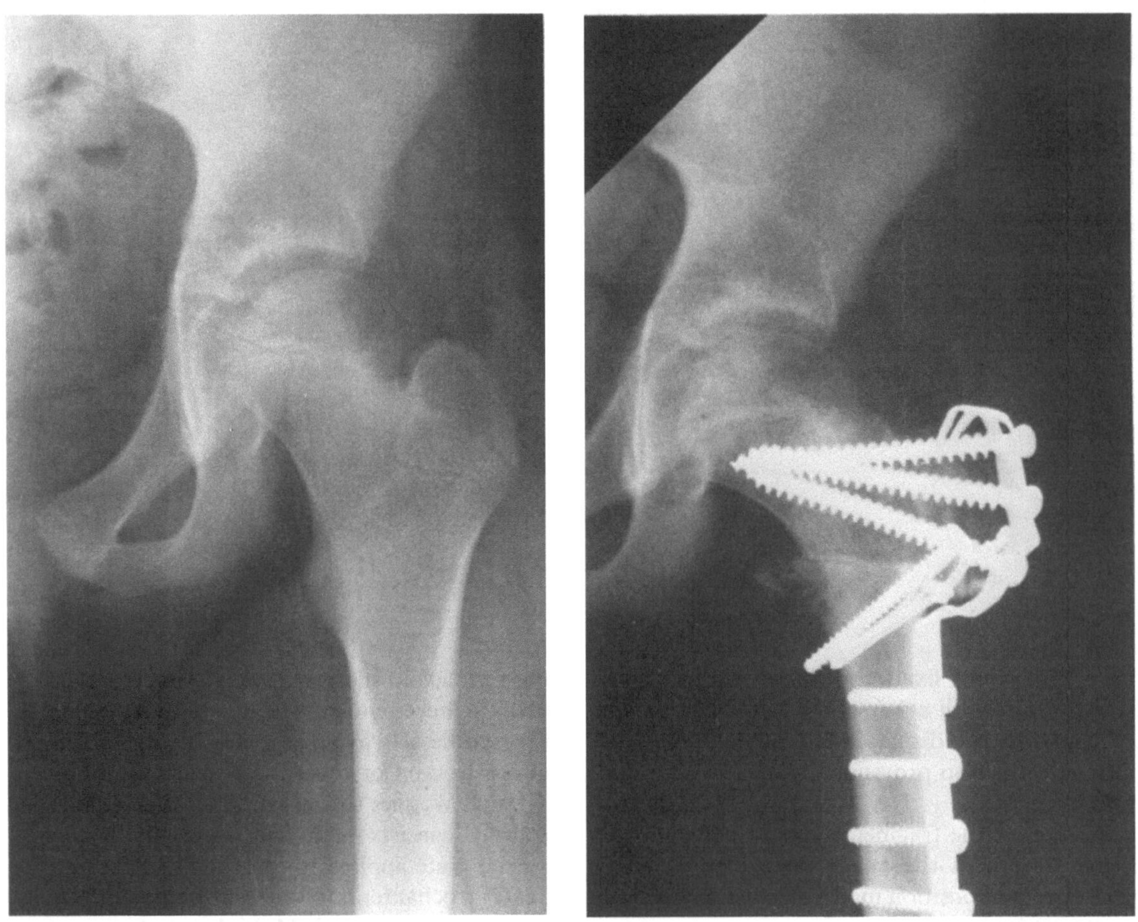

A B

FIG. 14–24 Double intertrochanteric osteotomy. **A** This 12-year-old female had a lateral arrest to the proximal femoral physis with eversion of the articular surface, shortening of the neck, and relative overgrowth of the greater trochanter. **B** Double intertrochanteric osteotomy allows simultaneous varization of the femoral articular surface and restoration of normal abductor mechanics (rather than increased elevation of the trochanter which simple varization would create).

the healing bone experiences some loading to facilitate early bony healing and remodeling along functional lines. Early function is felt to be as essential to normalization of the proximal femoral bony architecture as is the realignment itself. After surgery, two crutches are used for about 3 months, with about 15–20% of body weight being borne on the operated limb. One crutch is usually employed for an additional 3 months. Active abduction exercises should be avoided for at least the first 2 postoperative months.

Transfer of the Greater Trochanter

Relative overgrowth of the greater trochanter (always secondary to ischemic damage to the capital femoral physis) with secondary functional abductor insufficiency may be unaccompanied by other deformity serious enough to warrant surgery. This is an indication for simple trochanteric transfer, a relatively small but very efficient operation in terms of biomechanical and functional improvement gained (Fig. 14–25).

The transfer should normalize the length and orientation of the abductor lever arm by bringing the tip of the trochanter down to the level of the center of the femoral head and lateralizing it from the center of the femoral head by a distance of at least two times the radius of the head.

Edgren [17a] introduced the concept of the articulotrochanteric distance (ATD), which is a useful parameter in quantifying relative overgrowth of the greater trochanter. Langenskjold [41] and Gage [23] both suggested that if potential trochanteric overgrowth can be diagnosed early, before the trochanter has grown above the level of the femoral head, then secondary abductor insufficiency usually can be prevented by timely epiphysiodesis of the greater trochanter. They suggest that it is usually necessary to perform this growth arrest of the greater trochanter before age 8 for the procedure to prevent trochanteric overgrowth.

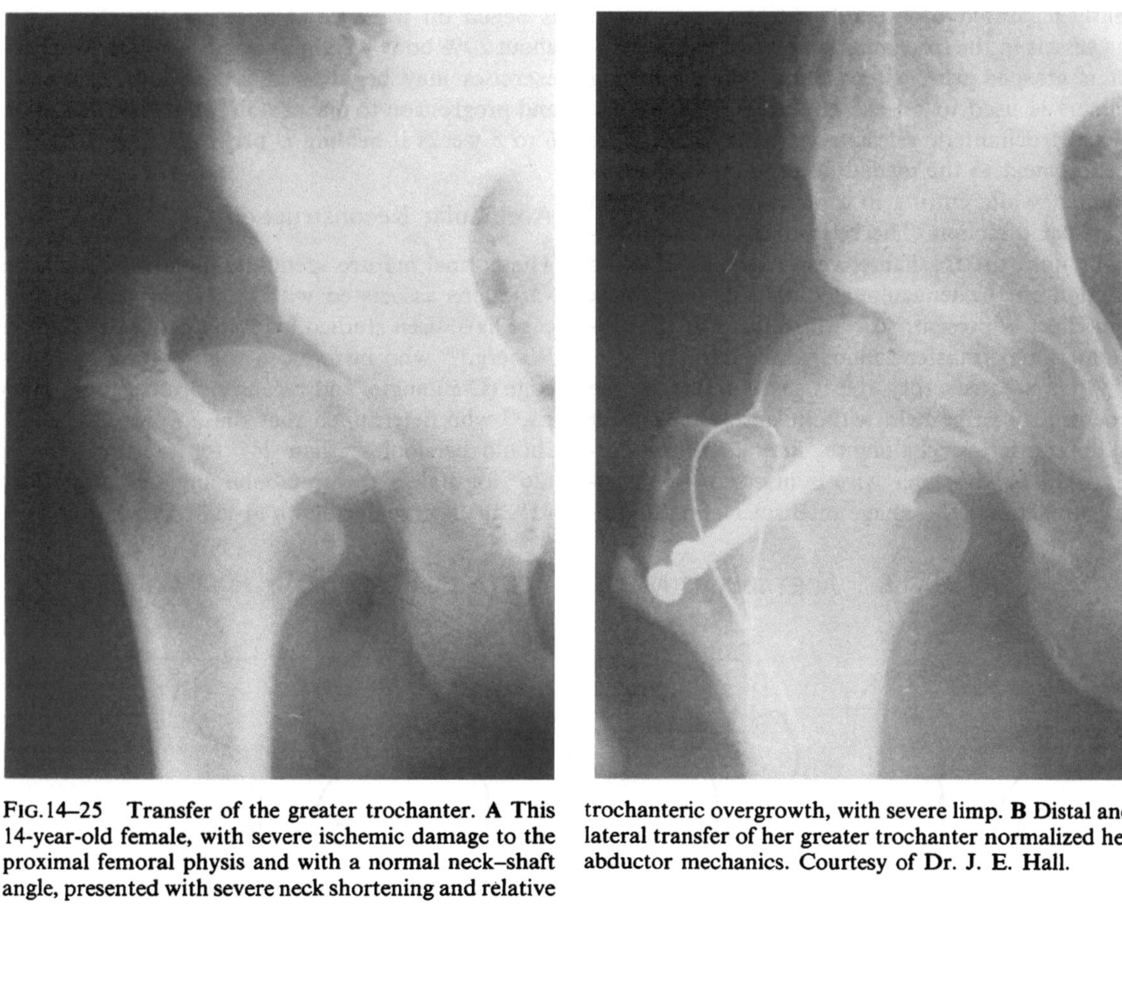

A B

FIG. 14–25 Transfer of the greater trochanter. **A** This 14-year-old female, with severe ischemic damage to the proximal femoral physis and with a normal neck–shaft angle, presented with severe neck shortening and relative trochanteric overgrowth, with severe limp. **B** Distal and lateral transfer of her greater trochanter normalized her abductor mechanics. Courtesy of Dr. J. E. Hall.

The technique is well described by Langenskjold [41] and probably does have a limited indication. We have preferred in such cases to wait until near skeletal maturity, at which time a precise relocalization of the trochanter can be done. In addition, a certain number of patients who in mid-childhood seem to be candidates for growth arrest of the greater trochanter will turn out to require double osteotomy, whether or not the trochanteric growth arrest is done early. It seems preferable, when possible, to carry out one operation of relatively definitive type at a time when deformity will not reoccur.

Technique A lateral surgical approach is used, with careful mobilization of the vastus lateralis origin. The leg is internally rotated enough to eliminate any anteversion, to allow precise radiographic control. A Kirschner wire is inserted along the line of the desired osteotomy, and an oscillating saw is used to cut along the Kirschner wire just to the medial trochanteric cortex, still using image intensifier control. The fragments then should be gently separated with a wide osteotome, to avoid the vessels in the trochanteric notch. The trochanter is grasped with a tenaculum while a strong scissors is used to release any medial adhesions.

The trochanteric release consists in keeping the scissors next to the medial periosteum of the trochanter, while cutting in a proximal rather than a medial direction. The release continues proximally until the trochanter responds elastically to traction on the tenaculum holding it. If a check rein effect is present, scar still tethers to the trochanter, and transfer cannot yet be done.[96]

After a satisfactory release is completed, the trochanter can be held without undue tension at an appropriate level along the lateral femoral cortex while a Kirschner wire is inserted for provisional fixation. The image intensifier should confirm that the position is as desired. Two cortical or cancellous screws, with washers, are inserted anterior and posterior to the Kirschner wire, which can then be removed. The screws should be directed distally and medially to oppose statically the abductor forces.

Trochanteric transfer may rarely be indicated in the presence of an open trochanteric apophysis when further trochanteric growth is desired. In such a situation, screw fixation should be avoided to prevent pressure damage to the growth center. Superomedially directed smooth Kirschner wires, rather than screws, should therefore be employed to provide the static internal fixation.

After any intertrochanteric transfer, the dynamic tension band effect of the vastus lateralis is as important as the character of the internal fixation. Advancing the vastus origin onto the transferred trochanter promotes good early function and healing.

After surgery, sitting is prohibited for at least 3 weeks to prevent rotatory forces from loosening the osteosynthesis. Ambulation with two crutches is begun on the second postoperative day, with about 20% body weight allowed. Active abduction exercises may be allowed after about 1 month, and progression to one crutch can be allowed after 6 to 8 weeks if healing is progressing well.

Acetabular Reconstruction

The normal mature acetabulum and its dysplastic variations associated with degenerative joint disease have been studied by many people, including Wiberg,[100] who introduced the important center-edge (C-E) angle, and recently, Stulberg and Harris,[82] who determined that the normal C-E angle should be no less than 24° for mature females (26° for males), the acetabular angle no more than 41°, the acetabular depth at least 14 mm (15 mm

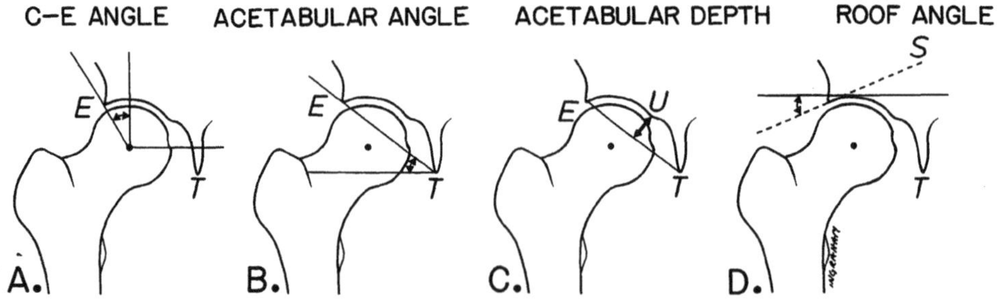

FIG. 14–26 Schematics of radiographic parameters of the mature hip.

TABLE 14–3 Center-edge Angle at Different Ages

Age (years)	Normal	Questionable	Dysplastic
20–35	>26°	20–26°	<20°
14–20	>26°	20–26°	<20°
6–13	≥20°	15–19°	<15°

From Severin.[70]

for males), and the roof angle should be greater than zero (lateral acetabular roof should slope downward) (Fig. 14–26; Tables 14–2 and 14–3).

Salter [69] and Lloyd-Roberts [45] have both emphasized the significance of acetabular anteversion in the pathology of the dysplastic hip. Radiographic determination of acetabular inclination and femoral head coverage in the lateral projection is done rarely, probably much too infrequently. We have found an oblique view, with the patient turned 45° from the supine toward the hip to be examined, valuable in assessing anterolateral coverage without undue radiation.

In certain situations, a single clinical and radiographic evaluation may be sufficient to allow formulation of a treatment program that includes surgery. Quite often, though, particularly in young children, the deformity may be mild enough to warrant determination of the tendency of the hip joint over time. If further development leads to spontaneous improvement in joint structure and function, then continued observation is more appropriate than immediate surgical intervention. Any worsening of structure or function certainly argues for timely reconstruction, lest the anatomy become so distorted that the patient falls into the salvage category.

Precipitous intervention is to be avoided, however, and preoperative training is important in obtaining the best result. The patient's understanding and motivation must be secured before admission. In addition, maximal range of motion and muscle strength should be achieved and skill with crutches learned prior to surgery.

Up to about 4 years of age, there is enough remodeling capacity in the undamaged acetabulum and proximal femur that normalizing alignment on one side of a hip with moderate dysplasia on both sides of the joint may lead to postoperative resolution of the dysplasia on the other side as well. In older patients, coincident persisting femoral and acetabular deformity usually requires both femoral and acetabular reconstruction.

Up to about 6 or 7 years of age, both acetabuloplasty and Salter innominate osteotomy are quite useful in the treatment of residual acetabular dysplasia, provided that good centering of the femoral head is achieved by simple appropriate positioning. If an irreducible subluxation is present, however, then one must choose between exploration of the hip joint (usually not rewarding in the child over about 3 years), in an effort to achieve a concentric reduction, or one must relegate the patient to the salvage category and consider those salvage procedures to be described below.

The principle is that carrying out reconstructive procedures in a salvage situation may hasten the onset of degenerative joint disease, just as may the performance of salvage procedures in the patient suited for reconstruction.

Arthrography may be a useful adjunct to simple examination of the patient under the image intensifier, to determine not only the articular dynamics by viewing the subchondral bony outlines, but also the articular surfaces. This may help one to decide whether acetabular realignment or change in acetabular contour is indicated, as well. We have little experience with CAT scanning in evaluating residual hip dysplasia, although others extol the virtues of the method after early experiences.[85]

Acetabuloplasty In the older child being considered for acetabuloplasty, some authors recommend previous or simultaneous femoral varization almost routinely to decrease the pressure on the femoral head. Even if such varization and psoas tenotomy are done to decrease the transarticular pressures, the abrupt change in acetabular contour effected by acetabuloplasty may damage the cartilage in the older child. Most authors suggest 6 years as the upper age limit for true acetabuloplasty, although good results have been reported up to about age 10 or more.[60] We feel the risks are too great to recommend routinely classic acetabuloplasty after about age 6. The Pem-Sal variation may be useful in the older child, with less risk for cartilage damage.[48] The technique for each of these procedures in the older child is virtually as described in the section on open reduction.

Innominate Osteotomy

Salter suggests innominate osteotomy as being indicated in the treatment of primary or residual reducible hip subluxation from 18 months of age to adulthood.[69] The prerequisites are full range of motion, good articular congruency, and a stable relationship between the femoral head and the acetabulum in flexion and abduction.

The main disadvantage of single innominate osteotomy is the limited degree of correction that is possible, particularly in the older patient.[29] The axis of rotation for this acetabular realignment procedure runs from the symphysis to the sciatic notch and correction is particularly sensitive to the age-dependent elasticity of the symphysis.[64] Rab has designed a geometrical model of the Salter procedure that suggests the upper limit of the acetabular reorientation to be about 25° of extension and 10° of adduction.

Rab suggests a specific radiographic study [65] to determine whether the Salter type of single innominate osteotomy will provide sufficient coverage. With the patient supine, the hip is flexed 25° and abducted 10° in neutral rotation. The x-ray beam is then directed 25° caudally for a radiograph which will approximate the AP radiograph after a well-done innominate osteotomy. A lateral radiograph may be taken with the lateral beam directed 50° rostrally, with the hip maintained in the position suggested above.

The Rab views reveal the probable maximum coverage one can expect after the Salter procedure. The older the patient, the less correction one will achieve reliably. We have noted an average change in acetabular index of 20° up to age 10, but only an improvement in acetabular index of 8° over age 10 [29] (Fig. 14–26). This correlates with the experience of others, whose average corrections in acetabular index after about age 10 have been in the neighborhood of about 10 to 12°.[50a,92a]

Morscher suggested an acetabular index of 40° and Chapchal 30° as the upper limit indications for correctability with single innominate osteotomy.[11a,50a,92a]

The principle to be emphasized is the inherently limited correction possible with the Salter procedure. This necessitates modifying Salter's procedure or employing an entirely different method in moderate to severe cases of reducible subluxation (congruous acetabular insufficiency), particularly in the older patient.

First, an element of femoral malalignment should be either ruled out or correction incorporated into the surgical plan. If a proximal femoral normalization can bring the joint's anatomical insufficiency to within the limits of correctability possible with an innominate osteotomy, then preliminary proximal femoral correction should probably precede innominate osteotomy. If the degree of acetabular insufficiency itself is too much for the Salter procedure, but a reconstructive indication exists, then either a modification of the innominate osteotomy [77–79,83] or a spherical acetabular osteotomy [19,86,95] should be considered.

If innominate osteotomy is performed in the older patient with an intact capsule, displacement of the osteotomy can be facilitated by placing the ipsilateral leg in the frog position after the osteotomy cut is made. The distal fragment may also be displaced a bit anterolaterally, to maximize correction, before the graft is interposed and fixed (see above for technical details).

Modifications of Innominate Osteotomy Kalamchi's modification of the innominate osteotomy [34] is useful if acetabular redirection with intrapelvic shortening is desired (indicated if the ipsilateral leg is the longer limb). He cuts a small notch in the inferior surface of the proximal iliac fragment, into which the posterior corner of the distal fragment is locked (Fig. 14–27B).

Transiliac limb lengthening [50] may be employed to achieve both acetabular redirection and intrapelvic compensation for a short ipsilateral limb. This is achieved by using a trapezoidal interposition graft, instead of the usual triangular graft described by Salter. When congruous acetabular dysplasia with an acetabular angle of up to about 60° is associated with ipsilateral limb shortening, transiliac limb lengthening (similar in principle to Wagner type II acetabular osteotomy, described below) offers advantages over simple acetabular redirection supplemented by a shoe lift. Transiliac limb lengthening can increase femoral head coverage by acetabular redirection as the pelvis is leveled, whereas a shoe lift would decrease coverage of the hip in this situation by producing relative hip adduction in stance (Fig. 14–27C).

Important technical points in this procedure include the following: (1) generous release of the tendinous portion of the psoas (as in all innominate osteotomies); (2) careful distraction of the osteotomy with a laminar spreader as manual traction is applied to the leg and distal pressure is applied to the iliac crest; (3) use of heavy threaded Steinmann pins to transfix the osteotomy fragments and graft; (4) crutch protection for at least 3 months; and (5) pins left in situ for at least 6 months.

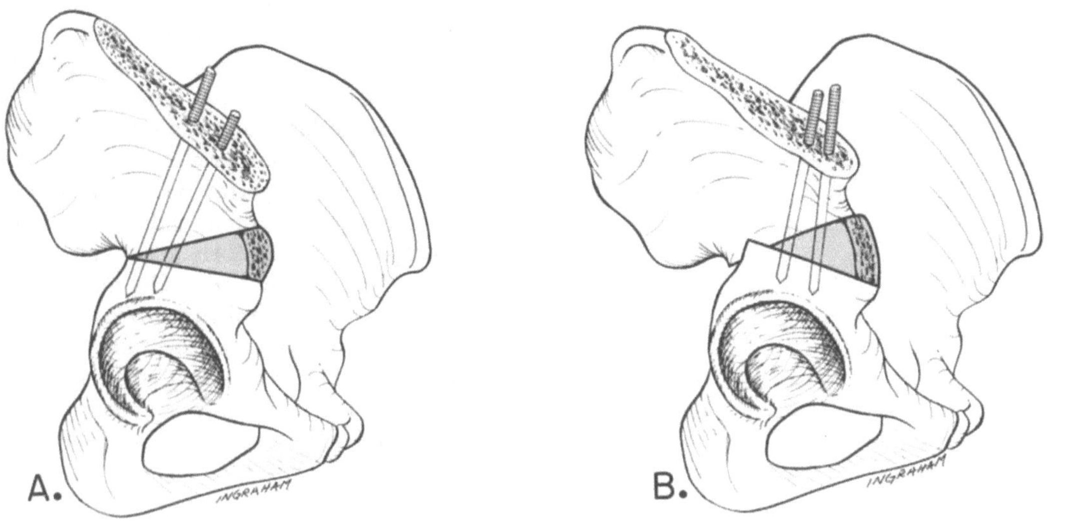

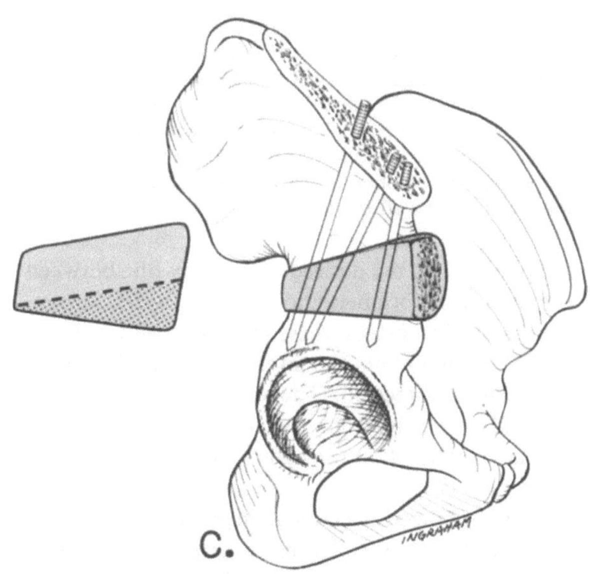

FIG. 14–27 Modified single innominate osteotomies. A Classic Salter type. B Kalamchi modification eliminates lengthening effect and increases stability. A notch is made in the inferior surface of the superior fragment. The posterior corner of the distal fragment is displaced anterosuperiorly to lock into the notch before interposition of graft and fixation. C The transiliac limb lengthening modification allows both acetabular redirection and intrapelvic lengthening effect of as much as 3 cm. Distraction is achieved before the trapezoidal graft is taken. Protected weight bearing is required for at least 3 months, and the pins are removed no earlier than 6 months after surgery.

Double Innominate Osteotomy

Sutherland [83,84] and Hopf [32] have described supplementing Salter's single innominate osteotomy with a second simultaneous pelvic cut, to allow greater mobilization and reduction of the acetabulum. Hopf's second osteotomy site is in the area of the tear drop. Sutherland's second osteotomy site is in the medial pubis, just lateral to the symphysis.

Sutherland's procedure allows more medialization of the joint. This second osteotomy is relatively easily visualized and has no risk of joint penetration, making his procedure preferable to that of Hopf for most surgeons.

Technique of Sutherland Procedure The innominate osteotomy cut is made first,[84] through the usual oblique groin incision, exactly as described by Salter (Fig. 14–28). The second Sutherland osteotomy line is made with a rongeur, through a separate midline suprapubic incision. A Foley catheter is inserted preoperatively to empty the bladder. The spermatic cord or round ligament is retracted laterally to allow sharp dissection of the rectus abdominis and pyramidalis muscles off the superior pubis just lateral to the symphysis. The adductor longus origin is stripped from the inferior pubis and the location of the symphysis is confirmed radiographically. A Kirschner wire is inserted into

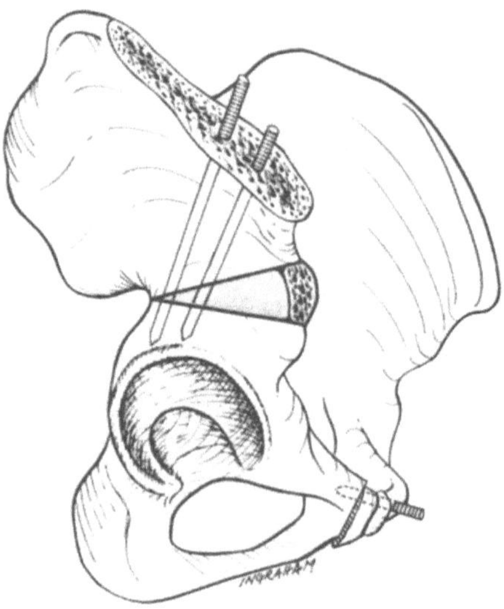

FIG. 14–28 Double innominate osteotomy. Sutherland's osteotomy employs a suprapubic supplementary incision to osteotomize the pubis just lateral to the symphysis. Removing a small wedge allows some joint medialization. The freed pelvic fragment is rotated anterolaterally with towel clips. The pubic osteotomy is pinned under direct vision, followed by routine fixation of the innominate osteotomy. Spica immobilization is routine for 4 to 6 weeks after surgery.

the pubis along the desired osteotomy line between the obturator foramen and the symphysis. A rongeur is used to osteotomize the pubis under direct vision, cutting along the lateral margin of the wire in a caudal direction. The urogenital diaphragm is freed carefully from the inferior pubic cortex in a lateral direction for about 2 cm after the osteotomy is complete.

The mobilized acetabular segment is realigned by using two towel clamps to grip the fragment, with one gripping the ilium below the Salter osteotomy, just superior to the acetabulum, and the second gripping the pubis, just lateral to the pubic osteotomy. The iliac clamp is rotated anteriorly and distally. The medial towel clamp is simultaneously pulled superiorly and medially. This rotates the acetabulum in an anterolateral direction and also medializes it as the gap at the pubic osteotomy is closed. Internal fixation is achieved first in the pubis under direct vision, with a 2.8-mm threaded Steinmann pin traversing the contralateral medial pubis, the symphysis, and passing into the superior pubic ramus across the osteotomy. The Salter iliac osteotomy is stabilized thereafter in the usual manner, with two or three threaded pins transfixing the appropriately shaped interposition bone graft. A spica is necessary for 4 to 6 weeks after surgery. Weight bearing is delayed until 8 weeks after surgery, at which time the pubic pin is removed. The iliac pins may be removed whenever healing is adequate. Sutherland suggests 4 to 6 months following surgery as appropriate.

Sutherland has reported postoperative average improvement in acetabular index of 21° and in center-edge angle of 21°. He noted an average hip joint medialization of 7 mm. His major reported complication was hip ankylosis following simultaneous double innominate osteotomy and double femoral osteotomy in a patient who had preoperative degenerative changes. He emphasizes the need for preoperative joint congruency if double osteotomy is to be successful.

Triple Innominate Osteotomy

LeCoeur,[42] Hopf,[32] Steel,[77-79] and Tönnis[91] have each described basically similar triple innominate osteotomies which supplement the Salter osteotomy with additional cuts through the superior and inferior pubic rami or ischium. The indication is high-grade acetabular maldirection in a joint with good congruence. Tonnis reported average improvements in the C-E angle of between 22 and 32° in three different patient groups. Triple innominate osteotomy theoretically allows more direction than Sutherland's procedure, although its added complexity may be a drawback. The Tonnis and Steel procedures are best described. Each requires an initial buttock incision for the posterior osteotomy.

Technique Tönnis osteotomizes the ischium with the patient prone, approaching the bone by blunt dissection through the gluteus maximus at the ischial tuberosity (Fig. 14–29). He divides the gemelli and obturator internus from their origins to expose the ischium from tuberosity to the sciatic notch. A blunt retractor is placed into the notch to retract the gluteal neurovascular bundle and sciatic nerve superolaterally. A special pair of retractors placed in the obturator foramen allows an oblique ischial osteotomy to be made to connect the ischium and obturator foramen. Tönnis then closes the gluteal wound and finishes the procedure with the patient supine. He osteotomizes the superior pubic ramus in its lateral portion, through an inguinal incision medial to the psoas, retracting the psoas and femoral neurovascular bundle later-

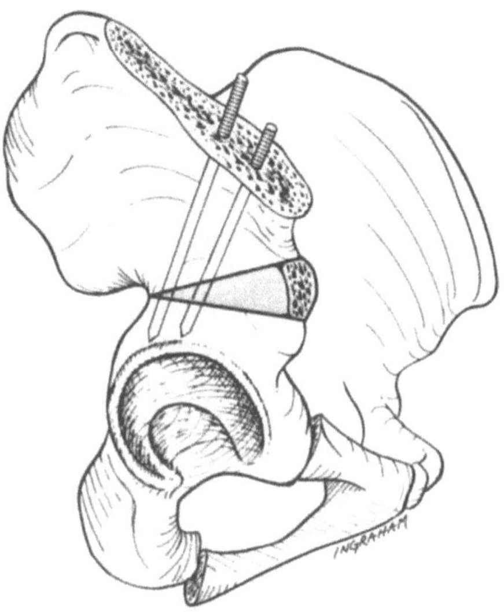

FIG. 14–29 Triple innominate osteotomy. Steele and Tonnis supplement Salter's osteotomy with two additional cuts. A superior pubic osteotomy is made through the medial portion of the anterior incision. The ischial osteotomy is made through a buttock incision. All three osteotomies are made under direct vision. Spica immobilization is routine for 6 to 10 weeks after surgery.

ally. A third incision, through the sartorius–tensor interval, is employed for the osteotomy from the sciatic notch to the anterior inferior iliac spine. This osteotomy ascends from outer to inner cortex, to allow easier rotation of the freed acetabular segment in a lateral and anterior direction.

Image intensifier monitoring is then done to check the correction and confirm that no lateralization of the joint has occurred. Any gaps between the fragments are filled with bone graft, and four Kirschner wires are inserted divergently from the ilium into the acetabular fragment above the joint. A spica is applied for 6 weeks before physical therapy and weight bearing are begun.

Steel also makes the ischial osteotomy through a buttock incision, but with the patient supine and the hip and knee flexed 90°. The ischial tuberosity is exposed subperiosteally, medial to the sciatic nerve, and a kidney pedicle forceps is passed around the ischium deep to the periosteum. This protects the pudendal neurovascular bundle in Alcock's canal. The ischium is then cut posteromedially to anterolaterally. The wound is closed and the patient reprepped and draped. The superior pubic ramus osteotomy is made through an anterior approach, exposing the ramus by flexing the hip and retracting the psoas medially. The psoas tendon can be divided if necessary for exposure. The Salter osteotomy then is made in routine fashion, through the same anterior incision. Interposing bone graft and divergent pinning of the iliac osteotomy are done before closure. Steel suggests at least 8 to 10 weeks of spica immobilization, with gradual rehabilitation to full weight bearing thereafter.

Steel has a large experience of over 200 cases, ranging from age 7 to 38, with a reported 86% incidence of satisfactory results.[79] He reports one important complication, postoperative hypertension, which persisted for 3 months in a patient whose osteotomy had lengthened her limb 2 inches.

Acetabular Osteotomy

The most elegant acetabular redirection is accomplished through spherical periacetabular osteotomy (Fig. 14–30). Blavier and Blavier,[6] Wagner,[95] Tagawa,[86] and Eppright [18,19] have described effective techniques. The amount of redirection possible is virtually unlimited. Several points deserve emphasis, however. First, the volume of the acetabulum remains unchanged, and any increase in anterolateral coverage is at the expense of posteromedial coverage. Second, this highest grade reconstructive procedure requires biological plasticity of the joint to adjust appropriately its microstructure to the large articular reorientation. This requirement may limit the application of this procedure to younger patients not much beyond skeletal maturity. Third, the area of the triradiate cartilage is disrupted by spherical acetabular osteotomy, contraindicating the use of this procedure before skeletal maturity. Last, this procedure demands not only special skill but also special instrumentation.

The proximity of the osteotomy to both the joint and neurovascular structures allows little margin for error. In addition, the indication for the procedure is good present function but poor prognosis. Much is demanded of the surgeon who accepts the responsibility of such extensive delicate hip surgery on the patient with little or no symptoms. Much is also demanded of the patient, in terms of understanding the rationale behind such prophylactic surgery.

From an anatomical point of view, spherical acetabular osteotomy has multiple advantages. Both the direction and the amount of acetabular reorientation are unlimited. The joint can be medialized. The rest of the pelvis is left undistorted. The anterior approach allows quick recovery of normal muscle function. The osteotomy surfaces are broad, congruent, and cancellous; therefore, the osteotomy is sufficiently stabilized by simple osteosynthesis to allow early protected weight bearing without external immobilization.

Acetabular osteotomy is a strictly reconstructive procedure and its indication is therefore quite limited. Its best indication is in a knowledgeable adolescent or young adult with a round femoral head and spherical but quite insufficient acetabulum. Range of motion should be normal, and the radiograph should show a normal cartilage space without any frank degenerative bony changes. Contraindications include an open triradiate cartilage and any characteristics which place the patient in the salvage category.

We prefer the method of Wagner,[95] utilizing his anterior approach and special chisels (Fig. 14–30A). Tagawa's approach [86] allows somewhat better visualization of the ischial portion of the osteotomy, but only at the expense of a much more extensive dissection (going both anterior and posterior to the abductor muscle mass).

There are three basic types of spherical acetabular osteotomy (Fig. 14–30) described by Wagner, the differences being in the manner in which the acetabular fragment is displaced. Type I involves simple rotation of the acetabulum within the congruent osteotomy cavity, usually in an anterolateral direction. Type II adds an element of transiliac lengthening by inferior displacement as well as anterolateral rotation. Either type I or type II osteotomy can add slight joint medialization by deepening the medial wall of the osteotomy cavity before final displacement and fixation. If much medialization is desired, however, type III should be employed.

Type III osteotomy supplements the periacetabular cut with a Chiari-like osteotomy with a Gigli saw, from sciatic notch to the region of the anterior inferior iliac spine. The biomechanical advantages of joint medialization offered by the Chiari procedure are thus combined with the physiological advantages of hyaline cartilage preservation.

Technique - A meticulous anterior approach is critical, with extensive exposure both medial and posterior to the capsule. The supine position allows the best intraoperative image intensifier control. The use of Wagner's spherical chisels is essential. The most serious orthopedic complication is penetration of the joint with the chisel, most likely to occur medially, or fracture of the acetabular fragment. Careful maintenance of at least 15 mm margin from the subchondral edge of the acetabulum and maintenance of capsular integrity will help prevent both these complications and ischemic necrosis of the acetabular fragment.

Surprisingly little rotation of the osteotomized acetabular unit is needed to achieve normalization of even severe malalignment. The partially self-stabilizing osteotomy is internally fixed by a simple osteosynthesis consisting of two specially fashioned semitubular plates, or in type III, by two fashioned Kirschner wires and a connecting special plate.

An atraumatic exposure and closure allow the patient to stand after the first or second postoperative day, and to be walking with partial weight bearing within the first week. Two crutches are maintained for at least 3 months and one crutch for at least 3 additional months. Physical therapy is functional, emphasizing a pain-free, supported gait and gentle isometrics rather than passive range of motion.

Wagner's results are spectacular.[95] In a report of 88 operations, 71 of which were done for a C-E angle of less than 10°, there was achievement of a C-E angle of greater than 20° in 85 hips. Complications were nonexistent except for one hip wound hematoma.

The spherical acetabular osteotomy seems to us the most nearly ideal acetabular reconstructive procedure in the mature patient, as regards both versatility and preservation of function after surgery. A skeletally immature patient, however, with an open triradiate cartilage and severe but congruent acetabular maldirection, must either await skeletal maturity or undergo the alternative double or triple osteotomy. The technical complexity of spherical acetabular osteotomy should greatly limit its use, despite the inherent appeal of the procedure (Fig. 14–31).

Salvage Procedures

The salvage category contains the patient in whom a normal hip prognosis is neither present nor achievable (Table 14–4). Irreversible hip deformation has already occurred. No urgency, therefore, exists, in the absence of symptoms, to institute

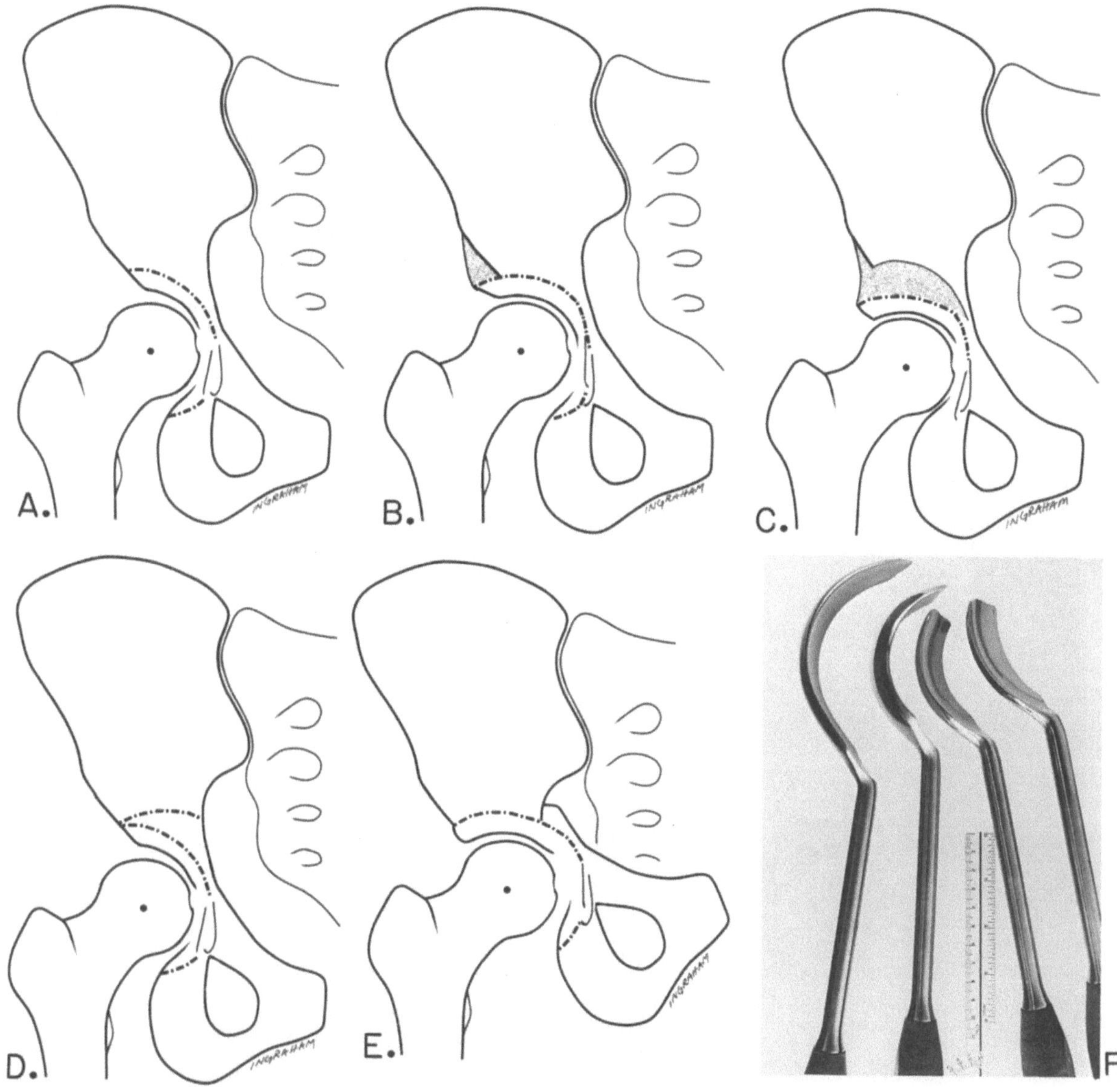

FIG. 14–30 Spherical acetabular osteotomy (Wagner). **A** A spherical periacetabular osteotomy is made 10 to 15 mm from the acetabular cartilage under image intensifier control. The teardrop is split medially. The capsule remains closed. **B** Type I osteotomy employs anterior and lateral acetabular redirection. **C** Type II osteotomy allows supplementary lengthening up to 2 cm. **D** Type III osteotomy employs a second supraacetabular cut to give a Chiari medialization effect in addition to acetabular redirection. **E** Medial displacement of the acetabular bony bed allows the acetabulum to be both redirected anterolaterally and medialized. **F** Wagner's special acetabular chisels.

operative salvage therapy. This is in marked contradistinction to the timing of reconstructive surgery, which must be done before irreversible degenerative changes appear. There is even some positive indication for withholding salvage surgery until the onset of symptoms, because of the limited duration of effectiveness of most salvage procedures.

There is a definite place for nonoperative treatment in the form of patient education, muscle training, avoidance of obesity, and intermittent gait support. A sound nonoperative program may

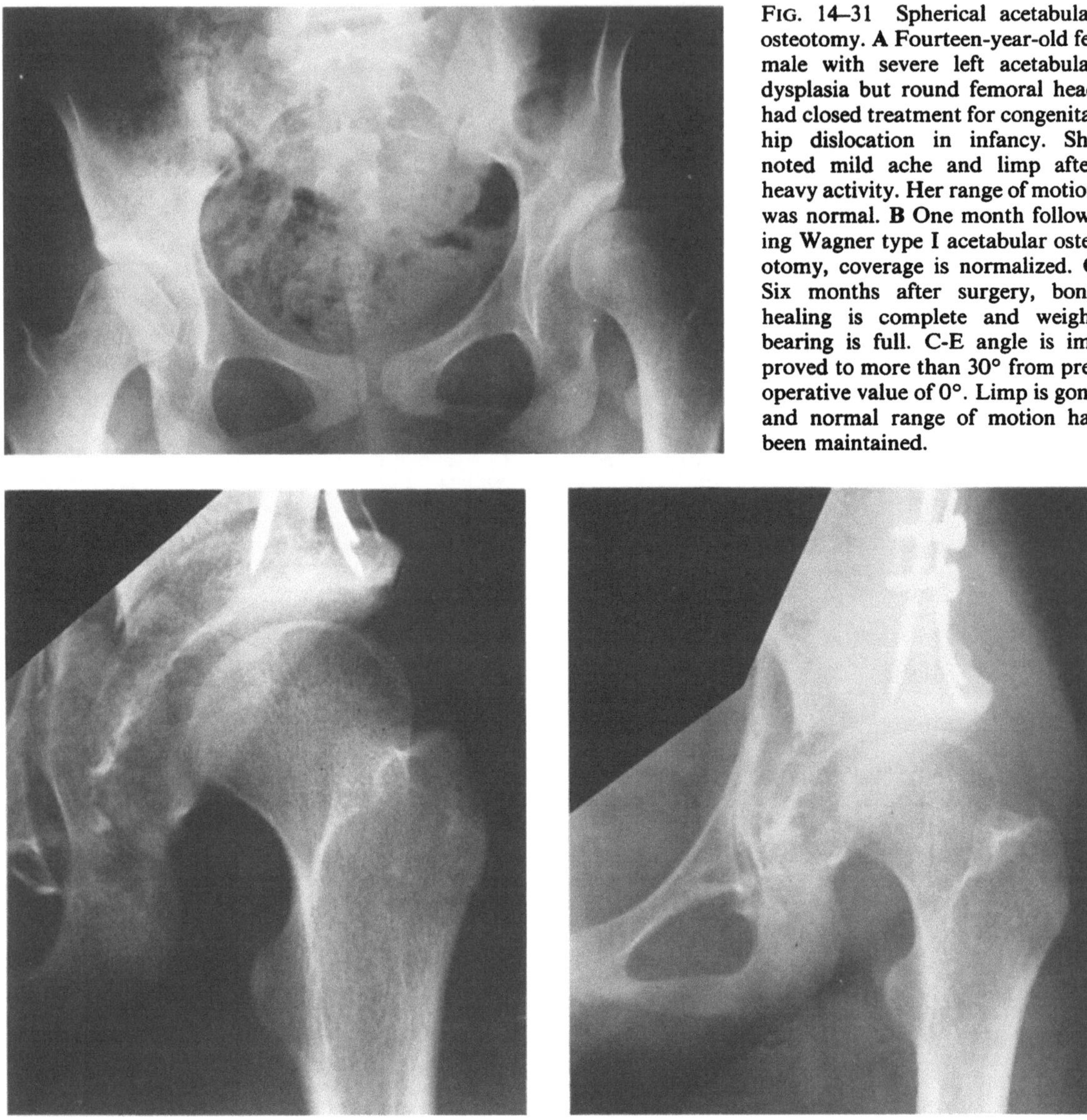

A B C

FIG. 14–31 Spherical acetabular osteotomy. **A** Fourteen-year-old female with severe left acetabular dysplasia but round femoral head had closed treatment for congenital hip dislocation in infancy. She noted mild ache and limp after heavy activity. Her range of motion was normal. **B** One month following Wagner type I acetabular osteotomy, coverage is normalized. **C** Six months after surgery, bony healing is complete and weight bearing is full. C-E angle is improved to more than 30° from preoperative value of 0°. Limp is gone and normal range of motion has been maintained.

improve function and alleviate symptoms enough to delay surgery for years. It is well recognized that residual deformity after CDH can place patients in the symptomatic salvage category at an age much too young to make arthroplasty a happy consideration. The several years gained by a nonoperative treatment program may allow a subsequent osteotomy to suffice for the altered demands of a later period of life.

The overriding principle in salvage osteotomy surgery is the relief of pain and improvement of function by reducing transarticular pressures. This is achieved by an increase in weight-bearing area and reduction in joint forces, often by further distortion of already abnormal anatomy, but without loss of bone stock. Salvage osteotomies usually presuppose at least 60° of flexion–extension and some motion in both the rotatory and abduction–adduction arcs. The patient must be content to remain on crutches for at least 6 months, which allows both the joint and the osteotomy to heal. The patient must also understand that pain relief will probably not be either immediate or complete and that further surgery may be required. He must understand that his active participation is absolutely essential for success.

TABLE 14–4 Osteotomies for Salvage

Procedure	Ideal Salvage Indication	Effect of Osteotomy
Chiari	Painful instability; slightly long limb; superior impingement; any C-E angle	Superior iliac fragment forms weight-bearing roof over capsule; acetabulum is medialized and slightly verticalized; limb is slightly shortened
Simple shelf	Congruent joint with moderate lack of coverage; equal limb lengths; more than 60° of flexion; C-E angle more than 0°	Increases coverage without change in acetabular orientation
Valgization (with or without extension)	Incongruence or impingement improved in adduction; more than 60° of flexion; more than 15° of adduction	Relief of superolateral impingement; possible formation of roof osteophyte; lengthening effect; valgus stress on knee
Varization (rare)	Nearly spherical head with valgus neck; well-developed superolateral acetabulum; incongruence or impingement improved in abduction; more than 60° of flexion; more than 15° of abduction	Limb shortening; initial relaxation of abductors, hamstrings, psoas; varus stress on knee
Trochanteric transfer (Rare)	Short femoral neck; more than 60° of flexion; no improvement of congruence in abduction or adduction	Improvement in abductor mechanics; secondary reduction in transarticular forces

Short-term satisfaction is certainly not so great for either the surgeon or the patient after salvage osteotomy as after replacement arthroplasty. Contemplation of the long-term result, however, is of utmost importance. Heinz Wagner spoke to the surgeon caring for the salvage hip patient when he said, "Consider not only the first operation on the hip, but also the second operation. Try to match the lifetime of the operation to the lifetime of the patient." [96] Maurice Muller also spoke eloquently: "The best hip replacement has an unknown but certainly finite life whereas a hip healed after osteotomy will often last a lifetime." [52]

Salvage procedures on the acetabular side consist of the various shelf operations. The pelvic osteotomy of Chiari is a special shelf procedure, which also medializes the entire joint. The best indication for the shelf procedure is hip pain associated with bony instability in the form of a reasonably normally shaped proximal femur under an insufficient acetabulum. In addition, loss of cartilage space is located superiorly and any incongruence persists with either abduction or adduction of the femur. If abduction or adduction creates better congruence, then varus or valgus intertrochanteric osteotomy should be considered instead of the shelf.

A supplemental shelf fashioned with an iliac graft applied to the anterolateral capsule may suffice for years of pain relief if the C-E angle is not less than 0°. More severe lack of coverage of femoral head deformity argues for a Chiari osteotomy, with or without a femoral osteotomy, to provide both medialization of the joint and a supplemental roof over the capsule.

All shelf procedures presume that extending the acetabulum laterally with bone graft applied to the superior surface of the joint capsule will promote capsular metaplasia into fibrocartilage. If such fibrocartilage forms and is in a position to bear weight, then the functional area of the acetabulum is increased and the joint pressures are reduced. Fibrocartilage must be presumed to have a limited life span, hence the probability of a limited period of pain relief (considered by some to be 15 to 20 years).

There are many different techniques for the shelf procedure in current use. Common to all effective procedures are (1) broad contact of the shelf with the capsule; (2) load sharing by the shelf without undue force concentration onto a small area of the shelf; and (3) postoperative functional treatment to encourage joint remodeling.

Technique of Shelf Procedure In the Zeiler–Wagner procedure,[103] an anterior approach allows good visualization of the superior capsule without injury to the abductors. The reflected head of the rectus femoris is dissected off the capsule in a distal direction. The capsule is meticulously peeled downward off the ilium to the thin prominence marking the edge of the true acetabulum. A single full-thickness iliac bone graft, roughly 5 × 7 cm, is removed from the ilium posterior and superior to the joint, leaving a 2-cm rim of ilium intact between graft site and crest. The concave side of the graft is laid on the hip capsule. A 1-cm-deep slot the thickness of the bone graft is cut into the ilium just above the subchondral edge of the superior acetabulum. The bone chips are saved for graft.

The iliac graft is appropriately trimmed with a rongeur and set into the slot, projecting anterolaterally and distally under the capsule. A Kirschner wire is drilled under image intensifier control medially through the graft and into the supraacetabular ilium for provisional fixation. Two special pronged plates are inserted to maintain the graft in position, and the Kirschner wire is then removed (Fig. 14–32). Range of motion is checked and the graft repositioned or trimmed as necessary. The bone chips taken from the slot are laid onto the shelf. A final radiograph is taken before closure.

The patient uses two crutches, bearing 20–25% of body weight, for 3 months, and one crutch for 3 months thereafter.

Other Shelf Procedure Techniques Staheli,[74] Wilson,[102] and Kumar [39] prefer to thin the thickened joint capsule to appose a partial-thickness cortical-cancellous iliac slab more closely to the femoral head. The slab is slotted into the ilium between the reflected rectus and the peeled-down capsule, and cancellous graft is applied on top of the iliac slab. The shelf should create a C-E angle of about 30°. The capsular flap is sutured partly over the graft, but no internal fixation is used by Staheli or Kumar. Wilson uses a single Kirschner wire for fixation of a supplemental triangular iliac strut to hold the shelf down.

Kumar uses spica immobilization for about 6 weeks, with progressive weight bearing thereafter.

Chiari Procedure The medial displacement pelvic osteotomy of Chiari [12,13,15] is indicated at almost any age as a salvage procedure when painful instability is severe, with a C-E angle less than zero, especially if slight adduction of the femur leads to greater joint congruence (Fig. 14–33). As with other salvage osteotomies, at least 60° of flexion–extension arc should be present, and some range in the other arcs of motion. When compared with simple shelf procedures, Chiari osteotomy has both advantages and disadvantages. Advantages include the relatively unlimited amount of displacement possible, with the full thickness of superior ilium coming to lie on the exposed capsule as the joint is medialized. The medialization of the joint also reduces the force across the joint. Disadvantages include the following: (1) The acetabular hyaline cartilage is verticalized as the joint is medialized, removing it partially from the weight-bearing function. This could be an advantage only if a superior point of impingement is removed from the femoral head by this acetabular verticalization. (2) Coverage is poorest anteriorly (because of the narrowness of the anterior ilium), where it is usually most needed.[15] This often necessitates supplemental interposition of iliac graft on the exposed capsule between the acetabular edge and the lateralized superior iliac shelf. (3) The osteotomy has a shortening effect on the limb.

We and others have modified Chiari's original technique to allow better anterolateral coverage and early postoperative ambulation without immobilization.

TECHNIQUE FOR MODIFIED CHIARI OSTEOTOMY The anterior approach allows complete pericapsular visualization and, after subperiosteal exposure to both sides of the ilium, safe retraction of the sciatic notch structures with Lane bone levers or a Hohmann retractor (Fig. 14–34).[27,96] As with any shelf procedure, adherent capsule must be peeled off the ilium down to the level of the joint and the desired osteotomy level confirmed radiographically. A Gigli saw is employed to start

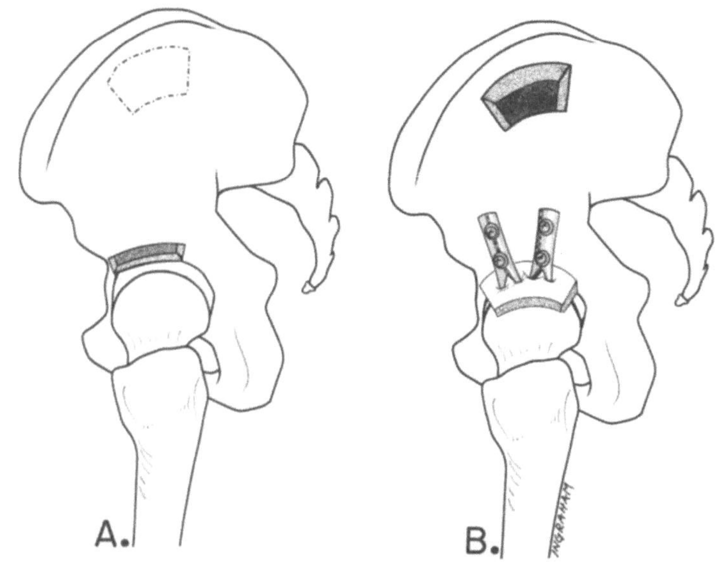

FIG. 14–32 Shelf procedure (Zeiler–Wagner). **A** The anterior and superior capsule is exposed meticulously. A 1-cm-deep slot is cut into the ilium at the level of the junction of the superior capsule with the true acetabular rim. Full-thickness iliac graft, about 5 × 7 cm, is taken from the ilium, just below the crest. **B** The bone graft is trimmed, pushed into the slot, and appropriately positioned for optimal contact with the capsule, concave side down. Provisional fixation is with Kirschner wires. Definitive fixation is with pronged plates and screws. **C** This 13-year-old male had multiple previous operations for congenital hip dislocation. He had mild limitation of motion, an abductor limp, and slight shortening. His aspherical femoral head was poorly covered, but he was free of pain. **D** A shelf procedure of Zeiler–Wagner type provided femoral head coverage without disturbing the reasonably congruous relationship between the acetabulum and the medial surface of the head.

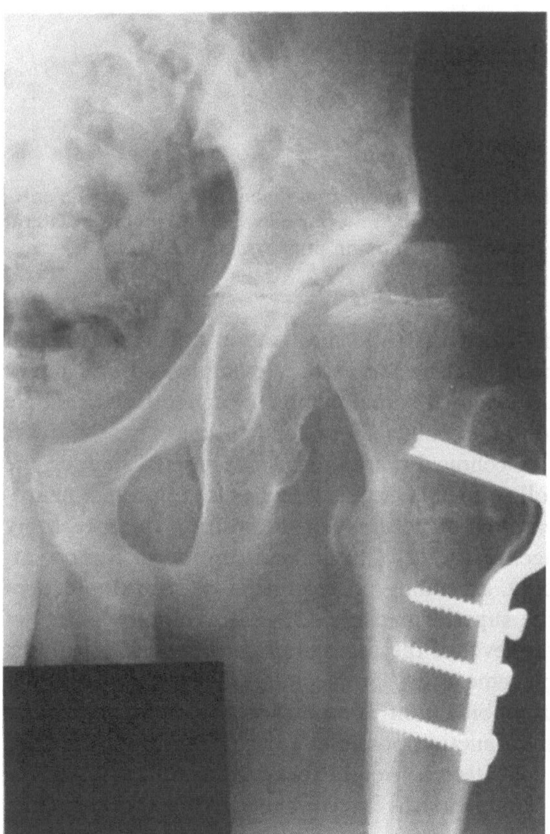

C.

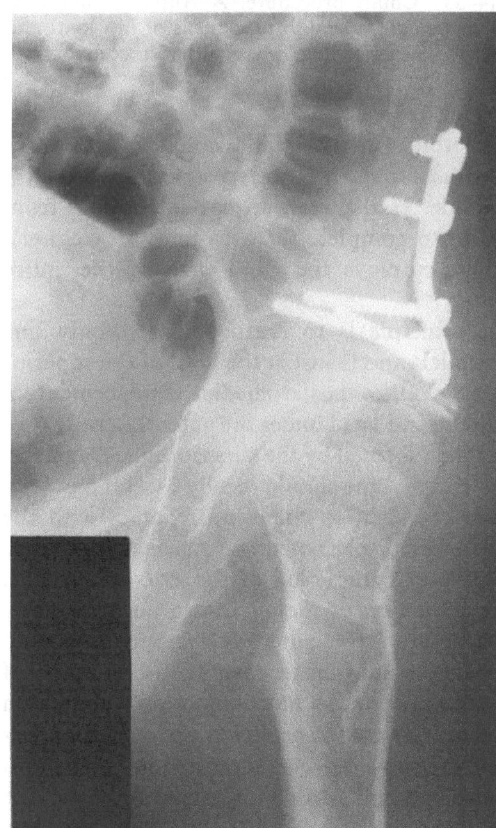

D.

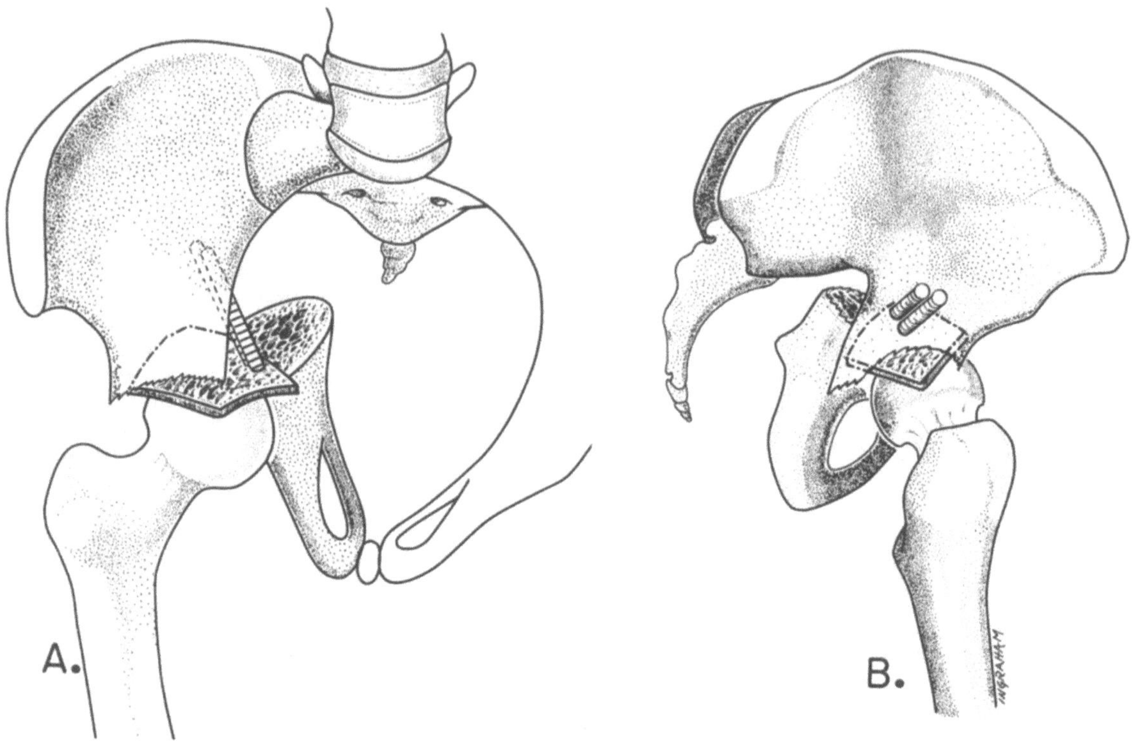

FIG. 14–33 Chiari procedure. **A** Anteromedial view shows the posteromedial displacement of hip joint and capsule. The superior iliac fragment lies in contact with the capsule. Supplemental iliac bone graft fills the anterior gap over the anterior capsule. **B** The anterolateral view shows Steinmann pins passing medial to the joint.

the osteotomy in the sciatic notch and to work forward as far as the posterosuperior corner of the capsule. Hall prefers to use osteotomes from this point to complete the osteotomy.[27] Wagner's technique employs the Gigli saw for the entire osteotomy.[96]

The principle is to create an osteotomy line that parallels and is just at the level of the superior capsule, to allow posteromedial displacement of the capsule and head under the anterolaterally projecting shelf formed by the superior iliac fragment. The osteotomy line should ideally ascend medially to allow the shelf to come into contact with the capsule after displacement. Displacement is easy to achieve at completion of the osteotomy, with simple abduction of the leg and a push medially on the greater trochanter. Displacement should be enough to normalize coverage (C-E angle of 30 to 40°), but not so much as to limit abduction or flexion. Areas of capsule left uncovered anteriorly are then covered with supplemental iliac graft. Medial displacement of more than 100% of the width of the ilium is possible and often desirable, provided that internal fixation and supplemental bone grafting are used. We employ several heavy threaded Steinmann pins; Wagner uses a single long cancellous screw for fixation.

Technical points to be emphasized include the following: (1) Extensive exposure to protect neurovascular structures and to position the osteotomy accurately. (2) Curvilinear attitude of the osteotomy, ascending posteromedially from the level of the superior capsule. (3) Radiographic control of the level of the osteotomy and the amount of displacement. (4) Stable internal fixation to render immobilization unnecessary and early postoperative function possible.

Protected weight bearing with crutches for about 6 months is recommended after surgery (Fig. 14–35).

Intertrochanteric Osteotomy for Salvage Intertrochanteric osteotomy (Fig. 14–36) is indicated occasionally as a salvage procedure in painful coxarthrosis secondary to hip dysplasia.[7] A good range of motion must always be present, and joint incon-

FIG. 14–34 Chiari osteotomy. **A** Chisels are directed superiorly, medially, and posteriorly along a curved osteotomy line exactly at the capsular insertion. **B** Following medial displacement of the joint, the raw inferior osteotomy surface covers and is in contact with the capsule. **C** Supplemental bone graft fills the anterior gap between the fragments. Steinmann pins fix the fragments and allow early protected ambulation.

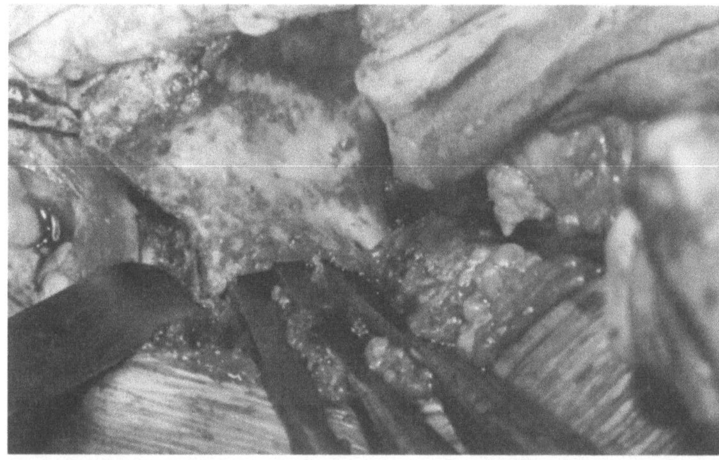

A

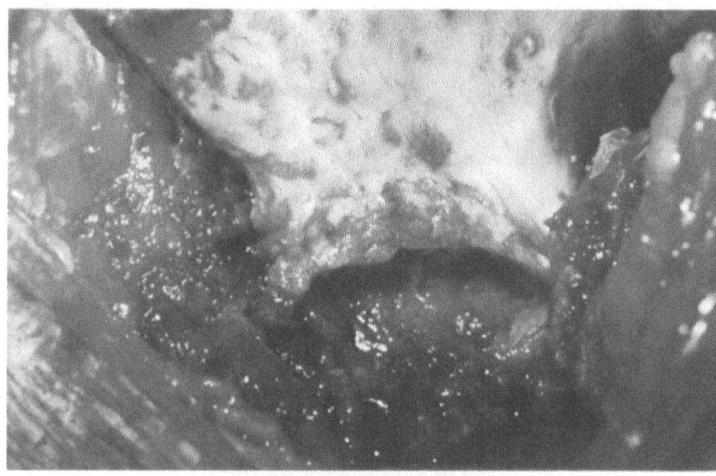

B

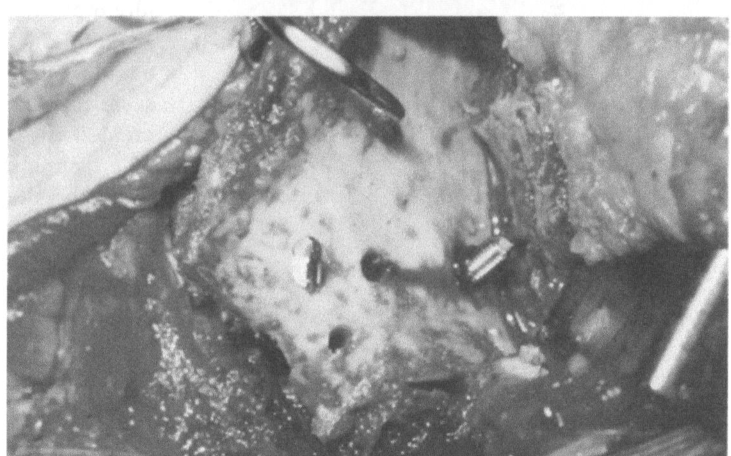

C

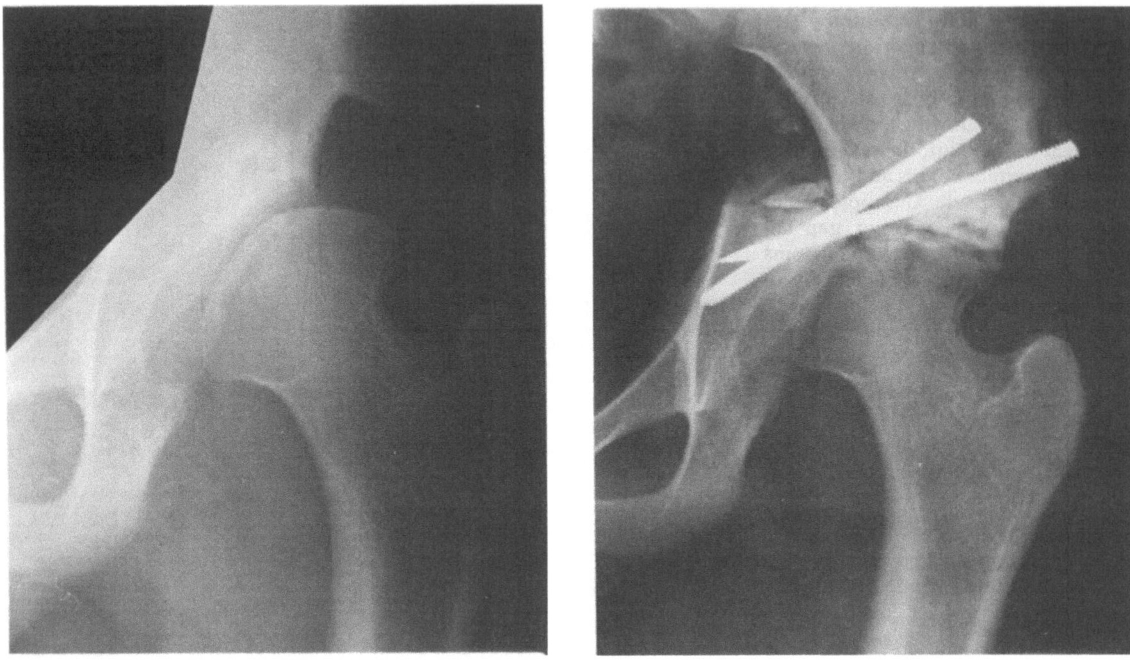

A

B

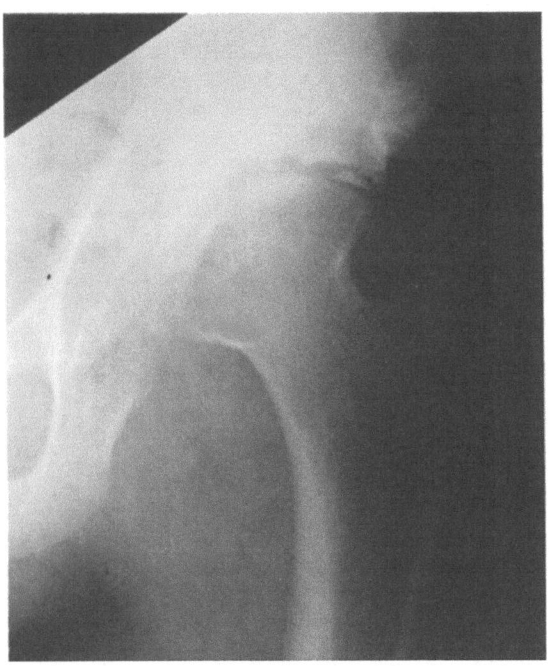

C

FIG. 14–35 **A** Chiari osteotomy. Fourteen-year-old female with painful, incongruent left hip subluxation. Ninety degrees of hip flexion is present. Operative photographs shown in Fig. 14–34. **B** Coverage shown 3 months following surgery. **C** Radiographic result at 1 year is shown. Limp and pain are gone, and range of motion has been preserved.

gruence should be ameliorated by some position of abduction or adduction.

If congruence is improved and areas of superolateral impingement are relieved in adduction, and flexion in adduction is comfortable, then valgus osteotomy has a good indication. With valgus osteotomy, lateralization of the distal fragment is usually indicated to avoid valgus stresses on the knee. In addition, enough bone should be removed to avoid a lengthening effect, because arthritic joints seem unusually sensitive to the increased stresses created by the lengthening effect of valgization. The technique of valgus osteotomy for salvage is basically the same as for reconstruction. The amount of valgization, by the method of Wagner, is judged to be that which renders the head and acetabulum most congruent with the leg in the weight-bearing position. Wagner employs a 95° condylar plate for osteosynthesis, with one long screw and blade in the proximal fragment.[96] In the dysplastic form of coxarthrosis, Bombelli has noted that valgus osteotomy is frequently indicated and varus osteotomy rarely indicated.[7] Bombelli considers valgus and some extension to be important in the usual case, and he considers increased congruence in adduction not decisive. He has noted the usual gradual improvement of congruence by hypertrophy of acetabular and femoral

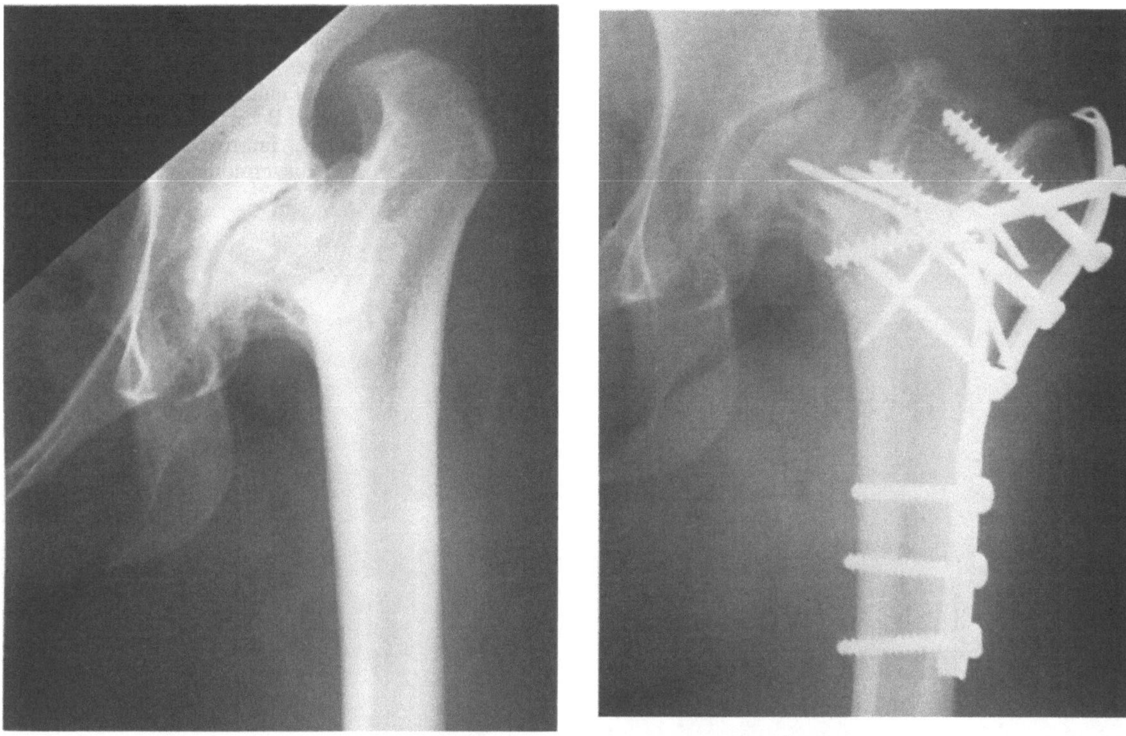

A B

FIG. 14–36 **A** Intertrochanteric osteotomy for salvage. This 25-year-old female with left hip pain, limp, and severe deformity had good range of motion, with flexion to 85° but limited abduction. **B** Valgus intertrochanteric osteotomy with supplemental trochanteric transfer relieved her symptoms and improved her gait by both improving abductor mechanics and reducing joint pressures by eliminating superolateral impingement.

head osteophytes after valgus extension intertrochanteric osteotomy, as long as more than 30° of flexion and 15° of adduction are present preoperatively. Bombelli employs a 130° angled blade plate for fixation. He routinely osteotomizes the tip of the greater trochanter and sections the iliopsoas. Gait is with two crutches for 6 months. Supplementary Chiari osteotomy may be indicated on occasion, if the desired amount of valgization renders the joint unstable.

VARUS OSTEOTOMY FOR SALVAGE Varus osteotomy seems rarely indicated as a *salvage* procedure after hip dysplasia, in contradistinction to its relatively frequent indication in early reconstruction. Bombelli limits its use to cases where osteophytes have not yet appeared, the acetabulum is sufficient (i.e., good lateral coverage), and the femoral neck is in a valgus attitude. In such rare cases, where a round femoral head that lies in valgus is in better contact and in more congruence with the acetabulum in abduction, varus osteotomy for salvage is indicated. In clinics where a relatively large number of osteotomies are carried out around the hip in salvage situations, only a small fraction of intertrochanteric osteotomies are of varization type.[7,96]

Operative technique for varus osteotomy in salvage situations is identical to that for reconstruction. Enough varization should be carried out to produce the attitude of best joint congruence with the leg in the weight-bearing position. The 90° trochanteric blade plate is used, with medial displacement of the distal fragment to avoid creation of pathological varus stresses across the knee and increased bending stresses in the femoral neck.

TROCHANTERIC TRANSFER FOR SALVAGE Transfer of the greater trochanter in a distal and lateral direction is a salvage procedure with rare but definite indications in the treatment of dysplastic coxarthrosis. In the salvage patient with no indication for either intertrochanteric osteotomy or arthroplasty, and pain persisting after nonoperative therapy, a distal and lateral greater trochanteric transfer may be useful if the femoral neck is short. It may reduce forces across the joint enough to relieve pain in this very specific situation

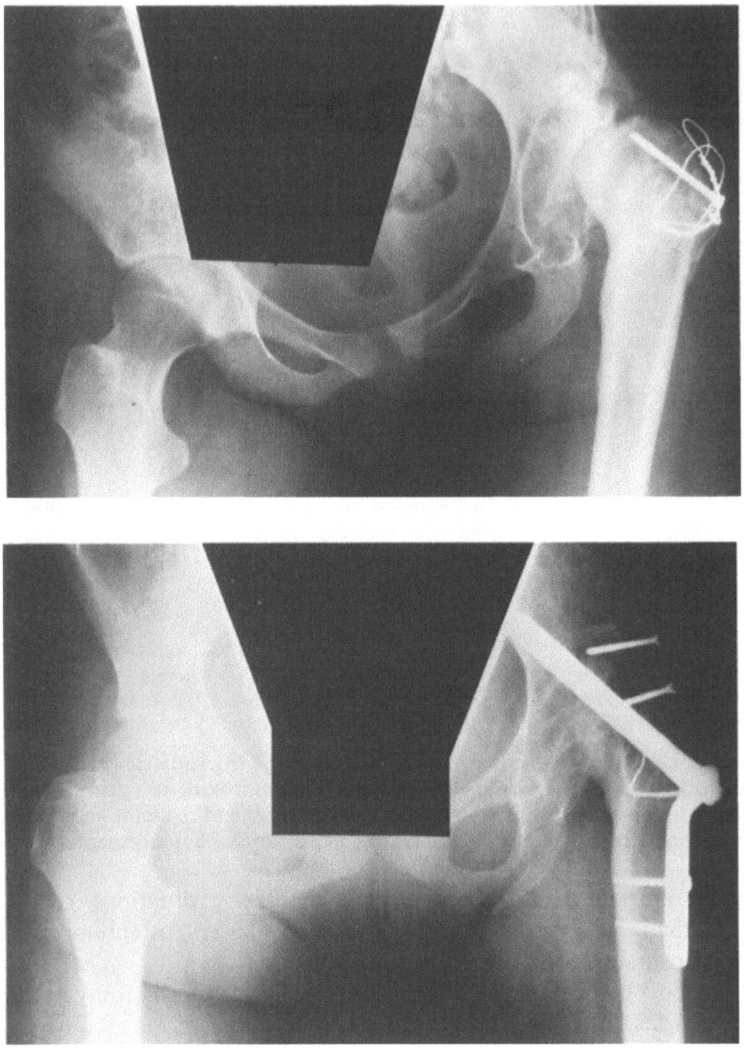

A

B

FIG. 14–37 **A** Seventeen-year-old female with painful adducted hip, severe subluxation, incongruity, loss of motion, and loss of cartilage space. **B** Arthrodesis normalized stance, improved gait, and eliminated symptoms.

where abductor efficiency can be increased mechanically.

Arthrodesis In the occasional unfortunate young patient, severe complications from treatment of hip dysplasia may lead to both destruction of function and of the relatively modest capacity for biological plasticity that is required for salvage osteotomies to be of use. The clinical setting is that of pain with hip function, great restriction of hip motion, irreversible joint incongruence, thinning of cartilage space, and subchondral sclerosis. Nonoperative therapy in the form of muscle training, achievement of ideal body weight, and a trial at protected weight bearing should have been tried.

In this clinical situation, even in this era of increasingly sophisticated arthroplasties, the hip arthrodesis is a very reasonable consideration, particularly in the male patient. If the lumbar spine and ipsilateral knee are normal, then a solid hip fusion in good position can provide many years of painless support (Fig. 14–37).

We have preferred combinations of intraarticular and extraarticular fusion techniques, employing moderately rigid internal fixation supplemented by a spica cast for the first 2 to 3 postoperative months. We have hesitated using the relatively massive rigid internal fixation offered by the Cobra plate for fear of damaging the abductor muscles. The integrity of the abductor muscles is of paramount importance if the hip arthrodesis should be taken down at a future date and converted to an arthroplasty.

Special Problems

Ischemic Necrosis

Ischemic damage incurred during early treatment of the congenitally dislocated hip is an all too frequent complication. Delay in appearance of the capital femoral secondary ossification center, broadening of the femoral neck, and fragmentation or irregularity of the epiphysis are a few of the early radiographic signs that such vascular insult has occurred.

In the presence of such signs, most authors suggest part-time abduction splinting in the young child, beyond what would be done for stability of the hip joint itself. The principle of containment is employed as in Perthes' disease. After epiphyseal reossification is complete, splinting is discontinued.

Late treatment awaits the development of deformity. Ogden [11] and Kalamchi [35] have both classified patterns of postischemic proximal femoral maldevelopment. The mildest deformity requiring surgical intervention consists of femoral neck shortening without much alteration of neck–shaft angle and relative trochanteric overgrowth. This requires either early trochanteric epiphysiodesis, or preferably, trochanteric transfer at maturity, when definitive proximal femoral realignment can be done.

Most severe deformity occurs after lateral physeal growth arrest (Ogden type II), when epiphyseal valgus orientation complicates neck shortening and relative trochanteric overgrowth. This deformity usually requires double intertrochanteric osteotomy, combining varization and distal and lateral transfer of the greater trochanter.

The most severe postischemic deformities follow the Ogden type III pattern. If the femoral head is round, then femoral reconstruction of the more complex Wagner double osteotomy type should be carried out.[94] Acetabular dysplasia is usually present in this situation and requires treatment as well.

Most patients who require hip surgery for postischemic deformity have measurable ipsilateral femoral shortening. Separate consideration of this problem is important, as well.

Leg Length Inequality

Ipsilateral limb shortening produces relative abduction of the hip in stance. Occasionally the extra femoral head coverage given by slight femoral shortening may be useful to preserve.

Particularly in cases with residual acetabular dysplasia accompanied by significant (1 inch or more) femoral shortening, we have found it useful to restore postural balance and stance by limb lengthening above the joint, rather than with epiphysiodesis on the contralateral side or an ipsilateral shoe lift. We have employed a modified innominate osteotomy,[50] utilizing a trapezoidal iliac graft to provide both acetabular redirection and up to 3 cm of effective limb lengthening. Such "transiliac limb lengthening" can also be achieved through a Wagner type II acetabular osteotomy,[95] and the technical details of both procedures are described above.

Contralateral epiphysiodesis is rarely indicated for secondary leg length inequality following complications of congenital hip dislocation treatment. We consider transiliac limb lengthening [50] usually preferable to epiphysiodesis if any limb length equalization surgery is needed.

Femoral lengthening is rarely indicated following treatment of idiopathic congenital hip dislocation, in contradistinction to congenital femoral hypoplasia or congenital coxa vara. In any case, only if the hip is anatomically and functionally normalized, and a femoral shortening of 4 cm or more persists, should femoral lengthening be considered.

Following the treatment of congenital hip dislocation, rarely will the ipsilateral leg be longer than a normal leg, although some overgrowth and coxa magna may be seen following open reduction. In bilateral cases, however, it is not so rare for therapy to be directed at the longer side, particularly since the longer leg tends to lie relatively adducted in stance. In the situation where increased femoral head coverage is needed, and yet shortening is an object, both varus intertrochanteric osteotomy and Chiari osteotomy should be considered, since both inherently shorten the limb. In addition, a modified innominate osteotomy can provide transiliac shortening, as has been described by Kalamchi.[34]

Acknowledgements

I am deeply grateful to Professors John Hall and Heinz Wagner for continuing guidance, support, and inspiration. The further assistance of Ms. D. Federman, Ms. B. Ingraham, and Mr. J. Koepfler is also appreciated.

Bibliography

1. Andren, L., and VonRosen, S.: The diagnosis of dislocation of the hip in newborn and the primary result of immediate treatment. Acta Radiol., 49:69, 1958.
2. Ashley, R. K., Larsen, L. J., and James, P. M.: Reduction of dislocation of the hip in older children. J. Bone Joint Surg., 54A:545, 1972.
3. Barlow, T. G.: Early diagnosis and treatment of congenital dislocation of the hip. J. Bone Joint Surg., 44B:292, 1962.
4. Becker, F.: Die Konservative Behandlung der HuftDysplasie und Huftverrenkung. Z. Orthop., 106:173, 1969.
5. Benson, M. K. D., and Evans, D. C. J.: The pelvic osteotomy of Chiari: An anatomical study of hazards and misleading radiographic appearances. J. Bone Joint Surg., 58B:164, 1976.
6. Blavier, L., and Blavier, J.: Traitement de la subluxation de la hanche. Chir. Orthop., 48:208, 1962.
7. Bombelli, R.: Osteoarthritis of the Hip. New York, Springer-Verlag, 1976.
8. Browning, W. H., Rosenkrantz, H., and Tarquinio, T.: Computed tomography in congenital hip dislocation. J. Bone Joint Surg., 64A:27, 1982.
9. Buchanan, J. B., Greer, R. B., and Cutler, J. M.: Management strategy for prevention of avascular necrosis during treatment of congenital dislocation of the hip. J. Bone Joint Surg., 63A:140, 1981.
10. Bucholz, R. W., Ezaki, M., and Ogden, J. A.: Injury to the acetabular triradiate cartilage. J. Bone Joint Surg., 64A:600, 1982.
11. Bucholz, R. W., and Ogden, J. A.: Patterns of ischemic necrosis of the proximal femur in nonoperatively treated congenital hip disease. In: The Hip, Vol. 6, St. Louis, Mosby, 1978, pp. 43–63.

11a. Chachal, G.: Indications for various types of pelvic osteotomy. Clin. Orthop. 98:111–115, 1974.

12. Chiari, K.: Ergebnisse mit Der Beckenosteotomie Als Pfannendachplastik. Z. Orthop., 87:14, 1955.
13. Chiari, K.: Medial displacement osteotomy of the pelvis. Clin. Orthop., 98:155, 1974.
14. Coleman, S. S.: Congenital dysplasia and dislocation of the hip. St. Louis, Mosby, 1978.
15. Colton, C. L.: Chiari osteotomy for acetabular dysplasia in young subjects. J. Bone Joint Surg., 54B:578, 1972.
16. Dega, W.: Development and clinical importance of the dysplastic acetabulum. Progr. Orthop. Surg., 2:47, 1978.
17. Dunn, P. M.: Perinatal observations on the etiology of congenital dislocation of the hip. Clin. Orthop., 119:11, 1976.

17a. Edgren, W.: Coxa plana. Acta Orthop. Scand. Suppl. 84, 1965.

17b. Eilert, R., Chang, F., Rosenberg, R.: The dynamic closed treatment of congenital dislocation of the hip. Exhibit, American Academy of Orthopaedic Surgeons Annual Meeting, 1983.

18. Eppright, R. H.: Dial osteotomy of the acetabulum in the treatment of dysplasia of the hip. In: International Symposium on Congenital Hip Pathology, Royal Oak, Michigan, 1974.
19. Eppright, R. H.: Dial osteotomy of the acetabulum in the treatment of dysplasia of the hip. J. Bone Joint Surg., 57A:1172, 1975.
20. Ferguson, A. B., Jr.: Primary open reduction of congenital dislocation of the hip using a medial adductor approach. J. Bone Joint Surg., 55A:681, 1973.
21. Ferguson, A. B., Jr.: Primary recognition and treatment of congenital dislocation of the hip. Pediar. Ann., 5:28, 1976.
22. Ferguson, A. B., Jr.: Treatment of congenital dislocation of the hip in infancy using the medial approach. In Tachdjian, M. O. (ed.): Congenital Dislocation of the Hip. New York, Churchill Livingstone, 1982, pp. 283–292.
23. Gage, J. R., and Cary, J. M.: The effects of trochanteric epiphyseodesis on growth of the proximal end of the femur following necrosis of the capital femoral epiphysis. J. Bone Joint Surg., 62A:785, 1980.
24. Gage, J. R., and Winter, R. B.: Avascular necrosis of the capital femoral epiphysis as a complication of closed reduction of congenital dislocation of the hip. J. Bone Joint Surg., 54A:373, 1972.
25. Gill, A. B.: An evaluation of present-day methods of dealing with congenital dislocation of the hip. J. Bone Joint Surg., 18:487, 1936.
26. Grech, P.: Hip Arthrography. Philadelphia, Lippincott, 1977.
27. Hall, J. E., and Bailey, T.: Chiari osteotomy. J. Bone Joint Surg., in press.
28. Hall, J. E., and Homes, J. C.: Late management of congenital hip disease. In: The Hip, Vol. 8. St. Louis, Mosby, 1980, pp. 245–277.
29. Hall, J. E., and Karlin, L.: Unpublished data.
30. Harris, H. H.: Acetabular growth potential in congenital dislocation of the hip and some factors

upon which it may depend. Clin. Orthop., 119:99, 1976.
31. Harris, N. H., Lloyd-Roberts, G. C., and Gallien, R.: Acetabular development in congenital dislocation of the hip. J. Bone Joint Surg., 57B:46, 1975.
32. Hopf, A. von: Huftpfannenverlagerung durch doppelte Beckenosteotomie zur Behandlung Huftgelenksdysplasie und Subluxation bei Jugendlichen und Erwachsenen. Z. Orthop., 101: 559, 1966.
33. Hughes, J. R.: Acetabular dysplasia and acetabuloplasty. In Tachdjian, M. O. (ed.): Congenital Dislocation of the Hip. New York, Churchill Livingstone, 1982, pp. 665–693.
34. Kalamchi, A.: Modified Salter osteotomy. J. Bone Joint Surg., 64A:183, 1982.
35. Kalamchi, A., and MacEwen, G. D.: Avascular necrosis following congenital dislocation of the hip. J. Bone Joint Surg., 62A:876, 1980.
36. Kalamchi, A., Schmidt, T., and MacEwen, G. D.: Congenital dislocation of the hip: open reduction by the medial approach. Clin. Orthop., 169:127, 1982.
37. Klisic, P.: Open reduction with femoral shortening and pelvic osteotomy. In Tachdjian M. O. (ed.): Congenital Dislocation of the Hip, New York, Churchill Livingstone, 1982, pp. 417–426.
38. Klisic, P., and Jankovic, L.: Combined procedure of open reduction and shortening of the femur in treatment of congenital dislocation of the hips in older children. Clin. Orthop., 119:60, 1976.
39. Kumar, S. J., and MacEwen, G. D.: Shelf operation. In Tachdjian, M. O. (ed.): Congenital Dislocation of the Hip. New York, Churchill Livingstone, 1982, pp. 695–704.
40. Lang, J., and Wachsmith, W.: Praktische Anatomie, Ister Band, 4er teil: Bein und Statik, Berlin, Springer-Verlag, 1972.
41. Langenskjold, A., and Salenius, P.: Epiphyseodesis of the greater trochanter. Acta Orthop. Scand. 38:199, 1967.
42. LeCoeur, P.: Osteotomie isthmique de bascule. In: Beckenosteotomie Pfannendachplastik. Stuttgart, Thieme, 1965, p. 112.
43. Liechti, R.: Hip Arthrodesis and Associated Problems. New York, Springer-Verlag, 1978.
44. Lindstrom, J. R., Ponseti, I. V., and Wenger, D. R.: Acetabular development after reduction in congenital dislocation of the hip. J. Bone Joint Surg., 61A:112, 1979.
45. Lloyd-Roberts, G. C., Harris, N. H., and Chrispin, A. R.: Anteversion of the acetabulum in congenital dislocation of the hip. Orthop. Clin. North Am., 9:89, 1978.
46. Ludloff, K.: The open reduction of the congenital hip dislocation by an anterior incision. Am. J. Orthop. Surg., 10:438, 1912.
47. Machasek, F., and Salzer, M.: Ergebnisse der OffenenHuftgelenks-repoisition nach Ludloff. Beitr. Orthop. Traumatol., 24:1, 1977.
48. Marafioti, R. G., and Westin, G. W.: Factors influencing the result of acetabuloplasty in children. J. Bone Joint Surg., 62A:765, 1980.
49. Mau, H., et al.: Open reduction of congenital dislocation of the hips by Ludloff's method. J. Bone Joint Surg., 53A:1281, 1971.
50. Millis, M. B., and Hall, J. E.: Transiliac lengthening of the lower extremity. J. Bone Joint Surg., 61A:1182, 1979.
50a. Morscher, E.: Our experiences with Salter's innominate osteotomy in the treatment of hip dysplasia. Progr. Orthop. Surg. 2:107, 1978.
51. Mubarak, S., et al.: Pitfalls in the use of the Pavlik harness for treatment of congenital dysplasia, subluxation, and dislocation of the hip. J. Bone Joint Surg., 63A:1239, 1981.
52. Muller, M.: Foreword. In Bombelli, R. (ed.): Osteoarthritis of the Hip. New York, Springer-Verlag, 1976.
53. Muller, M. E., Allgower, M., Schneider, R., and Willenegger, H.: Manual of Internal Fixation. New York, Springer-Verlag, 1979.
54. Ogden, J. A.: Changing patterns of proximal femoral vascularity. J. Bone Joint Surg., 56A:941, 1974.
55. Ogden, J. A.: Treatment positions for congenital dysplasia of the hip. J. Pediatr., 86:732, 1975.
56. Ogden, J. A., and Moss, H. L. Pathologic anatomy of congenital hip disease. Progr. Orthop. Surg., 2:3, 1978.
57. Ortolani, M.: Congenital hip dysplasia in the light of early and very early diagnosis. Clin. Orthop. 119:6, 1976.
58. Pauwels, F.: Biomechanics of the normal and diseased hip. New York, Springer-Verlag, 1976.
59. Pavlik, A.: Die Funktionelle Behandlungsmethode mittels Riembenbugel als Prinzip der konservativen Therapie bei angeborenen Huftgelelenksverrenkungen der Sauglinge. Orthop., 89: 341, 1957.
60. Pemberton, P.: Pericapsular osteotomy in the treatment of congenital dislocation of the hip. J. Bone Joint Surg., 47A:65, 1965.
61. Peterson, H. A., et al.: The use of computed tomography in dislocation of the hip and femoral neck anteversion in children. In Tachdjian, M. O. (ed.): Congenital Dislocation of the Hip. New York, Churchill Livingstone, 1982, pp. 263–282.
62. Ponseti, I. V.: Growth and development of the acetabulum in the normal child. J. Bone Joint Surg., 60A:575, 1978.
63. Ponseti, I. V.: Morphology of the acetabulum in

congenital dislocation of the hip. J. Bone Joint Surg., 60A:586, 1978.
64. Rab, G. T.: Biomechanical aspects of Salter osteotomy. Clin. Orthop., 132:82, 1978.
65. Rab, G. T.: Preoperative roentgenographic evaluation for osteotomies about the hip in children. J. Bone Joint Surg., 63A:306, 1981.
66. Ramsey, P., Lasser, S., and MacEwen, G. D.: Congenital dislocation of the hip. Use of the Pavlik harness in the child during the first six months of life. J. Bone Joint Surg., 58A:1000, 1976.
67. Roose, P. E., et al.: Open reduction for congenital dislocation of the hips using the Ferguson procedure. J. Bone Joint Surg., 61A:915, 1979.
68. Salter, R. B., and Dubos, J. P.: The first 15 years personal experience with innominate osteotomy in the treatment of congenital dislocation and subluxation of the hip. Clin. Orthop., 98:72, 1974.
69. Salter, R. B., Kostuik, J., and Dallas, S.: Avascular necrosis of the femoral head as a complication or treatment for congenital dislocation of the hip in children. A clinical and experimental investigation. Canad. J. Surg., 12:44, 1969.
70. Severin, E.: Contribution to the knowledge of congenital dislocation of the hip joint: Late results of closed reduction and arthrographic studies of recent cases. Acta Chir. Scand., 84:1, 1941.
71. Simons, G. W.: A comparative evaluation of the current methods for open reduction of the congenitally displaced hip. Orthop. Clin. North Am., 11:161, 1980.
72. Smith-Petersen, M. N.: A new supra-articular sub-periosteal approach to the hip joint. Am. J. Orthop. Surg., 15:592, 1917.
73. Somerville, E. W.: Displacement of the Hip in Childhood, New York, Springer-Verlag, 1982.
74. Staheli, L. T.: Shelf operation. AOA 1st International Symposium: Congenital Hip Dysplasia. Wilmington, 1980.
75. Staheli, L. T.: Medial approach open reduction for congenitally dislocated hips: Critical analysis of 40 cases. In Tachdjian, M. O. (ed.): Congenital Dislocation of the Hip. New York, Churchill Livingstone, 1982, pp. 295–303.
76. Stanisavljevic, S.: Congenital Hip Pathology in the Newborn. Baltimore, Williams & Wilkins, 1964.
77. Steel, H. H.: Triple osteotomy of the innominate bone. J. Bone Joint Surg., 55A:343, 1973.
78. Steel, H. H.: Triple osteotomy of the innominate bone. Clin. Orthop., 122:16, 1977.
79. Steel, H. H.: Triple osteotomy of the innominate bone. In Tachdjian, M. O. (ed.): Congenital Dislocation of the Hip. New York, Churchill Livingstone, 1982, pp. 566–594.
80. Strauss, H. J.: Chiari pelvic osteotomy for hip dysplasia in patients below age 20. Progr. Orthop. Surg., 2:121, 1978.
81. Strauss, H. J.: Comment on open reduction of the dislocated hip without preliminary attempt at closed reduction. In: Congenital Hip Dislocation: Avascular Necrosis. New York, Thieme-Stratton, 1982, pp. 97–98.
82. Stulberg, S. D., and Harris, W. H.: Acetabular Dysplasia and Development of Osteoarthritis of the Hip. In: Proceedings of the Second Open Scientific Meeting of the Hip Society. St. Louis, Mosby, 1974, pp. 82–93.
83. Sutherland, D. H.: Double innominate osteotomy in congenital hip dislocation or dysplasia. In Tachdjian, M. O. (ed.): Congenital Dislocation of the Hip. New York, Churchill Livingstone, 1982, pp. 595–608.
84. Sutherland, D. H., and Greenfield, R.: Double innominate osteotomy. J. Bone Joint Surg., 59A:1082, 1977.
85. Tachdjian, M. O.: Salter's innominate osteotomy to derotate the maldirected acetabulum. In Tachdjian, M. O. (ed.): Congenital Dislocation of the Hip. New York, Churchill Livingstone, 1982, pp. 525–541.
86. Tagawa, S.: Rotational Acetabular Osteotomy. American Academy of Orthopaedic Surgeons Film Library. Chicago, 1982.
87. Thomas, C. L., Gage, J. R., and Ogden, J. A.: Treatment concepts for proximal femoral ischemic necrosis complicating congenital hip disease. J. Bone Joint Surg., 64A:817, 1982.
88. Tönnis, D.: Normal values of the hip joint for evaluation of x-rays in children and adults. Clin. Orthop., 119:39, 1976.
89. Tönnis, D.: Triple osteotomy close to the hip joint. In Tachdjian, M. O. (ed.): Congenital Dislocation of the Hip. New York, Churchill Livingstone, 1982, pp. 555–565.
90. Tönnis, D. (ed.): Congenital Hip Dislocation: Avascular Necrosis. New York, Thieme-Stratton, 1982.
91. Tönnis, D., Behrens, K., and Tscharani, F.: Eine neue Technik der Dreifach-Osteotomie fur Schwenkung dysplasticher Huftpfannen bei Jugendlichen und Erwachsenen. Z. Orthop., 119: 253, 1981.
92. Tönnis, D., and Kuhlmann, G. P.: Untersuchungen uber die Haufigkeit von Huftkopfnekrosen bei Spreizhosenbehandlung und verschiedenen konservativen Behandlungsmethoden der angeborener Huftdysplasie und Huftluxation. Z. Orthop., 106:651, 1969.
92a. Utterback, T. D., MacEwen, G. D.: Comparison of pelvic osteotomies for the surgical correction of the congenital hip. Clin. Orthop., 98:110, 1974.

93. Wagner, H.: Osteotomies for congenital hip dislocation. In: The Hip: Proceedings of the Fourth Meeting of the Hip Society, 1976. St. Louis, Mosby, 1976, pp. 45–66.
94. Wagner, H.: Femoral osteotomies for congenital hip dislocation. Progr. Orthop. Surg., 2:85, 1978.
95. Wagner, H.: Experiences with spherical acetabular osteotomy for the correction of the dysplastic acetabulum. Progr. Orthop. Surg., 2:131, 1978.
96. Wagner, H.: Personal communication.
97. Weiner, D. S., Hoyt, W. A., and O'Dell, H. W.: Congenital dislocation of the hip: The relationship of premanipulation traction and age to avascular necrosis of the femoral head. J. Bone Joint Surg., 59A:306, 1977.
98. Weinstein, S., and Ponseti, I.: Congenital dislocation of the hip: Open reduction through a medial approach. J. Bone Joint Surg., 61:A:119, 1979.
99. Westin, G. W., Ilfeld, F. W., and Provost, J.: Total avascular necrosis of the capital femoral epiphysis in congenital dislocated hips. Clin. Orthop., 119:93, 1976.
100. Wiberg, G.: Studies on dysplastic acetabula and congenital subluxation of the hip joint. Acta Chir. Scand., 83(Suppl.):58, 1939.
101. Willis, B.: The natural history and treatment of extensive avascular necrosis following congenital dislocation of the hip. Transactions, 8th Annual Meeting, Pediatric Orthopaedic Study Group, Nashville, 1981.
102. Wilson, J. C., Jr.: Surgical treatment of the dysplastic acetabulum in adolescence. Clin. Orthop., 98:137, 1974.
103. Zeiler, G., and Wagner, H.: Personal communication.

CHAPTER 15

Neonatal and Infantile Septic Arthritis

EDUARDO A. SALVATI

Historical Review

In 1874 Thomas Smith [32] described, in a classic paper published in the *Saint Bartholomew's Hospital Reports,* the characteristics, evolution, and postmortem findings of septic arthritis of the hip. The severity of this pathology was emphasized: of 21 patients with pyogenic arthritis of the hip, 13 died. Only eight recovered, but with severe hip disability.

In 1935 Inge and Liebolt [14] reviewed the historical attitude and treatment for acute suppurative arthritis, suggesting that the chief concern of the eighteenth-century surgeon was to preserve life, that the nineteenth-century surgeon tried in addition to save the affected limb, and that only with the twentieth century came the idea of preserving the function of suppurative joints.

In 1936, Green and Shannon [9] pointed out the rarity of the recurrence of osteomyelitis under the age of 2 years. Infant bones are small, with large cancellous spaces and a loosely attached periosteum, which allows rapid escape of pus and decompression of the septic process. Reabsorption of dead bone is aided by the fast turnover of the surrounding bone. Thus sequestration and chronic draining sinuses usually do not occur.[3,30] Septic arthritis during infancy generally is not complicated by ankylosis (unless it is iatrogenically induced), the joint structures being cartilaginous. In older children ankylosis is a frequent outcome. Also in 1936, Harmon and Adams [12] in a study of the end results of 147 cases of septic arthritis of the hip, recognized the relatively more benign course of the infection under the age of 2 or 3 years.

In the same year, Badgley and coworkers [1a] reviewed the end results of 113 cases of septic arthritis of the hip in all ages. They emphasized that severe hip disability could be prevented by early diagnosis and arthrotomy. In addition they also pointed out the more favorable prognosis under the age of 2 years, and in cases of primary synovial infection, in comparison to those of osteomyelitic origin. The mortality was 12% and only 6.2% of the hips were normal at the end result.

Since the advent of antibacterial therapy the surgeon has become more aggressive in the treatment of bone infections. However, it is worthwhile emphasizing the number of deaths due to hematogenous osteomyelitis prior to the antibacterial era.* In 1933, Beekman and Sullivan reported the preceding 10 years' experience at Bellevue Hospital in the treatment of 218 cases of hematogenous osteomyelitis. Thirty-eight of these cases or 17.4% died, the majority due to septicemia. The mortality was 46% in cases with positive blood cultures. The mortality in staphylococcal and streptococcal osteomyelitis was 16.5 and 17%, respectively. A half century later the mortality almost has been eradicated. In fact our experience 50 years later

* "In no one of the inflammatory lesions in and about the hip is there a greater call for the employment of correct surgical principles. . . . If abscess forms, the pus should be promptly evacuated. . . . I made a diagnosis of periarthritis and advised an incision. The advice was not accepted by the attending surgeon. Two-and-a-half months later I saw the case again, and at that time the abscess extended throughout the whole of the gluteal region. It opened spontaneously; extensive sloughing followed and the patient finally, in an extreme degree of emaciation, found a home in one of the sea-side sanitariums. She died of exhaustion a year after the first appearance of the disease." From Gibney, V. P.: *The Hip and Its Disease,* 1884.

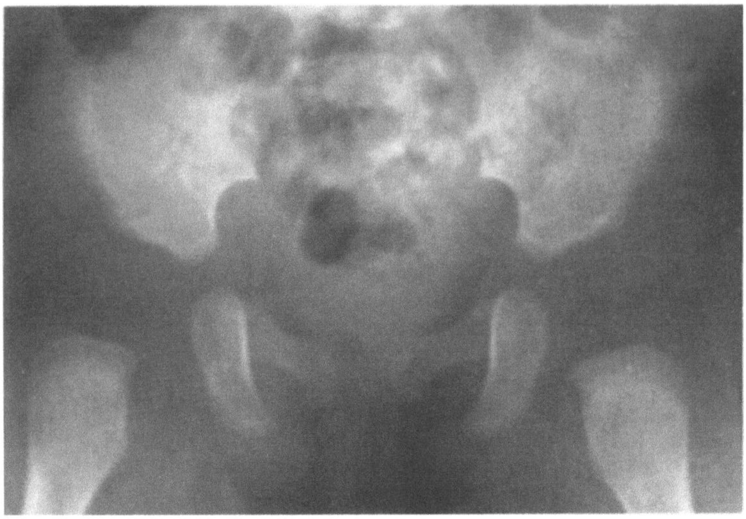
A

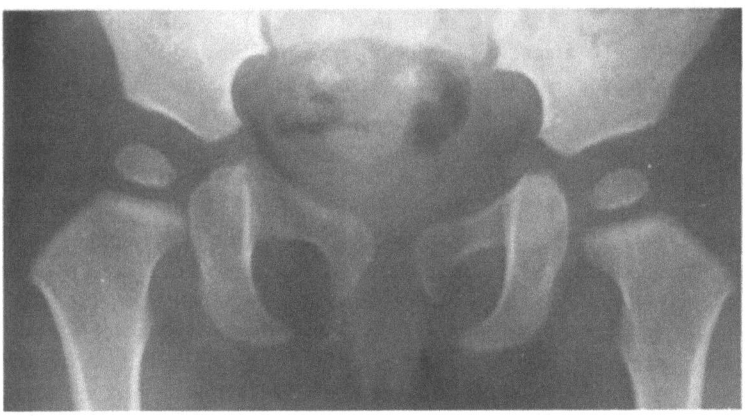
B

FIG. 15–1 **A** One-month-old baby girl with acute and early septic arthritis of the right hip (*Staphylococcus aureus*). The only radiographic finding is lateral displacement of the proximal femur. The hip was treated by incision and drainage as an emergency on the second day after the onset of symptoms, and immobilized for 3 weeks. Antibiotic therapy was continued for 6 weeks. **B** The right hip is normal 1 year after the episode of septic arthritis.

shows no mortality, but only 21% of normal hips at the completion of skeletal growth.[10] Thus we are still short of the twentieth-century goal of preserving function in all cases of suppurative arthritis, a goal that could be accomplished by early diagnosis and treatment (Fig. 15–1).

Most large series of septic arthritis identify the hip as the joint most frequently affected (about 40%), followed by the knee (30%), ankle (10%), shoulder, elbow, wrist, hand, sternoclavicular joint, and foot. Severe residual disability is observed most frequently after septic arthritis of the hip (43% of cases), followed by the shoulder (33%), ankle (15%), and knee (8%).[7,13,26–28]

Pathogenesis

Sepsis can originate from direct inoculation following femoral venipuncture,[5] from a hematogenous synovial infection (which carries a better prognosis), or from decompression of osteomyelitis of the proximal femur or, more rarely, of the ilium.[2a] Osteomyelitis of the proximal metaphysis of the femur will drain into the hip joint owing to its intracapsular location.

Bone and joint infections are dependent, as any other infection in general, on the interplay between the microorganism and the resistance of the host. Factors such as type, number and virulence of infecting bacteria, localization, cellular and humoral immune mechanisms, and so on play an essential role. Hematogenous osteomyelitis in children usually occurs in the metaphysis of long bones, particularly the femur and tibia. The microvascular anatomy in the metaphyseal area favors the localization of bacteria: the branches of the nutrient artery end as straight, narrow capillaries which sharply turn at the level of the growth plate. The veins are of a wider caliber, and eventually drain into the venous sinusoids of the marrow.

The sharp capillary turn and the wider venous caliber produce a significant slowing of the blood flow which favors localization and growth of bacteria. Frequent sources of infecting organisms are the umbilicus in the neonatal period, skin infections, and sepsis in other organ systems. In the first few years of life, the metaphyseal cortical bone is relatively thin; the periosteum is loosely attached and allows the inflammatory exudate to spread to the surrounding tissues.

Decreased host defense mechanisms have been identified as well. Prematurity and complicated deliveries seem to be predisposing factors in the neonatal period. The majority of affected infants had antecedent illnesses or were subjected to potentially infective procedures. Immunodeficiency, including abnormal immunoglobulins, complement, and phagocytosis, has been shown in some of these infants.[14a,16]

The increased intraarticular pressure resulting from the septic process may dislocate the femoral head and interrupt its intracapsular blood supply. These factors, combined with the chondrolytic activity of the pus, may lead to severe damage of the acetabulum, triradiate cartilage,[10a,34a] femoral head, and its intraarticular epiphyseal plate.

The effect of staphylococcal pus and other proteolytic enzymes on the structural integrity of articular cartilage is well documented. The hypercellular synovial fluid in septic arthritis, with a large preponderance of polymorphonuclear leukocytes, provides the basis for lysosomal enzymatic destruction of cartilage. In addition, fibrous deposition adheres to the cartilage surface, blocking its nutrition from the synovial fluid. The sequence of events is rather rapid, and if diagnosis and adequate treatment are not established within a very few days, permanent damage will occur.

Diagnosis

The importance of early diagnosis and treatment cannot be overemphasized. The hip joint, being deeply seated, is difficult to examine and aspirate. Thus the diagnosis of septic arthritis tends to be delayed, if not missed, particularly in the neonate and infant who cannot voice their complaint specifically.

In the newborn diagnosis can be difficult because the typical findings of fever, chills, elevated white blood count, and prostration may be absent. This is particularly so in the premature neonate with decreased immunological response. However, such newborns present irritability and crying on any attempted motion of the affected lower extremity. This is most obvious on diaper changes. There is lack of movement of the extremity, which is held in a position of slight flexion, abduction, and external rotation. This position allows the maximum capacity to the intraarticular space, decreasing the tension of the joint exudate. Palpation and movement of the hip joint are extremely painful. As time passes the lower extremity can develop swelling and edema. There is a general feeling that the infant is doing poorly: refusal or regurgitation of feeding, lethargy or irritability, and failure to maintain or gain weight are demonstrated. Not infrequently other skeletal areas can be affected.

Laboratory findings include an elevated erythrocyte sedimentation rate and a high white blood count with an elevated percentage of polymorphonuclear leukocytes and a shift to the left. Blood cultures can be positive in over 50% of the cases, particularly if taken during chills or high temperature.

To establish the diagnosis the procedure of choice is a hip aspiration, performed at the bedside or preferably under the image intensifier, with strict antiseptic precautions. The fluid aspirated is sent immediately to the bacteriology laboratory for direct smear (Gram's stain) and aerobic, anaerobic, myobacterial, and fungal cultures and sensitivities. The infecting organism may be a susceptible fragile bacteria. In order to increase the chances of growth the aspirate should be inoculated as soon as possible into the appropriate medium. The use of a transport system with a culture medium to support the bacteria during the time of transport can also be helpful. The phenomenon of "sterile" infections may well be due to the difficulty of recovering and growing this fragile type of bacteria.

A complete cell count and differential count of the hip aspirate should be done, for it may give valuable information. If the complete count shows more than 20,000 white blood cells/ml and the differential count more than 75% polymorphonuclear leukocytes, infection should be suspected. Obviously the higher the numbers, the greater the possibility of infection. If enough fluid is obtained, glucose and protein levels could also be helpful in making the diagnosis. The synovial glucose level will be less than half the blood glucose value because there is a decreased perfusion and an increased utilization of glucose by the inflamed synovial tissue, and by the higher number of cells and bacteria in the synovial fluid. On the other hand, the protein levels will be elevated: normal synovial fluid contains only one-third as much protein as does serum and none of the recognized factors in the blood clotting system. But in septic arthritis there is an augmented passage of plasma proteins into the joint, including clotting factors. This explains the formation of a large fibrinous clot soon after withdrawal of the exudative effusion. However, on rare occasions, the results of white blood cell and differential counts and glucose and protein levels in synovial fluid from inflammatory and septic arthritis can be similar. In these cases, only the positive results of direct smear and cultures can establish the diagnosis.

Elevated lactic acid in synovial fluid has been found to be useful in the diagnosis of septic arthritis, and of particular diagnostic value in patients in whom antibiotic therapy was started before joint aspiration. Sequential measurements can be helpful in assessing the response of septic arthritis to treatment.[31a]

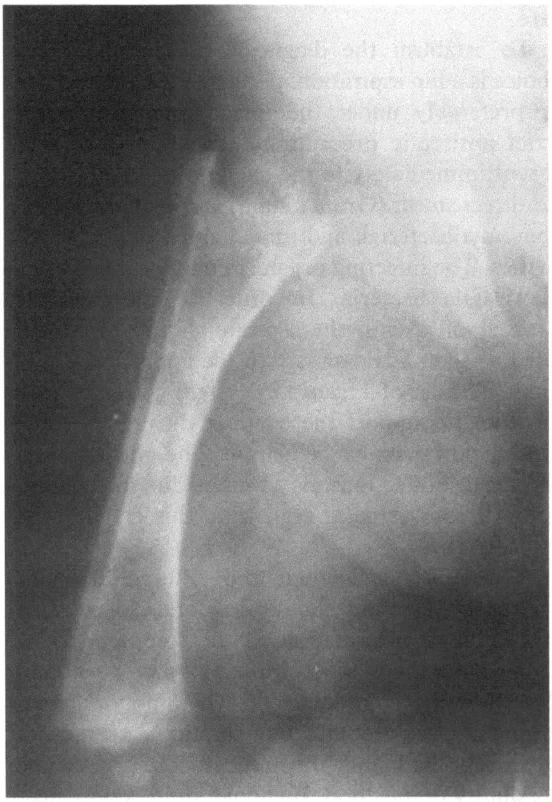

FIG. 15–2 Two months after septic arthritis the hip is dislocated with periosteal new bone formation around the femoral shaft.

Radiology should not be expected to establish an early diagnosis of septic arthritis. By the time there is radiographic evidence, the septic process will be well established. However, soft tissue swellings with obliteration of the adjacent fat planes due to edema and a slight lateral displacement of the proximal femur due to the exudate and synovial inflammation could be observed in the early stages (Fig. 15–1). Other radiographic findings, including periostitis, periarticular osteoporosis, and dislocation are late (Fig. 15–2).

Bone imaging by nuclear scanning can give valuable information in the early stages. Technetium-99 polyphosphate, gallium, and other radioactive agents have been used with variable success. Recently, the use of indium-111–labeled autologous polymorphonuclear leukocytes has been shown to be more specific and reliable in the diagnosis of infection. However, the only definite and conclusive diagnostic tool remains the isolation and identification of the infecting organism, which can be done best by prompt hip aspiration.

Acute Treatment

Once the diagnosis is established we feel that the treatment of choice is immediate surgical incision and drainage under adequate intravenous antibiotic therapy, followed by immobilization for a few weeks, until the joint becomes stable (Fig. 15–3).

Unless the infecting organism is highly sensitive, antibiotic therapy alone is insufficient in most instances in eradicating the infection without suffering permanent joint damage. It might suppress the symptoms and select resistant strains, while not resolving the underlying infection.

The effectiveness of antibiotic therapy is closely related to the intensity of the bacterial metabolism. Bacteria are killed promptly when penicillin is added early, during the logarithmic phase of bacterial growth, but this fails to occur if the addition of antibiotics is delayed until the stationary growth phase. In thick purulent exudates, penicillin exerts only a slow bactericidal effect. The bacteria tend to persist at a stationary growth phase.

Depending on the sensitivity of the infecting organism, bactericidal drugs of first choice should

FIG. 15–3 Diagnosis and treatment of acute septic arthritis of the hip.

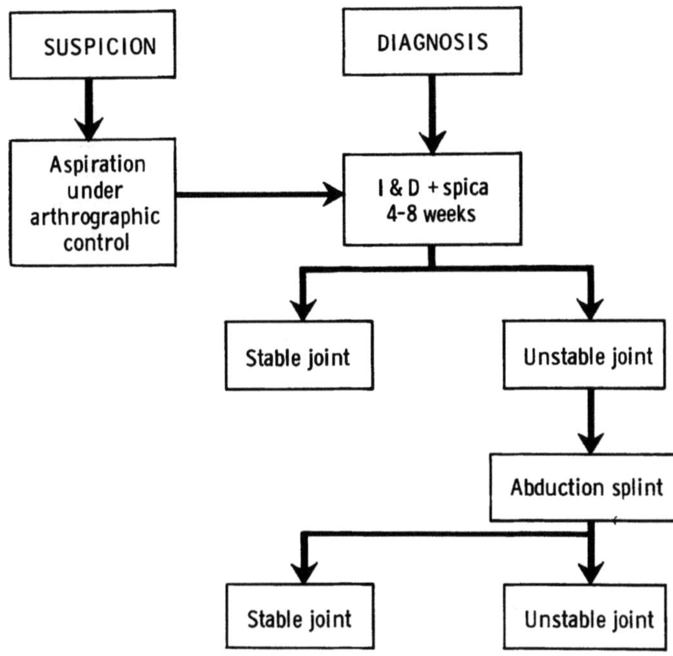

be given in high doses intravenously for at least 1 month. Although, ideally, selecting the drug of choice from the large number of antibiotics available should not be difficult, several factors limit the selection of the antibiotic, such as the drug resistance of the organism and the general health and tolerance of the infant.

All these factors should be thoroughly assessed prior to deciding what antibiotic regimen is to be used, and not infrequently we may have to resort to antibiotics of second choice. If they produce adverse effects, we are forced then to switch to a drug of third choice, narrowing the alternatives even further. The need for careful monitoring of infants on antibiotics should be kept in mind, considering the high doses and prolonged time necessary for adequate treatment.[14a]

Surgical Treatment

The most adequate decompression of the joint is obtained by surgical incision and drainage. We do not favor repeat aspirations. The posterior Ober approach, described in 1924, is preferred because it allows dependent drainage. However, a medial approach (Ludloff) or an anterior approach (Heuter) could be utilized (see below).

Attention should be given to the sciatic nerve, if the posterior approach is selected. The hip capsule should be incised parallel to the neck of the femur and over its posterior aspect, to avoid injury to the posterosuperior and posteroinferior retinacular vessels, and branches of the medial circumflex artery which are the main vascular supply to the proximal femoral chondroepiphysis.

Once the hip joint has been adequately exposed and debrided, the capsule is left open, and the fascia of the gluteus maximus is closed with a few interrupted sutures as well as the skin. Some authors prefer to place a Penrose drain. Others emphasize closed suction irrigation. However, this technique is only applicable in the older patient.

Immobilization in a spica cast is indicated, with the hip in slight flexion, abduction, and neutral rotation, maintaining the remnant of the proximal femur in the acetabulum until the hip is stable by clinical and radiographic examination. We do not favor traction, owing to the difficulty of maintaining it in a small infant, nor early mobilization, for fear of pathological subluxation or dislocation. Although the majority of the hips achieve a stable situation within a few weeks, some may require longer periods, particularly if the septic process has destroyed the femoral head and neck. In such situations it might be better to use abduction braces at night to prevent the development of fixed

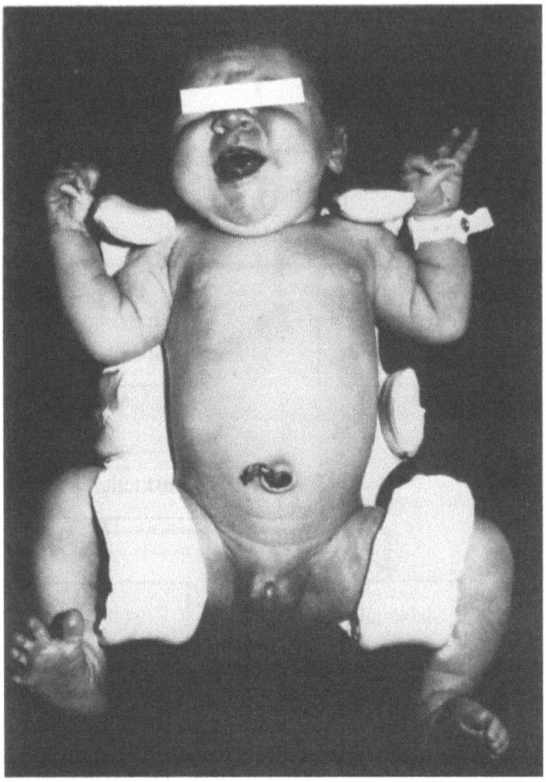

FIG. 15–4 Von Rosen splint maintaining the hips in gentle abduction and flexion.

adduction contractures, allowing free hip motion during the day (Fig. 15–4).

Sequelae

A good understanding of the natural history of the sequelae of septic arthritis of the hip in infancy seems essential in outlining a thoughtful plan of treatment, in order to assure the best possible hip when skeletal growth is completed. It is also important to obtain a favorable anatomical hip condition for a suitable biomechanical prosthetic reconstruction which may be required at a later date.

The femoral head damage may vary from simple delay of ossification to complete destruction (Fig. 15–5). If the damage is partial, the inferomedial portion of the femoral head and neck is the area most-likely preserved, resulting in a deformed small head and neck. Later growth potential will depend on the integrity of the epiphyseal plate. The damage to the triradiate cartilage will also play a significant role in the acetabular development.[10a,29,34a]

For treatment of the sequelae, a conservative approach and several operative procedures have been recommended, including open reduction; osteotomies, both femoral and pelvic; shelves; trochanteric arthroplasties; advancement of the greater trochanter or abductor mechanism; arthrodesis; epiphysiodesis of the distal contralateral femur; leg lengthening and shortening; and so on.

The literature is scarce in long-term follow-up studies and controversial in the treatment of choice for the sequelae, once the septic process is over.

In 1948 Bryson[4] reported 17 cases of suppurative arthritis of the hip complicated by pathological dislocation. One was treated by Colonna reconstruction, four by subtrochanteric osteotomy, and 11 by arthrodesis of the hip. After an average follow-up period of 10 years (a range of 1 to 18 years), he concluded that arthrodesis performed between 12 and 15 years of age was the treatment of choice.

In 1949 Nicholson[25] reported ten cases of septic arthritis of the hip, suggesting early closed or open reduction, non–weight-bearing braces, and if indicated, osteotomies at a later age. He was able to follow seven of these cases for an average of 17 years (a range of 1 to 28 years).

In 1960 Eyre-Brook[6] reviewed ten cases of septic arthritis of the hip in infants, seven with osteomyelitis of the upper end of the femur. He described four types of sequelae: (1) destruction of the capital epiphysis with dislocation of the hip; (2) destruction of the capital epiphysis with the femoral neck remaining in the acetabulum; (3) destruction of the epiphyseal plate with the femoral head remaining in the acetabulum and connected to the femoral neck by a fibrous union;[15] and (4) recovery with coxa magna but no other deformity. After following these cases for an average of 9 years (a range of 2 to 20 years), he concluded that controlled abduction osteotomy played a useful part in stabilizing the hip joint.

Although it is of only historical interest, in 1960 Mayer[21] briefly mentioned having implanted the fibular head in two hips with absent head and neck, following infantile septic arthritis of the hip suffered at 3 months of age. The results were unsatisfactory after 15 and 18 years' follow-up. It is obvious from this review that no consensus exists in the ideal treatment of the sequelae. To shed some light on this matter we will present our experience.

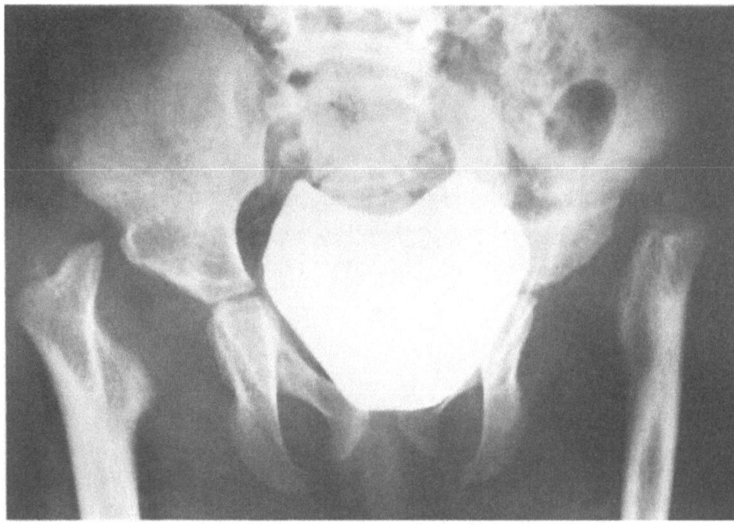

FIG. 15–5 Sequelae of bilateral septic arthritis at 2.5 years of age. Both hips are dislocated with an absent head and neck. The trochanteric apophysis is already present on the left. The bilateral septic arthritis was caused by *Staphylococcus aureus* and was diagnosed late in a 1-month-old baby girl, born after 29 weeks of gestation (birth weight, 930 g).

Clinical Material

We have followed 26 cases of infantile septic arthritis of the hip in 23 patients (three bilateral cases) occurring in the first 7 months of life.[10] There were 12 females and 11 males. Although the majority originally had osteomyelitis of the proximal metaphysis of the femur, two had osteomyelitis of the iliac bone as the source of the septic arthritis. Few had primary synovial infection. The patients' ages at follow-up ranged from 11 to 39 years with a mean of 17 years. These cases were managed at The Hospital for Special Surgery in New York. To our knowledge it represents the largest series with a long-term follow-up.

The radiographs taken at the last follow-up examination were used to determine the extent of damage to the hip. Earlier films could not be used adequately in most cases because, as a result of the acute septic process, the proximal femur may remain cartilaginous during the first years of life, thus providing little valuable information in terms of size, shape, and damage to the hip.

The septic hips were classified into three groups according to the radiographic evidence of damage to the femoral head. Group I included five hips with normal or slightly nonspherical femoral heads (Fig. 15–6); group II included nine hips with a deformed, small head and neck (Fig. 15–7); and group III included 11 hips with absent femoral head and neck (Fig. 15–8). In addition, one hip had an epiphyseal separation owing to destruction of the growth plate, with a normal relationship between the femoral head and acetabulum (Fig. 15–9).

In general the hips with more severe damage correlated well with one or more of the following factors: prematurity, late diagnosis, inadequate treatment, virulence of the organism (particularly if it was *Staphylococcus aureus*), and osteomyelitis.[20,24,36]

Treatment of the Sequelae

The ideal goal is to obtain a movable, stable, well-formed, and well-located hip. This goal can be obtained provided the damage to the hip joint is mild, the femoral head remains located within the acetabulum, and the growth potential is preserved. Following treatment of the acute septic process it is important to determine the location, stability, amount of damage, and growth potential of the proximal femur, which is not easy. Plain radiographs are of little assistance: owing to the infection the proximal femur may remain cartilaginous for a few years. Arthrography proved to be an unreliable method in establishing the extent of joint destruction, probably due to the severe intraarticular scarring as a consequence of the septic process. In our series, in only four of 11 arthrographic studies was the radiographic interpretation in agreement with the surgical findings at the time of open reduction or with the later development of the hip (Fig. 15–10), Glassberg and Ozonoff[8] found that arthrographic studies in several of their

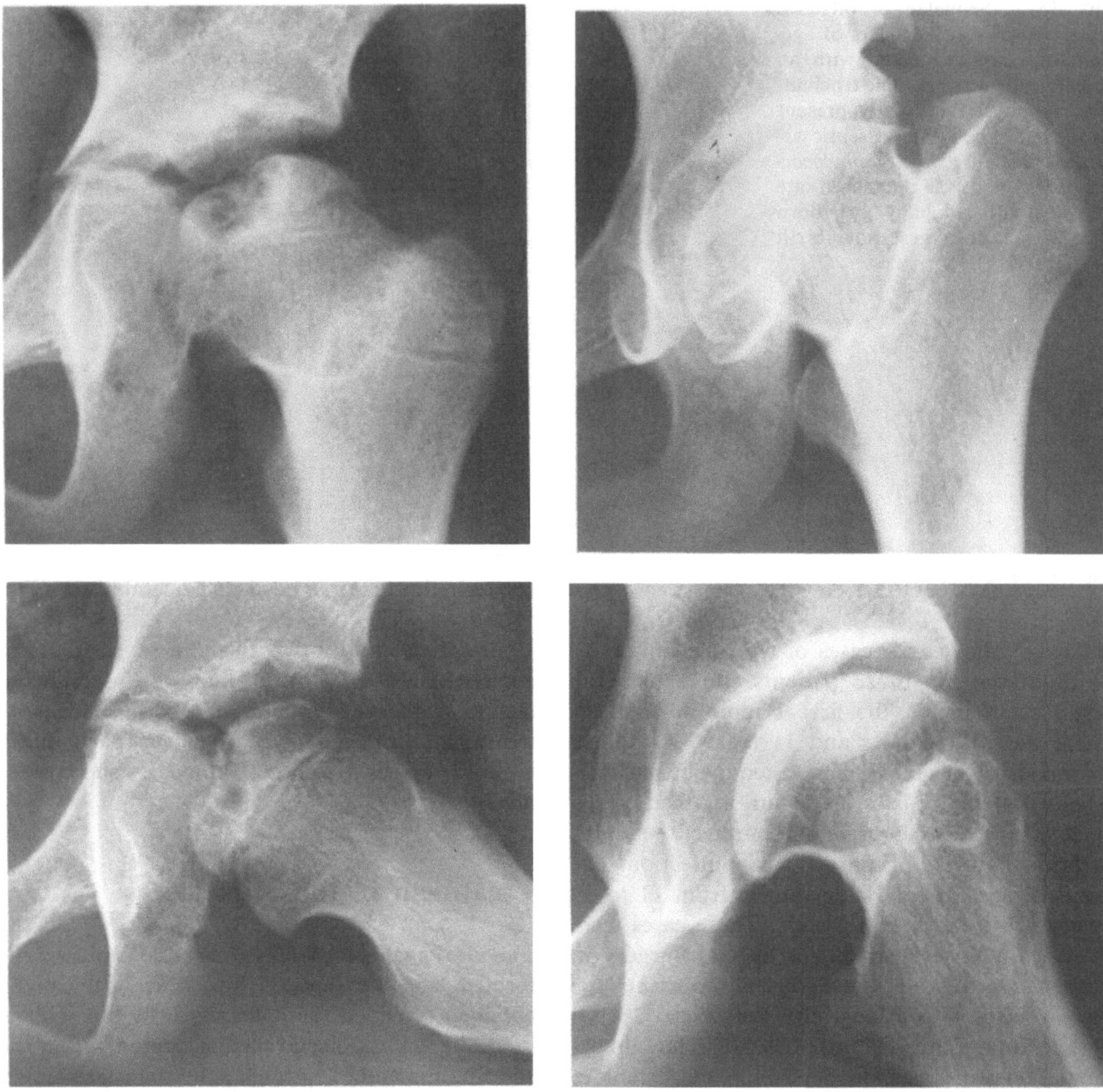

A B C D

FIG. 15–6 **A** This patient had septic arthritis in the neonatal period. Her evolution was satisfactory following early diagnosis and treatment. At 8 years of age she developed Perthes-like changes. **B** The lateral radiograph shows most of the involvement affecting mostly the posterior aspect of the proximal femoral epiphysis. This location is unusual for Perthes' disease, which usually affects the anterior and middle third of the proximal femoral epiphysis. **C** and **D** Residual deformity at 16 years of age.

septic hips were technically difficult to perform, probably because of contraction of the joint capsule. In addition, synovial adhesions and marked distortion of the normal anatomy made interpretation difficult.

The most reliable indication of whether the hip was well located during the first several months after infection was to test the stability of the joint by push-pull clinical and radiographic examination.

If after 1 year of conservative treatment the hip still remains unstable or in a dislocated position, surgical exploration is indicated. Opening the joint is the only reliable way of fully appraising the extent of damage. As mentioned previously, the chances of recurrence of infection in this age group are rare, particularly after adequate treatment. Open reduction is likely to give a successful result provided a well-preserved femoral head is found. If there is a very small remnant of head

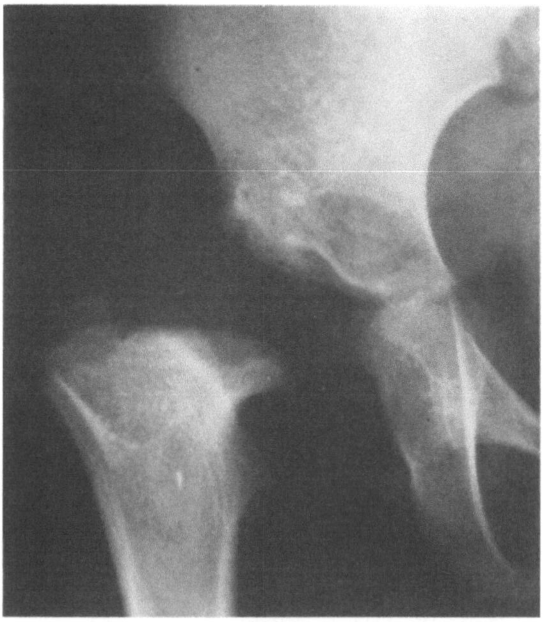

FIG. 15–7 Deformed, small head and neck following septic arthritis of the hip.

and neck, the chances of obtaining and maintaining an adequate, stable reduction are poor. Thus the alternatives remain a trochanteric arthroplasty or accepting the dislocation without attempting any reconstruction (Fig. 15–11).

Trochanteric Arthroplasty

Trochanteric arthroplasties have been suggested by several previous authors. L'Episcopo [18] in 1936 and Harmon [11,12] in 1942 described a Y-type osteotomy of the proximal femur, inserting the medial limb of the Y into the acetabulum (Figs. 15–12 and 15–13). The follow-up reported was 4 months for the first case and 5 years for the second. In 1946 Leveuf [19] described a trochanteric arthroplasty based on the Whitman reconstruction, which was performed through a transtrochanteric approach, according to Ollier (Fig. 15–14). It was followed by a varus osteotomy 3 months later. Leveuf reported on 14 cases with variable follow-

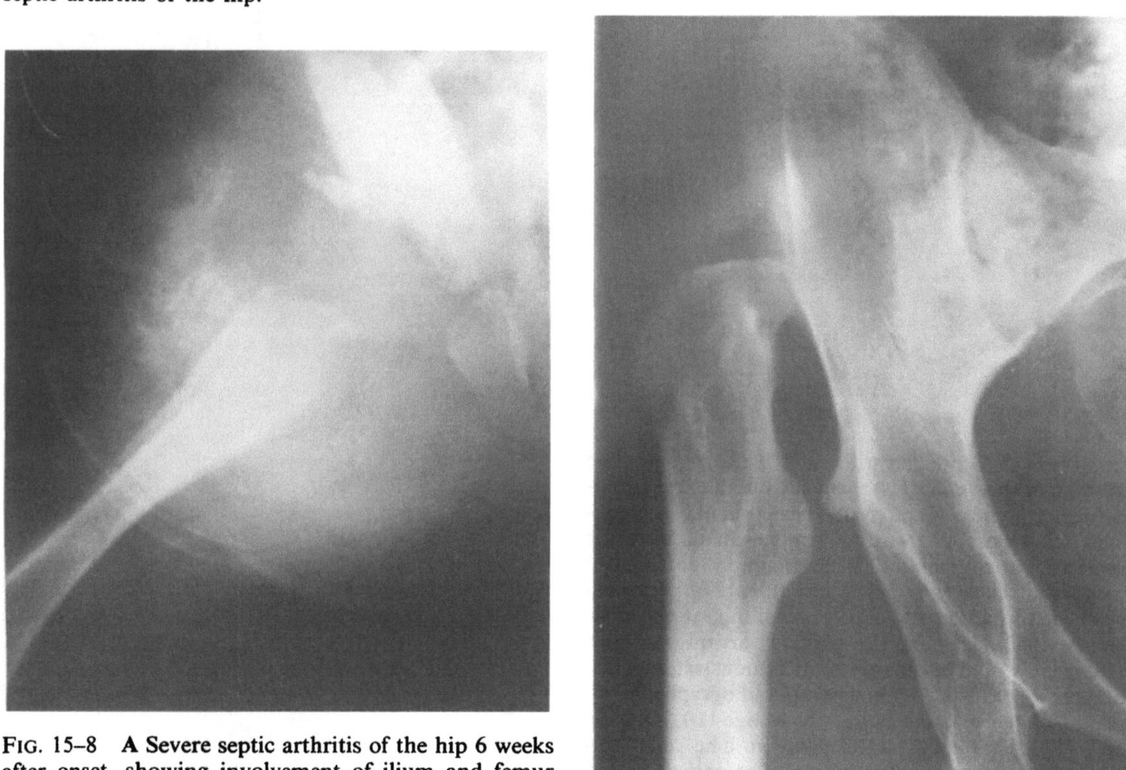

A

B

FIG. 15–8 **A** Severe septic arthritis of the hip 6 weeks after onset, showing involvement of ilium and femur with severe periosteal new bone formation and soft tissue swelling. **B** Last follow-up at 17 years of age. High iliac dislocation and poorly developed acetabulum. Nevertheless, the patient was pain free, walked as far as needed, though with a marked abductor lurch, and was functionally unlimited. His range of motion demonstrated 120° of flexion, 45° each of abduction and adduction, 85° each of internal and external rotation, and 7.5 cm of shortening.

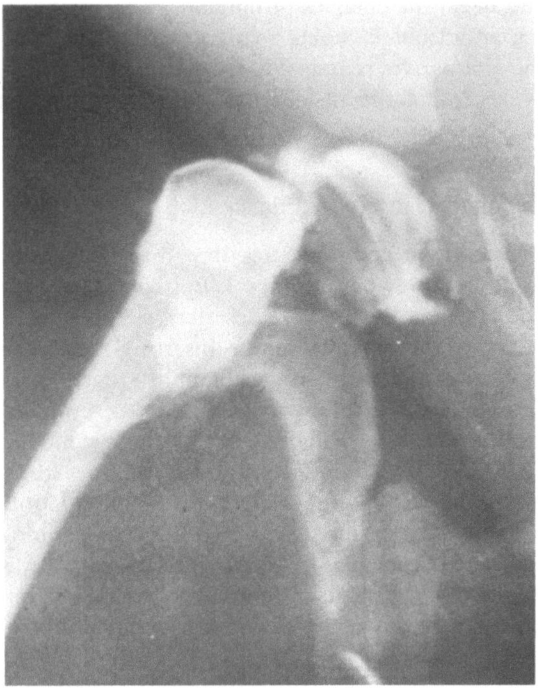

A

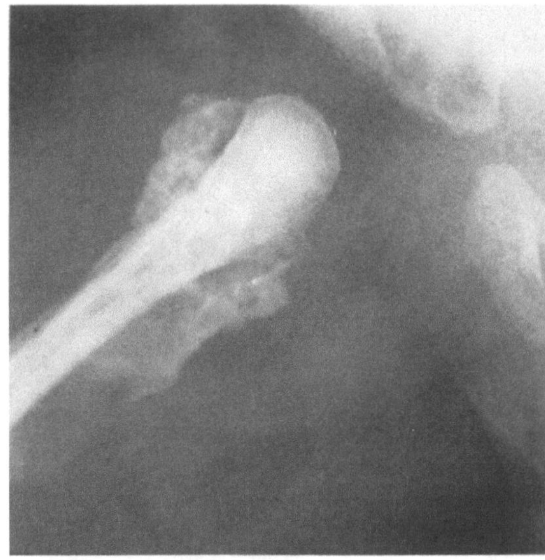

B

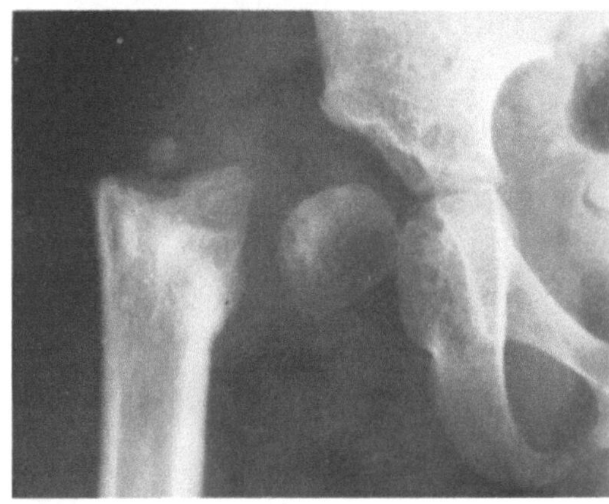

D

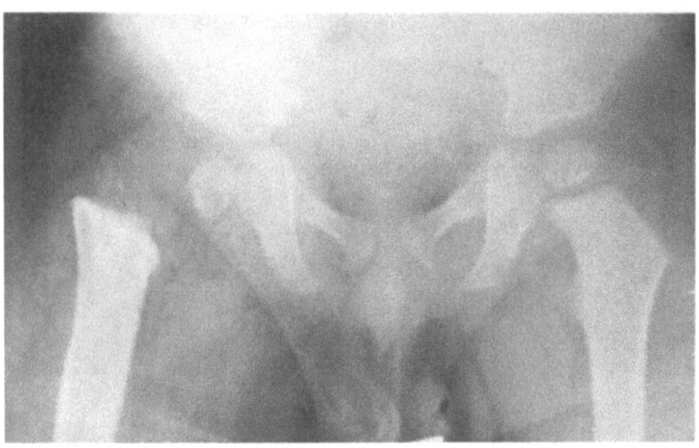

C

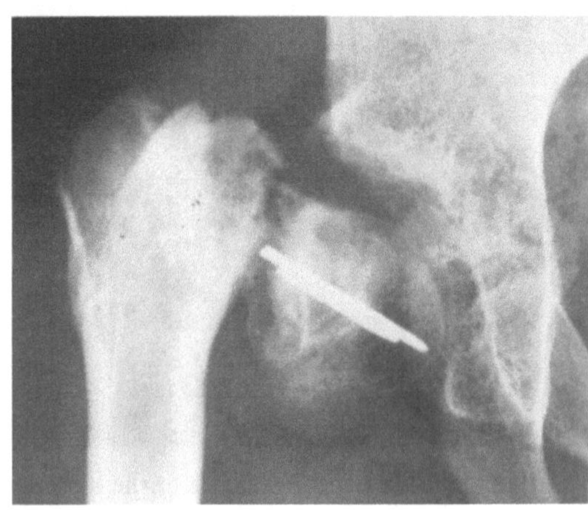

E

FIG. 15–9 **A** Septic arthritis at 1 week of age. The arthrogram shows contrast agent surrounding the proximal femoral chondroepiphysis, located in the acetabulum. It is separated from the femoral shaft, which is displaced superolaterally. **B** Radiograph obtained 2 weeks after the arthrogram. There is marked periosteal new bone formation and superolateral migration of the femoral shaft. Without the previous arthrogram this radiograph would be interpreted as demonstrating a dislocated hip. **C** and **D** Follow-up radiographs at 10 months of age **(C)** and 37 months of age **(D)**, showing the pathological epiphyseal separation. The small trochanteric apophysis is already seen. The patient underwent autologous bone graft and internal fixation at 4 years of age. **E** Radiograph at 10 years of age showing healing of the pathological separation with varus deformity owing to breakage of internal fixation. A valgus osteotomy has been recommended.

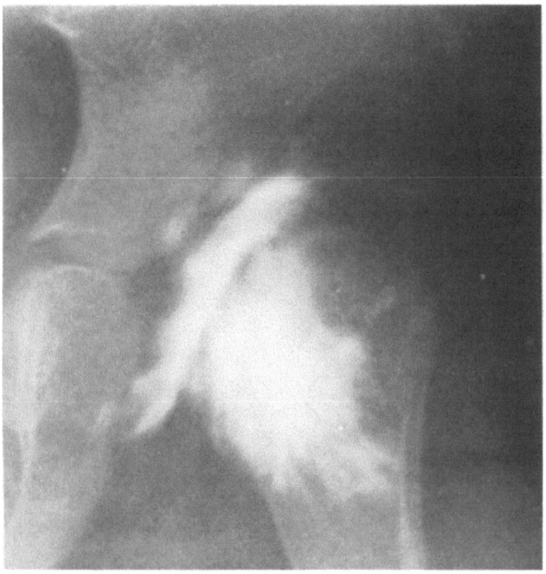

FIG. 15–10 Arthrogram obtained at 15 months of age, following septic arthritis. The arthrographic interpretation of absent head and neck was confirmed at surgery.

up and results. Trochanteric arthroplasty as performed on our patients was mentioned by Tachdjian.[34] Weissman[35] utilized this technique in a 3.5-year-old patient and Stetson et al.[33] in a 3-year-old patient. In both cases a varus subtrochanteric osteotomy was added. They published their results with a follow-up of 6.5 and 11 years, respectively. Both patients had a well-located hip, with only 3 cm of limb shortening in the first case and equal legs, following epiphysiodesis, in the second. However, their joints were ankylosed.

In 1973 Rigault and coworkers[31] reported their experience with ten trochanteric arthroplasties, six of which were performed for sequelae of infantile septic arthritis. Two of these six hips had almost no motion, two had a fair range of motion, and in the remaining two the follow-up period was too short to assess motion. Freeland et al.[6a] have reported 17 trochanteric arthroplasties, labeling them "stick femur reconstructions," six of which were performed for sequelae of infantile septic arthritis. Menelaus[22] performed a similar operation on a 2.5-year-old patient. Owing to progressive flexion contracture, an extension osteotomy was required at 6 years of age.

In our two trochanteric arthroplasties performed at 1.5 and 2.5 years of age, in which the hip remained located, the shape of the trochanteric apophysis eventually resembled that of the femoral head, as described in other published cases (Fig. 15–15). However, four other trochanteric arthroplasties, although located after surgery, progressively subluxated, dislocated, or ankylosed (Figs. 15–16 and 15–17).

Surgical Technique The technique of the trochanteric arthroplasty, indicated in those cases in which no femoral head and neck is found at the time of surgical exploration, consists of a lateral approach with detachment of the abductor mechanism, iliopsoas, and short external rotators from the proximal femur. This is followed by cleaning the acetabulum of scar tissue and deepening it by reaming at the level of the triradiate cartilage. Identifying the acetabulum can be difficult, as it will be completely covered by fibrous tissue. The

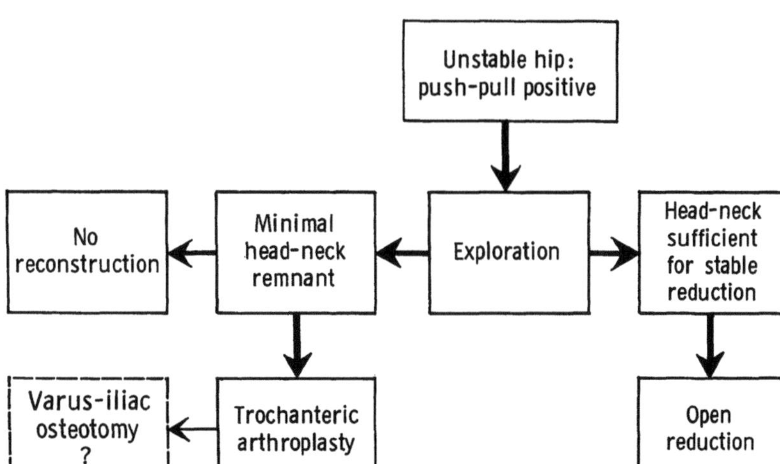

FIG. 15–11 Treatment of unstable hip following septic arthritis at 1 to 3 years of age.

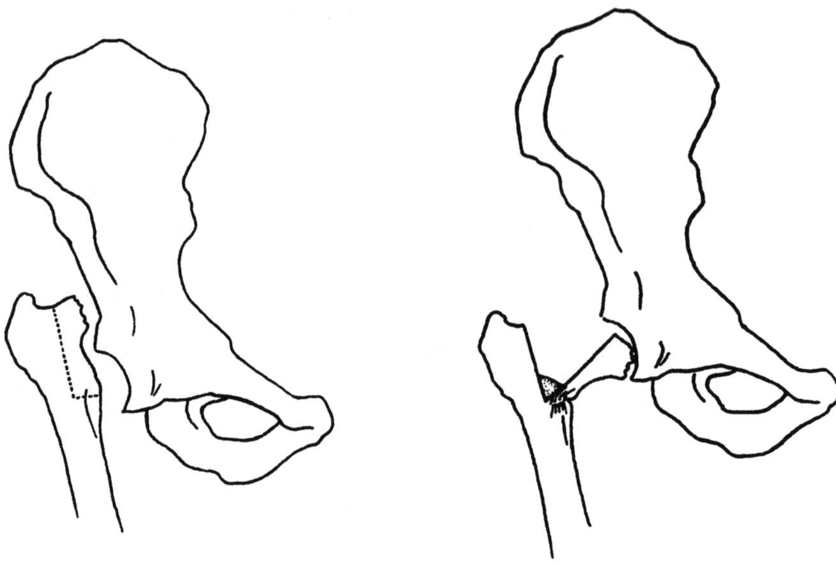

FIG. 15–12 Osteotomy of the proximal femur to stabilize a pathological dislocation following septic arthritis, according to L'Episcopo.

following anatomical landmarks can be helpful in locating the acetabulum: the obturator foramen inferiorly, the iliopectineal line anteriorly, and the ilioischiatic column posteriorly; retractors should be placed around the mentioned anatomical landmarks.

It is important to identify the sciatic nerve and other neurovascular structures that can be entrapped in scar tissue. Only when these anatomical structures have been well identified is it advisable to start deepening the acetabulum. As suggested by Rigault and coworkers,[31] reaming should be directed toward the vertical part of the triradiate cartilage so as to stay in the proper anteroposterior plane. One must remain below the horizontal part of the triradiate cartilage to prevent proximal migration.

The proximal femur must be reshaped to conform to the newly created acetabulum and must be seated in its depth. Once a stable reduction is achieved, the abductors are reattached distally on the lateral aspect of the proximal femur. The reduction should be stable in flexion, extension, abduction, adduction, and internal and external rotation. The prominence of the lesser trochanter should be excised if it impinges in adduction against the inferior pelvis, subluxating the joint. If a stable reduction cannot be obtained, a varus osteotomy might be of benefit. The hip is immobilized in a spica cast in a position of abduction,

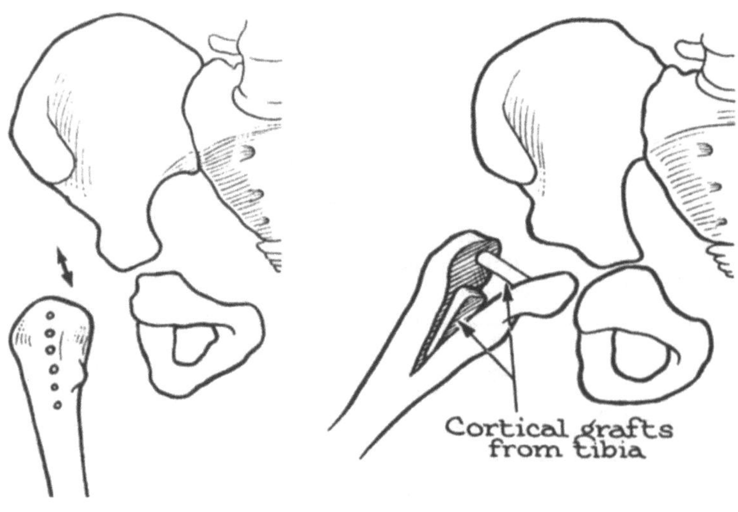

FIG. 15–13 Osteotomy and grafting as suggested by Harmon in 1942.

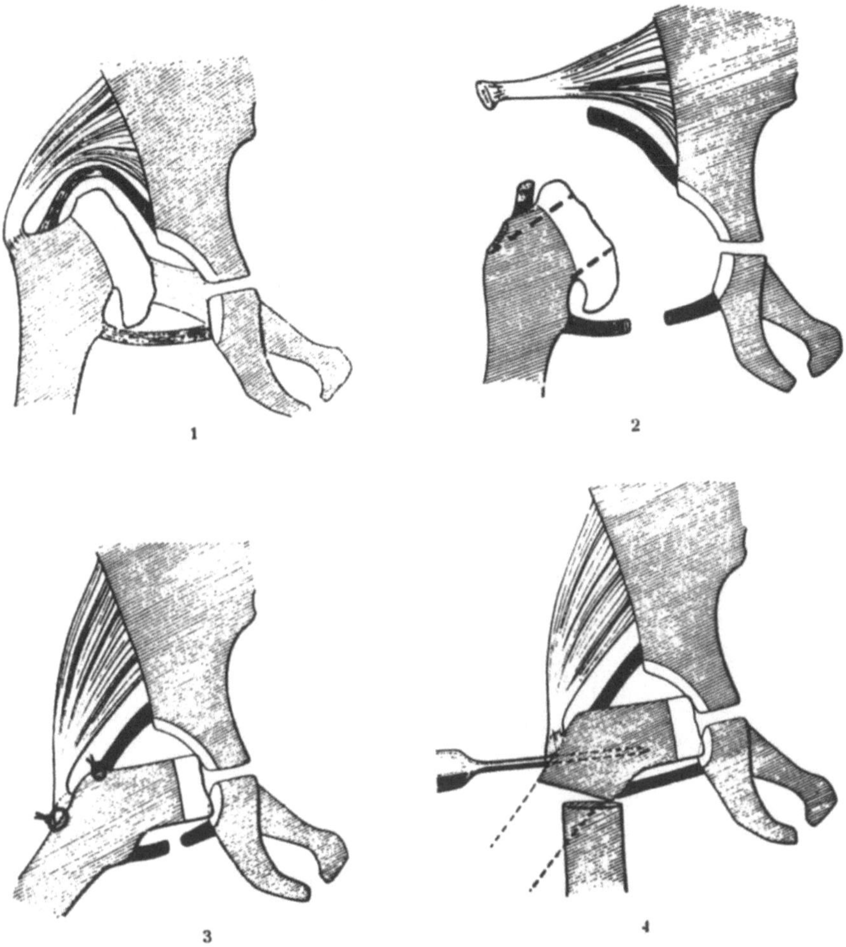

FIG. 15–14 Trochanteric arthroplasty with varus osteotomy as suggested by Leveuf in 1946.

slight flexion, and neutral rotation for about 2 to 3 months. Following this period of immobilization the child is allowed to mobilize the hip progressively.

Axer[1] recently described a new technique of greater trochanteric arthroplasty in which the femur is divided at the subtrochanteric level and the upper fragment is rotated 180° to place the greater trochanter deeply in the acetabulum. The author reports a successful result in one patient after a follow-up of 16 years.

Advantages of a trochanteric arthroplasty as compared to a complete dislocation are stability, a less conspicuous abductor lurch, a lesser leg length discrepancy, and a better anatomical condition for a late prosthetic reconstruction. The disadvantages are a restricted range of motion, including the possibility of ankylosis; increased chance of pain owing to bony contact; and secondary degenerative changes. The predictability of a trochanteric arthroplasty is also questionable, as some may progress into subluxation or even dislocation in spite of adequate surgery, postoperative immobilization, and rehabilitation. In these cases an adequately timed varus and/or iliac osteotomy might prevent the migration.

The results of the trochanteric arthroplasty, although generally modest, are most encouraging when it is performed during the first few years of life. The potential of the cartilaginous trochanteric apophysis to undergo spherical remodeling when it is reduced and maintained with the acetabulum in the first few years of life has been observed by various authors and ourselves. If the

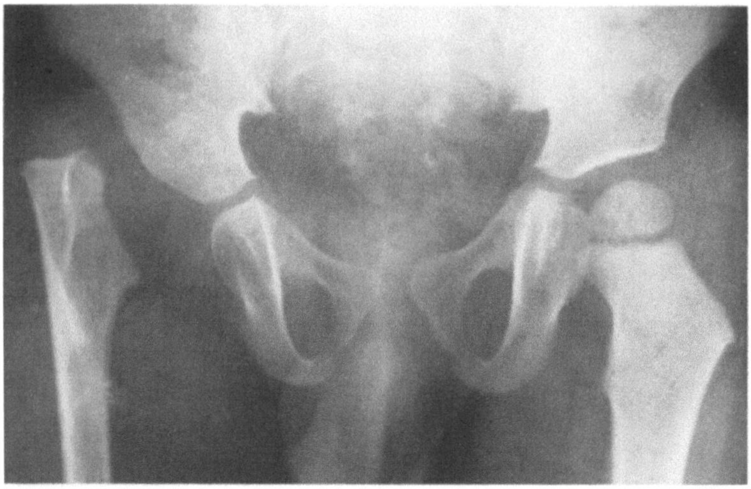

A

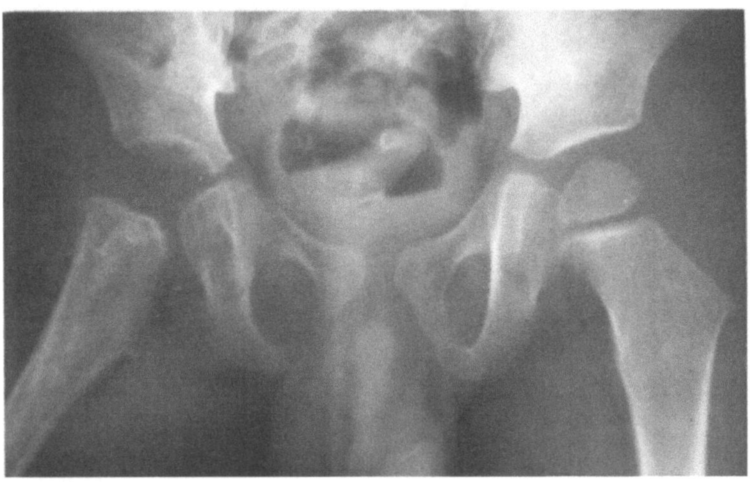

B

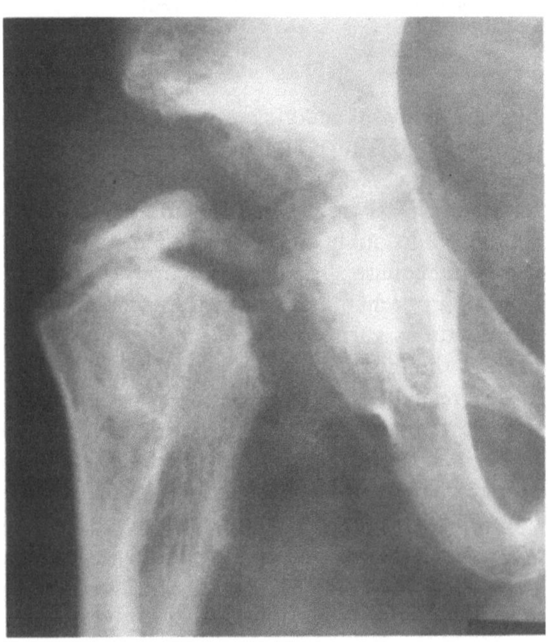

C

FIG. 15–15 **A** Dislocation of the right hip following septic arthritis in a 2.5-year-old child. **B** Three months after trochanteric arthroplasty performed at 2.5 years of age. The trochanteric apophysis is within the acetabulum. **C** Four years after trochanteric arthroplasty, the trochanteric apophysis is remodeled, resembling a femoral head. The acetabulum is developing as well.

arthroplasty is performed after the age of 4 or 5 years, the chances for adequate remodeling are marginal because the trochanteric apophysis is already quite ossified and less likely to yield a satisfactory result.

If the proximal femur is kept within the acetabulum, an acceptable acetabular development and satisfactory anatomical relationship occur, which are most useful for later prosthetic reconstruction. Ponseti [29] has reported that the acetabulum develops following the model given by the femoral head. In trochanteric arthroplasties it is the trochanteric apophysis that remodels, based on the acetabular form.

Overgrowth of the Greater Trochanter

Hips with a deformed, small head and neck showed a consistent pattern in their evolution, pro-

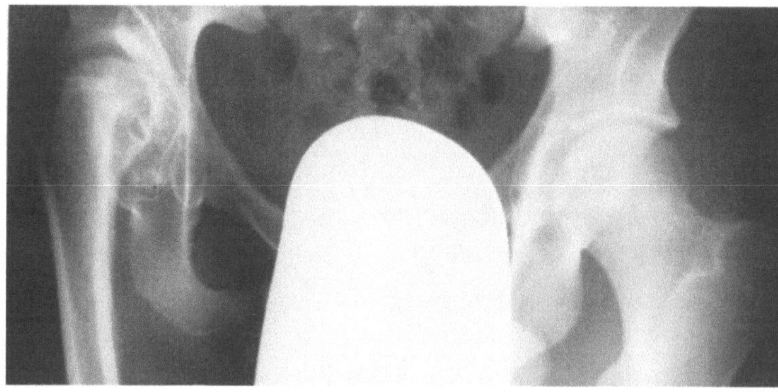

FIG. 15–15 (*cont.*). **D** Last follow-up at 18 years of age. The hip is well located. The patient has no pain, walks as far as needed with a mild abductor lurch, and is functionally unlimited. The mobility of the hip is limited (45–75° of flexion, 5° of abduction, 20° of adduction, and 10° of internal and external rotation). He has 2 cm of shortening following epiphysiodesis on the contralateral distal femur at 12 years of age.

vided they remained reduced in the acetabulum. They developed proximal overgrowth of the greater trochanter due to the arrested growth of the femoral head and neck while the greater trochanteric apophysis, still intact, continued to grow. The trochanteric apophysis is extracapsular and is not damaged by the septic process. This overgrowth of the greater trochanter became more notable toward the end of the first decade of life and caused progressive abductor weakness and lurch, pain in extreme abduction, and increasing limitation of abduction owing to impingement of the greater trochanter on the ilium.

Serial follow-up x-ray studies of patients with this deformity are necessary to establish the ideal time to perform an epiphysiodesis of the greater trochanter, although it is usually about 8 to 10 years of age.[17] If the problem is recognized late, advancement of the greater trochanter is indicated. Some authors have recommended subtrochanteric abduction osteotomies,[2] and in our series three hips were treated in this fashion (Fig. 15–18). This procedure eliminated the pain, providing a better abductor mechanism. However, we do not favor this approach because the small head is further uncovered from the already deficient acetabulum

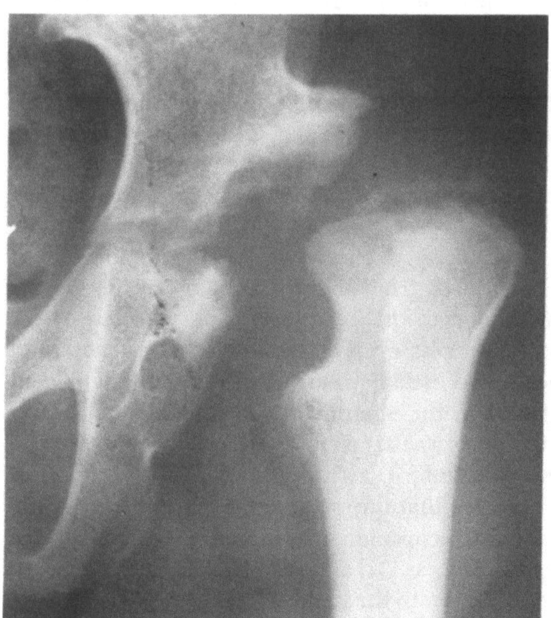

A

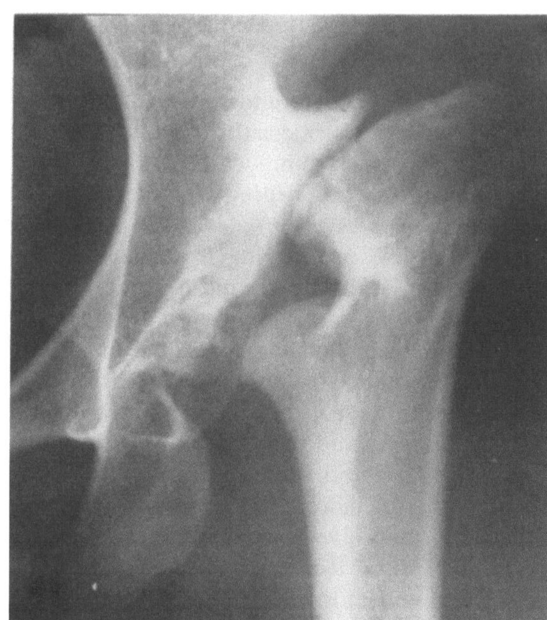

B

FIG. 15–16 **A** Failed trochanteric arthroplasty at 10 years of age. The hip has progressively subluxated. **B** At 18 years of age the subluxation is severe. However, the patient is still pain free and functionally unlimited. The range of motion is limited with 30–90° of flexion, 20° of abduction, 10° of adduction, no rotation, and 5 cm of shortening.

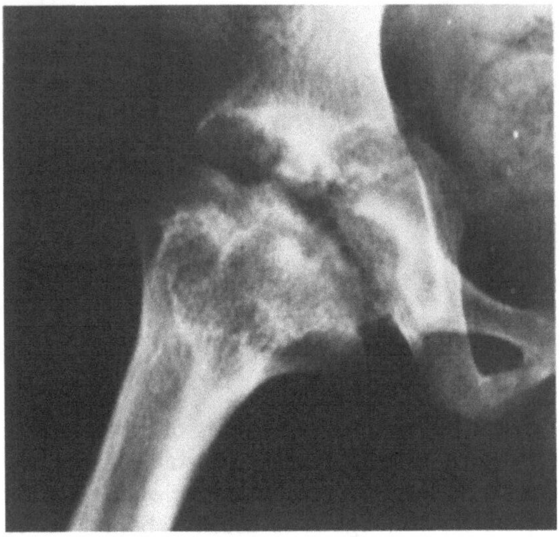

FIG. 15–17 Fibrous ankylosis of the hip 4 years after trochanteric arthroplasty, performed at 2 years of age following infantile septic arthritis.

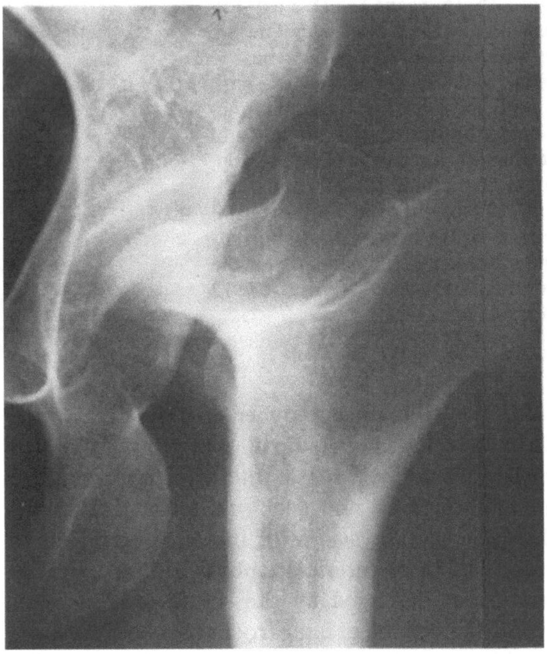

FIG. 15–18 Deformed, short head and neck. This patient had subtrochanteric abduction osteotomy at 9 years of age for a sequela of septic arthritis. At age 24 she was pain free and walked as needed with no abductor lurch. The range of motion was 120° of flexion, 30° of adduction, 0° of abduction, 5° of external and 15° of internal rotation, with 4 cm of shortening.

by the abduction osteotomy. We also condemn advancing the abductor mechanism alone, leaving the trochanter in place, because it will continue to grow and the deformity will not be prevented (Fig. 15–19).

Leg Length Discrepancy

All patients with moderate to severe involvement of the hip following septic arthritis in infancy will develop femoral shortening, which can vary from 1 to 9 cm in our experience. The shortening is associated with arrested or delayed growth of the femoral head and neck owing to damage to the proximal epiphyseal plate (the mean femoral shortening in our cases was 3.4 cm, with a range of 2 to 5 cm), in association with proximal migration if the hip is subluxated or dislocated (mean, 6 cm; range, 3 to 9 cm).

Up to 2 cm of shortening are acceptable and often helpful, facilitating the abductor gait. Femoral shortening of more than 2 cm was observed in 16 cases. Only five had epiphysiodesis of the contralateral distal femur. With the exception of one, all were undercorrected (mean, 3.5 cm; range, 1 to 7.5 cm), suggesting the epiphysiodesis was done too late. Annual scanograms and charting of bone growth according to skeletal age are essential to establish the projected height, femoral length discrepancy, and ideal time for epiphysiodesis if the expected shortening exceeds 2.5 cm. If the patient will be of short stature, femoral lengthening might be considered, although we prefer epiphysiodesis of the opposite distal femur owing to its technical simplicity. For the same reason we do not suggest contralateral femoral shortening.

Interestingly, the length of the femoral shaft as measured from the proximal tip of the greater trochanter to the knee joint is not affected by the septic process even if there is total destruction of head and neck.[23] Nor is there any significant change in the amount of growth following introduction of the trochanter into the acetabulum in the trochanteric arthroplasties. This is explained by the fact that the trochanteric part of the epiphysis is extracapsular and thus not affected by the septic process. It also emphasizes its significant contribution to the longitudinal growth of the femoral shaft.

High Iliac Dislocation

Acceptance of a high iliac dislocation without further treatment remains a possibility. As pointed

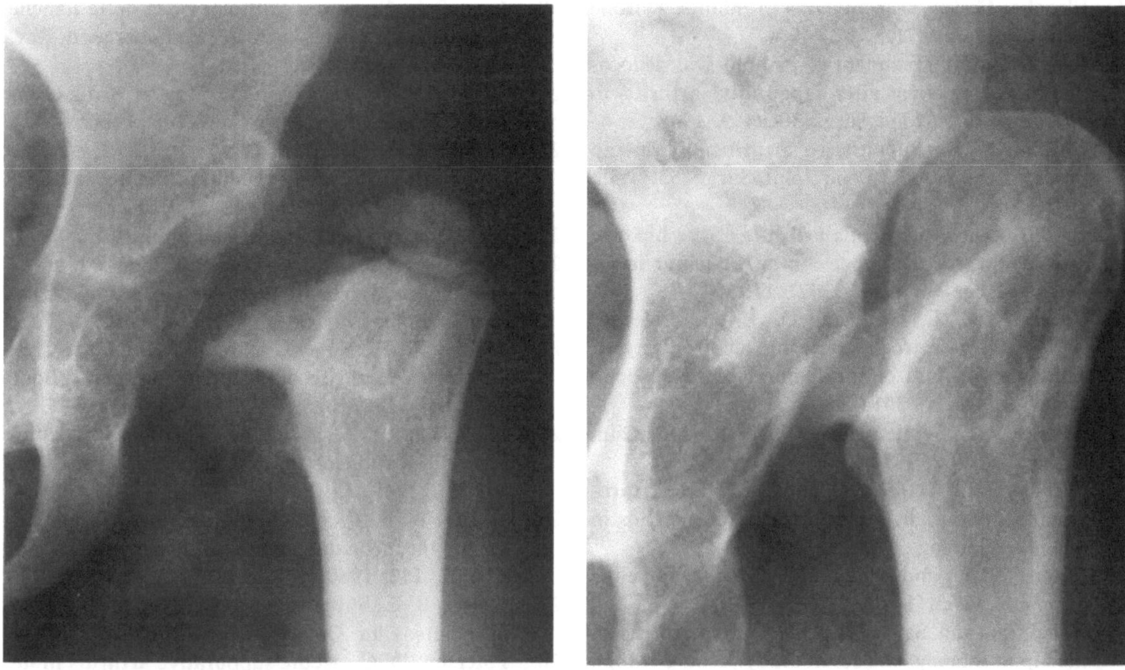

FIG. 15–19 **A** Deformed, short head and neck at 4.5 years of age. At 6.5 years of age she had an advancement of the abductor mechanism. **B** Last follow-up at 15 years of age. The hip was located but with a marked overgrowth of the greater trochanter. She had some pain on exertion, a moderate abductor lurch, 30–110° of flexion, 5° of abduction, 40° of adduction, 10° of external rotation, and 5° of internal rotation. She had some degree of functional limitation and a shortening of 3.5 cm.

out by Obletz,[26,29] these hips are the childhood counterpart of the Girdlestone operation of resection of the femoral head and neck in the adult. In our experience the majority of patients are pain free and surprisingly able to cope with normal daily activities up to adulthood. They usually have an excellent range of motion. However, they all have severe abductor lurch and limb shortening (mean, 7 cm; range, 5 to 9 cm). It is likely that as they grow older they might develop early degenerative changes of the lumbosacral spine due to the added strain of the severe abductor lurch during ambulation. In addition, if these hips require prosthetic reconstruction, the hypoplastic acetabulum will need autogenous iliac bone graft or allografting, as the femoral head is absent.

Prosthetic Reconstruction A significant number of these hips, following septic arthritis, will require joint replacement arthroplasty later in life. The risk of recurrence of infection seems to be remote, as the pathological process occurred very early in life. For the same reason they generally have severe anatomical abnormalities and special prosthetic components are likely to be necessary (extra-small cups, custom-made stems, extra-short necks, and so on). Adequate exposure is mandatory with careful dissection to prevent injury to neurovascular structures that may be surrounded and hidden by scar tissue. We feel that, in order to obtain an ideal biomechanical reconstruction, osteotomy and advancement of the greater trochanter are essential.

Bibliography

1. Axer, A., and Aner, A.: A new technique for greater trochanteric hip arthroplasty. J. Bone Joint Surg., 66B:331, 1984.

1a. Badgley, C. E., et al.: Study of the end results in 113 cases of septic hips. J. Bone Joint Surg., 18:1047, 1936.

2. Banks, S. W., Krigsten, W., and Compere, E. L.: Degeneration of epiphyseal centers of ossification, J.A.M.A., 114(1):23, 1940.

2a. Beaupré, A., and Carroll, N.: The three syndromes of iliac osteomyelitis in children. J. Bone Joint Surg. 61A:1087–1092, 1979.

3. Blanche, D. W.: Osteomyelitis in infants. J. Bone Joint Surg., 34A:71, 1952.
4. Bryson, A. F.: Treatment of pathological dislocation of the hip joint after suppurative arthritis in infants. J. Bone Joint Surg., 30B:449, 1948.
5. Chacha, P. B.: Suppurative arthritis of the hip joints in infancy. J. Bone Joint Surg., 53A:538, 1971.
6. Eyre-Brook, A. L.: Septic arthritis of the hip and osteomyelitis of the upper end of the femur in infants. J. Bone Joint Surg., 42B:11, 1960.
6a. Freeland, A. E., Sullivan, D. J., and Westin, G. W.: Greater trochanteric hip arthroplasty in children with loss of the femoral head. J. Bone Joint Surg., 62A:1351, 1980.
7. Gillespie, R.: Septic arthritis of childhood. Clin. Orthop., 96:152, 1973.
8. Glassberg, G. B., and Ozonoff, M. B.: Arthrographic findings in septic arthritis of the hip in infants. Radiology, 128:151, 1978.
9. Green, W. T., and Shannon, J. G.: Osteomyelitis of infants. Arch. Surg., 32:462, 1936.
10. Hallel, T., and Salvati, E. A.: Septic arthritis of the hip in infancy: end result study. Clin. Orthop., 132:115, 1978.
10a. Hallel, T., Salvati, E. A.: Premature closure of the triradiate cartilage: a case report and animal experiment. Clin. Orthop., 124:278, 1977.
11. Harmon, P. H.: Surgical treatment of the residual deformity from suppurative arthritis of the hip occurring in young children. J. Bone Joint Surg., 24:576, 1942.
12. Harmon, P. H., and Adams, C. O.: Pyogenic coxitis: end results and considerations of diagnosis and treatment. Surg. Gynecol. Obstet., 78:371, 1944.
13. Heberling, J. A.: A review of 201 cases of suppurative arthritis. J. Bone Joint Surg., 23:917, 1941.
14. Inge, A. L., and Liebolt, F. L.: Treatment of acute suppurative arthritis: report of 36 cases treated by operation. Surg. Gynecol. Obstet., 60:86, 1935.
14a. Jackson, M. A., and Nelson, J. D.: Etiology and medical management of acute suppurative bone and joint infections in pediatric patients. J. Pediat. Orthop. 2:313–323, 1982.
15. Kaye, J. J., Winchester, P. H., and Freiberger, R. H.: Neonatal septic dislocation of the hip: true dislocation or pathological epiphyseal separation? Radiology, 114:671, 1975.
16. Kuo, K. N., et al.: Immunodeficiency and infantile bone and joint infection. Arch. Dis. Child., 50:51, 1975.
17. Langenskjöld, A., and Salenius, P.: Epiphysiodesis of the greater trochanter. Acta Orthop. Scand., 38:199, 1967.
18. L'Episcopo, J. B.: Stabilization of pathological dislocation of the hip in children. J. Bone Joint Surg., 18:737, 1936.
19. Leveuf, J.: Luxations pathologiques de la hanche consecutives a l'osteo-arthrite due nourrisson. Rev. Orthop., 32:213, 1946.
20. Lloyd-Roberts, G. C.: Suppurative arthritis of infancy. J. Bone Joint Surg., 42B:706, 1960.
21. Mayer, L.: Discussion. In Obletz, B. E.: Acute suppurative arthritis of the hip in the neonatal period. J. Bone Joint Surg., 42A:150, 1960.
22. Menelaus, M. B.: Personal communication, 1977.
23. Morgan, J. D., and Somerville, E. W.: Normal and abnormal growth at the upper end of the femur. J. Bone Joint Surg., 42B:264, 1960.
24. Morrey, B. F., Bianco, A. J., and Rhodes, K. H.: Suppurative arthritis of the hip in children. J. Bone Joint Surg., 58A:388, 1976.
25. Nicholson, J. T.: Pyogenic arthritis with pathologic dislocation of the hip in infants. J.A.M.A., 141:826, 1949.
26. Obletz, B. E.: Acute suppurative arthritis of the hip in the neonatal period. J. Bone Joint Surg., 42A:23, 143, 1960.
27. Obletz, B. E.: Suppurative arthritis of the hip joint in infants. Clin. Orthop., 22:27, 1962.
28. Paterson, D. C.: Acute suppurative arthritis in infancy and childhood. J. Bone Joint Surg., 52B:474, 1970.
29. Ponseti, I. V.: Growth and development of the acetabulum in the normal child. J. Bone Joint Surg., 60A:575, 1978.
30. Potter, C. M. C.: Osteomyelitis in the newborn. J. Bone Joint Surg., 36B:578, 1954.
31. Rigault, P., et al.: La trochanteroplastie: operation de sauvetage dans les mutilations de la tete et du col du femur chez l'enfant. Indications, technique, et resultats a propos de 10 cas. Rev. Chir. Orthop., 59:565, 1973.
31a. Riordan, T., et al.: Synovial fluid lactic acid measurements in the diagnosis and management of septic arthritis. J. Clin. Pathol., 35:390, 1982.
32. Smith, T.: On the acute arthritis of infants. St. Bartholomew's Hosp. Rep., 10:189, 1874.
33. Stetson, J. W., DePonte, R. J., and Southwick, W. O.: Acute septic arthritis of the hip in children. Clin. Orthop., 56:105, 1968.
34. Tachdjian, M. O.: Pediatric Orthopaedics. Philadelphia, Saunders, 1972, p. 674.
34a. Weintroub, S., Lloyd-Roberts, G. C., and Fraser, M.: The prognostic significance of the triradiate cartilage in suppurative arthritis of the hip in infancy and early childhood. J. Bone Joint Surg., 63B:190–193, 1981.
35. Weissman, S. L.: Transplantation of the trochanteric epiphysis into the acetabulum after septic arthritis of the hip. J. Bone Joint Surg., 49A:1647, 1967.
36. Whitesides, T. E., and Shufflebarger, H.: Septic dislocation of the hip in infants. J. Bone Joint Surg., 53A:1245, 1971.

Index

MIX
Papier aus verantwortungsvollen Quellen
Paper from responsible sources
FSC® C105338

If you have any concerns about our products,
you can contact us on
ProductSafety@springernature.com

In case Publisher is established outside the EU,
the EU authorized representative is:
Springer Nature Customer Service Center GmbH
Europaplatz 3, 69115 Heidelberg, Germany

Printed by Libri Plureos GmbH
in Hamburg, Germany